DATE DUE

OC 15 '98		
OC 1 '98		
AR 1 1 '99		
AP 1 '99		
AP 27 '99		
'99		
DE 1 '00		
AP 15 02		
NO 17 04		
DE 9 04		
JE 13 05		
DE 1 05		
JE 8 07		

The Medical Management of AIDS

Fifth Edition

MERLE A. SANDE, M.D.
Professor and Chairman
Department of Medicine
University of Utah
Salt Lake City, Utah

PAUL A. VOLBERDING, M.D.
Professor, Department of Medicine
University of California, San Francisco
Director, AIDS Program
San Francisco General Hospital
San Francisco, California

W. B. SAUNDERS COMPANY
A Division of Harcourt Brace & Company
Philadelphia, London, Toronto, Montreal, Sydney, Tokyo

Library of Congress Cataloging-in-Publication Data

The medical management of AIDS / [edited by] Merle A. Sande, Paul A.
   Volberding.–5th ed.
       p.   cm.
   Includes bibliographical references and index.
   ISBN 0-7216-6908-5
   1. AIDS (Disease)—Treatment.   I. Sande, Merle A.
II. Volberding, Paul.
   [DNLM: 1. Acquired Immunodeficiency Syndrome.   2. HIV Infections.
WC 503 M489 1997]
RC607.A26M43   1997
616.97′92—dc20
DNLM/DLC
                                                                   96-28911

THE MEDICAL MANAGEMENT OF AIDS   ISBN 0–7216–6908–5

Last digit is the print number: 9   8   7   6   5   4   3   2

Dedication

This edition is dedicated to Dr. Connie Wofsy, who passed away this year after a long illness. Connie's life of dedication and commitment to medicine, infectious diseases, and for the last 15 years to AIDS, was without parallel in our field. As one of the original founders of the AIDS program at San Francisco General Hospital, Connie initiated many of the early studies dealing with diagnosis and treatment of infectious complications of HIV infection, and represented all of us, but especially women, on many national councils. Connie was particularly effective in raising awareness of HIV infection in grade schools, high schools, and colleges, as well as corporations, business groups, and whoever would listen around the country and the world. She spoke clearly and with great sensitivity about the importance of safe sex but also about the lack of danger of transmission from casual contact with infected persons. She was clearly our most articulate spokesperson.

Connie's life, both professional and private, exemplified great caring of family, patients, and colleagues, remarkable personal courage, and a palpable sense of dignity and integrity. She was a wonderful role model and we will all miss her dearly.

CONTRIBUTORS

DONALD I. ABRAMS, MD
Professor of Clinical Medicine, University of California, San Francisco; Assistant Director, AIDS Program, San Francisco General Hospital, San Francisco, California

Alternative Therapies for HIV

TIMOTHY G. BERGER, MD
Associate Clinical Professor, University of California, San Francisco; Chief, Dermatology Service, San Francisco General Hospital, San Francisco, California

Dermatologic Care in the AIDS Patient

GAIL BOLAN, MD
Assistant Clinical Professor of Medicine, University of California, San Francisco; Staff Physician, San Francisco General Hospital; Director, STD Prevention and Control, San Francisco Department of Public Health, San Francisco, California

Management of Syphilis in HIV-Infected Persons

LISA CAPALDINI, MD
Associate Clinical Professor of Medicine, University of California, San Francisco; Ralph K. Davies Hospital, San Francisco, California

HIV Disease: Psychosocial Issues and Psychiatric Complications

ANDREW CARR, MD
Senior Lecturer in Medicine, University of New South Wales; Staff Specialist in HIV Medicine/Immunology, St. Vincent's Hospital, Sydney, Australia

Primary HIV Infection

JOHN P. CELLO, MD
Professor of Medicine and Surgery, University of California, San Francisco; Chief, Gastroenterology, San Francisco General Hospital, San Francisco, California

Gastrointestinal Tract Manifestations of AIDS

MELVIN D. CHEITLIN, MD
Professor of Medicine, University of California, San Francisco; Chief, Cardiology Division, San Francisco General Hospital, San Francisco, California

Cardiovascular Complications of HIV Infection

DAVID A. COOPER, DSc, MD, FRACP, FRCPA
Professor of Medicine, National Centre in HIV Epidemiology and Clinical Research, University of New South Wales; Director, HIV Medicine Unit, St. Vincent's Hospital, Sydney, Australia

Primary HIV Infection

ALEJANDRO DORENBAUM, MD
Assistant Clinical Professor of Pediatrics, University of California, San Francisco, San Francisco, California

Pediatric AIDS: Perinatal Transmission and Early Diagnosis

W. LAWRENCE DREW, MD, PhD
Professor of Laboratory Medicine and Medicine, University of California, San Francisco; Director, Clinical Microbiology and Infectious Diseases, Mt. Zion Medical Center of the University of California, San Francisco, San Francisco, California
Management of Herpesvirus Infections (CMV, HSV, VZV)

KIM S. ERLICH, MD
Assistant Clinical Professor of Medicine, University of California, San Francisco, San Francisco, California; Consultant in Infectious Diseases, Northern Peninsula Infectious Diseases, Seton Medical Center, Daly City, California
Management of Herpesvirus Infections (CMV, HSV, VZV)

MARK B. FEINBERG, MD, PhD
Medical Officer, Office of AIDS Research, National Institutes of Health, Bethesda, Maryland
Natural History and Immunopathogenesis of HIV-1 Disease

JULIE LOUISE GERBERDING, MD, MPH
Associate Professor of Medicine (Infectious Diseases) and Epidemiology and Biostatistics, University of California, San Francisco; Director, Epidemiology and Preventive Interventions Center, San Francisco General Hospital, San Francisco, California
Limiting the Risks of Health Care Workers

PHILIP C. GOODMAN, MD
Professor of Radiology, Chief of Thoracic Imaging, Department of Radiology, Duke University Medical Center, Durham, North Carolina
The Chest Film in AIDS

WARNER C. GREENE, MD, PhD
Professor of Medicine, Microbiology, and Immunology, University of California, San Francisco; Director, Gladstone Institute of Virology and Immunology, San Francisco, California
Molecular Insights Into HIV-1 Infection

DEBORAH GREENSPAN, BDS, DSc, FDS, ScD(hon)
Clinical Professor, Department of Stomatology, and Clinical Director, Oral AIDS Center, School of Dentistry, University of California, San Francisco, San Francisco, California
Oral Complications of HIV Infection

JOHN S. GREENSPAN, BSc, BDS, PhD, FRCPath, ScD(hon)
Professor and Chair, Department of Stomatology, and Director, Oral AIDS Center, School of Dentistry; Professor of Pathology and Director, AIDS Clinical Research Center, School of Medicine, University of California, San Francisco, San Francisco, California
Oral Complications of HIV Infection

CARL GRUNFELD, MD, PhD
Professor of Medicine, University of California, San Francisco; Co-Director, Special Diagnostic and Treatment Unit, Department of Veteran's Affairs Medical Center, San Francisco, California
Endocrinologic Manifestations of HIV Infection

JULIE HAMBLETON, MD
Assistant Adjunct Professor of Medicine, University of California, San Francisco, San Francisco, California
Hematologic Manifestations of HIV Infection

HARRY HOLLANDER, MD

Professor of Clinical Medicine, University of California, San Francisco; Director, HIV Clinic; Director, Categorical Internal Medicine Residency Program, University of California, San Francisco, California

Initiating Routine Care for the HIV-Infected Adult

PHILIP C. HOPEWELL, MD

Professor of Medicine, University of California, San Francisco; Chief, Division of Pulmonary and Critical Care Medicine, San Francisco General Hospital, San Francisco, California

Tuberculosis in Persons with Human Immunodeficiency Virus

LAURENCE HUANG, MD

Assistant Professor of Medicine, University of California, San Francisco; Medical Director, San Francisco General Hospital, Inpatient AIDS Unit; Chief, San Francisco General Hospital AIDS Chest Clinic, San Francisco, California

Pneumoncystis carinii Pneumonia

MICHAEL H. HUMPHREYS, MD

Professor of Medicine, School of Medicine, University of California, San Francisco; Chief, Division of Nephrology, San Francisco General Hospital, San Francisco, California

Renal Complications of HIV Infection

MARK A. JACOBSON, MD

Associate Professor of Medicine in Residence, University of California, San Francisco; Attending Physician, San Francisco General Hospital, San Francisco, California

Disseminated Mycobacterium avium Complex and Other Bacterial Infections

HAROLD W. JAFFE, MD

Instructor in Medicine, Emory University School of Medicine, Grady Memorial Hospital, Atlanta, Georgia

Current Trends in the Epidemiology of HIV/AIDS

DIANE JONES, RN

Head Nurse, AIDS/Oncology Special Care Unit, San Francisco General Hospital, San Francisco, California

HIV Nursing Care

LAWRENCE D. KAPLAN, MD

Associate Professor of Medicine, University of California, San Francisco; Director, AIDS-Oncology Clinical Services San Francisco General Hospital, San Francisco, California

Malignancies Associated with AIDS

JANE E. KOEHLER, MD

Assistant Professor of Medicine, University of California, San Francisco, San Francisco, California

Bacillary Angiomatosis and Other Unusual Infections in HIV-Infected Individuals

DANIEL V. LANDERS, MD

Associate Professor, Department of Obstetrics, Gynecology, and Reproductive Sciences, University of Pittsburgh; Director, Reproductive Infectious Diseases, University of Pittsburgh; Associate Scientist, MAGEE Womens Hospital, Pittsburgh, Pennsylvania

Management of Pregnant Women with HIV Infection

BELLE L. LEE, Pharm.D.
Assistant Professor of Medicine and Pharmacy, University of California, San Francisco; Director of Clinical Pharmacology Antimicrobial Laboratory, San Francisco General Hospital, San Francisco, California
Drug Interactions and Toxicities in Patients with AIDS

J. B. MOLAGHAN, RN, ANP
Guest Lecturer, University of California, San Francisco; Administrative Nurse, AIDS/Oncology Special Care Unit, San Francisco General Hospital, San Francisco, California
HIV Nursing Care

MEG D. NEWMAN, MD
Assistant Professor of Medicine, University of California, San Francisco; Director, AIDS Education Program, (SFGH), San Francisco, California
Gender-Specific Issues in HIV Disease

DONALD W. NORTHFELT, MD
AIDS Oncologist, Pacific Oaks Medical Group, Palm Springs, California
Malignancies Associated with AIDS

LYLE R. PETERSEN, MD, MPH
Robert Koch Institute, Berlin, Germany
Current Trends in the Epidemiology of HIV/AIDS

RICHARD W. PRICE, MD
Professor of Neurology, University of California, San Francisco; Neurology Service Chief, San Francisco General Hospital, San Francisco, California
Management of the Neurologic Complications of HIV-1 Infection and AIDS

JACK S. REMINGTON, MD
Professor of Medicine, Stanford University School of Medicine, Stanford, California; Palo Alto Medical Foundation, Palo Alto, California
AIDS-Associated Toxoplasmosis

MICHAEL S. SAAG, MD
Associate Professor of Medicine, and Director, AIDS Outpatient Clinic, University of Alabama at Birmingham, Birmingham, Alabama
Quantitation of HIV Viral Load: A Tool for Clinical Practice?; Cryptococcosis and Other Fungal Infections (Histoplasmosis, Coccidioidomycosis)

MORRIS SCHAMBELAN, MD
Professor of Medicine, University of California, San Francisco; Chief, Division of Endocrinology, and Program Director, General Clinical Research Center, San Francisco General Hospital, San Francisco, California
Endocrinologic Manifestations of HIV Infection

DEBORAH E. SELLMEYER, MD
Endocrine Fellow, Division of Endocrinology, University of California, San Francisco, California
Endocrinologic Manifestations of HIV Infection

MAUREEN T. SHANNON, CNM, FNP, MS
Associate Clinical Professor, University of California, San Francisco; Coordinator Womens Services, Bay Area Perinatal Center, San Francisco General Hospital, San Francisco, California
Management of Pregnant Women with HIV Infection

JOHN D. STANSELL, MD
Assistant Professor of Medicine, University of California, San Francisco; Medical Director, AIDS Program, San Francisco General Hospital, San Francisco, California

Pneumocystis carinii Pneumonia

SILVIJA I. STAPRANS, PhD
Assistant Adjunct Professor, University of California, San Francisco, San Francisco, California

Natural History and Immunopathogenesis of HIV-1 Disease

MARY JEAN STEMPIEN, MD
Director, Medical Research, Roche Global Development, Palo Alto, California

Management of Herpesvirus Infections (CMV, HSV, VZV)

CARLOS S. SUBAUSTE, MD
Research Associate, Research Institute, Palo Alto Medical Foundation; Consultant in Infectious Diseases, Palo Alto Veterans Affairs Medical Center, Palo Alto, California

AIDS-Associated Toxoplasmosis

PAUL A. VOLBERDING, MD
Professor of Medicine, University of California, San Francisco; Director, AIDS Program, San Francisco General Hospital, San Francisco, California

Antiretroviral Therapy

JOHN W. WARD, MD
Chief, Surveillance Branch, Division of HIV/AIDS Prevention, National Center for HIV, STD, TB Prevention, Centers for Disease Control and Prevention, Atlanta, Georgia

Current Trends in the Epidemiology of HIV/AIDS

DIANE W. WARA, MD
Professor of Pediatrics, University of California, San Francisco, San Francisco, California

Pediatric AIDS: Perinatal Transmission and Early Diagnosis

CONSTANCE B. WOFSY, MD*
Professor of Medicine, University of California, San Francisco; Co-Director, AIDS Program, and Associate Director, Infectious Disease, San Francisco General Hospital, San Francisco, California

Gender-Specific Issues in HIV Disease

SIN YEW WONG, MD
Postdoctoral Fellow, Stanford University, Stanford, California; Palo Alto Medical Foundation Research Institute, Palo Alto, California

AIDS-Associated Toxoplasmosis

---

* Deceased

PREFACE

Fifteen years after it was first recognized, AIDS continues to spread across this planet at frightening speed. As we publish our 5th edition of *The Medical Management of AIDS* it is disheartening to note that except for some isolated instances, there have been few successes in slowing the spread of this viral infection. Most cases are still found in sub-Saharan Africa; however, spread continues to accelerate in Southeast Asia, South America, and Eastern Europe. In the United States, heterosexual sex is the fastest growing method of transmission, particularly among women in minority populations. The epidemiology is becoming that of other sexually transmitted diseases and crack cocaine use appears to be an important facilitator of transmission as it is for other STD's. A study conducted in Tanzania demonstrated that aggressive STD control programs can reduce HIV transmission by nearly 50 per cent. Unfortunately, there is little evidence to suggest that major support for these efforts is forthcoming from international agencies or the governments of the affected countries. Worrisome trends are also occurring in some groups of young gay men: Up to one third of gay men in San Francisco between the ages of 17 and 23 years admitted to practicing unprotected receptive anal intercourse. HIV infection rates are now again on the increase in this population. Although attempts to alter sexual behavior on a global scale have, not surprisingly, been unsuccessful, it has been particularly devastating that to date, no effective vaccine has been developed to slow or prevent transmission. It appears that we are at least a decade away from having a tested vaccine available. There is therefore, at this time, little reason to be optimistic that the spread of this devastating infection will slow in the near future. The number of AIDS patients will undoubtedly continue to rise.

In the first six months of 1996, several new antiretroviral drugs and tests for quantifying viral load have been approved that will have a major impact on the care of patients. These new drugs certainly appear, at this time, to have the potential to significantly slow the progression of HIV infection and prolong survival. In addition, the use of quantitative viral endpoints to measure the therapeutic effect of therapy adds greatly to our ability to maintain the fine balance between effective treatment and toxicity. Consequently, as new strategies for care are developed and an increasing body of clinical information becomes available, we think frequent updates of this textbook, now in its fifth edition in 8 years, are critical. We believe this edition is particularly timely since guidelines for the use of the three new protease inhibitors and the one new reverse transcriptase inhibitor (3TC), in concert with the tests for viral quantitation are just being developed.

Other important advances that are covered in this edition include management of needlestick injuries after the release by the CDC in late 1995 that use of antiretroviral drugs after exposure markedly reduces HIV transmission, review of the 1995 recommendations for preventing opportunistic infections which were published by the Infectious Diseases Society of America and the CDC, and new observations on the pathophysiology of the viral infection. Therefore, marked changes in AIDS/HIV care have recently taken place and guidelines written over 6 months ago are likely out of date.

We hope this text will continue to fill an important role in providing a user-friendly book that provides clinicians with relevant up-to-date information that allows them to provide cutting edge AIDS care. All of the chapters have been updated to reflect the most current information as of early 1996. By continuing these efforts to keep precious AIDS care givers updated, we hope to help make caring for the HIV infected patient more effective and rewarding.

We thank The Hoffmann-La Roche and Glaxo Wellcome Companies for continued educational support for the "Clinical Care of the AIDS Patient" conference which is held in San Francisco in early December each year, and from which this publication results. Special thanks are due to Alice Fishman and her staff at the Department of Medicine, SFGH/UCSF and Kathy Mello, Susan Rogers, and staff from the Department of Medicine's Office of Continuing Education. A special thank you is also extended to Pamela Derish, our editor, who put this all together.

MERLE A. SANDE, MD

CONTENTS

SECTION III
SPECIFIC INFECTIONS AND MALIGNANT CONDITIONS

SECTION IV
SPECIAL ASPECTS OF AIDS

COLOR PLATE IA. Maculopapular rash on trunk of an individual with acute HIV infection. (See page 90.)

COLOR PLATE IB. Hairy leukoplakia on tongue. (See page 174.)

COLOR PLATE IC. Giemsa stain of induced sputum demonstrating cysts and trophozoites of *Pneumocystis carinii*. There is no uptake of stain by cyst wall; therefore, walls appear as clear-to-white circles. Trophozoites appear as dark dots. (×960.) (See page 276.)

COLOR PLATE ID. Acid-fast stain of lymph node tissue demonstrating large numbers of red-staining *Mycobacterium avium-intracellulare*. (See page 301.)

COLOR PLATE IE. Severe edema complicating advanced lower extremity cutaneous Kaposi's sarcoma. (See page 415.)

COLOR PLATE IF. Cytomegalovirus-associated retinitis. Note characteristic hemorrhages and exudates. (See page 381.)

COLOR PLATE IG. Widespread cutaneous Kaposi's sarcoma in a Caucasian individual: typical violaceous appearance of skin lesions. (See page 415.)

COLOR PLATE IH. Typical appearance of early Kaposi's sarcoma involving the palate. (See page 415.)

PLATE I

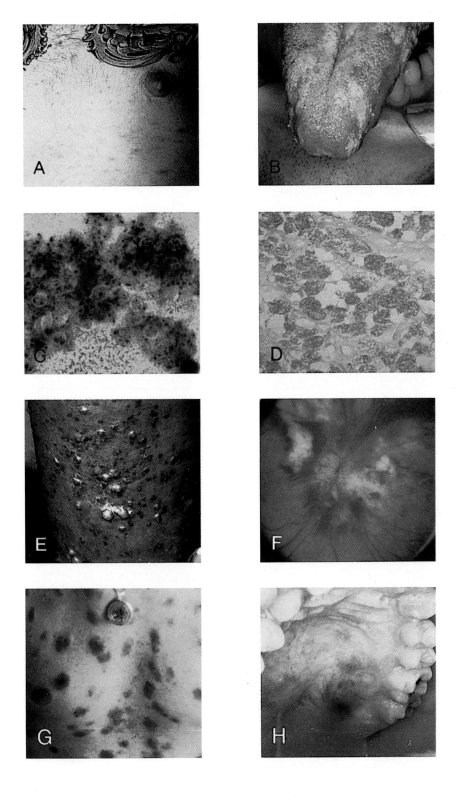

PLATE II

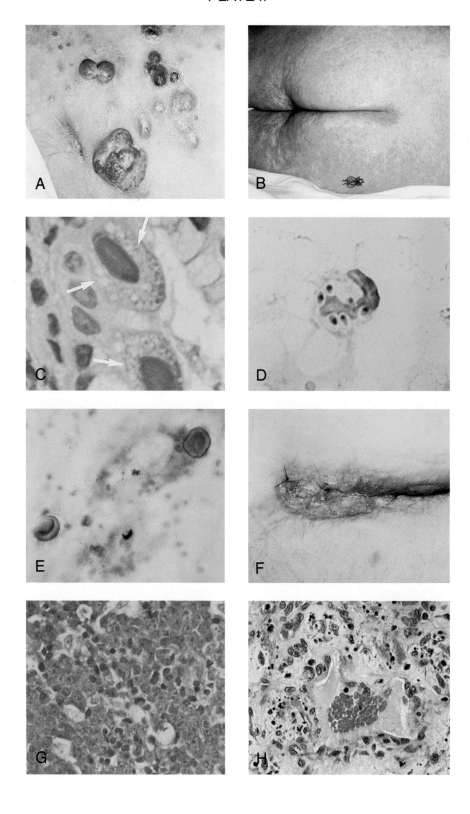

COLOR PLATE IIA. Bacillary angiomatosis of the upper thigh in an AIDS patient who was seen initially 6 months earlier with subacute cellulitis. (See page 162.)

COLOR PLATE IIB. Widespread maculopapular eruption typical of rashes seen with trimethoprimsulfamethoxazole and other antibiotics. (See page 163.)

COLOR PLATE IIC. Ampullary biopsy—AIDS papillary stenosis. Note large cells with intranuclear inclusions characteristic of cytomegalovirus *(arrows)*. (See page 185.)

COLOR PLATE IID. Wright-Giemsa stain of circulating phagocyte with intracellular *Histoplasma capsulatum*. (See page 337.)

COLOR PLATE IIE. Papanicolau stain of sputum demonstrating spherules (one intact, one partially collapsed) of *Coccidioides immitis*. (See page 339.)

COLOR PLATE IIF. Atypical chronic HSV infection at the gluteal cleft in a patient with AIDS. Note the clinical resemblance to a pressure decubitus. (See page 390.)

COLOR PLATE IIG. Small noncleaved-cell Burkitt's lymphoma involving lymph node. (Original magnification, × 100.) (See page 415.)

COLOR PLATE IIH. Hematoxylin and eosin staining of a biopsied cutaneous BA lesion demonstrating a dermal vessel. The vessel is lined with protuberant endothelial cells surrounded by myxoid connective tissue containing neutrophils and amphophilic granular material in close proximity to the vascular lumen. (See page 369.) (From Koehler JE, LeBolt PE, Eghert BM, et al: Cutaneous vascular lesions and disseminated cat-scratch disease in patients with the acquired immunodeficiency syndrome (AIDS) and AIDS-related complex. Ann Intern Med 109:449–455, 1988.)

Section I

THE VIRUS:
ITS TRANSMISSION
AND INFECTION

Chapter *1*

Current Trends in the Epidemiology of HIV/AIDS

JOHN W. WARD, LYLE R. PETERSEN,
and HAROLD W. JAFFE

In this chapter, we examine current trends in the epidemiology of the human immunodeficiency virus/acquired immunodeficiency syndrome (HIV/AIDS) epidemic in both the United States and the rest of the world. For the United States, we will consider the current magnitude of the epidemic, the effect of the epidemic on mortality trends, and the extent to which populations at highest risk for HIV infection are now changing. For the rest of the world, we will also consider the magnitude of the epidemic, how HIV transmission patterns vary in different parts of the world, HIV-2 infections, and some recent advances in prevention.

UNITED STATES

Data on the HIV/AIDS epidemic in the United States come from a variety of sources. AIDS case surveillance data provide well-standardized information about persons with late-stage HIV infection. Vital statistics data add information about HIV/AIDS as a cause of death. For data on earlier stage HIV infection, we rely on HIV seroprevalence surveys. Together these data sources provide a reasonably accurate picture of the HIV/AIDS epidemic.

AIDS Case Surveillance

The reporting of AIDS is based on standard case definitions for adults and children <13 years of age developed by the Centers for Disease Control and Prevention (CDC) in collaboration with state and local health departments. The AIDS surveillance case definition was revised in 1985, 1987, and 1993 to incorporate additional severe illnesses found to be associated with HIV infection, and to reflect changes

in medical management of persons with AIDS.[9,11,13] The 1993 revision also included HIV-infected adults and adolescents with CD4+ T-lymphocyte counts <200 cells/μl or a percentage of total lymphocytes <14.[13] These immunologic criteria were rapidly implemented by local AIDS reporting sources and were the basis for almost half of the AIDS cases reported in 1993 and 1994.[14,18]

In 1993, the number of AIDS cases reported increased over 100% to 106,618 compared with the 49,016 cases reported in 1992. This large increase was primarily a result of the reporting of the accumulated number of HIV-infected persons diagnosed in earlier years with low CD4+ T-lymphocyte counts. In 1994, 80,691 AIDS cases were reported, reflecting the persistent but waning effect of the expansion of AIDS surveillance criteria.[18]

AIDS cases reported based on only the immunologic criteria represent persons less immunosuppressed than persons with AIDS-defining opportunistic illnesses (OIs) and are reported at an earlier stage of HIV illness.[14] Thus, following the expansion of the case definition, some of the increase in AIDS cases included HIV-infected persons who would have been reported with AIDS-OIs in later years. To take the expanded surveillance criteria into account for analysis of temporal trends in AIDS incidence, a statistical adjustment is required to estimate when persons who were reported using the CD4+ criteria will develop an AIDS-OI.[16] (Fig. 1–1). This adjustment is necessary so that annual changes in AIDS incidence can be compared based on the diagnosis of AIDS-OIs, as was done before the surveillance definition was revised. Estimated AIDS-OIs can then be used to describe the growth of the AIDS epidemic nationally and among different populations.

From 1990 through 1994, the estimated diag-

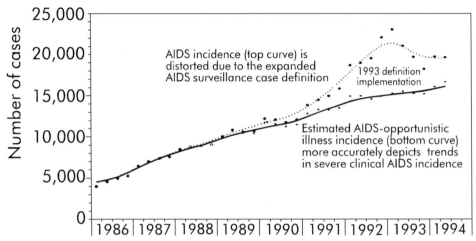

FIGURE 1–1. AIDS incidence and estimated AIDS–opportunistic illness incidence adjusted for delays in reporting, by quarter-year of diagnosis, January 1986 through June 1994, United States.

nosis of all AIDS-related OIs increased 40% (Fig. 1–1). In 1993 and 1994, however, the annual increase slowed to approximately 5%. This slowing suggests that the national epidemic is approaching a plateau. Additional analyses indicate the plateau is largely the result of decreasing AIDS incidence among white homosexual/bisexual men, particularly in large cities. For example, in New York City, from 1989 through 1994, the rate of AIDS-OIs decreased 20% among white homosexual/bisexual men.[20]

This trend among white homosexual/bisexual men has resulted in a smaller increase in the incidence of AIDS-OIs among all homosexual/bisexual men than among male injecting drug users (IDUs), and men with het-

erosexually acquired AIDS (Fig. 1–2). For women, AIDS-OIs are increasing fastest among those with heterosexually acquired AIDS-OIs, and the number of women in this category has surpassed the number related to injecting drug use (Fig. 1–3). From 1990 through 1994, the increase in AIDS-OI incidence among Hispanics (49%) and blacks (73%) was three and four times, respectively, more than the increase among whites (17%) (Fig. 1–4). If this trend continues, the number of blacks reported annually with AIDS will exceed the number of whites reported annually with AIDS. The AIDS-OI trends also indicate the shift in the geographic areas of highest AIDS incidence from the North and West to the South (Fig. 1–5).

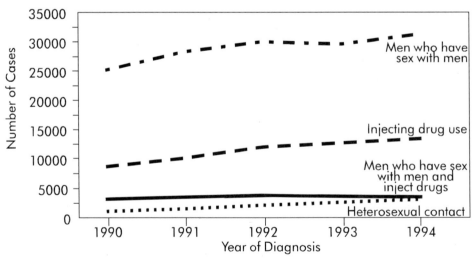

FIGURE 1–2. Estimated AIDS–opportunistic illness incidence for men, by exposure category, and year of diagnosis, 1990 through 1994, United States.

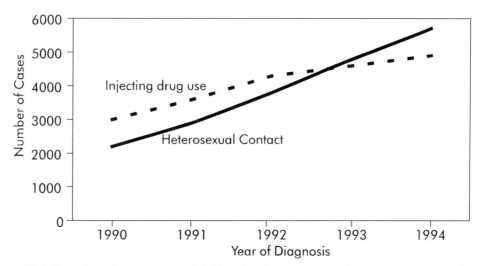

FIGURE 1–3. Estimated AIDS–opportunistic illness incidence for women, by exposure category, and year of diagnosis, 1990 through 1994, United States.

The rate of AIDS and the profiles of risks for HIV transmission also differ among racial/ethnic communities in different parts of the country. Overall, blacks and Hispanics in the Northeast and Florida have the highest rates of AIDS.[15] Blacks tend to have higher rates of AIDS than whites in most geographic areas. The incidence of AIDS and the risks for HIV infection among Hispanics and Asian/Pacific Islanders may vary by their country of origin.[32,55] In the states that border Mexico, the AIDS rate among Hispanics is less than the rate among whites.[32] It is important to recognize, however, that race and ethnicity are not risk factors for HIV infection. Rather, race and ethnicity are surrogates for behavioral, socioeconomic, and other factors that influence HIV transmission. For example, black women with AIDS have lower income and educational levels than other black women, and minority communities with the highest AIDS case rates have the lowest socioeconomic indicators.[33,45,75]

The AIDS surveillance case definition for children <13 years of age did not change in 1993. Through October 1995, 6817 children <13 years of age have been reported with AIDS. In 1994, 1017 children were reported with AIDS, an 8% increase from the number re-

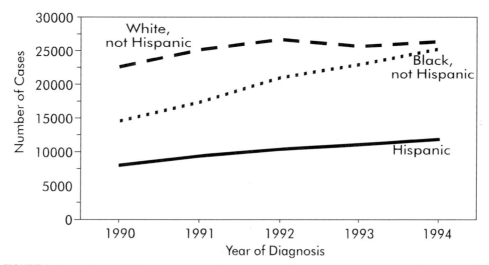

FIGURE 1–4. Estimated AIDS–opportunistic illness incidence by race/ethnicity, and year of diagnosis, 1990 through 1994, United States.

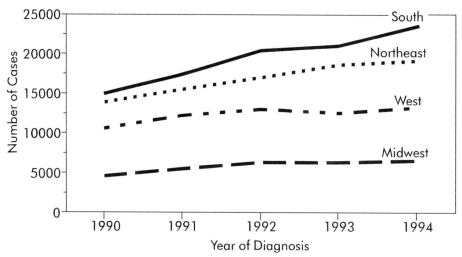

FIGURE 1–5. Estimated AIDS–opportunistic illness incidence by region of residence and year of diagnosis, 1990 through 1994, United States.

ported in 1993. Of the cases reported in 1994, 933 (92%) were infected through perinatal transmission, 506 (50%) were female, 631 (62%) were black, and 236 (23%) were Hispanic.

In 1994, a regimen of zidovudine given to HIV-infected mothers before and at the time of birth and to infants following birth was shown to reduce the risk of perinatal HIV transmission by approximately two thirds.[27] If the use of zidovudine is widely accepted by HIV-infected pregnant women and the effect found in the study is similar for all pregnant women, the number of children with AIDS should begin to decrease in the near future.[17]

AIDS-Related Morbidity and Mortality

Over 95% of HIV-infected persons in clinical care will develop AIDS-OIs before death.[25] *Pneumocystis carinii* pneumonia (PCP) is the leading OI diagnosed among persons with AIDS.[47] The reported frequency of AIDs-OIs may differ among persons with different modes of HIV transmission, gender, and different geographic exposures (Table 1–1).[38,47] Toxoplasmosis, isoporiasis, and extrapulmonary tuberculosis are more common among Hispanics and foreign-born persons than among white or black Americans.[44,76] The frequency of PCP, candidiasis, and cryptococcosis has decreased among homosexual/bisexual men, probably due in part to the increasing use of prophylactic medications to prevent these illnesses.[48,74]

Of 501,310 persons reported with AIDS through October 1995, 311,381 (61%) are known to have died.[22] The median survival for persons reported with AIDS-OIs is 17 months, and the median is 27 months for all persons with AIDS-defining conditions, reflecting the reporting of persons through the use of the CD4+ criteria (CDC, unpublished data).

National vital statistics data are a useful measure of HIV-related mortality and how HIV-related deaths have increased over the course of

TABLE 1–1. PERCENTAGE OF AIDS–OPPORTUNISTIC ILLNESSES ≥ 1 YEAR FOLLOWING INITIAL AIDS DIAGNOSIS AMONG HOMOSEXUAL MEN AND INJECTING DRUG USERS FROM THE ADULT/ADOLESCENT SPECTRUM OF DISEASE (ASD) PROJECT, 1990–1992

AIDS Conditions	Homosexual/ Bisexual (*N* = 1428)	Injecting Drug Users (*N* = 324)
Pneumcystis carinii pneumonia	56.7	63.6
Kaposi's sarcoma	27.0	3.7
Disseminated *Mycobacterium avium*	22.9	13.9
Esophageal candidiasis	22.3	32.7
Wasting syndrome	20.5	18.8
Cytomegalovirus retinitis/disease	15.0	4.9
HIV encephalopathy	11.1	8.3
Extrapulmonary cryptococcosis	9.7	6.2
Toxoplasmosis of brain	6.4	3.7
Chronic cryptosporidiosis	5.1	3.4
Extrapulmonary tuberculosis	4.8	10.5
Chronic herpes simplex	<1	4.3

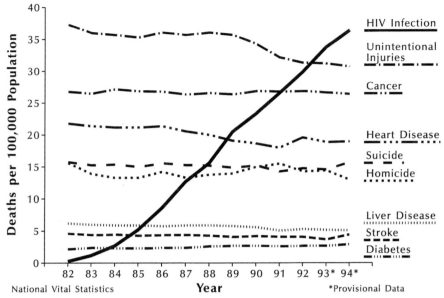

FIGURE 1-6. Death rates per 100,000 population for leading causes of death among persons 25 to 44 years of age, by year, United States, 1982 through 1994.

the HIV epidemic. In 1994, over 42,000 persons died with HIV infection.[57] HIV is the fourth leading cause of years of potential life lost among all Americans before age 65 years and is the leading cause of death for Americans between 25 and 44 years of age (Fig. 1–6). Racial minorities share a disproportionate burden of the HIV-related mortality. In 1994, HIV was the cause of death for 32% of black men and 22% of black women 25 to 44 years of age with mortality rates of 178 and 51 per 100,000 population, respectively. For this age group, HIV was also the leading cause of death for white men with a rate of 47/100,000 and was the fifth leading cause for white women (6/100,000). Since not all HIV-related deaths are indicated on death certificates, the magnitude of HIV mortality in the United States is even greater than indicated by vital statistics data.[5,6]

HIV Serosurveillance

Beginning in 1988, a U.S. national HIV serosurveillance system[34,64] sponsored by the CDC has gathered seroprevalence data from sexually transmitted disease (STD) clinics,[54,62,82] drug treatment centers,[3,49,72] women's reproductive health clinics,[2,79,80] tuberculosis clinics,[61] adolescent and young adult clinics,[83] and sentinel hospitals.[46,78] In addition, a survey using filter paper specimens collected for newborn metabolic screening conducted in 45 states, the District of Columbia, Puerto Rico, and the U.S. Virgin Islands allows estimation of HIV seroprevalence among childbearing women[41,42,56, 59,60,65,81] and children.[29] All of these surveys utilize anonymous, unlinked (blinded) HIV testing in which personally identifying information is removed from the blood specimen; only basic demographic and HIV risk behavior information is retained. In addition, national HIV seroprevalence data are available from routine screening of applicants for military service,[7,8, 12,39] blood donors,[35,51,66–68] and residential Job Corps entrants.[28,77] (Job Corps is a training program for rural and urban disadvantaged youth from 16 to 21 years of age.)

The available serosurveillance data suggest that by the late 1980s and early 1990s, HIV prevalence among U.S. men stabilized and may have begun to decrease in some groups, and in women, has probably stabilized overall. HIV seroprevalence has not significantly increased nationally in any monitored population after the late 1980s.

The STD clinic surveys provide most of the national data about HIV infection prevalence among gay and bisexual men. In 1993, HIV prevalences among gay and bisexual men attending STD clinics were the highest (median clinic prevalence 29.6%) of any group surveyed as part of the CDC's National Serosurveillance Program.[23,24] HIV prevalence exceeded 15% in

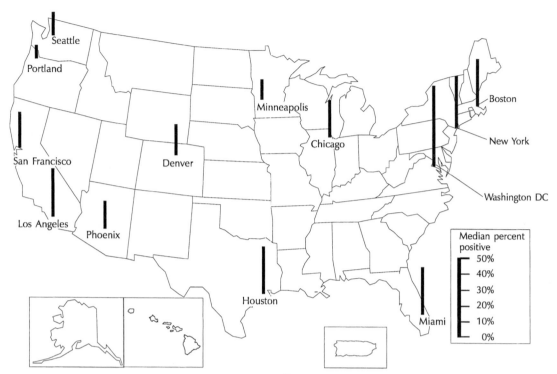

FIGURE 1–7. HIV seroprevalence among men having sex with men, sexually transmitted disease clinics, 1993.

nearly every participating U.S. city (Fig. 1–7). Nevertheless, HIV prevalence from 1988 through 1992 decreased overall among gay and bisexual men attending STD clinics. This decrease was particularly pronounced among young men, non-Hispanic whites, and Hispanics.[82] Among non-Hispanic white men 15 to 29 years old, seroprevalence decreased from 32% in 1989 to 22% in 1992. The high seroprevalence among young men who had sex with men suggests that new HIV infections (incidence) continue to occur. However, the trends toward decreasing HIV seroprevalence, particularly among young persons, suggest that the incidence also was decreasing over time.

Drug treatment centers are the primary sources of national HIV seroprevalence data for IDUs. In 1993, the seroprevalence among IDUs entering drug treatment programs (median 5.4%) was the second highest of any group surveyed.[23,24] In contrast with men who had sex with men, the geographic HIV seroprevalence among IDUs was markedly diverse, with prevalences from 15% to 40% in most cities along the Atlantic Coast and in Puerto Rico, and generally low prevalences (<7%) elsewhere (Fig.

1–8). From 1988 through 1993, seroprevalence remained stable in all groups except for decreases among non-Hispanic whites.[72] These data suggest that in most cities HIV seroprevalence among IDUs increased to a certain level before 1989 and since then has remained relatively constant. The reasons for the persistent geographic heterogeneity in seroprevalence are unknown. The stable seroprevalences over time do not mean that new infections were not occurring, but rather that the incidence was roughly equal to the rate that HIV-infected persons were leaving the population of IDUs, either through long-term cessation of drug use, illness, or death.

Compared with men who have sex with men and IDUs, the seroprevalence among high-risk heterosexuals, such as persons attending STD clinics, is low. In STD clinics in 1993, the median prevalences among persons who did not acknowledge male homosexual contact or injecting drug use were 2.1% among men and 1.1% among women.[24] These figures probably overestimated the prevalences among noninjecting heterosexuals because some gay and bisexual men or some IDUs probably did not acknowledge these behaviors and were

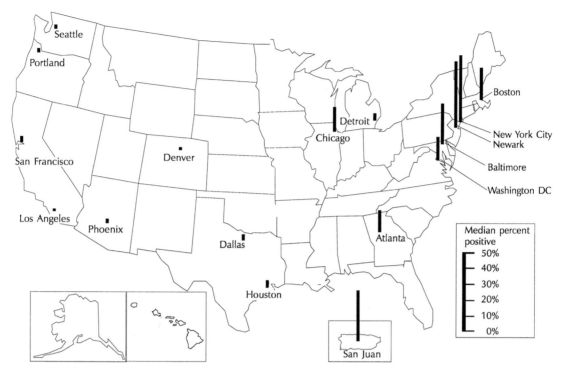

FIGURE 1–8. HIV seroprevalence among injecting drug users entering drug treatment programs, 1993.

misclassified. From 1988 through 1992, among heterosexual STD patients without reported injecting drug use, HIV seroprevalence decreased among whites and, to a lesser degree, Hispanics, but remained essentially stable among blacks.[82]

Consistent with the stable HIV seroprevalence in STD clinics among persons with neither male homosexual contact nor injecting drug use, other serosurveillance data also suggest that seroprevalence may have stabilized among heterosexuals. Although HIV seroprevalence among young women who entered the Job Corps doubled between 1988 and 1990, seroprevalence has remained stable since that time[24,28] (Fig. 1–9). The initial increase was probably due to heterosexual transmission because other data indicate that few seropositive women entering the Job Corps had injected drugs.

Among childbearing women, national HIV seroprevalence from 1988 through 1993 has remained between 0.16% and 0.17%.[24] However, reliance on these national data may mask important regional trends. For example, regional data indicate that prevalence is decreasing in the Northeast and increasing in the South.[19] Although the Survey of Childbearing Women does not collect HIV risk behavior information, data from pediatric AIDS case surveillance suggest that, particularly in the South, an increasing proportion of HIV-infected mothers acquired their infection heterosexually.[58]

Data from the Survey of Childbearing Women provide precise information to estimate pediatric HIV incidence. In 1993, HIV seroprevalence was 0.17%, which corresponded to nearly 7000 births to HIV-seropositive women per year. Based on a perinatal transmission rate of between 20% and 30%, approximately 1400 to 2100 newborns were infected that year.[23,24] Estimates using data from the Survey of Childbearing Women and from AIDS case surveillance indicated that in 1993 approximately 10,000 children were living with HIV infection.[29]

HIV seroprevalence substantially decreased among young men entering the Job Corps[24,28] and applying for military service[23,24] (Figs. 1–9 and 1–10). Although recruiting policies with respect to HIV did not substantially change through 1993, it is possible that the decreasing HIV prevalence trend was due to fewer men with behavioral risks for HIV applying for entrance in the military or Job Corps rather than a true change in the population-at-large. However, decreasing prevalence among these young men was consistent with decreasing HIV seroprevalence among young gay and bisexual men

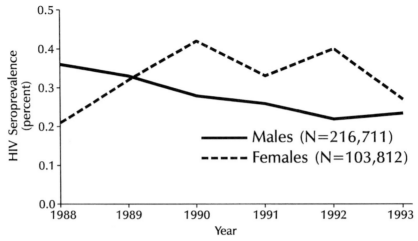

*Annual prevalences were adjusted for differences in age, race/ethnicity, region, and MSA.

FIGURE 1–9. HIV seroprevalence among Job Corps entrants, by sex and date of entrance, 1988 through 1993.

attending STD clinics[82] and among young, non-Hispanic white IDUs entering drug treatment.[72] Importantly, because of their recent initiation of sexual activity or injecting drug use, HIV prevalence trends among youth may closely reflect recent HIV incidence trends.

Data from national HIV serosurveillance also provide substantial information about geographic variations in HIV prevalence in the population-at-large. Among sentinel populations not chosen because of specific HIV risk behaviors, HIV seroprevalences had marked geographic heterogeneity, suggesting enormous differences in the impact of the HIV epidemic among U.S. communities. For example,

HIV seroprevalence in sentinel hospital patients ranged nearly 60-fold among similar demographic groups at hospitals in different cities.[23,24,78] Although the relationship between HIV seroprevalence in the sample population and that of the hospital's catchment population was unknown, the extremely high seroprevalence observed at some hospitals indicated a substantial HIV impact in some inner city communities, particularly in the Northeast. At one hospital in the Northeast, 7.3% of the black women admitted to that hospital for conditions not associated with HIV infection nor with conditions related to HIV risk behaviors were HIV seropositive.[24] Data from this survey also indi-

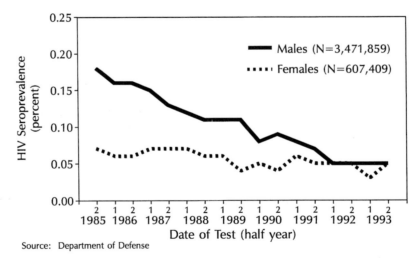

Source: Department of Defense

FIGURE 1–10. HIV seroprevalence among civilian applicants for military service, by test date and sex, October 1985 through December 1993.

cated that HIV seroprevalence was generally higher in metropolitan than in rural areas; however, an exception to this pattern was the high seroprevalence observed among childbearing women in the rural South.[81] A similar observation was seen among Job Corps applicants.

HIV serosurveillance data also indicate the persistence of marked racial and ethnic disparities in HIV seroprevalence. Blacks had a substantially higher seroprevalence than non-Hispanic whites in nearly every serosurveillance population.[24] For example, among STD clinic attendees in 1992, black men who had sex with men had nearly twice the median HIV prevalence (40%) than non-Hispanic whites (22%).[82] Similarly, black IDUs entering drug treatment had seroprevalences two to six times higher than non-Hispanic whites.[72] The data from Hispanic IDUs were less geographically consistent. In the western states, HIV seroprevalence was similar in Hispanic and non-Hispanic white IDUs, while in states along the Atlantic Coast, seroprevalence was higher in Hispanics than non-Hispanic whites and was similar to rates among blacks. The geographic seroprevalence variation among Hispanics is likely due to high seroprevalence among persons of Puerto Rican origin who mainly reside along the Atlantic Coast and lower prevalences among persons of Mexican origin who mainly reside in the West.[73] HIV seroprevalence[23,24] and AIDS case incidence[73] are high in Puerto Rico.

INTERNATIONAL ASPECTS

Magnitude of the Epidemic

For surveillance purposes, a variety of AIDS case definitions are used throughout the world.[4] The definitions vary mainly as a result of variation in the availability of diagnostic tests and procedures, but all definitions basically include persons with late-stage HIV infection. Through June 1995, a cumulative total of about 1 million AIDS cases had been reported to the Global Programme on AIDS of the World Health Organization (WHO).[85] Taking into account the incompleteness of diagnosis and reporting of AIDS cases in many countries, the WHO estimates the true cumulative case total is about 4.5 million adults and children with AIDS. Of these cases, more than 70% are estimated to have occurred in Africa, where AIDS is the leading cause of death for adults in cities

such as Abidjan, Ivory Coast.[31] The United States accounts for <10% of cases globally.

The World Health Organization also estimates that a cumulative total of about 20 million persons have been infected with HIV, including 18.5 million adults and 1.5 million children. Among adults, the ratio of infected men to women is about 3:2. More than half of all infected adults have lived in sub-Saharan Africa (Fig. 1–11). As summarized by Piot and Laga,[70] seroprevalence data from Africa indicate infection rates as high as 25% to 30% among childbearing women from Kigali, Rwanda; Kampala, Uganda; and Lusaka, Zambia. More than 85% of female prostitutes in Abidjan, Ivory Coast, and Nairobi, Kenya, were found to be infected. Another area of great concern is south and southeastern Asia, where the epidemic has spread rapidly in recent years.[85]

Transmission Patterns

Although the basic routes of HIV transmission are the same worldwide, local practices or circumstances influence HIV transmission. For example, HIV-infected women in the United States are advised not to breastfeed their infants,[10] but in sub-Saharan Africa breastfeeding is routine for such women. Dunn et al estimated that breastfeeding adds an additional 14% risk of mother-to-infant HIV transmission for women who have been infected before or during pregnancy.[36] For women who become HIV infected postnatally, the transmission risk for breastfeeding is estimated to be 29%. Another example concerns transmission in residential or hospital settings. In institutionalized populations of abandoned infants and children in Romania, medical injections using unsterilized needles and syringes transmitted HIV.[43] A nosocomial outbreak of HIV infection in the former Soviet Union was also attributed to improper reuse of syringes.[71]

Overall patterns of HIV transmission also vary throughout the world. In Europe, for example, the majority of reported AIDS cases in Scandinavia and the United Kingdom have occurred among homosexual men, while in Spain and Italy most persons with AIDS have been IDUs.[37] In sub-Saharan Africa, the spread of HIV has occurred primarily through heterosexual contact, although transfusion-related infections continue to occur in areas that transfuse unscreened or inadequately screened blood.[69] The most recent epidemic, that seen in Asia, is a mixture of

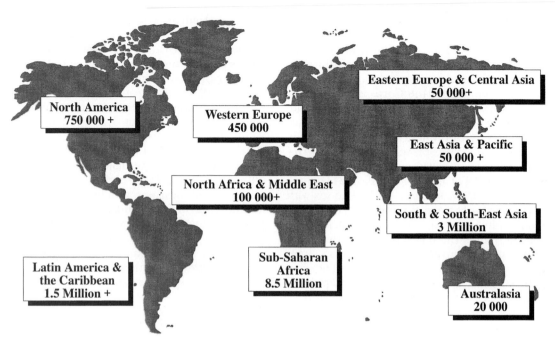

FIGURE 1–11. Estimated distribution of total adult HIV infections from late 1970s/early 1980s until mid-1995. Cumulative total: 18.5 million. (Source: World Health Organization.)

epidemics occurring as a result of heterosexual transmission and injecting drug use.

The Thailand Example

By studying the example of Thailand, we can learn much about the potential for the rapid spread of HIV in a developing country. Because the Thai Ministry of Public Health initiated surveillance for HIV infection in 1987, the Thai epidemic was extraordinarily well documented.

As summarized by Weniger et al, very little HIV infection had been identified in Thailand until early 1988, when the virus began to spread explosively among IDUs in Bangkok.[84] Seroprevalence rose from 1% at the start of the year to between 30% and 40% at the end of the year, with a peak incidence of 5% per month. A year later a second "wave" of the epidemic was then documented among female prostitutes, particularly brothel-based prostitutes in northern Thailand. A third epidemic "wave" was then seen among sexually active heterosexual men. By 1990, HIV seroprevalence had risen to over 10% among 21-year-old men who had been conscripted for military service in some northern Thai provinces.

The appearance of these sequential "waves" of infection suggested a very simple epidemio-logic model, in which male IDUs transmitted HIV to female prostitutes who, in turn, transmitted the infection to other partners. However, this model appears to be too simple. Genetic sequencing studies of HIV isolates collected throughout Thailand indicated the existence of two distinct strains, one found predominantly in Bangkok IDUs and the other among persons infected heterosexually in northern Thailand.[63] Thus, two different HIV strains entered Thailand in the late 1980s and established parallel epidemics in different populations.

By 1995, there were 16,000 reported AIDS cases and an estimated 700,000 HIV-infected persons in Thailand, a country of between 57 and 60 million persons (Thai Ministry of Public Health, unpublished data). Thus, in less than 8 years, HIV prevalence in Thailand rose from essentially zero to a rate that is now about four to five times higher than that found in the United States.

HIV-2

The presence of a second AIDS-related retrovirus, HIV-2, creates an additional dimension to the AIDS epidemic in some parts of the world. This virus was first isolated from two West Afri-

nodeficiency syndrome in Romania. Lancet 338: 645, 1991

44. Hu DJ, Fleming PL, Castro KG, et al: How important is race/ethnicity as an indicator of risk for specific AIDS-defining conditions? J Acquir Immune Defic Syndr 10:347, 1995

45. Hu DJ, Frey R, Costa SJ, et al: Geographical AIDS rates and socio-demographic variables in the Newark, New Jersey metropolitan area. AIDS Public Policy J 9:20, 1994

46. Janssen RS, St. Louis ME, Satten G, et al: HIV infection among patients in U.S. acute-care hospitals: Strategies for the counseling and testing of hospital patients. N Engl J Med 327:445, 1992

47. Jones JL, Hanson DL, Chu SY, et al: Surveillance of AIDS defining conditions in the United States. AIDS 8:1489, 1994

48. Jones J, Hanson DL, Chu SY, et al: Incidence trends in AIDS-related opportunistic illnesses. In Abstracts of the 35th Interscience Conference on Antimicrobial Agents and Chemotherapy (Abstract I121). San Francisco, 1995

49. Jones TS, Allen DM, Onorato IM, et al: HIV seroprevalence surveys in drug treatment centers. Public Health Rep 105:125, 1990

50. Kanki PJ, DeCock KM: Epidemiology and natural history of HIV-2. AIDS 8 (Suppl 1):S85, 1994

51. Lackritz EM, Satten GA, Aberle-Grasse J, et al: Estimated risk of transmission of the human immunodeficiency virus by screened blood in the United States. N Engl J Med 333(6):1721, 1995

52. Marlink R, Kanki P, Thior I, et al: Reduced rate of disease development after HIV-2 infection as compared to HIV-1. Science 265:1587, 1994

53. Mastro TD, Limpakarnjanarat K: Condom use in Thailand: How much is it slowing the HIV/AIDS epidemic? AIDS 9:523, 1995

54. McCray E, Onorato IM, Field Services Branch: Sentinel surveillance of human immunodeficiency virus infection in sexually transmitted disease clinics in the United States. J Sex Transm Dis 19:235, 1992

55. Metler R, Hu DJ, Fleming PL, Ward JW: AIDS among Asians and Pacific Islanders (A/PI) reported in the USA. In Abstracts of the Xth International Conference AIDS/International Conference on STD, vol 12 (Abstract PCO325). Yokohama, 1994

56. Morse DL, Medvesky MG, Glebatis DM, Novick LF: Geographic distribution of newborn HIV seroprevalence in relation to four sociodemographic variables. Am J Public Health 81(Suppl):25, 1991

57. National Center for Health Statistics: Annual summary of births, marriages, divorces, and deaths: United States, 1994. Hyattsville, Maryland: U.S. Department of Health and Human Services, Public Health Service, CDC (Monthly vital statistics report; vol 43, no 13), 1995, p 18

58. Neal JJ, Fleming PL, Ciesielski C: Distribution and patterns of heterosexually acquired AIDS in the United States. In Abstracts of the First National Conference on Human Retroviruses and Related Infections (Abstract 667). Washington, DC, 1993

59. Novick LF, Berns D, Stricof R, et al: HIV seroprevalence in newborns in New York State. JAMA 261: 1745, 1989

60. Novick LF, Glebatis DM, Stricof RL, et al: Newborn seroprevalence study: Methods and results. Am J Public Health 81(Suppl):15, 1991

61. Onorato IM, McCray E: Prevalence of human immu-

nodeficiency virus infection among patients attending tuberculosis clinics in the United States. J Infect Dis 165:87, 1992

62. Onorato IM, McCray E, Pappaioanou M, et al: HIV seroprevalence surveys in sexually transmitted disease clinics. Public Health Rep 105:119, 1990

63. Ou C-Y, Takebe Y, Weniger BG, et al: Independent introduction of two major HIV-1 genotypes into distinct high-risk populations in Thailand. Lancet 341: 1171, 1993

64. Pappaioanou M, Dondero TJ, Petersen LR, et al: The family of HIV seroprevalence surveys: Objectives, methods, and uses of sentinel surveillance for HIV in the United States. Public Health Rep 105:113, 1990

65. Pappaioanou M, George JR, Hannon WH, et al: HIV seroprevalence surveys of childbearing women—objectives, methods, and uses of the data. Public Health Rep 105:147, 1990

66. Petersen LR, Dodd R, Dondero TJ: Methodologic approaches to surveillance of HIV infection among blood donors. Public Health Rep 105:153, 1990

67. Petersen LR, Doll L, HIV Blood Donor Study Group: Human immunodeficiency virus type 1 infection in United States blood donors: Epidemiologic, laboratory, and donation characteristics. Transfusion 31: 698, 1991

68. Petersen LR, Doll LS, White CR, et al: Heterosexually acquired human immunodeficiency virus infection and the U.S. blood supply: Considerations for screening of potential blood donors. Transfusion 334:552, 1993

69. Petersen LR, Simonds RJ, Koistinen J: HIV transmission through blood, tissues, and organs. AIDS 7(Suppl 1):S99, 1993

70. Piot P, Laga M: Epidemiology of AIDS in the developing world. In Broder S, Merigan TC Jr, Bolognesi D (eds): Textbook of AIDS Medicine. Baltimore, Williams & Wilkins 1994, p 112

71. Pokrovsky VV, Eramova EU: Nosocomial outbreak of HIV infection in Elista, USSR. In Abstracts of the Fifth International Conference on AIDS (Abstract WAO5). Montreal, 1989

72. Prevots DR, Allen DM, Lehman JS, et al: Trends in HIV seroprevalence among injection drug users entering drug treatment centers, United States, 1988–1993. Am J Epidemiol 143:733, 1996

73. Selik RM, Castro KG, Pappaioanou M: Birthplace and the risk of AIDS among Hispanics in the United States. Am J Public Health 79:836, 1989

74. Selik RM, Chu SY, Ward JW: Trends in infectious diseases and cancers among persons dying of HIV infection in the United States from 1987 to 1992. Ann Intern Med 123:933, 1995

75. Simon PA, Hu DJ, Diaz T, Kerndt PR: Income and AIDS in Los Angeles County. AIDS 9:281, 1995

76. Slutsker L, Castro KG, Ward JW, et al: Epidemiology of extrapulmonary tuberculosis among persons with AIDS in the United States. Clin Infect Dis 16:513, 1993

77. St. Louis ME, Hayman CR, Conway GA, et al: Human immunodeficiency virus infection in disadvantaged adolescents: Findings from the U.S. Job Corps. JAMA 266:2387, 1991

78. St. Louis ME, Rauch KJ, Petersen LR, et al: Seroprevalence rates of human immunodeficiency virus infection at sentinel hospitals in the United States. N Engl J Med 323:213, 1990

79. Stricof RL, Nattell TC, Novick LF: HIV seroprevalence in clients of sentinel family planning clinics. Am J Public Health Suppl 41:81, 1991

80. Sweeney PA, Onorato IM, Allen DM, et al: Sentinel surveillance of HIV infection in women seeking reproductive health services in the United States, 1988–1989. Obstet Gynecol 79:503, 1992

81. Wasser SC, Gwinn M, Fleming P: Urban-nonurban distribution of HIV in childbearing women in the United States. J Acquir Immune Defic Syndr 6:1035, 1993

82. Weinstock HS, Sidhu J, Gwinn M, et al: Trends in HIV seroprevalence among persons attending sexually transmitted disease clinics in the United States, 1988–1992. J Acquir Immune Defic Syndr 9:514, 1995

83. Wendell D, Onorato IM, McCray E, et al: Youth at risk: Sex, drugs, and human immunodeficiency virus. Am J Dis Child 146:76, 1992

84. Weniger BG, Limpakarnjanarat K, Ungchusak K, et al: The epidemiology of HIV infection and AIDS in Thailand. AIDS 5(Suppl 2):S71, 1991

85. World Health Organization: The current global situation of the HIV/AIDS pandemic. 3 July 1995.

Chapter 2

Molecular Insights into HIV-1 Infection

WARNER C. GREENE

Human immunodeficiency virus type 1 (HIV-1) has been clearly identified as the primary cause of the acquired immunodeficiency syndrome (AIDS).[5,46] The magnitude of the mounting AIDS problem is sobering. In the United States, more than 470,000 cases have been reported to the Centers for Disease Control and Prevention (CDC) through June of 1995.[14] The World Health Organization (WHO) now estimates that more than 18 million adults and 1.5 million children worldwide have been infected with HIV.[130] This virus has now spread to all of the continents including the major population centers in India and Asia. The most conservative estimates suggest that 38 million people will be infected by the year 2000.

HIV-1 is spread by sexual contact, exposure to infected blood or blood products, and through perinatal transmission from mother to child.[24] Although the incidence of AIDS in the homosexual population has received great public attention, worldwide more than 60% of the cases of HIV-1 infection have been heterosexually acquired. The rational design and development of drug therapies to control the virus and the preparation of an effective vaccine to prevent infection represent public health goals of the highest priority. However, substantial progress in these areas will likely hinge on achieving a more complete understanding, in molecular and biochemical terms, of this pathogenic retrovirus and the nature of its cytopathic interplay with its cellular host. In the following sections, I review our current understanding of the molecular biology of HIV-1 infection, highlighting the stages in the life cycle of the retrovirus that appear particularly amenable to therapeutic intervention.

HIV GENOMIC STRUCTURE

HIV-1 is the prototypical member of the Lentivirinae subfamily of retroviruses affecting humans. The lentiviruses characteristically cause indolent infections in their animal hosts notable for involvement of the nervous system, long periods of clinical latency, and weak humoral immune responses complicated by persistent viremia.[81] Other lentiviruses include the visna and maedi viruses, which cause severe demyelinating encephalomyelitis and interstitial pneumonia in sheep, the simian immunodeficiency virus (SIV), which causes an AIDS-like disease in Asian monkeys, the caprine arthritis-encephalitis virus, the equine infectious anemia virus, and the feline immunodeficiency virus.

One feature that distinguishes the lentiviruses from other retroviruses is the remarkable complexity of their viral genomes. Most retroviruses that are capable of replication contain only three genes—namely, *gag, pol,* and *env.*[122] The *gag* and *env* genes encode the core nucleocapsid polypeptides and surface-coat proteins of the virus, respectively, whereas the *pol* gene gives rise to the viral reverse transcriptase and other enzymatic activities (Fig. 2–1). HIV-1, however, contains within its 9-kilobase RNA genome not only these three essential genes but at least six additional genes (*vif, vpu, vpr, tat, rev,* and *nef*) (Fig. 2–1). It is the distinct but concerted actions of these additional genes that probably underlie the profound pathogenicity of HIV-1. From a therapeutic standpoint, this same genomic complexity may also be the "Achilles heel" of the virus should effective antagonists specific for these HIV-1 gene products be successfully isolated.

THE HIV-1 VIRION

High-resolution electron microscopy has revealed the HIV-1 virion as an icosahedral struc-

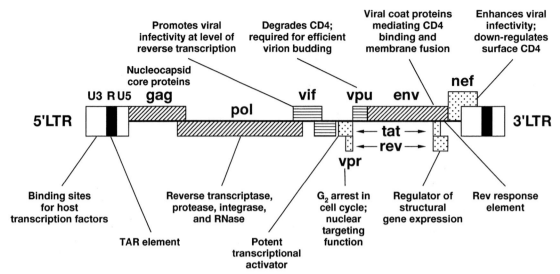

FIGURE 2–1. Genomic structure of HIV-1. The nine known genes of HIV-1 are shown, and their recognized primary functions are summarized. The 5′ and 3′ long terminal repeats (LTRs) containing regulatory sequences recognized by various host transcription factors are also depicted, and the positions of the Tat and Rev RNA response elements—transactivation response (TAR) element and Rev response element (RRE)—are indicated.

ture[50] containing 72 external spikes (Fig. 2–2). These spikes are formed by the two major viral envelope proteins, gp120 and gp41. The HIV-1 lipid bilayer is also studded with a number of host proteins, including class I and class II histocompatibility antigens, acquired during virion budding. The core of HIV-1 contains four nucleocapsid proteins, p24, p17, p9, and p7, each of which is proteolytically cleaved from a 53-kD Gag precursor by the HIV-1 protease. The phosphorylated p24 polypeptide forms the

chief component of the inner shelf of the nucleocapsid (Fig. 2–2), whereas the myristylated p17 protein is associated with the inner surface of the lipid bilayer and probably stabilizes the exterior and interior components of the virion. The p7 protein binds directly to the genomic RNA through a zinc-finger structural motif and, together with p9, forms the nucleoid core. Importantly, this retroviral core also contains two copies of the single-stranded HIV-1 genomic RNA that are associated with the various preformed viral enzymes, including the reverse transcriptase, RNase H, integrase, and protease (Fig. 2–2).

THE LIFE CYCLE OF HIV-1

Attachment of the Virion

The human CD4+ T lymphocyte and monocyte are the major cellular targets for HIV-1 infection in vivo.[35] HIV-1 specifically infects these cells because the CD4 membrane antigen present on each represents the principal high-affinity cellular receptor for this retrovirus (Fig. 2–3).[26,76] The HIV-1 gp120 envelope protein binds to CD4 with an affinity of approximately 4×10^{-9} M. This role of CD4 as the HIV-1 receptor has prompted considerable interest in the therapeutic use of soluble forms of the CD4

FIGURE 2–2. Schematic diagram of the HIV-1 virion. Each of the virion proteins making up the envelope (gp120env and gp41env) and nucleocapsid (p24gag, p17gag, p9gag, and p7gag) is identified. In addition, the diploid RNA genome is shown associated with reverse transcriptase, an RNA-dependent DNA polymerase.

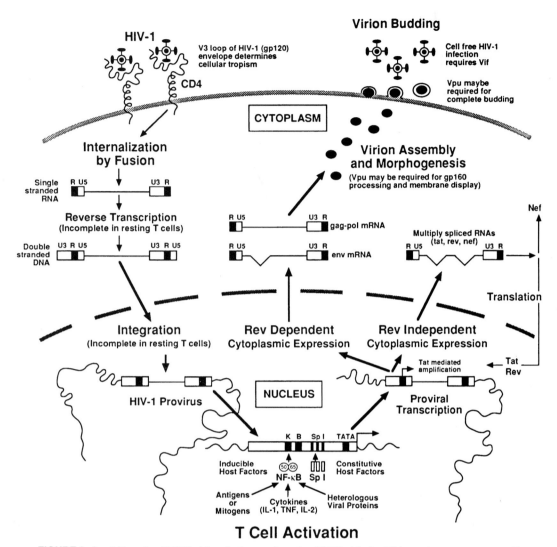

FIGURE 2–3. Life cycle of HIV-1. After the interaction of gp120^{env} with the CD4 membrane receptor, gp41-mediated membrane fusion occurs, leading to the entry of HIV-1 into the cell. After uncoating, reverse transcription of viral RNA begins, resulting in the production of the double-stranded DNA form of the virus in the presence of the appropriate host factors. In turn, the HIV-1 integrase promotes the insertion of this viral DNA duplex into the host genome, thereby giving rise to the HIV-1 provirus. The expression of the HIV-1 gene is stimulated initially by the action of select inducible and constitutive host transcription factors with binding sites in the long terminal repeat, which then leads to the sequential production of various viral mRNAs. The first mRNAs produced correspond to the multiply-spliced species of approximately 2.0 kilobases encoding the Tat, Rev, and Nef regulatory proteins. Subsequently, the viral structural proteins are produced, allowing the assembly and morphogenesis of virions. The free HIV-1 virions that are produced by viral budding from the host cell can then reinitiate the retroviral life cycle by infecting other CD4+ target cells.

protein as receptor decoys to block HIV-1 infection.[40,114] Subsequent studies, however, revealed that primary viral isolates, in contrast to laboratory-adapted strains of HIV, are rather resistant to such soluble CD4 analogs.[25] Further problems with short biologic half-life and poor tissue penetration have limited the overall therapeutic usefulness of this class of antiviral agents.

The progressive loss of the critical CD4+ subset of human T cells that is induced by HIV-1 infection squarely underlies the profound immunodeficiency characteristic of advanced AIDS.[35] These CD4+ T cells serve as both essential regulators and effectors of the normal immune response. HIV-1 infects monocytes and macrophages[47,62] as well but has much less pronounced cytopathic effects in these cells. Infected monocytes may, in fact, serve as a cellular reservoir for HIV-1, allowing further dissemination of the pathogen to the brain and other organs of the body. Besides T cells and monocytes, HIV-1 also may infect other types of cells, including glial cells, gut epithelium, and bone marrow progenitors.[13] Infection of these target cells may well contribute, respectively, to the progressive dementia, diarrhea-wasting syndrome, and hematologic abnormalities frequently observed in patients infected with HIV-1. Whether HIV-1 infection of these diverse cell types is mediated exclusively through CD4 or involves alternative cellular receptors, including the glycolipid galactosylceramide, remains an area of active investigation. Remarkably, certain strains of HIV-1 preferentially infect monocytes and macrophages, whereas others display selectivity for T cells.[13,38,47,62] Studies suggest that a particular subregion of the HIV-1 envelope, termed the V3 loop, plays a dominant role in determining these restricted patterns of infectivity.[38,133] In fact, single amino acid changes within this V3 loop may suffice to alter completely the tropic pattern of infection by this virus.[20] Similarly, differences in the V3 loop contribute to resistance to the effects of soluble CD4.[103] Recent evidence indicates that the initial infecting virus displays a lack of syncytia-inducing potential and preferential tropism for monocytes and T cells, whereas isolates obtained later in the course of the disease are often syncytia-inducing.[135]

Internalization of the Virion

Receptor-bound HIV-1 virions are internalized by pH-independent membrane fusion mediated by the gp41 Env protein.[6,123] This gp41 polypeptide contains a single membrane-spanning region that anchors both envelope proteins (gp41 and gp120) in the lipid bilayer and an N-terminal fusogenic domain resembling the F proteins of the paramyxoviruses (e.g., mumps and parainfluenza[107]). Activation of this domain leads to fusion of the viral and host cell membranes, perhaps by conformational changes induced by gp120/CD4 interaction. So far, no effective drugs have been identified that impair this apparently vulnerable stage of the life cycle of HIV-1.

Reverse Transcription and Integration

After internalization, the HIV-1 virion is partially uncoated in preparation for the replicative phase of its life cycle.[122] Viral replication in a cytoplasmic particle retaining nucleocapsid proteins begins with the generation of a first-strand DNA copy of the viral RNA mediated by the HIV-1–encoded reverse transcriptase (Fig. 2–3). Second-strand DNA synthesis is also controlled by the reverse transcriptase but proceeds only after the action of a second *pol* gene product, ribonuclease H, which partially degrades the original RNA template. After completion of two strand switches whereby reverse transcriptase jumps from one strand of the diploid RNA genome to the other, a double-stranded DNA replica of the original RNA genome is made that contains tandem long terminal repeats at each end of the DNA. This viral DNA duplex is then imported into the nucleus and inserted into the host genome by the viral integrase, another enzymatic product of the *pol* gene (Fig. 2–3). Considerable quantities of unintegrated viral DNA often persist in cells infected with HIV-1,[83] a finding also noted with other cytopathic retroviruses.[70] Recently, the p17 Gag and Vpr gene products have been shown to be associated with the preintegration complex and to contain nuclear localization signals. These nuclear localization signals likely permit nuclear import of the preintegration complex in nondividing cells such as macrophages.[11,59,125] The p17 Gag protein has also been shown to undergo tyrosine phosphorylation[44] and to interact with integrase,[45] events that are likely central to successful nuclear uptake and integration of the double-stranded viral DNA complex. Candidate inhibitors of HIV integrase are now entering clinical trials. Certainly, additional drugs that would act proximal to incorporation of HIV into the cellular genome would be welcome additions to the pharmaceutical armamentarium.

The greatest therapeutic attention has been on the clinical use of dideoxynucleosides, agents that specifically inhibit the action of the viral reverse transcriptase (see Chapter 8).[132] Among others, these compounds include 3′-azido-2′, 3′-dideoxythymidine (zidovudine[74,124]); 2′, 3′-dideoxycytidine (ddC, zalcitabine[37]); 2′, 3′-dideoxyinosine (ddI, didanosine[68]); d4T (stavudine); and 3TC (lamivudine). Each is phosphorylated to an active triphosphate form after entry into the cell and then acts either as a chain terminator of the nascent DNA strand produced by the reverse transcriptase or as a simple competitor blocking the incorporation of the respective normal deoxynucleoside 5′-triphosphate. The viral reverse transcriptase appears to incorporate these dideoxynucleoside analogs preferentially, which probably underlies their therapeutic effectiveness. The principal toxic effect of zidovudine is bone marrow suppression, frequently manifested as anemia and macrocytosis. All these compounds are active when administered orally but show variable central nervous system (CNS) penetration (zidovudine, good; d4T/3TC, intermediate; ddI/ddC, poor). Since these drugs often exhibit patterns of toxicity that do not overlap (e.g., peripheral neuropathy with ddC and ddI, pancreatitis with ddI, and bone marrow suppression with zidovudine), combination therapies are under active evaluation with the hope of enhancing antiviral effectiveness without unacceptable toxicities. Unfortunately, the error-prone nature of the HIV reverse transcriptase (at least one mistake per replication cycle) leads to the generation of a swarm of HIV mutants.[34,43,101] Certain mutants exhibit resistance to these nucleoside antagonists and rapidly become the preponderant virus in the population. Recently, since resistance to the antiviral agents is encoded at different amino acid sites in the reverse transcriptase, combinations of reverse transcriptase inhibitors have been tested. For example, increased therapeutic benefit has been noted with combinations of AZT plus ddI,[68] or AZT plus ddC.[37] Particularly exciting effects of combinations of AZT and 3TC have been observed with 3TC preventing AZT resistance or restoring sensitivity to this agent.

Viral Latency

After entry into the CD4+ cell, HIV-1 may establish a latent or persistent form of infection. With sensitive techniques of DNA and RNA amplification based on the polymerase chain reaction, it has been found that approximately 1 in 1000 peripheral blood CD4+ T cells from patients with AIDS expresses HIV-1 RNA.[112] In contrast, approximately 1 in every 100 of these CD4+ T cells contains detectable HIV-1 DNA. Thus, if one assumes comparable sensitivity for the two techniques of amplification, for every T cell actively producing virus, nine other T cells contain latent virus. A similar pattern of HIV latency in lymph node tissue recently has been described by Haase et al.[33] The biochemical basis of this apparent viral latency is poorly understood but may be determined by the overall state of cellular activation.[93] Many viruses, including HIV-1, do not replicate in resting T cells, presumably because critical host factors are ab-

sent.[22] However, activation of these T cells by antigens, mitogens, select cytokines (tumor necrosis factor-α or interleukin-1), or various gene products of different viruses (human T-cell leukemia virus type I, herpes simplex virus, Epstein-Barr virus, cytomegalovirus, hepatitis B virus, and human herpesvirus type 6) creates a permissive cellular environment that promotes a high level of HIV-1 replication.[110] Many of these activating agents induce the expression of select host transcription factors, notably the NF-κB/Rel family of enhancer-binding proteins.[52,79] These NF-κB/Rel proteins, which normally regulate the expression of various T-cell genes involved in growth, including interleukin-2[63] and the alpha subunit of the interleukin-2 receptor,[8] bind to and activate the two κB enhancer elements present in the U3 region of the HIV-1 proviral long terminal repeat.[100] It seems likely that the induced expression of NF-κB/Rel, which accompanies T-cell activation, may play an important part in the initial stimulation of latent or persistent proviral forms of HIV-1. Various constitutively expressed host transcription factors such as Sp1[66] and TFIID (TATA factor) also are required for expression of the various HIV-1 genes.

Although certain cells may contain latent viral genomes, recent studies have suggested a very dynamic pattern of HIV replication and CD4 T-cell turnover during the period of clinical latency that follows primary infection and antedates the development of disease. When sensitive measurements of viral RNA load[12,105] were used after treatment with antiviral agents, the plasma $T_{1/2}$ of HIV was determined to be approximately 2 days.[61,128] Indeed, roughly 1 billion new virions are produced on a daily basis, likely reflecting replication in lymph tissue.[61] The immune system counters by the daily production of 1 to 2 billion new CD4 cells needed to replenish the HIV-induced losses. Thus, while this infective process follows a chronic course, the actual infection and host response are remarkably dynamic. It is a true testament to the power of the host immune system that it is able to contain this "virologic mayhem" over several years. These findings also argue for intensive early treatment of HIV infection.[18,60]

Early Expression of HIV-1 Regulatory Genes

The binding of inducible and constitutive host transcription factors to sites in the HIV-1 long terminal repeat stimulates a low but important level of expression of the HIV-1 genes (Fig.

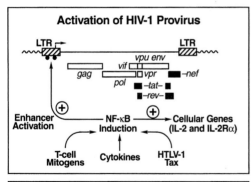

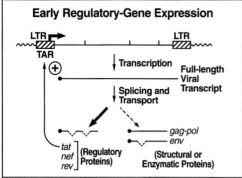

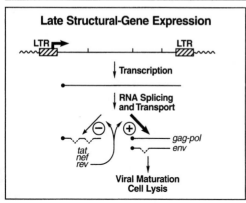

FIGURE 2–4. Stages in the expression of the HIV-1 proviral gene. The first stage of expression of the HIV-1 gene involves activation of the provirus by various T-cell mitogens, cytokines (tumor necrosis factor-α or interleukin-1), or other viral gene products, including the Tax protein of the human T-cell leukemia virus type I (HTLV-I) (*top*). IL-2 denotes interleukin-2, and IL-2Rα denotes the alpha subunit of the high-affinity IL-2 receptor. Among the many other transcriptional events, the NF-κB family of DNA-binding proteins is induced, binds to the HIV-1 enhancer present in the long terminal repeat (LTR), and augments the expression of the HIV-1 genes. The resultant low-level transcription of HIV-1 allows early synthesis of the products of the HIV-1 regulatory genes, including the HIV-1 Tat protein (*middle*). Tat, acting through the transactivation response (TAR) element, functions as a potent amplifier of viral gene expression, leading to a high level of expression of all sequences linked to the HIV-1 long terminal repeat. The HIV-

2–4). Analyses of one-step HIV-1 growth curves reveal that the initial population of genomic-length viral messenger RNA (mRNA) molecules reaches the cytoplasm exclusively as fully spliced, approximately 2-kilobase viral transcripts.[72] These viral mRNAs uniquely encode the various regulatory proteins of HIV-1, including Tat, Rev, and Nef. Tat corresponds to an 86–amino acid nuclear protein that is essential for the replication of HIV-1.[28,39] Tat potently *trans*-activates the expression of all viral genes.[3,118] The Tat protein appears to contain three primary structural domains, including a proline-rich N-terminus, a cysteine-rich central portion, and a positively charged distal segment.[111] The cysteine-rich domain probably mediates dimerization of this *trans*-activator,[41] whereas the positively charged distal segment is responsible for both RNA binding and nuclear–nucleolar localization.[57] So far, no clear function has been ascribed to the proline-rich domain.

Tat acts through binding to an RNA stem-loop structure termed the *trans*-activation response (TAR) element, located at the beginning of all HIV-1 mRNAs.[104,113] Both Tat[32] and various cellular proteins[48,49] have been found to bind directly to the *trans*-activation response element, but the precise function of Tat remains controversial. The preponderance of evidence suggests that it acts primarily at the level of transcription elongation, initiation, or both.[21,78] A principal effect of Tat is to stimulate effective RNA elongation by the already bound RNA polymerase, giving rise to full-length HIV-1 transcripts rather than the short, truncated transcripts that are formed in the absence of Tat.[69] This action of Tat likely requires its interaction with one or more cellular cofactors whose identity remains unknown.

The product of the HIV-1 *nef* gene (Nef) is a second regulatory protein expressed early in the course of HIV-1 infection.[51] However, in contrast to the essential role of Tat in HIV-1 replication, the 27-kD Nef protein is dispensable for viral growth in many T-cell lines. Early studies suggested that this myristylated cytoplasmic protein[55] actually inhibited the replica-

FIGURE 2-4. *Continued.* 1 Rev protein then activates the expression of the HIV-1 structural and enzymatic genes while simultaneously inhibiting the production of regulatory proteins, thus allowing viral maturation, the assembly of infectious virions, and cell lysis (*bottom*). Rev is thus important in governing the transition from the expression of early regulatory genes to that of late structural genes.

tion of HIV-1 (hence Nef, for "negative factor"[86,120]) by down-regulating the transcriptional activity of the HIV-1 long terminal repeat.[1,102] However, later reports failed to confirm these proposed negative effects of Nef.[56,73] Emerging evidence now indicates that Nef acts as a positive factor serving to enhance HIV infectivity.[17,30,98,99,106] In both SIV-infected adult rhesus macaques[71] and HIV-infected humans,[65,75] the defects in the *nef* gene have been associated with the absence of disease development in infected individuals.[31] These results emphasize the urgent need to identify effective Nef antagonists.

Late Expression of HIV-1 Structural and Enzymatic Genes

As noted, the early phase of expression of the HIV-1 genes is characterized by cytoplasmic expression of the multiply-spliced 2.0-kilobase class of viral mRNAs uniquely encoding the HIV-1 regulatory proteins.[72] For the assembly of infectious HIV-1 virions, however, the retroviral structural and enzymatic proteins also must be produced. These proteins are translated from incompletely processed viral transcripts, including the unspliced *gag-pol* mRNA and the singly spliced *env* mRNA. The transition between the synthesis of early regulatory gene products and late structural gene products appears critically dependent on the HIV-1 Rev protein (Fig. 2–4). Rev is a 19-kD nuclear phosphoprotein,[23] which, like Tat, is essential for the replication of HIV-1.[36,116] The Rev protein appears to exert its regulatory activity at a posttranscriptional level by activating the cytoplasmic expression of the unspliced and singly spliced forms of HIV-1 RNA that encode the products of the *gag, pol,* and *env* genes.[90] In the absence of Rev, these incompletely spliced viral mRNAs remain sequestered in the nucleus, where they are either degraded or completely spliced. Rev produces these posttranscriptional effects likely by both inhibiting viral RNA splicing[15] and activating nuclear export of these incompletely spliced mRNA species.[7,42,91]

Like Tat, Rev functions through a highly structured RNA stem-loop structure, termed the Rev response element. This RNA motif is located in the *env* gene, and, because of the pattern of HIV-1 splicing, is present only in those mRNA species whose expression is regulated by Rev.[91] Mutational analyses of both Rev[89] and the Rev response element[29,58,92] have revealed that a positively charged, arginine-rich domain in the Rev protein mediates its direct binding to the Rev response element.[27,134] Rev also contains a second peptide domain that is uniquely required for its functional activity.[89] Mutations in this putative activation domain result in dominant negative mutant proteins that not only lack intrinsic Rev biologic activity but also block the action of the wild-type Rev protein.[4,89] The potential use of such *trans*-dominant *rev* mutants as a genetic therapy to attenuate HIV infection is now in clinical trials.

Morphogenesis of the HIV-1 Virion

The products of the HIV-1 *gag* and *pol* genes form the core of the mature HIV-1 virion, whereas the products of the *env* genes are the principal exterior coat proteins (Fig. 2–2). These coat proteins are synthesized as a gp160 precursor that is subsequently cleaved by a cellular protease in the Golgi apparatus to yield gp120 and gp41. Although gp160 is extensively modified by glycosylation, these sugars are not essential for subsequent CD4 ligation. Similarly, the HIV-1 Gag proteins are derived from a 53-kD precursor protein that is specifically cleaved by the HIV-1-derived protease, yielding the p24, p17, p9, and p7 Gag proteins. Of potential therapeutic interest is the observation that inhibiting the myristylation of the p17 Gag protein appears to abrogate the assembly of the HIV-1 virion and viral infectivity.[10] As with the *rev* gene, dominant negative mutants of the HIV-1 *gag* gene have been identified and shown to inhibit the replication of HIV-1 in tissue culture.[121]

The HIV-1 Pol protein is translated from the same transcript as the Gag precursor by a novel ribosomal frame-shifting mechanism with a −1 nucleotide change of frame.[64] In general, approximately 20-fold more Gag protein than Pol protein is produced, reflecting the relative inefficiency of this frame-shifting process. Inhibition of this ribosomal frame-shifting reaction also would be an attractive approach to therapy, but agents with such activity have not been identified. Once translated, the *pol* gene precursor is cleaved to produce several critical viral enzymes, including reverse transcriptase, integrase, ribonuclease, and an aspartyl protease. Both the HIV-1 reverse transcriptase and protease proteins have been crystallized, and data have been collected regarding their intrinsic three-dimensional structures.[85,94,129] In the case of the HIV-1 protease, this structural information has permitted exciting progress in the rational development of specific inhibitors.[95,96] One such HIV protease inhibitor, saquinavir, has now received U.S. Food and Drug Administration (FDA) approval for use in HIV-infected individuals.

Assembly of the infectious HIV virion proceeds in a stepwise manner, initially involving aggregation of the ribonucleoprotein cores beneath the plasma membrane. These retroviral cores are composed of the HIV-1 RNA, Gag proteins, and the various enzymes encoded by the *pol* gene. Once assembled, these cores bud through the plasma membrane, where they acquire their lipid membranes, complete with the two protein products of the HIV-1 *env* gene. It is only after this final budding process that the cleavage events mediated by HIV-1 protease occur, leading to maturation of the viral particle.

The protein products of two additional HIV-1 genes, *vpu* and *vif,* appear to have important functional roles during these late stages of virion morphogenesis. Specifically, the Vpu protein promotes the efficient release of the budding virions from the surface of the cell.[77] Remarkably, mutations within the *vpu* gene result in viruses that remain loosely tethered to the host cell. The *vpu* gene product may also, with Nef, serve to down-regulate CD4. Vpu binds to the cytoplasmic tail of intracellular CD4, targeting it for proteolysis.[9,15,131] The product of the *vif* gene also appears to be necessary for full infectivity of the released HIV-1 virions,[117,119] since mutations in this gene substantially impair both cell-free and cell-associated transmission of HIV[126] and proviral DNA synthesis.[126]

CYTOPATHIC EFFECTS OF HIV-1

The ability of HIV-1 to produce cytopathic effects within the CD4+ subset of human T lymphocytes underlies the profound state of immunodeficiency clinically manifested as AIDS. Despite considerable investigative efforts, the precise mechanism (or mechanisms) by which HIV-1 kills CD4 cells remains unknown. The recent finding of high-level dynamic viral replication argues in favor of a direct effect of the virus on cell viability. One clear in vitro mechanism of HIV-1–induced killing involves cell fusion and the formation of syncytia mediated by the gp41 Env protein after the gp120 Env pro-

tein interacts with "CD4.[84,115] This fusion process requires only the presence of the HIV-1 Env proteins on the surface of infected cells and thus may involve uninfected CD4-expressing cells that inadvertently come in contact with virally infected cells expressing HIV-1 Env proteins. Subsequent fusion of these cells leads to the formation of multinucleated syncytia that ultimately die. It is noteworthy that cells expressing low levels of CD4 receptors appear less susceptible to this form of cell death, a finding that may underlie the relative paucity of cytopathic effects produced by HIV-1 in monocytes and macrophages. Recent studies have demonstrated that HIV Vpr expression leads to arrest of cells in the G_2 phase of the cell cycle.[67,108] Whether such cell cycle arrest ultimately leads to the death of CD4 cells or a change in this state of cellular differentiation[82] is currently under investigation. HIV *env* has also been proposed to alter cell cycle progression by causing inappropriate phosphorylation of p34[cdc2], thus leading to "mitotic catastrophe."[19] Other mechanisms of cytopathicity induced by HIV-1 include apoptosis (programmed cell death),[53,97] high-level replication of the virus with associated membrane injury,[80] accumulation of unintegrated HIV-1 DNA,[83] altered second-messenger production, and changes in membrane permeability,[54,88] and autoimmune destruction of T cells infected with HIV-1 by both antibody-dependent and cytotoxic T-cell–dependent mechanisms.[87,109,127] Which if any of the potential processes contribute markedly to the cytopathic effects of HIV-1 in vivo remains to be determined.

SUMMARY

Although AIDS remains incurable at present, remarkable progress has been made in our overall understanding of this fatal immunodeficiency syndrome and its retroviral cause. The application of modern techniques of molecular and cellular biology has yielded unprecedented information regarding the structural, enzymatic, and regulatory genes of HIV-1 and the nature of its frequently lethal interplay with its cellular host. These studies have identified several promising points of attack to interdict the HIV-1 life cycle, including the attachment and internalization of the virion, reverse transcription, integration, viral transcription, viral RNA splicing and transport, and virion morphogenesis and budding. The clear challenge now is to translate this basic information into effective pharmacologic therapies and an efficacious vaccine capable of halting the spread of this pathogenic human retrovirus.

REFERENCES

1. Ahmad N, Venkatesan S: Nef protein of HIV-1 is a transcriptional repressor of HIV-1 LTR. Science 241:1481–1485, 1988
2. Aiken C, Trono D: Nef stimulates human immunodeficiency virus type 1 proviral DNA synthesis. J Virol 69(8):5048–5056, 1995
3. Arya SK, Guo C, Josephs SF, et al: Trans-activator gene of human T-lymphotropic virus type III (HTLV-III). Science 229:69–73, 1985
4. Baltimore D: Intracellular immunization. Nature 335:395–396, 1988
5. Barre-Sinoussi F, Chermann JC, Rey F, et al: Isolation of a T-lymphotropic retrovirus from a patient at risk for acquired immune deficiency syndrome (AIDS). Science 220:868–8671, 1983
6. Bedinger P, Moriarty A, von Borstel RC Jr, et al: Internalization of the human immunodeficiency virus does not require the cytoplasmic domain of CD4. Nature 334:162–165, 1988
7. Bogerd HP, Fridell RA, Madore S, et al: Identification of a novel cellular cofactor for the Rev/Rex class of retroviral regulatory proteins. Cell 82(3):485–494, 1995
8. Bohnlein E, Lowenthal JW, Siekevitz M, et al: The same inducible nuclear protein(s) regulate mitogen activation of both the interleukin-2 receptor-alpha gene and type I human immunodeficiency virus. Cell 53:827–836, 1988
9. Bour S, Schubert U, Strebel K: The human immunodeficiency virus type 1 Vpu protein specifically binds to the cytoplasmic domain of CD4: Implications for the mechanism of degradation. J Virol 69(3):1510–1520, 1995
10. Bryant ML, Heuckeroth RO, Kimata JT, et al: Replication of human immunodeficiency virus 1 and Moloney murine leukemia virus is inhibited by different heteroatom-containing analogs of myristic acid. Proc Natl Acad Sci U S A 86(22):8655–8659, 1989
11. Bukrinsky MI, Haggerty S, Dempsey MP, et al: A nuclear localization signal within HIV-1 matrix protein that governs infection of non-dividing cells. Nature 365:666–669, 1993
12. Cao Y, Ho D, Todd J, et al: Clinical evaluation of branched DNA signal amplification for quantifying HIV type 1 in human plasma. AIDS Res Hum Retroviruses 11(3):353–361, 1995
13. Castro BA, Cheng-Mayer C, Evans LA, et al: HIV heterogeneity and viral pathogenesis. AIDS 2(Suppl 1):S17–S27, 1988
14. Centers for Disease Control and Prevention: MMWR AIDS Update—United States. 44(64):66–67, 1994
15. Chang DD, Sharp PA: Regulation by HIV Rev depends upon recognition of splice sites. Cell 59:789–795, 1989
16. Chen MY, Maldarelli F, Karczewski MK, et al: Human immunodeficiency virus type 1 Vpu protein induces degradation of CD4 in vitro: The cytoplasmic domain of CD4 contributes to Vpu sensitivity. J Virol 67(7):3877–3884, 1993
17. Chowers MY, Spina CA, Kwoh TJ, et al: Optimal infectivity in vitro of HIV-1 requires an intact nef gene. J Virol 68:2906–2914, 1994
18. Coffin JM: HIV population dynamics in vivo: Implications for genetic variation, pathogenesis, and therapy. Science. 267:483–489, 1995
19. Cohen DI, Tani Y, Tian H, et al: Participation of tyrosine phosphorylation in the cytopathic effect of human immunodeficiency virus-1. Science. 256:542–545, 1992
20. Cordonnier A, Montagnier L, Emerman M: Single amino-acid changes in HIV envelope affect viral tropism and receptor binding. Nature 340:571–574, 1989
21. Cullen BR: Trans-activation of human immunodeficiency virus occurs via a bimodal mechanism. Cell 46(7):973–982, 1986
22. Cullen BR, Greene WC: Regulatory pathways governing HIV-1 replication. Cell 58(3):423–426, 1989
23. Cullen BR, Hauber J, Campbell K, et al: Subcellular localization of the human immunodeficiency virus trans-acting art gene product. J Virol 62(7):2498–2501, 1988
24. Curran JW, Jaffe HW, Hardy AM, et al: Epidemiology of HIV infection and AIDS in the United States. Science 239:610–616, 1988
25. Daar ES, Li XL, Moudgil T, et al: High concentrations of recombinant soluble CD4 are required to neutralize primary human immunodeficiency virus type 1 isolate. Proc Natl Acad Sci U S A 87(17):6574–6578, 1990
26. Dalgleish AG, Beverley PCL, Clapham PR, et al: The CD4 (T4) antigen is an essential component of the receptor for the AIDS retrovirus. Nature 312:763–767, 1984
27. Daly TJ, Cook KS, Gray GS, et al: Specific binding of HIV-1 recombinant Rev protein to the Rev-responsive element in vitro. Nature 342:816–819, 1989
28. Dayton AI, Sodroski JG, Rosen CA, et al: The trans-activator gene of the human T cell lymphotropic virus type III required for replication. Cell 44(6):941–974, 1986
29. Dayton ET, Powell DM, Dayton AI: Functional analysis of CAR, the target sequence for the Rev protein of HIV-1. Science 246:1625–1629, 1989
30. de Ronde A, Klaver B, Keulen W, et al: Natural HIV-1 Nef accelerates virus replication in primary human lymphocytes. Virology 188(1):391–395, 1992
31. Deacon NJ, Tsykin A, Solomon A, et al: Genomic structure of an attenuated quasi species of HIV-1 from a blood transfusion donor and recipients. Science 270:988–991, 1995
32. Dingwall C, Ernberg I, Gait MJ, et al: Human immunodeficiency virus 1 tat protein binds trans-activation-responsive region (TAR) RNA in vitro. Proc Natl Acad Sci U S A 86(18):6925–6929, 1989
33. Embretson J, Zupancic M, Ribas JL, et al: Massive covert infection of help T lymphocytes and macro-

phages by HIV during the incubation period of AIDS. Nature 362:359–362, 1993

34. Emini E, Graham D, Gotlib L, et al: HIV and multidrug resistance. Nature 364:679, 1993

35. Fauci AS: The human immunodeficiency virus: Infectivity and mechanisms of pathogenesis. Science 239:617–622, 1988

36. Feinberg MB, Jarrett RF, Aldovini A, et al: HTLV-III expression and production involve complex regulation at the level of splicing and translation of viral RNA. Cell 46(6):807–817, 1986

37. Fischl MA, Stanley K, Collier AC, et al: Combination and monotherapy with zidovudine and zalcitabine in patients with advanced HIV disease. Ann Intern Med 122(1):24–32, 1995

38. Fisher AG, Ensoli B, Looney D, et al: Biologically diverse molecular variants within a single HIV-1 isolate. Nature 334:444–447, 1988

39. Fisher AG, Feinberg MB, Josephs SF, et al: The transactivator gene of HTLV-III is essential for virus replication. Nature 320:367–371, 1986

40. Fisher RA, Bertonis JM, Meier W, et al: HIV infection is blocked in vitro by recombinant soluble CD4. Nature 331:76–78, 1988

41. Frankel AD, Bredt DS, Pabo CO: Tat protein from human immunodeficiency virus forms a metal-linked dimer. Science 240:70–73, 1988

42. Fritz CC, Zapp ML, Green MR: A human nucleoporin-like protein that specifically interacts with HIV Rev. Nature 376:530–533, 1995

43. Frost S, McLean A: Quasispecies dynamics and the emergence of drug resistance during ziduvudine therapy of HIV infection. AIDS 8(3):323–332, 1994

44. Gallay P, Swingler S, Aiken C, et al: HIV-1 infection of nondividing cells: C-terminal tyrosine phosphorylation of the viral matrix protein is a key regulator. Cell 80(3):379–388, 1995

45. Gallay P, Swingler S, Song J, et al: HIV nuclear import is governed by the phosphotyrosine-mediated binding of matrix to the core domain of integrase. Cell 83:569–576, 1995

46. Gallo RC, Salahuddin SZ, Popovic M, et al: Frequent detection and isolation of cytopathic retroviruses (HTLV-III) from patients with AIDS and at risk for AIDS. Science 224:500–503, 1984

47. Gartner S, Markovits P, Markovitz DM, et al: The role of mononuclear phagocytes in HTLV-III/LAV infection. Science 233:215–219, 1986

48. Gatignol A, Kumar A, Rabson A, et al: Identification of cellular proteins that bind to the human immunodeficiency virus type 1 trans-activation-responsive TAR element RNA. Proc Natl Acad Sci U S A 86(20):7828–7832, 1989

49. Gaynor R, Soultanakis E, Kuwabara M, et al: Specific binding of a HeLa cell nuclear protein to RNA sequences in the human immunodeficiency virus transactivating region. Proc Natl Acad Sci U S A 86(13):4858–4862, 1989

50. Gelderblom HR, Hausmann EH, Ozel M, et al: Fine structure of human immunodeficiency virus (HIV) and immunolocalization of structural proteins. Virology 156(1):171–176, 1987

51. Green WC: Regulation of HIV-1 gene expression. Ann Rev Immunol 8:453–475, 1990

52. Greene WC, Bohnlein E, Ballard DW: HIV-1, HTLV-1 and normal T-cell growth: Transcriptional strate-

gies and surprises. Immunol Today 10(8):272–278, 1989

53. Groux H, Torpier G, Monte D, et al: Activation-induced death by apoptosis in CD4+ T cells from human immunodeficiency virus-infected asymptomatic individuals. J Exp Med 175(2):331–340, 1992

54. Gupta S, Vayuvegula B: Human immunodeficiency virus-associated changes in signal transduction. J Clin Immunol 7(6):486–489, 1987

55. Guy B, Kieny MP, Riviere Y, et al: HIV F/3' orf encodes a phosphorylated GTP-binding protein resembling an oncogene product. Nature 330:266–269, 1987

56. Hammes SR, Dixon EP, Malim MH, et al: Nef protein of human immunodeficiency virus type 1: Evidence against its role as a transcriptional inhibitor. Proc Natl Acad Sci U S A 86:9549, 1989

57. Hauber J, Perkins A, Heimer EP, et al: Trans-activation of human immunodeficiency virus gene expression is mediated by nuclear events. Proc Natl Acad Sci U S A 84(18):6364–6368, 1987

58. Heaphy S, Dingwall C, Ernberg I, et al: HIV-1 regulator of virion expression (Rev) protein binds to an RNA stem-loop structure located within the Rev response element region. Cell 60(4):685–693, 1990

59. Heinzinger NK, Bukinsky MI, Haggerty SA, et al: The Vpr protein of human immunodeficiency virus type 1 influences nuclear localization of viral nucleic acids in nondividing host cells. Proc Natl Acad Sci U S A 91(15):7311–7315, 1994

60. Ho D: Time to hit HIV, early and hard (Editorial). N Engl J Med 333(7):450–451, 1995

61. Ho DD, Neumann AU, Perelson AS, et al: Rapid turnover of plasma virions and CD4 lymphocytes in HIV-1 infection. Nature 373:123–126, 1995

62. Ho DD, Rota TR, Hirsch MS: Infection of monocyte/macrophages by human T lymphotropic virus type III. J Clin Invest 77(5):1712–1715, 1986

63. Hoyos B, Ballard DW, Bohnlein E, et al: Kappa B-specific DNA binding proteins: Role in the regulation of human interleukin-2 gene expression. Science 244:457–460, 1989

64. Jacks T, Power MD, Masiarz FR, et al: Characterization of ribosomal frameshifting in HIV-1 gag-pol expression. Nature 331:280–283, 1988

65. Jamieson BD, Aldrovandi GM, Planelles V, et al: Requirement of human immunodeficiency virus type 1 nef for in vivo replication and pathogenicity. J Virol 68(6):3478–3485, 1994

66. Jones KA, Kadonaga JT, Luciw PA, et al: Activation of the AIDS retrovirus promoter by the cellular transcription factor, Sp1. Science 232:755–759, 1986

67. Jowett JB, Planelles V, Poon B, et al: The human immunodeficiency virus type 1 vpr gene arrests infected T cells in the G2 + M phase of the cell cycle. J Virol 69(10):6304–6313, 1995

68. Kahn JO, Lagakos SW, Richman DD, et al: A controlled trial comparing continued zidovudine with didanosine i human immunodeficiency virus infection. N Engl J Med 327(9):581–587, 1992

69. Kao SY, Calman AF, Luciw PA, et al: Anti-termination of transcription within the long terminal repeat of HIV by tat gene product. Nature 330:489–493, 1987

70. Keshet E, Temin HM: Cell killing by spleen necrosis virus is correlated with a transient accumulation of spleen necrosis virus DNA. J Virol 31(2):376–388, 1979

71. Kestler HW III, Ringler DJ, Mori K, et al: Importance of the *nef* gene for maintenance of high virus loads and for development of AIDS. Cell 65(4):651–662, 1991

72. Kim SY, Byrn R, Groopman J, et al: Temporal aspects of DNA and RNA synthesis during human immunodeficiency virus infection: Evidence for differential gene expression. J Virol 63:3708, 1989

73. Kim SY, Ikeuchi K, Byrn R, et al: Lack of a negative influence on viral growth by the nef gene of human immunodeficiency virus type 1. Proc Natl Acad Sci U S A 86:9544, 1989

74. Kinloch-de Loes S, Hirschel BJ, Hoen B, et al: A controlled trial of zidovudine in primary human immunodeficiency virus infection. N Engl J Med 333:408–413, 1995

75. Kirchhoff F, Greenough TC, Brettler DB, et al: Brief report: Absence of intact nef sequences in a long-term survivor with nonprogressive HIV-1 infection. N Engl J Med 332(4):228–232, 1995

76. Klatzmann D, Champagne E, Chamaret S, et al: T-lymphocyte T4 molecule behaves as the receptor for human retrovirus LAV. Nature 312:767–768, 1984

77. Klimkait T, Strebel K, Hoggan MD, et al: The human immunodeficiency virus type 1-specific protein vpu is required for efficient virus maturation and release. J Virol 64(2):621–629, 1990

78. Laspia MF, Rice AP, Mathews MB: HIV-1 Tat protein increases transcriptional initiation and stabilizes elongation. Cell 59(2):283–292, 1989

79. Lenardo MJ, Baltimore D: NF-kappa B: A pleiotropic mediator of inducible and tissue-specific gene control. Cell 58(2):227–229, 1989

80. Leonard R, Zagury D, Desportes I, et al: Cytopathic effect of human immunodeficiency virus in T4 cells is linked to the last stage of virus infection. Proc Natl Acad Sci U S A 85(10):3570–3574, 1988

81. Letvin NL: Animal models for AIDS. Immunol Today 11(9):322–326, 1990

82. Levy DN, Fernandes LS, Williams WV, et al: Induction of cell differentiation by human immunodeficiency virus 1 vpr. Cell 72(4):541–550, 1993

83. Levy JA, Kaminsky LS, Morrow WJ, et al: Infection by the retrovirus associated with the acquired immunodeficiency syndrome: Clinical, biological, and molecular features. Ann Intern Med 103(5):694–699, 1985

84. Lifson JD, Reyes GR, McGrath MS, et al: AIDS retrovirus induced cytopathology: Giant cell formation and involvement of CD4 antigen. Science 232:1123–1127, 1986

85. Lowe DM, Aitken A, Bradley C, et al: HIV-1 reverse transcriptase: Crystallization and analysis of domain structure by limited proteolysis. Biochemistry 27(25):8884–8889, 1988

86. Luciw PA, Cheng-Mayer C, Levy JA: Mutational analysis of the human immunodeficiency virus: The orf-B region down-regulates virus replication. Proc Natl Acad Sci U S A 84:1434, 1987

87. Lyerly HK, Matthews TJ, Langlois AJ, et al: Human T cell lymphotropic virus IIIB glycoprotein (gp120) bound to CD4 determinants on normal lymphocytes and expressed by infected cells serve as target for immune attack. Proc Natl Acad Sci U S A 84(13):4601–4605, 1987

88. Lynn WS, Tweedale A, Cloyd MW: Human immunodeficiency virus (HIV-1) cytotoxicity: Perturbation of the cell membrane and depression of phospholipid synthesis. Virology 163(1):43–51, 1988

89. Malim MH, Bohnlein S, Hauber J, et al: Functional dissection of the HIV-1 Rev trans-activator—derivation of a trans-dominant repressor of Rev function. Cell 58(1):205–214, 1989

90. Malim MH, Hauber J, Fenrick R, et al: Immunodeficiency virus rev trans-activator modulates the expression of the viral regulatory genes. Nature 335:181–183, 1988

91. Malim MH, Hauber J, Le SY, et al: The HIV-1 rev trans-activator acts through a structured target sequence to activate nuclear export of unspliced viral mRNA. Nature 338:254–257, 1989

92. Malim MH, Tiley LS, McCarn DF, et al: HIV-1 structural gene expression requires binding of the Rev trans-activator to its RNA target sequence. Cell 60(4):675–683, 1990

93. McCune J: Viral latency in HIV disease. Cell 82(2):183–188, 1995

94. McKeever BM, Navia MA, Fitzgerald PM, et al: Crystallization of the aspartylprotease from the human immunodeficiency virus, HIV-1. J Biol Chem 264(4):1919–1921, 1989

95. McQuade TJ, Tomasselli AG, Liu L, et al: A synthetic HIV-1 protease inhibitor with antiviral activity arrests HIV-like particle maturation. Science 247:454–456, 1990

96. Meek TD, Lambert DM, Dreyer GB, et al: Inhibition of HIV-1 protease in infected T-lymphocytes by synthetic peptide analogues. Nature 343:90–92, 1990

97. Meyaard L, Otto SA, Jonker RR, et al: Programmed death of T cells in HIV-1 infection. Science 257:217–219, 1992

98. Miller MD, Feinberg MB, Greene WC: The HIV-1 nef gene acts as a positive viral infectivity factor. Trends Microbiol 2(8):294–298, 1994

99. Miller MD, Warmerdam MT, Page KA, et al: Expression of the human immunodeficiency virus type 1 (HIV-1) *nef* gene during HIV-1 production increases progeny particle infectivity independent of gp160 or viral entry. J Virol 69(1):579–584, 1995

100. Nabel G, Baltimore D: An inducible transcription factor activates expression of human immunodeficiency virus in T cells. Nature 326:711–713, 1987

101. Najera I, Holguin A, Quinones MM, et al: Pol gene quasispecies of human immunodeficiency virus: Mutations associated with drug resistance in virus from patients undergoing no drug therapy. J Virol 69(1):23–31, 1995

102. Niederman TM, Thielan BJ, Ratner L: Human immunodeficiency virus type 1 negative factor is a transcriptional silencer. Proc Natl Acad Sci U S A 86:1128, 1989

103. O'Brien WA, Chen IS, Ho DD, et al: Mapping genetic determinants for human immunodeficiency virus type 1 resistance to soluble CD4. J Virol 66(5):3125–3130, 1992

104. Pavlakis GN, Felber BK: Regulation of expression of human immunodeficiency virus. New Biol 2(1):20–31, 1990

105. Piatak MJ, Saag MS, Yang LC, et al: High levels of HIV-1 in plasma during all stages of infection de-

termined by competitive PCR. Science 259: 1749–1754, 1993

106. Rhee SS, Marsh JW: HIV-1 Nef activity in murine T cells: CD4 modulation and positive enhancement. J Immunol 152(10):5128–5134, 1994

107. Richardson CD, Choppin PW: Oligopeptides that specifically inhibit membrane fusion by paramyxovirus studies on the site of action. Virology 131(2): 518–532, 1983

108. Rogel ME, Wu LI, Emerman M: The human immunodeficiency virus type 1 vpr gene prevents cell proliferation during chronic infection. J Virol 69(2):882–888, 1995

109. Rook AH, Lane HC, Folks T, et al: Sera from HTLV-III/LAV antibody-positive individuals mediate antibody-dependent cellular cytotoxicity against HTLV-III/LAV-infected T cells. J Immunol 138(4): 1064–1067, 1987

110. Rosenberg ZF, Fauci AS: Activation of latent HIV infection. J NIH Res 2:41–45, 1990

111. Sadaie MR, Benter T, Wong-Staal F: Site-directed mutagenesis of two trans-regulatory genes (tat-III,trs) of HIV-1. Science 239:910–913, 1988

112. Schnittman SM, Psallidopoulos MC, Lane HC, et al: The reservoir for HIV-1 in human peripheral blood is a T cell that maintains expression of CD4. Science 245:305–308, 1989

113. Sharp PA, Marciniak RA: HIV TAR: An RNA enhancer? Cell 59(2):229–230, 1989

114. Smith DH, Byrn RA, Marsters SA, et al: Blocking of HIV-1 infectivity by a soluble, secreted form of the CD4 antigen. Science 238:1704–1707, 1987

115. Sodroski J, Goh WC, Rosen C, et al: Role of the HTLV-III/LAV envelope in syncytium formation and cytopathicity. Nature 322:470–474, 1986

116. Sodroski J, Goh WC, Rosen C, et al: A second post-transcriptional trans-activator gene required for HTLV-III replication. Nature 321:412–417, 1986

117. Sodroski J, Goh WC, Rosen C, et al: Replicative and cytopathic potential of HTLV-III/LAV with sor gene deletions. Science 231:1549–1553, 1986

118. Sodroski J, Patarca R, Rosen C, et al: Location of the trans-activating region on the genome of human T cell lymphotropic virus type III. Science 229: 74–77, 1985

119. Strebel K, Daugherty D, Clouse K, et al: The HIV 'A' (sor) gene product is essential for virus infectivity. Nature 328:728–730, 1987

120. Terwilliger E, Sodroski JG, Rosen CA, et al: Effects of mutations within the 3' orf open reading frame region of human T cell lymphotropic virus type III (HTLV/LAV) on replication and cytopathogenicity. J Virol 60(2):754–760, 1986

121. Trono D, Feinberg MB, Baltimore D: HIV-1 Gag mutants can dominantly interfere with the replication of the wild-type virus. Cell 59(1):113–120, 1989

122. Varmus H: Retroviruses. Science 240:1427–1435, 1988

123. Veronese FD, DeVico AL, Copeland TD, et al: Characterization of gp41 as the transmembrane protein coded by the HTLV-III/LAV envelope gene. Science 229:1402–1405, 1985

124. Volberding PA, Lagakos SW, Grimes JM, et al: A Comparison of immediate with deferred zidovudine therapy for asymptomatic HIV-infected adults with CD4 cell counts of 500 or more per cubic millimeter. N Engl J Med 333:401–407, 1995

125. von Schwedler U, Kornbluth RS, Trono D: The nuclear localization signal of the matrix protein of human immunodeficiency virus type 1 allows the establishment of infection in macrophages and quiescent T lymphocytes. Proc Natl Acad Sci U S A 91(15):6992–6996, 1994

126. von Schwedler U, Song J, Aiken C, et al: Vif is crucial for human immunodeficiency virus type 1 proviral DNA synthesis in infected cells. J Virol 67(8): 4945–4955, 1993

127. Walker BD, Chakrabarti S, Moss B, et al: HIV-specific cytotoxic T lymphocytes in seropositive individuals. Nature 328:345–348, 1987

128. Wei X, Ghosh SK, Taylor ME, et al: Viral dynamics in human immunodeficiency virus type 1 infection. Nature 373:117–122, 1995

129. Wlodawer A, Miller M, Jaskolski M, et al: Conserved folding in retroviral proteases: Crystal structure of a synthetic HIV-1 protease. Science 245:616–621, 1989

130. World Health Organization: The HIV/AIDS pandemic: 1994 overview. WHO/GPA/TCO/SEF, 1994, p 4

131. Yao XJ, Friborg J, Checroune F, et al: Degradation of CD4 induced by human immunodeficiency virus type 1 Vpu protein: A predicted alpha-helix structure in the proximal cytoplasmic region of CD4 contributes to Vpu sensitivity. Virology 209(2): 615–623, 1995

132. Yarchoan R, Mitsuya H, Broder S: Immunologic issues in anti-retroviral therapy. Immunol Today 11(9):327–333, 1990

133. York-Higgins D, Cheng-Mayer C, Bauer D, et al: Human immunodeficiency virus type 1 cellular host range, replication, and cytopathicity are linked to the envelope region of the viral genome. J Virol 64(8):4016–4020, 1990

134. Zapp ML, Green MR: Sequence-specific RNA binding by the HIV-1 Rev protein. Nature 342:714–716, 1989

135. Zhu T, Mo H, Wang N, et al: Genotypic and phenotypic characterization of HIV-1 patients with primary infection. Science 261:1179–1181, 1993

Natural History and Immunopathogenesis of HIV-1 Disease

SILVIJA I. STAPRANS and MARK B. FEINBERG

Infection with the human immunodeficiency virus type 1 (HIV-1) leads to a protracted disease course that culminates in the near complete destruction of the CD4+ T-lymphocyte population. The essential clinical features of HIV-1 disease derive from how HIV-1 interacts with host cells and tissues during the course of virus infection. The application of new sensitive methods to quantitate HIV-1 replication in infected individuals has demonstrated that plasma HIV-1 RNA levels reflect active ongoing virus replication. Thus, recent observations strengthen the notion that the cytopathic (cell damaging) consequences of ongoing viral replication cause the progressive immune deterioration (immunopathogenesis) of HIV-1 disease. Further progress in understanding the mechanisms by which HIV-1 causes disease will depend upon an improved understanding of fundamental aspects of HIV-1 replication, both within individual cells and tissues, as well as within infected people. This chapter summarizes our current understanding of basic principles of HIV-1 replication as it relates to the pathogenic potential of the virus.

Several features of the biology of HIV-1 are important in the consideration of how and why infection leads to AIDS, and why the derivation of durably effective treatments for infection has been so difficult. First, HIV-1 targets CD4+ cells, focusing virus-induced pathology on essential components of the immune system. Target cells of HIV include: CD4+ helper T cells that provide signals for the activation and regulation of multiple limbs of the immune response, and macrophages which perform phagocytosis and presentation of antigens for recognition by antigen-specific T cells. Second, virus replication depends upon the HIV-1 reverse transcriptase, an imprecise enzyme that results in variant viruses. Such variants, produced during each round of virus replication, may differ in important ways, such as in their sensitivity to drugs, in their antigenicity, or in their cell tropism. Third, the ability of HIV-1 to productively infect CD4+ T lymphocytes depends on the target cell being activated and proliferating. As a result, HIV-1 infections are preferentially focused on cells that are responding to antigenic stimulation or those T cells that are proliferating, in response to as yet unidentified signals, as the host's immune system attempts to compensate for T cells that have been depleted as a result of virus-induced damage. Thus, cell populations that are the preferred targets of HIV-1 infection represent those that may be the most essential in maintaining normal immune function. Fourth, HIV-1 possesses specific genetic functions that allow it to productively infect mature nondividing macrophages. Macrophage tropism may be important for the ability of HIV-1 to establish chronic infection that cannot be cleared, although the precise mechanisms by which HIV-1 causes persistent infection despite a strong host immune response are still poorly understood.

VIRAL TRANSMISSION

Epidemiologic studies indicate that semen, cervical and vaginal secretions, breast milk, and blood and blood products appear to be the predominant, if not exclusive, vehicles for viral transmission.[22] Thus, HIV-1 is transmitted via sexual intercourse, injection drug use, transfusion of virus-contaminated blood or blood products, and between mother and infant either before or at the time of birth, or breast feeding. Currently the factors that determine the ability of an HIV-1–infected person to transmit the virus are incompletely understood. HIV-1 can be transmitted via the transfer of infected cells, free virus, or both, although the precise contribution of these components to a given infection probably depends upon the nature and route of exposure. If a virus-transmitting donor is in the midst of his or her own episode of primary HIV-1 infection or has advanced HIV-1 disease, the recipient may be more likely to become infected.[82,123] In both of these instances, plasma and cell-associated virus loads are often high.[34,142] Some studies have indicated that HIV-1 RNA is present in greater quantities in the semen of men with lower CD4+ T cell counts, although the variations that may exist in concentrations of HIV-1 in semen across the course of HIV-1 infection have not been clearly deliniated[112] (see Viral Load studies, and Fig. 3–1 below). Thus, increased transmissibility may be due to increased viral load in the transmitter or to increased virulence of the transmitted strains of HIV-1 or to both. Infection by an advanced-stage donor is associated with a higher incidence of symptomatic acute HIV-1 infection, which may portend a more rapid progression to AIDS, again possibly the result of increased viral loads or virulence

in the transmitter.[184] Certain isolates of HIV-1 are known to induce cell fusion in culture, resulting in the formation of multinucleated giant cells called "syncytia." The presence of cytopathic syncytium-inducing (SI) viral phenotypes in donors with advanced disease has been associated with an increased risk of rapid disease progression in recipients when such SI viruses are transmitted and establish infection within the new host.[153,162] Regardless of the stage of HIV-1 in a male virus donor, the presence of genital inflammatory states such as urethritis and epididymitis appear to result in increased concentrations of infected lymphocytes in the semen, which may result in higher levels of infectiousness. It is likely that inflammatory states affecting vaginal and cervical tissues may also result in increased local concentrations of HIV-1 and hence the ability of an HIV-1–infected woman to transmit the virus to her sexual partner; however, standardized, reproducible techniques to quantitate the levels of HIV-1 present in the female genital tract are not yet available to address these questions.

The variables that influence a person's susceptibility to HIV-1 infection following exposure have yet to be clearly defined. HIV-1 is much more efficiently transmitted (approximately 20 times greater) from men to women than from women to men as a result of a single

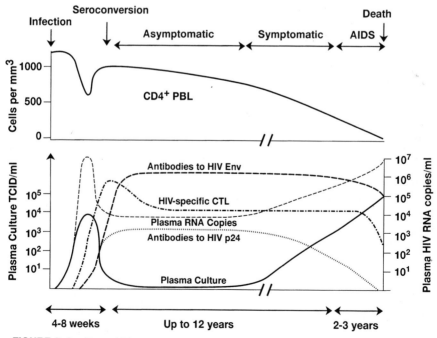

FIGURE 3–1. Natural history of HIV-1 infection. (Data from Piatak et al[142] and Weiss.[187])

episode of vaginal intercourse. The biologic basis of this differential susceptibility to infection is not known. However, the surface area of the mucosal tissues of the female reproductive tract that are exposed to virus or virus-infected cells present in the semen is significantly greater than that of the male urethra exposed to infected vaginal fluid. Furthermore, the duration of exposure to virus-containing fluids is also greater for women. Sexual transmission is facilitated by compromise of the integrity of mucosal surfaces and the presence of other sexually transmitted diseases (STDs), such as syphilis and chancroid that result in genital ulcerations, particularly in the recipient.[24] As a result, the prevalence of sexually transmitted disease in a population of persons at risk for HIV-1 infection can significantly alter the efficiency of viral spread.[42,148] Although the biologic mechanism for this enhanced susceptibility to infection has not been rigorously established, it is believed to result from the structural compromise of the epithelial lining of the mucosal surface and the presence of inflammatory processes that serve to increase the local concentration of activated T cells and antigen-presenting cells that likely represent the target cells for the first cycles of virus propagation in the new host.

Although changes in the female reproductive tract that occur in the course of the menstrual cycle might potentially result in transient increases or decreases in relative susceptibility to HIV-1 infection at different stages of the menstrual cycle, these have not yet been defined. One recent study reports that implantable or injectable progesterone-based contraceptives significantly increase the risk of infection following vaginal inoculation of simian immunodeficiency virus (SIV) in rhesus macaques.[104] The observed increased susceptibility to infection correlates with the progesterone-induced thinning of the epithelial lining of the vagina. Should similar effects of progesterone-based, long-acting contraceptive methods be demonstrated for HIV-1 infection of humans, it will have significant implications for HIV-1 prevention strategies and birth control practices, particularly in developing countries where use of these methods is common.

Studies of the simian acquired immunodeficiency syndrome (AIDS) model show that mucosa-associated macrophages appear to be the predominant cells infected in the vaginal mucosa following intravaginal inoculation of SIV.[116] SIV DNA has also been detected in presumptive dendritic cells just beneath the uterine mucosa of monkeys that were acutely infected with the virus intravaginally.[171] These observations are consistent with evidence that HIV-1 isolated early after transmission is more macrophage-tropic than later isolates, and further suggests that virus replication in macrophages is important after sexual transmission.[191] Elucidation of HIV-1 or SIV genetic determinants of sexual transmission efficiency would indicate whether HIV-1 antigens may be usefully included in candidate vaccines designed to prevent sexual transmission of HIV-1.

HIV-1 Subtypes and Sexual Transmission

Genetic or biologic features that may affect the efficiency with which individual strains of HIV-1 may be transmitted have yet to be clearly identified. It is not known whether individual viral gene products play specific roles that may modulate virus transmission or the early course of infection in the new host. Furthermore, little information is available concerning whether the pronounced genetic variation seen in HIV-1 quasispecies present in infected individuals affects the efficiency of virus transmission or the course of the initial stages of the establishment of the infection.

It has been recently suggested that an HIV-1 subtype, clade E, prevalent in Asia, may spread more easily through the vaginal mucosa, perhaps accounting for the greater efficiency of heterosexual spread of the virus in that part of the world.[95,128] This is in contrast to most transmissions of HIV-1 in the United States and Europe, which have been associated with male homosexual (receptive anal intercourse) or injection drug use (contaminated blood). HIV-1 subtype E viruses have been reported to replicate much better in tissue culture obtained than the American subtype B does on Langerhans' cells (LCs) from vaginal mucosa or penile foreskin, linking. Such LCs are found in high density and close to the mucosal surface in the penile foreskin, the vagina, and cervix. A potentially alarming conclusion of these studies is that if viruses such as HIV-1 E were introduced into the West, they might pose a greater threat for heterosexual transmission than HIV-1 B.[170] However, these data have been challenged on both virologic and epidemiologic grounds and additional studies will be needed to resolve these important issues.

Mother-to-Child Transmission

The observed rates of transmission of HIV-1 from mother to infant have varied from 13% to 45% in cohort studies conducted in Europe and Africa, respectively, with an average of approximately 25% reported.[17,50,121,177] The reasons for this variation are not known but they are likely to relate to differences in the stage of the maternal HIV-1 disease and in the adequacy of prenatal and perinatal medical care. A variety of factors associated with advanced HIV-1 disease in the mother, including p24 antigenemia, high levels of HIV-1 RNA in the plasma, and low CD4+ T cell counts are associated with an increased risk of infection in the neonate. Additional risk factors in perinatal transmission include: high maternal CD8+ lymphocyte counts, placental membrane inflammation, and maternal fever.[177]

Transmission of HIV-1 from a mother to her infant may occur in utero through placental passage of virus, during delivery, or postnatally through breast-feeding. Reports have described HIV-1 in the thymus, spleen, and peripheral blood mononuclear cells (PBMCs) of aborted fetuses from HIV-1–infected women, suggesting that HIV-1 infection can occur in utero.[35] New methods for early diagnosis of HIV-1 infection of infants have helped elucidate the timing of vertical transmission. A subset of neonates with detectable virus at birth is hypothesized to be infected in utero, whereas those with virus first detected 1 week or more after birth are thought to have been infected perinatally.[115] It is likely that many infant HIV-1 infections are acquired through contact with contaminated blood or secretions that occur at the time of birth.[123] Among twins, higher risk of HIV-1 infection is reported for the firstborn, even for twins delivered by cesarean section, suggesting that factors related to delivery affect the risk of infection.[60] Recent data indicate that prolonged duration of rupture of fetal membranes prior to delivery is independently associated with risk of transmission.

Although certain recent studies have found a strong correlation between elevated maternal plasma HIV-1 RNA levels and an increased risk of neonatal infection, instances of transmission have been reported across the spectrum of virus load, including the infants born to women with low plasma RNA levels.[19,51,186] Further analyses are needed to define whether a threshold exists for significantly increased risk of transmission, or whether antiviral therapy aimed at interrupting maternal-to-infant HIV-1 transmission must suppress viral replication in the mother below a threshold level in order to be effective.

An important recent study demonstrated that when zidovudine is administered to pregnant women during the second and third trimesters of pregnancy, is continued intrapartum, and is then administered to their infants during the first 6 weeks of life, the risk of maternal-to-infant transmission of HIV-1 can be reduced by approximately two thirds.[33,152] This study involved pregnant women with mildly symptomatic disease and little or no prior use of zidovudine; it is not known whether similar results can be obtained in women at other stages of disease and to what extent zidovudine resistance will limit the efficacy of this intervention. The reduction in perinatal transmission does not appear to be explained on the basis of reduced maternal viremia alone, suggesting that other factors might be important, such as the prophylactic effect of treating newborns with an antiretroviral. Indeed, it is surprising that a relatively weak antiviral drug like zidovudine can exert such a significant protective effect. Zidovudine therapy results in only modest decrease in HIV-1 replication in treated individuals, and these decreases are not durable. It will be important to determine whether the protective effect of zidovudine is manifest in the mother, or whether the drug is simply acting to effect postexposure prophylaxis against infection in the neonate. If the latter proves to be the case, the treatment regimen might be able to be simplified significantly. Future studies should help define the optimal timing for delivery of antiviral therapy to limit maternal-to-infant transmission, the mechanism of the protective effect of antiviral therapy and whether other antiviral drugs or alternative treatment strategies may be even more effective.

Attachment to and Infection of Target Cells

The HIV-1 envelope glycoprotein subunit gp120 mediates binding to the CD4 molecule found on cells, including T helper (Th) cells, monocytes/macrophages, and dendritic cells.[97,187] As CD4 is expressed at early stages of T cell development, CD4 T cells may be susceptible to HIV infection and destruction at all stages in their differentiation. After binding to CD4, the lipid bilayers of HIV-1 and the target-cell plasma membrane fuse, resulting in the release of the viral core into the cytoplasm.[52] The events that result in fusion have not been delineated clearly, but it appears that binding to CD4 alone is insufficient; one or more additional cellular cofactors are required.[27] Recent studies have revealed the identity of these essential cofactors for HIV-1 fusion and entry. Interestingly, these cofactors, which mediate a post-binding fusion event, are members of the chemokine receptor family, suggesting that recently identified HIV-1 suppressive chemokines may act by inhibiting HIV-cell fusion[53] (see below).

Virtually all HIV-1 isolates, including both primary patient-derived isolates and laboratory-adapted strains, grow in activated peripheral blood lymphocytes. Envelope glycoproteins of HIV-1 isolates adapted to growth in immortalized T-cell lines are unable to mediate efficient entry into macrophages, and envelope glycoproteins of macrophage-tropic strains cannot mediate entry into immortalized T-cell lines. These variations in tropism usually are not absolute but instead are manifested as the relative ability of different isolates to grow in different cell types. Observations suggest that the expression of cofactors involved in the initial stages of infection may vary between different target cells and that interactions with specific genetically determined components of the envelope glycoprotein are a key determinant of cell tropism.[81] Other viral genetic determinants may also influence the initial virus–host interaction after virus entry into cells.

It has been demonstrated that mixtures of T cells and dendritic cells (DCs) placed together in tissue culture support significant levels of HIV-1 replication.[146,147] Extending these observations, HIV-1 replication has been observed in dendritic cell-derived syncytia at the mucosal surface of the adenoid or tonsil.[56] In trying to identify important sites of HIV-1 replication in the body, it may be important to focus on tissues that contain interacting DCs and T cells, such as the lymphoid tissues of the pharynx or the extralymphoid sites in inflamed genital surfaces.

Selection for HIV-1 Strains During Primary Infection

Analysis of HIV-1 isolates from identified donor-recipient transmission pairs indicates that the highly heterogeneous viral populations present in the donors are subject to a potent process of selection that allows established infection only by minor virus subsets.[190,191] In the newly infected host, viruses that are homogeneous in their envelope sequences predominate, indicating selection based on *env* characteristics. Such viruses are largely macrophage-tropic and nonsyncytium-inducing (NSI). In contrast to strong selective pressure to conserve sequences within the envelope region, there exists a higher degree of sequence variability found in the other regions of the genome such as *gag* p17.[191]

It is unclear what mechanisms confer advantage to a subpopulation of viruses on primary infection, but this selection occurs in recipients infected through sexual, injection, and vertical transmission.[190] Two models can be postulated to account for these observations: (1) Preferential replication of virus subsets occurs in the newly infected host. Such selective amplification could result from a specific biologic phenotype of the virus that is advantageous in the immunocompetent host; for instance, macrophage-tropic viruses might be less easily cleared by the immune response. (2) Transmission of a limited subset of HIV-1 variants from the virus transmitter to the recipient occurs during the earliest stages of primary infection.

Outgrowth of predominantly macrophage-tropic viruses early in infection suggests that HIV-1 replication in macrophages is favored in the newly infected host. This finding further implicates macrophages as the virus-transmitting cells, or the first target cells likely to encounter HIV-1 during infection, or as sanctuaries for viral persistence once an immune response emerges.

Migration of HIV-1 to Lymph Nodes

At its entry point, be it mucous membrane or intravenous introduction into the bloodstream, free HIV-1 or HIV-1–infected cells are presumably cleared from interstitial spaces and delivered into the lumina of the blood or lymphatic vessels. Entry of HIV-1 or HIV-1–infected cells into the lymph nodes and other lymphoid tissues, where active immune responses to antigens occur, may lead to new cycles of HIV-1 replication and target-cell infection. The immunologically activated lymphoid tissue environment is ideal for perpetrating viral spread to additional T cells and macrophages. Entry of HIV-1 into the central nervous system can also occur during the primary infection period.

TARGET ORGANS AND LOCALIZATION OF VIRAL BURDEN

CD4+ cells at sites of immune activation represent the major target cells for active HIV-1 replication in infected persons. However, with increasing age and maturation of the immune system, the primary sites where CD4+ cells, particularly CD4+ T cells, are produced, change from thymus to peripheral lymphoid organs. The target organs for HIV-1 infection and consequent damage change correspondingly. The bulk of CD4+ T cells in the first-trimester fetus are found in the thymus. After 16 gestational weeks, fetal lymph nodes are seeded with CD4+ T cells. After birth, the thymus decreases in size. Following its significant involution during puberty, the largest reservoir of CD4+ T cells is found in the peripheral lymphoid organs—the lymph nodes, adenoids, and tonsils.[106] Because with time CD4 cells are distributed from the thymus to peripheral lymphoid organs, the host age at the time of HIV-1 infection, particularly of transplacental infection, may determine the extent of targeting of HIV-1 to the thymus versus peripheral lymph nodes.

Cells of the monocyte/macrophage lineage also are important targets of HIV-1 infection in vivo.[47] Tissue macrophages in the lymph nodes, lung, and central nervous system (CNS) are likely to be significant reservoirs of HIV-1 and may, based on in vitro studies, support HIV-1 production for long periods of time without being killed. It is not known how long HIV-1–infected macrophages can persist in vivo, but this is likely determined both by their sensitivity to the cytopathic consequences of viral infection and by their susceptibility to clearance by an antiviral immune response. Based on recent studies, cells that may be chronically infected with HIV-1 do not contribute to any great extent (<1%) to the total daily production of virus.[76,139,185] It remains to be determined whether long-lived chronically virus-producing macrophages do, in fact, exist in infected persons. However, should such cells provide a persistent reservoir of HIV-1 infection, they need not be numerous to have an important role in maintenance of the infection in the host. In contrast to T-cell infection, macrophage infec-

tion results in the localization of most viral products to intracellular vacuoles. In effect, much of the virus might remain potentially insulated from the host immune response.[111] Precursors of macrophages, the peripheral blood monocytes, appear to be rare targets of infection.[7]

Development of the Thymus and Response to HIV-1 Infection

Among HIV-1–infected children, a bimodal pattern of the rates of disease progression has been observed, and the timing of HIV-1 transmission is the likely reason for these different clinical outcomes.[143] Children with rapid disease progression may have detectable levels of virus at birth, manifest symptoms at a younger age, have impaired in vitro lymphocyte proliferative responses, lack anti–HIV-1 antibodies, and frequently, but not always, have lower CD4+ cell counts.[46] One study compared vertically infected children likely to have been infected by HIV-1 perinatally with children with hemophilia who acquired their HIV-1 infection later in life via HIV-1–contaminated clotting factor preparations. HIV-1–specific CTL responses were deficient in the perinatally infected group, with no apparent relationships between CD4+ cell counts, CD8+ cell counts, or p24 antigen levels.[100] High-level viremia also has been observed in perinatally infected children who have normal CD4+ T-cell counts.[155] Such high-level viral expression and lack of virus-specific host immune responses may result from thymic infection and consequent induction of immunologic tolerance to HIV-1 antigens. These phenomena occur in laboratory model infections of neonatal animals with the lymphocytic choriomeningitis virus[127] and the thymotropic Gross murine leukemia virus.[92] Children manifesting slow HIV-1 disease progression presumably were infected late in the development of their immune systems; that is, when thymic maturation is relatively complete and CD4+ T-cell distribution to the peripheral lymphoid organs resembles that of adults.

A model for HIV-1 infection of the human fetal thymus is the severe combined immunodeficiency (SCID)-hu mouse, a genetically immunodeficient mouse that has received transplants of human fetal thymus and liver and can sustain the human cellular processes of hematopoiesis and differentiation of functionally competent T cells.[106] HIV-1 can infect and replicate in the human thymus present in the SCID-hu mouse, leading to disruption of thymopoiesis, cortical thymocyte depletion, and compaction of the thymic epithelium.[18,172] These latter two structural changes have been noted in some instances in fetuses aborted from HIV-1–infected women.[135]

HIV-1 infection of the adult thymus has been described, but these observations have involved only late-stage disease postmortem specimens.[163] In the SIV-infected rhesus macaque model, which resembles HIV-1 infection of humans, SIV can be detected clearly in the thymus early after infection.[13,14] Bone marrow stem cells do not appear to be a significant site of HIV-1 infection in humans.[38]

Role of Lymphoid Organs in HIV-1 Infection of Adults

In the early and intermediate stages of HIV-1 disease, the greatest concentration of HIV-1–infected cells, both CD4+ lymphocytes and macrophages, is found in the lymphoid organs (lymph nodes, adenoids, tonsils, spleen), the primary sites for generation of immune responses. In situ hybridization and polymerase chain reaction (PCR) analyses detect about 5 to 10 times more HIV-1 on a per-cell basis in lymphoid organs than in the peripheral blood. In all stages of HIV-1 disease, RNA PCR for HIV-1 demonstrates that HIV-1–infected lymphocytes in the lymphoid organs express more HIV-1 RNA than do their counterparts in the peripheral blood.[131]

Follicular dendritic cells (FDCs) present a major antigen-trapping mechanism of the lymphoid tissue. They bind antigens, usually in the form of antigen–antibody complexes. Antigen bound to FDCs may persist within lymph nodes for long periods of time.[90] In situ hybridization and electron microscopy locate HIV-1 particles trapped within the network of FDCs in the germinal centers of lymph nodes.[47,131] FDC-associated HIV-1 can be detected in the early and intermediate stages of the disease. At the late stage, an impaired FDC network apparently loses virus- and antigen-trapping ability. FDCs themselves probably are not infected but rather simply trap HIV-1 particles present in immune complexes via receptors for complement or the Fc fragment (constant region) of immunoglobulin.[131]

In vitro HIV-1 bound to dendritic cells obtained from the peripheral blood can greatly potentiate viral infection of CD4+ T cells. The precise relationship between peripheral blood-derived dendritic cells and FDCs in the lymphatics is unclear. FDCs in the lymph nodes similarly may facilitate infection of CD4+ lymphocytes migrating through lymphoid follicles in the course of an immune response or normal circulation.[25] The recent demonstration of HIV-1 replication in dendritic cell-derived syncytia at the mucosal surface of the adenoid and tonsil support an in vivo role for the interaction of dendritic cells and T cells in mucosa leading to substantial levels of virus production.[56]

PRIMARY INFECTION AND IMMUNE RESPONSE TO HIV-1

Although variable, the natural history of HIV-1 infection can be divided into several phases (Fig. 3–1). The range and severity of symptoms in primary HIV-1 infection varies considerably, with an acute mononucleosis-like viral syndrome developing in about 40% of patients.[97] Based on analyses of symptomatic primary infection, symptoms include fever, headache, lymphadenopathy, myalgia, rash, and transient intense viremia with 10^3 to 10^4 median tissue culture infectious doses ($TCID_{50}$) of infectious HIV-1 or $\geq 10^6$ HIV-1 genomic RNA copies per milliliter of plasma.[142] (An apparent disparity exists between the levels of cultivable virus and viral RNA in the plasma throughout HIV-1 infection. It is unclear whether this disparity derives from the insensitivity of culture methods or the predominance of replication-defective viral particles.) Events accompanying the intense viremia of primary infection presumably include efficient cell–cell spread of HIV-1 and the seeding of multiple lymph nodes, a likely prelude to the generalized lymphadenopathy common in HIV-1 infection.[132] Up to 1% of peripheral blood CD4+ T cells are infected during this acute syndrome. The number of CD4+ T cells in peripheral blood falls acutely. It is not known if this drop represents a loss or a redistribution to extravascular sites.[52]

We know less about the underlying virology or immunology of asymptomatic primary infection. One comparison of persons reporting either symptomatic or asymptomatic primary HIV-1 infection showed no significant differences in HIV-1 RNA levels and CD4+ counts at the time of seroconversion, although subsequent establishment and maintenance of low steady-state plasma HIV-1 RNA levels was seen more frequently following asymptomatic versus symptomatic primary infection.[71]

Coincident with the resolution of acute clinical symptoms, generally within 1 month, the magnitude of plasma viremia and the number of infected CD4 + T lymphocytes in the peripheral blood fall sharply.[52] The magnitude of decline in virus concentration following acute HIV-1 infection appears to vary substantially between patients from less than 10-fold to over a 1000-fold decline.[88] These values likely represent underestimates, as it is unlikely that true peak viremia measures were obtained. The decline in viremia may occur before overt seroconversion, suggesting that a cellular immune response that first appears around the time that the levels of plasma virus and infected cells begin to decline may be responsible for this diminished level of HIV-1 replication.[156]

Recipients with severe clinical presentations of primary HIV-1 infection before seroconversion appear more likely to progress rapidly to AIDS than those who experience asymptomatic primary infections.[86] A predominant concept emerging from natural history studies is that circumstances surrounding early primary HIV-1 infection may either determine or foreshadow the subsequent disease course. With the resolution of the acute syndrome, different patients display different steady-state levels of viral replication as manifest by different levels of plasma HIV-1 RNA. Several studies now suggest that the plateau concentration of plasma viral RNA (the so-called set-point) achieved 6 to 12 months after primary HIV-1 infection is predictive of the long-term clinical outcome. Thus, individuals who display higher steady-state levels of plasma HIV-1 RNA following resolution of their primary infection are at significantly greater risk for disease progression (see below).[72,78,83,109,110,157,158]

The determinants of the set-point of plasma viral load are not known but may include the effectiveness of the antiviral immune responses, the numbers of target cells available for infection, or the degree of immune activation extant in a given individual. It is also conceivable that a small viral load after seroconversion is related to a small virus inoculum and/or low pathogenicity of the infecting HIV-1 strain, circumstances of inoculation, or some combination of factors. What role the host genetic background might play in this initial interaction needs to be determined. Intervention with antiviral drugs during this period may have a significant impact on the rate of disease progression if key features of the initial host–virus interaction can be favorably altered.[75,88] Thus, the role of antiretroviral therapy in modulating this initial virus–host interaction, and possibly the associated disease course, is an important area for further investigation.[183]

In children infected through their mothers, the progression of HIV-1 disease follows two patterns.[46,164] In the first year of life, severe immunodeficiency develops in approximately 20% of infected infants and is frequently accompanied by HIV-1–associated CNS complications. The remainder of infected children manifest a more slowly progressive disease course similar to that seen in adults. The risk of developing early and severe disease is higher in newborns who test positive at birth for HIV-1 by viral culture, PCR, or serum p24 core antigen assay, which indicates they were likely infected in utero. The risk that rapid disease progression will occur is significantly greater for an infant of a mother with advanced HIV-1 disease at the time of the infant's birth. It is not yet known whether the increased risk results from a greater maternal viral load or the presence of more virulent viruses in a person with late-stage disease.

The Immune Response and Initial Control of Primary Viremia: Role of CD8 in Primary Infection

Immunologic control of viremia early after infection may be critical in determining the subsequent clinical course of HIV-1 infection.[71,109] There is a temporal association of HIV-1–specific CD8 + cytotoxic T lymphocytes (CTLs) with initial control of viremia in primary HIV-1 infection.[191] CTL precursors specific for cells expressing HIV-1 Gag, Pol, and Env antigens have been detected within 3 weeks of presentation of primary HIV-1 syndrome.[93] It cannot be rigorously ascertained what role CTLs have in reducing primary HIV-1 viremia; modeling of the dynamics of early HIV-1 infection predicts that reductions in virus concentration can be achieved in the absence of a specific immune response, and could be due to a decline in the availability of activated, uninfected CD4 + T cells.[141] Serum anti-gp120 antibodies are detected after virus titers have declined manyfold, suggesting that such antibodies do not play a major role in clearance of initial viremia, and neutralizing antibodies appear even later in the course of infection.[119]

In a study of a limited number of patients, major expansions of restricted subsets of CD8 + T cells determined by the usage of certain variable domains (V) of the beta (β) chain of the T-cell receptor (TCR) appeared to be associated with a less effective immune response in primary HIV-1 infection. These restricted expansions of Vβ subsets were oligoclonal and appeared to represent HIV-1–specific immune responses with cytolytic T-cell activity.[129,130] One interpretation of these studies is that an inability to mount a broad repertoire of T-cell responses to HIV-1 infection limits the host's ability to inhibit virus replication. Furthermore, there appears to be evidence of disappearance of the responding subsets of T cells over time, suggesting the possibility of clonal exhaustion of the responding CD8 + T cells, as has been reported for other viral infections.[120]

Evidence has also been presented for CD8 + T-lymphocyte control of virus infection by a noncytolytic, non–MHC-restricted HIV-1 suppressor activity.[102] This appears to be mediated by the release of HIV-1 suppressive factors. The chemokines RANTES, MIP-1-α, and MIP-1β were recently identified as major suppressor factors produced by CD8 + T cells in culture.[31] It is not yet clear how the secretion of these factors by CD8 + T cells in vivo may relate to the course of HIV-1 disease progression.

Thus the vigor of the initial immune response to HIV-1 appears to influence significantly the clinical outcome of HIV-1 disease. The absence of a serologic response to HIV-1 core protein and an impaired cellular immune response are associated with more rapid progression to AIDS.[86,140,153]

There are reports of HIV-1–seronegative individuals that are thought to have been exposed multiple times to HIV-1. Several publications have reported the presence of HIV-1–specific T-cell responses in these individuals (reviewed in references 154 and 167). Possible mechanisms explaining the detection of HIV-1–specific T-cell immunity in HIV-1–seronegative individuals exposed to HIV-1 include exposure to non-infectious HIV-1, infection with a defective HIV-1 strain, infection with a replicating HIV-1 that is killed or kept under control by T-cell–mediated immune responses or relative host cell resistance to infection. Nonhuman primate studies suggest that an established infection with an attenuated virus may induce robust immunity protective against subsequent infection with virulent virus.[37,137] It will be important to study these examples of apparent natural immunization of exposed individuals, as well as the SIV macaque model, in order to develop a strategy for immunization against HIV-1 infection. There is also a suggestion, based on epidemiologic data, that preexisting HIV-2 infection offers some relative protection against HIV-1 infection, suggesting that cross-protection is possible.[181] However, contrary reports have also been presented. It will be important to establish the veracity of these observations and to define the immunologic correlates of such protection.

In addition to a CD8 + lymphocyte anti–HIV-1 activity, a recent study also demonstrated the relative resistance to HIV-1 infection of CD4 lymphocytes from persons who had experienced multiple high-risk sexual exposure yet remained uninfected. This resistance was also associated with the chemokines RANTES, MIP-1-α, and MIP-1-β.[138] Thus some hosts may be more resistant to HIV-1 infection based on genetically determined features of their CD4 target cells.

Although a vigorous immune response to HIV-1 infection appears to occur in most individuals, containing the virus for varying periods of time, eventually the ability to contain virus replication is lost, resulting in immune compromise. Possible reasons for the inability to clear or contain HIV-1 replication include virus mutation and escape from the immune response, a latent virus reservoir, or a high rate of virus replication that the immune response is unable to catch up with and clear. There has been relatively little strong evidence to support the hypothesis of viral immune escape, although it was recently demonstrated that HIV-1 mutations arise that help HIV-1–infected cells evade the immune response. This appears to occur by the MHC I presentation of mutated peptides that vary slightly from the target peptide and which act to inactivate or anergize the specific anti–HIV-1 CTL response.[108,180] A putative role for a latent virus reservoir awaits the application of sensitive methods for virus detection in lymphoid tissues, particularly in the face of potent combination antiviral therapy that may reduce plasma viremia to undetectable levels. Finally, a rapid replication rate of HIV-1 that the immune response cannot catch up with does not explain why the immune system cannot clear poorly replicating viruses like the nef deletion mutants.[137]

Clinical Latency

Once the symptoms of primary infection subside and an antiviral immune response appears, patients usually enter a chronic, clinically asymptomatic or minimally symptomatic state that typically lasts for 7 to 11 years before the development of overt immunodeficiency. Studies clearly demonstrate that a high rate of viral replication continues in the lymph nodes throughout this period, clearly indicating that HIV-1 disease is active and progressive.[47,131] During this stage, there are low levels of infectious HIV-1 in the plasma and only a small fraction of CD4+ T cells in the peripheral blood are infected (between 1 in 10,000 and 1 in 100,000).[52] However, many patients have significant amounts of viral RNA in the plasma, ranging from 10^3 to 10^6 HIV-1 RNA copies per milliliter.[142]

VIRAL LOAD AND DISEASE PROGRESSION

As discussed above, individual patients display different steady-state levels of plasma HIV-1 RNA, the magnitude of which correlates with risk for disease progression. Thus patients with $\geq 10^5$ copies of HIV-1 RNA per milliliter of plasma are considered to be at significantly greater risk of disease progression than those with $<10^4$ copies/ml. These studies extend previous observations that showed that increasing viral burden in the plasma and elevated levels of HIV-1 DNA and RNA in peripheral blood cells correlated with depletion of CD4+ T cells. Clearly, plasma HIV-1 RNA levels have emerged as a strong, CD4+ T-cell–independent predictor of disease progression and should be a powerful tool for the stratification of patients for risk of disease development.[109] Recent studies also link increased expression of HIV-1 mRNA in PBMCs with more rapid progression to AIDS.[65,157,158]

Plasma HIV-1 RNA measurements are also useful for the assessment of therapeutics, and as a predictor of clinical response to therapy.[124] It will be important to better determine, through clinical trials, the correlation between changes in virus load and clinical outcome, so as to offer guidelines for physicians in the clinical use of HIV-1 quantitation assays.

The correlation of high viremia with short times to disease progression, and low viremia with longer survival, suggest the potential role of a cumulative virus replication burden in determining disease progression. Such a putative cumulative effect of ongoing virus replication may be a reflection of a finite capacity of the CD4+ T-cell system for renewal in the face of ongoing lymphocyte destruction (see HIV-1 Replication Kinetics below). Ongoing studies promise to elucidate the relationship between HIV-1 replication and T-cell destruction, which eventually results in frank immunodeficiency.

HIV-1 Disease Progression

Progression of HIV-1 disease to AIDS is presaged by an increase in the rate of loss of CD4+ lymphocytes and, in at least 50% of cases, the appearance of a more virulent SI virus phenotype.[91] Profound immunodeficiency is manifest clinically by opportunistic infections, as well as a variety of malignancies and wasting and neurologic disorders as described in other chapters. Increasing viral burden in the plasma and elevated levels of HIV-1 DNA and RNA in peripheral blood cells correlate with depletion of CD4+ T cells. As CD4+ T-cell numbers fall, the percentage of infected CD4+ T cells may reach 1 in 10.[6] In many instances, the increasing levels of plasma viremia exceed 10^4 $TCID_{50}$ and 10^5 to 10^6 HIV-1 genomic RNA copies/ml.[142]

Considerable variation exists in the time it takes for clinical disease to develop in different persons. A minority of persons succumb to an accelerated disease course, which may result in full-blown AIDS in 1 to 2 years.[142] At the other end of the spectrum, small cohorts of HIV-1–infected persons have been described who have sustained long-term (>10 years), symptom-free HIV-1 infection.[98] Studies have reported an association between HLA type and the course of HIV-1 infection, but there has been a lack of consistency between HLA types identified. Recently it was shown that combinations of human major histocompatibility complex genes appear to influence the course of HIV-1 infection.[84] Further epidemiologic linkage of specific HLA markers with longer or shorter AIDS-free intervals can focus the search for the immunologic mechanisms underlying this variability.

Changes in Viral Phenotype During HIV-1 Disease Progression

HIV-1 disease is an evolutionary process marked by changes from characteristic early to late viral phenotypes of distinct cellular tropism and cytopathic potential. The phenotype of viral isolates obtained during asymptomatic infection is notable for the great predominance of NSI isolates compared to SI isolates, slow- versus fast-growing viruses, and a preferential tropism for macrophages and inability to infect immortalized T-cell lines in tissue culture. NSI strains of HIV-1 are presumably less pathogenic, whereas SI strains appear more pathogenic and may replicate more efficiently. The prevalence of NSI strains in early and intermediate stages of disease may be due to the more rapid clearance of SI isolates at times when an effective antiviral immune response is present. As disease progresses, the more highly replicative, T-cell line-tropic SI viruses predominate.[34,91] These phenotypic differences can be reproduced at the level of the genotype with molecular clones, and studies with chimeric viruses have identified the envelope gene as the major determinant of cell tropism and cytopathogenicity.[3,55,66,94] It is unclear whether the postinfection increase in cytopathicity of HIV-1 isolates with time is the cause or the consequence of progressive immune system deterioration. The appearance of SI viruses is clearly not a prerequisite for the development of severe immunodeficiency, since approximately one half of individuals with AIDS harbor only NSI viruses. Furthermore, it is unclear how HIV-1 may be evolving in its passage from one host to the next, potentially giving rise to more or less pathogenic variants.

Long-Term Survivors of HIV-1 Infection

Small cohorts of HIV-1–infected persons have been described who have sustained long-term, symptom-free HIV-1 infection. About 5% of all HIV-1–infected people appear to experience nonprogressing HIV-1 infection, defined by 10 to 15 years of infection, good health, and stable CD4 + peripheral blood T-cell levels.[10,70] Some of these people represent the tail of the distribution of normal responses to HIV-1 infection. Only time and additional characterization will tell what percentage of these people represent truly unique host–virus relationships different from the vast majority of others. Nonetheless, study of the causes of nonprogressive or less aggressive HIV-1 infection is beginning to elucidate underlying features of nonprogressive infection.

Nonprogressors are a heterogeneous group with respect to viral load and antiviral immune responses. In general, they appear to have lower levels of plasma HIV-1 RNA levels and high pe-

ripheral blood CD8 + MHC class I–restricted anti–HIV-1 CTL levels (reviewed in references 10 and 70), although it is clear that exceptions exist. Nonprogressors have low concentrations of serum and cellular markers of immune activation, and, in limited numbers of individuals studied, the structure and function of lymph node germinal centers appear to be maintained and the follicular dendritic cells preserved. Individuals with exceptionally low viral loads and strong anti–HIV-1 CTL responses after prolonged HIV-1 infection appear to represent stable long-term nonprogressing infection, while those with higher viral loads and less vigorous anti–HIV-1 CTL responses are at higher risk of disease progression. Virus from some nonprogressors may grow less well, although viruses from asymptomatic people generally replicate less well than those from patients with late-stage disease, making it difficult to precisely discern the role of relative viral replicative fitness in nonprogressing infection.

A minority of nonprogressors appears to be infected with less pathogenic virus variants.[39,89] In particular, it was found that HIV-1 from a blood donor and a group of blood transfusion recipients from that donor did not exhibit evidence of HIV-1 disease progression despite 10 to 14 years' infection, and harbored viruses with deletions in the *nef* gene and the U3 region of the long-terminal repeat. These results parallel findings in monkeys infected with simian immunodeficiency viruses harboring *nef* deletions. In these experimental SIV infections, infection of adult monkeys with *nef*-deleted viruses causes nonprogressing SIV infection.[37,87] The *nef* alterations do not appear to account for most cases of nonprogressive HIV-1 infection.[79] It is conceivable that other lesions exist in viral strains from nonprogressors and that a low level of replication due to debilitating mutations is responsible for at least some cases of nonprogression.

HIV-1 REPLICATION KINETICS

Recent studies have demonstrated that high concentrations of virus are present in lymphoid tissues and plasma throughout the course of HIV-1 infection.[97,132,187] The magnitude of these measurements of viral concentration do not, however, indicate the rate of turnover of the virus population. Measurement of virus turnover requires some perturbation of the steady-state system, such as that provided by initiation of effective antiviral therapy, to allow measurement of viral clearance and the longevity of virus-producing cells.[32] The half-life of the clearance of plasma virions, estimated from the slope of the initial fall in viremia using simple mathematical models, was calculated to be very short (~6 hours).[139] Because the antiviral effects of the drugs prevent de novo infection of cells rather than affecting the clearance of virus or virus-producing cells, the estimates of clearance are expected to be valid for the pretreatment period as well. Furthermore, these studies indicate that the steady-state level of HIV-1 present in the plasma represents the product of numerous rounds of de novo infection of T cells. With the definition of such a short (and apparently constant [see below]) half life of HIV-1 virions in the circulation, it was realized that the major determinant of the steady-state level of virions present in the plasma is an accurate reflection of the amount of virus being produced at a given time in an infected individual. Thus, plasma HIV-1 RNA measures reflect active contemporary virus replication. In order to maintain the plasma viral loads usually found in the latter stages of HIV-1 infection, as many as 10^8 to 10^9 virions (or more) must be produced and cleared every day. At least 99% of this large pool of virus is produced by recently infected cells, rather than from long-lived, chronically infected cells or recently activated latently infected cells. The half-life of plasma virus varies little between patients with different viral loads or at different stages of the disease. Although the mechanism of clearance of plasma virions is not understood, the observed lack of correlation between plasma viral clearance and the initial CD4 count suggests that viral clearance may not be dependent on specific host immune responses. Rather, virions may be cleared in the reticuloendothelial system or due to inherent thermodynamic instability of the virus.

The rate and magnitude of the reduction of plasma virus seen in these studies also permits the estimation of how long infected cells produce virus and how long they live following HIV-1 infection.[32,63,76,139,185] Such calculations indicate that the lifespan of an infected cell is quite short, averaging less than 2 days. Thus, a very active process of infection of CD4 + T cells represents the fuel for HIV-1 replication in vivo, and like other types of fuel, the susceptible target cells for virus replication are consumed in the process. Surprisingly, the estimated lifespans of productively infected cells were not

markedly different between patients with differing initial CD4 T-cell counts, even though individuals with low CD4 counts are commonly believed to have less vigorous antiviral immune responses. Thus, it remains unclear whether and to what extent the host immune response can effectively interrupt HIV-1 replication by targeting newly infected cells for destruction before they produce infectious progeny virus.

Earlier comparisons of HIV-1 envelope sequences found in plasma viral RNA to those found in PBMC-associated proviral populations demonstrated significant envelope sequence differences,[168] indicating that virus circulating in the plasma must be produced by infected cells other than the HIV-1 DNA–positive lymphocytes present in the peripheral circulation. More recent studies have shown that HIV-1 DNA–containing cells in the peripheral blood appear to harbor largely defective, as opposed to infectious proviruses, reemphasizing the concept that such HIV DNA–positive cells represent a proviral "graveyard" of past infection events.[185]

Viral Variation

One feature of HIV-1 that is of particular importance to the biology of the virus and the development of effective therapeutic interventions is the high degree of nucleotide sequence variation between different viral strains.[32] HIV-1 variants generated during the course of an individual's infection may display variable cell tropism and cytopathic potential, as well as variable sensitivity to antiviral drugs. Much of this variation is the consequence of the manner in which HIV-1 replicates its genome, and is introduced by the retroviral reverse transcriptase, which lacks a so-called proofreading activity. Additional variation is introduced into viral genomic sequences by recombination. The probability that new viral mutants will arise increases with the number of cumulative cycles of virus replication. Thus, the numerous cycles of HIV-1 replication known to occur during the course of HIV-1 infection and the known infidelity of the reverse transcriptase result in the rapid emergence of variant viruses and a great genetic diversity of the virus population. Viral diversity may reflect the selection of immune escape mutants.

Viral diversification underlies the development of resistance to antiviral drugs. Increasing viral diversity leading to the crossing of an antigenic diversity threshold, whereby the immune system can no longer control the viral population, has been invoked as a cause of immune collapse in AIDS.[122]

IMMUNE ACTIVATION AND HIV-1 REPLICATION

Antigen presentation to T cells leads to activation of cytokine production, proliferation, and effector functions. A link between T-cell activation and HIV-1 infection occurs at three levels: (1) Early events, including viral entry and reverse transcription, are limited in resting T cells. (2) Integration of the HIV-1 genome into the host T-cell chromosome depends on an intracellular T-cell environment in which DNA synthesis is activated.[52] (By contrast, in macrophages, HIV-1 infection is not dependent on cell DNA synthesis but may be facilitated by the differentiation of monocytes into macrophages.[150]) (3) Expression of the integrated provirus is enhanced by cellular activation via the presence of DNA sequences within the long terminal repeat (LTR) of the integrated HIV-1 proviral genome that bind host–cell transcription factors that are induced during T-cell activation and lead to increased levels of viral RNA transcription.

The regulatory mechanisms that govern gene expression of the integrated HIV-1 provirus are complex and likely play important roles in the virus' ability to establish persistent infection, avoid clearance by the host immune system, and in determining the immunopathogenic consequences of viral infection. In T cells, the inducible host cell transcription factors, NF-κB play a major role in controlling the cellular response to antigenic stimulation.[5] Similarly, a number of important macrophage functions depend on NF-κB–mediated transcriptional activation. By incorporating NF-κB-mediated regulation in its regulatory repertoire, HIV-1 is intimately linked to the state of activation of lymphocytes and macrophages that provide targets for virus infection. Circumstances that lead to activation of the immune response may thus also result in activation of HIV-1 production. The lymphatic tissues (such as lymph nodes) that serve as sites of initiation of immune responses and are laden with activated cells and rich in cytokines display the highest density of virus-infected and virus-producing cells found in vivo. HIV-1 has thus effectively coopted important host regulatory functions by exploiting the activation of NF-κB to enhance viral RNA transcription and hence, replication.

While HIV-1 replication in culture is known to be greatly facilitated by T-cell activation, the ability of specific antigenic stimulation to augment HIV-1 replication in vivo has only recently been studied. Several reports have linked vaccination with transient increases in viremia in HIV-1–infected individuals.[21,74,125,173,174,188] Vaccination of HIV-1–infected individuals appears to lead to transient activation of virus replication in infected persons with preserved ability to immunologically respond to vaccine antigens. Increased levels of virus replication seen following immunization are likely the result of vaccine-induced increases in the size of the pool of target cells that are susceptible to HIV-1 infection, strengthening the concept that the pool of susceptible cells may be an important determinant of steady-state virus replication levels. It will be important to determine whether vaccination targets antigen-responsive T cells for cytopathic effects of virus infection.

Although the relationship between potentially immune-stimulating intercurrent or opportunistic infections and HIV-1 replication has not been systematically studied, emerging evidence suggests that such infections are associated with increases in HIV-1 viral load.[23,40,114,165] Furthermore, in HIV-1–infected individuals, it is reported that acyclovir therapy for those with a prior history of herpesvirus infection, and isoniazid therapy in tuberculin skin test–positive individuals, confer survival advantage and delay disease progression, respectively.[134,175] These observations suggest that reducing the chronic immune stimulation caused by these pathogens is beneficial. However, further study is needed to determine whether opportunistic infection–induced virus activation leads to a faster rate of disease progression. It will also be important to determine whether antigen-driven constriction in the repertoire of T-cell antigen recognition occurs, and if so, whether such constriction is irreversible. Given the demonstrated ability of antigenic challenge to activate virus replication, the effects of immune stimulation, due either to vaccines or intercurrent infections, are important topics for study. The role of antiretrovirals during known periods of immune stimulation and potential associated increased HIV-1 replication also need to be investigated.

MODULATION OF THE VIRUS–HOST INTERACTION BY HIV-1 GENE PRODUCTS

HIV-1 belongs to the lentivirus subfamily of retroviruses, characterized by the ability to cause persistent infection and slowly progressive disease. Lentiviruses have unusually complex genome structures that apparently underlie the ability of these viruses to engage in a highly modulated host–virus interaction, perhaps to permit avoidance of immune clearance. In trying to elucidate the evolutionary and functional significance of the complex genome structure of HIV-1, it is important to remember that HIV-1 likely evolved in and emerged from a nonpathogenic host–virus relationship. Such a nonpathogenic relationship between a T-cell tropic lentivirus and its natural host is exemplified by healthy, naturally SIV-infected sooty mangabeys in West Africa. Persistent SIV infection is prevalent in mangabeys, in the absence of any disease. Sooty mangabeys are the source of pathogenic SIV infection in macaques and HIV-2 infection in humans where disease appears in new, unnatural hosts following zoonotic (cross-species) transmission of virus. HIV-1 disease is also likely the result of transfer of HIV-1 from an "equilibrium" host to a "non-equilibrium" host.[9]

This section describes the role of HIV gene products in modulating the host–virus interaction. The role of HIV accessory genes *vpr, nef, vpu,* and *vif* in maximizing virus infectivity in vivo is elucidated by experimental infections of macaques with SIV variants that are unable to express specific accessory proteins.

Unlike simple retroviruses like murine leukemia virus, HIV-1 is able to infect nondividing cells such as macrophages. This is accomplished by active nuclear transport of the viral preintegration complex, mediated by the nucleophilic structural protein Gag matrix and the accessory viral protein Vpr.[8,69] Vpr, well conserved among the immunodeficiency viruses, is present in virus particles, consistent with its described function early in the virus life cycle. Later in the virus life cycle, Vpr induces cell-cycle arrest of infected cells. In HIV-2 and SIV, the two distinct functions of the HIV-1 Vpr are divided between two viral proteins, Vpr and Vpx. HIV-2 Vpr is responsible for the arrest of infected cells, while Vpx functions in permitting the nuclear transport of the viral preintegration complex.

The role of Vpr-induced cell cycle arrest in the biology of HIV-1 is unclear, but recent data indicate that infected cells that are arrested in the G_2 phase of the cell cycle produce greater quantities of virus. Some have postulated that cell cycle arrest leads to immune functional impairment and possible death of CD4+ lymphocytes.[12,43,144,151] However, *vpr* mutants of SIV still induce AIDS, suggesting that cell cycle arrest in simian lentivirus infection is not, in and of itself, necessary for disease induction.[58,77,96] Furthermore, the fact that natural SIV infection of its natural hosts, sooty mangabeys and African green monkeys, does not produce disease, suggests that cell cycle arrest is not sufficient for pathogenesis in vivo. Thus it appears that Vpr may facilitate virus persistence and/or viral production by interfering with the cell cycle of CD4+ cells and impairing immune surveillance of these cells or maximizing their virus production.[12]

Nef is one of the first viral proteins made in infected cells, and its expression continues throughout later stages of the viral life cycle.[52] Nef (1) acts to down-regulate cell-surface CD4, (2) acts as a positive factor for viral infection and replication in primary lymphocytes and macrophages, and (3) may alter the state of cell activation or the process of signal transduction via the TCR.[45,57,117,118]

The role of Nef-induced down-regulation of cell surface CD4 receptor expression is not completely understood. Nef may, via degradation of CD4, augment virus infectivity by rescuing viral Env glycoproteins from entrapment in intracellular complexes with CD4. Thus, Nef may increase the concentration of Env glycoproteins on virus particles. Nef also acts within infected cells to enhance infectivity of virus particles via a CD4-independent, but poorly understood mechanism.[61,117,118] These data support the concept that HIV-1 *nef* plays an important role in establishing a fulminant form of viral infection in vivo. Nef-induced enhancement of virus replication likely affects the balance between virus and host immune response. In the absence of *nef,* the immune response may prevail.

It has been suggested that Nef-elicited perturbations in T-cell signaling may play an important role in the viral life cycle in vivo.[99,169] Characterization of an SIV *nef* allele that causes lymphocyte activation provides suggestive evidence of a role for HIV-1 *nef* in signal transduction and cellular activation.[45]

Although not absolutely necessary for in vitro replication, *nef* clearly plays an essential role in the pathogenesis of HIV-1 and SIV infection. Infection of macaques with SIV with a deletion of *nef* does not replicate effectively or cause disease but instead protects animals from disease on subsequent infection with a pathogenic *nef*+ virus.[37] Furthermore, HIV-1 *nef* alterations are associated with nonprogressing HIV-1 infection.[39,89]

Vpu, a transmembrane protein, disrupts the formation of intracellular CD4-envelope gp160 complexes by inducing degradation of CD4 trapped in the endoplasmic reticulum by gp160. This may ensure sufficient cell surface expression of gp160 for incorporation into virions, and perhaps prevent the accumulation of toxic viral proteins or intracellular virion budding, reducing cytopathic effects. Independent of CD4 degradation, Vpu also mediates an increased rate of particle release; the net result of these activities appears to be enhanced virion production from infected cells.[161] The absence of a distinct *vpu* homologue in SIV, and thus the lack of an animal model to study *vpu* function, makes it difficult to assess the importance of *vpu* for pathogenicity. The detrimental effect of Vpu on CD4 appears to be redundant in that two other viral gene products result in down-modulation of CD4: Nef and the gp160 envelope glycoprotein. The net benefit of *vpu* may simply be an increased rate of virus production and prolonged output of virus from infected cells.[189]

The *vif* gene, encoded by all primate lentiviruses, appears to function as a virion component. The *vif* gene is essential for the production of infectious virus particles from primary peripheral blood lymphocytes or macrophages, consistent with the failure of *vif*-mutated SIV to replicate in vivo.[182]

The HIV-1 *rev* gene plays an essential role in ensuring that the appropriate balance of viral regulatory and structural proteins are produced throughout the virus life cycle in a coordinated fashion.[136] Although the role that Rev plays in the in vivo biology of HIV-1 infection is not known, Rev may act to coordinate HIV-1 assembly and production within a brief period of time so as to limit the capacity of the host immune system to identify and kill infected cells before the release of viral progeny. Alternatively, Rev may act to limit the cytopathic consequences of expression of the cytopathic Env protein to a precise time after infection so as to maximize HIV-1 production prior to death of the infected cells.

PATHOGENICITY OF HIV-1: POTENTIAL MECHANISMS

Recent studies have dramatically highlighted that appreciable viral expression and replication continue throughout the course of HIV-1 disease, including the clinically latent period, and argue that the direct cytopathic (cell damaging) effects of viral replication are responsible for progressive loss of CD4+ T cells and immune deterioration. However, indirect mechanisms of T-cell depletion can also be envisioned. This section describes potential cytopathic outcomes resulting from HIV-1 infection.

Direct HIV-1–Mediated Cytopathic Effects

HIV-1–induced cytopathology presumably arises from the interaction of HIV-1 gene products and host cells. Cytopathic effects of the virus occur in vitro and likely have relevance in vivo. Moreover, the recent demonstrations that the half-life of HIV-1–infected cells in vivo is extraordinarily short, and similar to the length of the viral life cycle (~2 days), further support the notion that HIV-1 infection leads to cytopathic depletion of CD4+ T cells.[139] However, extrapolation from in vitro observations to the in vivo situation must be performed cautiously. For example, high levels of viral replication in tissue culture and consequent cytopathic processes proceed unimpeded by the immunologic containment mechanism extant in vivo. Potential mechanisms for direct HIV-1–induced cytopathicity include single-cell killing, syncytia formation and cell killing, and suppression of immune cell function and modulation of the virus–host cell interaction by HIV-1 gene products.

Single-Cell Killing

HIV-1 can cause extensive cell death during in vitro infection of CD4+ T cells, and it is likely that this cytopathic effect is relevant in vivo. The newly synthesized HIV-1 envelope glycoprotein, gp160, interacts with the host cell CD4 molecule, retaining it in the endoplasmic reticulum.[36] The cytopathic consequences of this interaction appear to be disruption of cell membrane integrity, leading to cell lysis.[26] Accumulation and budding of HIV-1 particles may further disturb the structural and functional integrity of cellular components such as the plasma membrane. In addition to HIV-1 gene products, the accumulation of unintegrated viral DNA may potentially contribute to impairment of cell function and cell death.[132]

Syncytia Formation and Cell Killing

The HIV-1 envelope glycoprotein expressed on the surface of infected cells can interact with CD4 molecules present on the surface of other CD4+ cells—an event which, in tissue culture, results in fusion of the cells and the formation of multinucleated giant cells, or syncytia. Syncytia formation is a mechanism by which a few HIV-1–infected cells might fuse with and eliminate many uninfected CD4+ cells.[26,132] Significant levels of dendritic cell–derived syncytia have recently been observed at the mucosal surface of the adenoid.[56] Previously, syncytia formation had rarely been observed directly in vivo (except in the CNS, as seen in postmortem brain tissue), perhaps due to the rapid clearance of such aberrant multinucleated giant cells from the circulation. As discussed before, the in vitro phenotype of viral isolates changes with the course of disease progression from predominantly NSI viruses to SI viruses in at least 50% of cases.[179]

Indirect Virally Mediated Suppression of Immune Cell Function and Anergy

Immune dysregulation may be caused by soluble factors, such as cytokines, released by infected cells and affecting the ability of uninfected cells to mount an immune response. One potential mechanism for CD4+ cell dysfunction is raised by the observation that in vitro incubation of normal PBMCs with gp120 and anti-gp120 antibody down-regulates surface CD4 expression and depresses lymphocyte proliferative responses to anti-CD3 (antibody against the TCR). These same impairments are found in T cells taken directly from AIDS patients, supporting the hypothesis that epitopes present on the CD4 molecule are masked by gp120 and anti-gp120 antibody complexes, which would exist in vivo.[2] Inappropriate cell signaling caused by the binding of gp120 or gp120–antibody complexes to CD4 has been

hypothesized to cause anergy, an impairment in the immune response capacity of CD4+ cells in patients with advanced HIV-1 disease.[132] Alternatively, or in addition, the relative increase of anergic cells may simply result from the resistance of nonproliferative cells to the cytopathic effects of HIV-1, which targets activated T cells.

Apoptosis

The chronic immune stimulation caused by HIV-1 infection may indirectly contribute to the loss of uninfected CD4+ T cells by sensitizing them to initiate apoptosis, or programmed cell death. Apoptosis is an active process that requires protein and RNA synthesis and is implemented in part by activating cellular endonucleases. Apoptosis is a normal mechanism for eliminating certain classes of cells that might otherwise have a harmful effect; for example, lymphocytes capable of reacting with host antigens and triggering autoimmune phenomena. Two events may be necessary for apoptosis: The first event, the priming, sensitizes the lymphocyte for apoptosis, but the process of programmed cell death is initiated only after the second event—an activation stimulus that, in the absence of priming, would initiate lymphocyte activation and proliferation and not apoptosis. For lymphocytes, a priming signal may be generated when specific lymphocyte surface molecules from the same cell are cross-linked (i.e., simultaneously form a complex with an external molecule, such as a specific antigen, or an antigen–antibody complex). Normally, activation occurs when the TCR of a lymphocyte encounters a specific antigen, leading to cellular activation and proliferation.

Apoptosis is not unique to HIV-1 infection. Activated T cells from patients with acute viral infections, such as infectious mononucleosis or chickenpox, also undergo apoptosis, probably as part of the normal down-regulation of the immune response following acute infection.[149] Apoptosis is observed following activation in tissue culture of T cells from HIV-1–positive patients.[67,113] In HIV-1–infected people, the majority of cells undergoing apoptosis are uninfected, and only rarely have HIV-1–infected cells been observed to be apoptotic.[54] Both CD4 and CD8+ T cells are subject to apoptosis. Antigen–antibody complexes comprised of gp120 and anti-gp120 or gp120 alone that may complex with and cross-link T-cell CD4 surface receptors have been proposed as potential priming signals for apoptosis of CD4+ T lymphocytes. At some future time, binding of a specific antigen to the TCR of the primed cell might initiate apoptosis.[11] It has yet to be determined what is the in vivo extent of, and contribution to CD4+ T cell depletion, of apoptosis in HIV-1 infection.[54]

Superantigens

The possibility that the immune response to specific HIV-1–derived antigens may contribute directly to the immunopathogenesis of AIDS was raised by the discovery of virus-encoded superantigens within the genomes of two mouse retroviruses, mouse mammary tumor virus and the murine AIDS virus.[62,80] Superantigens were first recognized in relation to a number of bacterial toxins that activate T lymphocytes expressing certain TCR variable beta (V) genes. As superantigens bind to a TCR region located outside the antigen-binding domain, they activate all T cells bearing a given V region, regardless of antigenic specificity.[73]

Reports claiming that T cells expressing specific V receptors are preferentially infected or depleted in AIDS led to speculation that HIV-1 may encode a superantigen, but such reports are now generally discounted. An alternative and perhaps more likely model by which HIV-1 may cause immunodeficiency proposes that the exposure of HIV-1–infected individuals to environmental superantigens leads to the activation of V-beta–specific classes of T cells, promoting cytopathic HIV-1 infection or apoptotic cell death in the superantigen-responding T cells. It is worth mentioning that both cytomegalovirus and tuberculosis, common pathogens in HIV-1 infection, have recently been reported to encode superantigens.[44,126]

Infection of T-Cell Precursors

A puzzling aspect of HIV-1 infection is the apparent failure of T-cell regeneration to repopulate the helper cells that are depleted following viral infection. HIV-1 infection of T-cell precursors and thymic epithelial cells has been proposed as a mechanism for this irreversible depletion. Studies have found intrathymic T-cell precursors, namely the triple-negative CD3 CD4 CD8 thymocyte population, susceptible to HIV-1 infection.[159] In the human thymus in the SCID-hu mouse, HIV-1 infects CD4+CD8+

double-positive as well as single-positive cells, leading to thymocyte depletion.[18] Additionally, human thymic epithelial cells may be infected by or destroyed by the presence of HIV-1.[172] Thus, it is possible that Th cell precursors as well as thymic stromal elements thought to serve a critical role in thymic education are adversely affected by HIV-1 infection. Another important precursor under investigation is the bone marrow CD34+ stem cell. Although it appears that HIV-1 can infect this cell in tissue culture, such infection in vivo appears rare, even in the more advanced stages of AIDS.[38] It may not be necessary to invoke direct effects of HIV-1 infection on T-cell precursors to explain the failure of T-cell regeneration. Inexorable HIV-1 depletion of mature peripheral T cells may simply push the T-cell immune system to its natural limit with respect to regenerative capacity.

Virus-Specific Immune Responses

Immunologic responses may have a protective role in HIV-1 infection as well as pathogenic effects as a consequence of the elimination of cells, such as CD4+ T cells, macrophages, and FDCs, that are associated with HIV-1 antigens. HIV-1–specific CTLs, antibody-dependent cellular cytotoxicity, and natural killer (NK) cells could conceivably contribute to this immune system deterioration, although it is not known whether this actually occurs in vivo. The binding of gp120 to uninfected CD4+ cells may cause inappropriate targeting of the antiviral immune response to these cells. One can imagine that CD4+ T lymphocytes responding to coinfecting pathogens may be destroyed selectively by gp120-specific CTLs as a consequence of gp120 binding by their own surface CD4 molecules. This innocent-bystander effect could contribute to the depletion of Th cells.[27]

Cellular Proteins Bound to HIV-1

B_2-Microglobulin and human lymphocyte antigen (HLA) class I and class II proteins appear to be present on viral particles.[4] Presumably these cell proteins are acquired during virus assembly and budding from infected cells. Their presence raises the possibility that inappropriate signaling of T cells, for example, by virus-associated HLA class II binding to the TCR on

CD4+ cells may result in cellular activation, which could sensitize cells to undergo apoptosis.

Autoimmune Mechanisms of HIV-1 Pathogenesis

Autoimmune models of T-cell depletion propose that HIV-1 induces deleterious immune responses that may attack CD4 cells and the immune system itself. Limited structural homology between gp120 and HLA class II molecules has been suggested as a possible means by which crossreactive antibodies to class II molecules might be produced and alloactivation initiated.[133,187] The HIV-1–infected immune system is perturbed in global, poorly understood ways (e.g., the polyclonal activation of B cells), but no clear evidence currently exists to support suggestions that direct autoimmune mechanisms contribute to T-cell depletion in the setting of HIV-1 infection. The administration of HIV-1 antigens, most notably the HIV-1 envelope protein in the course of vaccine trials, has shown no evidence of inducing or exacerbating autoimmune phenomena.

Th1 and Th2 Lymphocyte Phenotypes

Imbalance in regulation of specific lymphocyte effector populations may contribute to progressive deterioration of the immune system. Such imbalance may explain the polyclonal B-cell activation and autoimmune phenomena observed in HIV-1 disease.[187] Studies of T-cell function in vitro have defined specific subsets of human helper T cells designated Th0, Th1, and Th2. Th1 cells manifest functions associated with cellular immune responses. T-lymphocyte clones specific for most viral and intracellular bacterial antigens are Th1 phenotype. Th2 cells manifest functions that contribute to humoral immune responses. They are helpers for B-cell antibody production. Factors that determine which phenotype a lymphocyte will express are not completely known but may include properties and dose of encountered antigens and cytokines and the nature of signaling generated when an antigen encounters the TCR.

During progression of HIV-1 disease, predominant immune responses and associated T-cell phenotypes have been proposed to switch from Th1 to Th2, resulting in depressed cellular and activated humoral responses.[30] However, analyses of cytokine expression patterns in HIV-1–infected individuals at different stages of disease did not provide evidence for a switch from the Th1 to the Th2 cytokine phenotype during disease progression.[64]

Cytokine Production and Effects

Cytokines are involved in the complex homeostatic regulation of immune responses, and disruption of cytokine networks during HIV-1 infection may have profound effects on responding cells.[68] Tumor necrosis factor-α (TNF-α), in particular, has attracted attention as a critical cytokine, the elevation of which in AIDS may have pathogenic effects.[105] As cytokines likely exhibit their most physiologically relevant actions within the lymphoid organ environment, perturbations of systemic cytokine levels must be carefully interpreted.[48] Proinflammatory cytokines such as TNF-α, interleukin-1, and interleukin-6 have been implicated in promoting HIV replication and spread.[15,145] Given the complex milieu of cytokine factors found in vivo, it is not trivial to identify the key cytokines involved in the pathogenesis of HIV-1 infection.

Effect of HIV-1 Infection on Macrophages and Antigen Presentation

Numerical or functional changes that occur in macrophages during HIV-1 infection have not been well defined. Most studies document normal numbers of monocytes in the peripheral bloodstream during HIV-1 infection.[111] However, mature macrophages resident in lymphoid and extralymphatic tissues are the ones that are active in antigen presentation, and these are not readily accessible for study. Macrophages as well as antigen-presenting dendritic cells present antigens to T cells. Antigen presentation does not seem affected in asymptomatic HIV-1 infection but is compromised in patients with severe disease.[29] The mechanism of HIV-1–induced antigen-presenting cell dysfunction is unclear but may be related to aberrant cytokine secretion that results in the selective dysregulation of T-cell subsets.[187]

IMMUNOPATHOGENIC OUTCOMES OF HIV-1 INFECTION IN VIVO

HIV-1 infection of the CD4+ T-cell immune system should be considered in the context of T-cell population dynamics (i.e., the balance between production and destruction of T cells). Unfortunately, the capacity of the T-cell immune system for self-renewal is poorly understood. Self-renewal, which may differ in adults and children, could arise from the maturation of progenitors. Another possibility, not mutually exclusive, is that self-renewal is based on clonal expansion of previously existing mature T cells. Delineation of the exact basis of self-renewal holds critical implications for HIV-1–induced thymic and lymphoid organ-associated T-cell pathology.

Loss of CD4+ T Cells and Disruption of T-Cell Homeostasis

The recent recognition that appreciable HIV-1 replication takes place throughout the course of the disease supports the view that the direct cytopathic effects of viral replication are responsible for much of the observed immune system compromise. Furthermore, recent interventional studies using potent antiviral drugs provide direct evidence that increasing levels of HIV-1 replication correlate with accelerated rates of destruction of the CD4+ T-cell population. In these studies, a surge in circulating CD4 cells was observed in patients who had rapid declines in plasma virus load. This surge in CD4 cells likely represents cells that were spared death from viral replication and proliferated to restore appropriate levels of host T-cell population. Surges in CD4+ cells in the peripheral blood could also be partly due to redistribution of lymphocytes due to decreased trapping of cells in lymphoid tissue as the amount of HIV-1 decreases during therapy; direct studies of CD4 cell turnover are necessary to address this possibility. The finding that the capacity for brisk CD4 cell recovery is at least partially preserved in AIDS patients suggests that the decline in CD4+ T-cell numbers that precedes ultimate immune collapse may be due to increases in viral replication rather than decreases in the host's capacity for lymphocyte proliferation.

The depletion of CD4+ T cells that is seen after HIV-1 infection must be considered in the context of T cell population dynamics (i.e., the balance between the production and the destruction of T cells). Unfortunately, the T-cell population's capacity for self renewal and the mechanisms by which the human immune system regulates the size of the T-cell population are not understood. Recent data suggest that rather than independently regulate the numbers of T cells of each subset (CD4 and CD8), the host immune system strives to maintain homeostasis of T-cell numbers based on a poorly understood gauge that senses total T-cell numbers (all CD3+ T cells).[103] This type of regulation has been referred to as "blind homeostasis." In the setting of HIV-1 infection where continuous virus replication results in the ongoing destruction of CD4+ T cells, the CD4+ cells dying due to HIV-1 replication would be replaced by CD8+ cells as well as some CD4+ cells. As the immune system's homeostatic sensors are set due to total T cell numbers, the result appears to be preferential expansion of the CD8+ T-cell compartment, which is not targeted for cytopathic effects of HIV-1 infection. Indeed, total CD3+ T cell counts in early and asymptomatic HIV-1 infection have been shown to be nearly stable due to increases in CD8+ cells compensating for losses of CD4+ cells.[103]

Blind T-cell homeostasis eventually breaks down approximately 18 months prior to the development of AIDS, resulting in a net loss of total T-cell numbers in peripheral blood.[103] The failure of homeostasis may represent the limit of compensatory increases in lymphocyte proliferation, which likely results from several processes. Most simply, T-cell proliferation may fail due to CD4+ depletion associated with "blind homeostasis" itself when CD4+ cell help becomes insufficient to maintain T-cell proliferation. Other processes contributing to the failure of T-cell homeostasis probably include the progessive deterioration of the architecture of the lymphoid organs that support the function and proliferation of mature T cells, the preferential loss of naive CD8+ T lymphocytes relative to memory cells seen in HIV-1–infected persons, increases in viral replication due to viral mutations that allow escape from immune responses, development of especially pathogenic viral variants, such as viruses that induce syncytia, or loss of T cells that carry out essential regulation functions.

It is not known to what extent the peripheral expansion of mature T cells or the maturation of new T cells from progenitors contributes to the maintenance of the total T-cell pool in adults; recent evidence suggests, however, that the contribution of the thymus to maintaining T-cell levels is greatly limited by approximately 20 years of age.[101] T-cell production after chemotherapy is more rapid in younger persons, who have larger thymic mass, as estimated from computed tomography (CT) scans, suggesting that thymic maturation of T-cell precursors is an important contributor in this setting.[101] In older persons, the thymus appears to contribute little, if anything, to maintenance of total T-cell numbers, which are presumably supported by the proliferation of the mature T-cell pool that circulates through peripheral lymphoid tissues. Decreased capacity for lymphocyte reconstitution may account for the more rapid progression of disease observed in older HIV-1–infected persons.[28] In any event, HIV-1 infection probably compromises both sources of T-cell production, so that cell replenishment does not match cell loss. The thymus is known to be an early target of HIV-1 infection and cytopathology, thus likely limiting the continuation of effective T-cell production even in younger individuals.[106] In the absence of adequate T-cell replacement, an inexorable decline in total CD4+ T-cell numbers may proceed.

Chronic Immune Stimulation and Activation

Persistence of virus in lymphoid organs causes a chronic stimulation of the immune system.[130] This immune activation is most marked in the CD8+ cell subsets of infected hosts where high level CD38 antigen expression is a strong prognostic marker for AIDS development and death.[59]

Thymus

THE FETAL THYMUS. The fetal thymus plays a central role in development of the T-cell immune system before birth. The thymus is seeded with fetal liver-derived CD4 T-lymphocyte precursors, which evolve through a CD4, CD8 double-negative stage, followed by a CD4+, CD8+ double-positive (DP) stage, which is followed by a process that actively eliminates or selects for T cells based on their antigenic specificity. Only a small fraction of the original thymocyte pool successfully matures into CD4+ and CD8+ single-positive cells.[1] HIV-1 infection of a progenitor before or at the DP stage could be expected to have drastic effects. In the SCID-hu mouse model, where thy-

mocytes are infected by HIV-1, the DP compartment is ablated, the normal CD4/CD8 ratio is inverted, and degeneration of thymic epithelial cells is observed.[18,172] About 10% of HIV-1–infected children have an inverted CD4/CD8 ratio at or before 3 months of age,[107] which could be consistent with a similar thymocyte depletion. Even without initial CD4/CD8 inversion, HIV-1 disease in a subset of children runs a rampant course, with rapid decline in CD4+ cell counts.[46] This finding suggests that HIV-1 may have a more pathogenic effect on the ability of the developing thymus to produce or renew CD4+ T cells than is evident when infection occurs later in life.

Several possible pathogenic mechanisms could be envisioned following HIV-1 infection of the thymus. Thymocytes or their precursors or both could be killed directly by viral infection or indirectly by some virus-induced signal. Thymic macrophages, dendritic cells, and epithelial cells could be susceptible to direct or indirect cytopathic effects of HIV-1 infection, resulting in stromal ablation or compromised capacity for thymopoiesis.[172] During intrathymic migration, some cells proliferate rapidly after entering the thymic cortex, and many cells die there as a result of thymocyte selection. A rapidly proliferating T-cell environment might stimulate HIV-1 infection, with direct cytopathic consequences. Further analysis of the HIV-1–infected SCID-hu mouse and simian immunodeficiency virus (SIV) –infected monkey models should elucidate the precise mechanisms of virus-induced pathology, providing a better understanding of the dynamics of T-cell loss and renewal and why self-renewal does not keep pace with the loss. In addition to T-cell depletion, T-cell dysfunction might result from HIV-1 infection. Finally, either HIV-1 infection or presentation of viral antigens on thymic stromal elements known to play key roles in thymocyte development[85] could lead to the development of tolerance to HIV-1 antigens, which would be perceived as "self." Thus HIV-1–reactive cells would be made tolerant or deleted. The identification of HIV-1–positive children with high-level viremia or deficient anti–HIV-1 CTL activity or both in the face of normal CD4+ cell counts suggests that the induction of tolerance by HIV-1 infection of the fetal thymus should be considered.[155]

THE ADULT THYMUS. The functional role and capacity of the adult thymus for T-cell production remains unclear. That neonatal thymectomy is well tolerated suggests the existence of extrathymic sites of postnatal T-cell development. Following puberty, the thymus greatly decreases in size, and the largest reservoir of CD4+ T cells is the peripheral lymphoid organs. Limited thymopoiesis may occur in the adult.[176] In the face of inexorable destruction of CD4+ T cells, a minor thymopoietic role of the thymus might take on greater significance, but only if it is functionally competent. If the thymus is necessary or helps to regenerate peripheral Th cells under these circumstances, its infection by HIV-1 might have pathogenic outcomes similar to those proposed for infection of the fetal thymus.

The Lymph Nodes and T-Cell Activation

The link between T-cell activation and HIV-1 expression is likely to play a role in the immunopathogenesis of HIV-1 infection. Localization of most of the viral burden to lymphatic tissue that is involved in the immune response suggests that immunologically activated T cells bear the brunt of the pathologic consequences of HIV-1 infection.[132] Continued immune stimulation may lead to the eventual depletion of the responding T cells.[52] Immune abnormalities in HIV-1–positive patients support this conclusion. Before a decline in CD4+ T-cell numbers, asymptomatic infected patients demonstrate specific defects in T-cell function. Such defects are most pronounced in memory T cells involved in recognition of and response to a secondary antigenic exposure.[166] Memory T cells appear to represent fertile targets for HIV-1 infection, and their preferential depletion occurs both in vitro and in vivo.[160] Studies of cell-mediated and humoral immune responses in HIV-1–infected children also provide evidence for loss of antigen-specific Th-cell activity as a function of time and, perhaps, immunizations[20] (B. Hamilton, personal communication). Assuming that memory Th cells recognize and proliferate in response to antigens that are common in the environment, their frequent activation in the context of an HIV-1 infection paradoxically may lead to their selective infection and destruction by HIV-1. Antigenic stimuli that could drive such a process include environmental antigens, vaccines, environmental superantigens, HIV-1 antigens, and, if they exist, HIV-1 superantigens. An inability to regenerate Th cells could lead to the loss of antigen-specific T-cell clones, in effect, a reduction of the T-cell repertoire.[36] As described previously, some of the Th-cell defects associated with late stages of disease may result from defective antigen presentation.[29]

Lymphadenopathy was one of the first recognized syndromes of early HIV-1 disease, and early reports described the detection of HIV-1 within lymph nodes, as well as the destruction of lymph nodes.[16,178] Studies of lymph nodes reveal many more infected CD4+ T cells in the lymph nodes than in the peripheral bloodstream. Furthermore, because they are in an environment favoring activation by antigens, these HIV-1–infected lymph node cells are more likely to express HIV-1 actively than are their counterparts in the peripheral blood.[133]

Starting early postinfection, FDCs within germinal centers trap viral particles, probably in a form that is likely to be infectious for CD4+ T cells circulating through these organs. Follicular hyperplasia and the expansion of the FDC network are associated with the early localization of HIV-1–infected cells to the lymph nodes. Pathologic alterations in lymph node architecture can be seen even in early disease stages. As disease progresses, obvious changes occur in the distribution pattern of HIV-1 in the nodes. Gradual destruction of the FDC network takes place, resulting in loss of virus-trapping and antigen-trapping ability.[133] Antigen retention on FDCs is probably important in continually stimulating and thus maintaining T- and B-cell memory. One functional consequence of FDC network destruction might be the selective loss of memory cells that is observed in HIV-1–infected patients before their CD4+ cell numbers decline.[90] In late-stage disease, lymph node architecture is disrupted markedly, with most of the germinal centers involuted, concomitant with the loss of virus-trapping ability. Degeneration and death of the FDC network usually is associated with an increase in peripheral viral load and disease progression.[133] It is unknown whether FDC network disruption results from a direct toxic effect of HIV-1 infection or from the observed influx of activated CD8+ cytotoxic T lymphocytes into germinal centers near the sites of FDC destruction. Such CD8+ cells are reported to produce high levels of interferon-γ, which may be involved in the anti–HIV-1 T-cell immune response, contributing to both control of viral spread and concomitant lymphoid follicular lysis.[49]

SUMMARY

The study of basic aspects of the life cycle of HIV-1 and the virologic and immunologic aspects of the pathogenesis of AIDS has been extremely productive over the past several years. Analyses of HIV-1 expression during the course of infection support the direct role of HIV-1 expression and cumulative viral burden in the immunopathogenesis of HIV-1 disease. Substantial plasma virus load is found throughout infection and is associated with direct cytopathic effects. Viral infection of immunologically activated T cells in the lymph nodes may deplete the responding cells. This work has laid the necessary foundation for improving the effectiveness of therapies to delay disease progression and prolong life following HIV-1 infection.

We are challenged with taking current hypotheses, and designing thoughtful experiments to further analyze immunopathogenic processes in vivo. This will require continued observation of HIV-1 infection in humans and the use of relevant animal models, such as the SIV-infected macaque. What are the precise mechanisms of CD4+ T cell depletion in vivo? Are antigen-specific T cells targeted for infection and depletion in vivo? What are the dynamics of and capacities for T-cell replenishment? What is the role of viral diversification in disease progression? What is the underlying pathophysiology of lymph node disruption in HIV-1 disease?

Although the lack of a precedent for natural protective immunity in HIV-1 infection of humans is daunting for vaccine development, natural and experimental models exist that are likely to be relevant to correlating resistance to HIV-1 infection and disease to the mechanisms of HIV-1 pathogenesis. These models include long-term asymptomatic HIV-1 infection of a few humans, the extensive SIV infection of sooty mangabeys and African green monkeys in the wild without manifestation of disease,[41] and the apparent resistance of certain individuals to infection by HIV-1, despite repeated exposures to virus.[138] It will be critical to determine which host or viral factors are responsible for a lack of or reduction in pathogenicity. A better understanding of the processes underlying the pathogenesis of HIV-1 infection will lead to improved strategies for therapeutic intervention.

REFERENCES

1. Abbas A, Lichtman A, Pober J: Cellular and Molecular Immunology, 2nd ed. Saunders Text and Review Series. Philadelphia, WB Saunders Co, 1994, p 457
2. Amadori A, et al: CD4 epitope masking by gp120/anti-gp120 antibody complexes. J Immunol 148:2709–2716, 1992
3. Andeweg A, et al: Genetic and functional analysis of a set of HIV-1 envelope genes obtained from biological clones with varying syncytium-inducing capacities. AIDS Res Hum Retroviruses 8: 1803–1813, 1992
4. Arthur L, et al: Cellular proteins bound to immunodeficiency viruses: Implications for pathogenesis and vaccines. Science 258:1935–1938, 1992
5. Baeuerle P, Henkel T: Function and activation of NF-kappa B in the immune system. Ann Rev Immunol 12:141, 1994
6. Bagasra O. et al: Detection of human immunodeficiency virus type 1 provirus in mononuclear cells by in situ polymerase chain reaction. N Engl J Med 326:1385–1391, 1992
7. Bagasra O, Pomerantz R: Human immunodeficiency virus type 1 provirus is demonstrated in peripheral blood monocytes in vivo: A study utilizing an in situ polymerase chain reaction. AIDS Res Hum Retroviruses 9:69–76, 1993
8. Balotta C, et al: Antisense phosphorothioate oligodeoxynucleotides targeted to the vpr gene inhibit human immunodeficiency virus type 1 replication in primary human macrophages. J Virol 67: 4409–4414, 1993
9. Baltimore D: The enigma of HIV infection. Cell 82: 175–176, 1995
10. Baltimore D: Lessons from people with nonprogressive HIV infection. N Engl J Med 332:259–260, 1995
11. Banda N, et al: Crosslinking CD4 by human immunodeficiency virus gp120 primes T cells for activation-induced apoptosis. J Exp Med 176:1099–1106, 1992
12. Bartz S, Rogel M, Emerman M: Human immunodeficiency virus type 1 cell cycle control: vpr is cytostatic and mediates G2 accumulation by a mechanism which differs fro DNA damage checkpoint control. J Virol 70:2324–2331, 1996
13. Baskin G, et al: Thymus in simian immunodeficiency virus-infected rhesus monkeys. Lab Invest 65: 400–407, 1991
14. Baskin GB, et al: Distribution of SIV in lymph nodes of serially sacrificed rhesus monkeys. AIDS Res Hum Retroviruses 11(2):273–285, 1995
15. Belec I, et al: Differential elevation of circulating interleukin-1 beta; tumor necrosis factor alpha, and interleukin-6 in AIDS-associated cachectic studies. Clin Diagn Immunol 1:177–190, 1995
16. Biberfeld P, et al: Histopathology and immunohistology of HTLV-III/LAV-related lymphadenopathy and AIDS. Acta Pathol Microbiol Immunol Scand [A] 95:47–65, 1987
17. Blanche S, et al: A prospective study of infants born to women seropositive for human immunodeficiency virus type 1. N Engl J Med 320:1643, 1989

18. Bonyhadi M, et al: HIV-1 induces thymus depletion in vivo. Nature 363:728–732, 1993

19. Borkowsky W, et al: High maternal viral titer measured by quantitative cell culture correlates with transmission. J Pediatr 125:345–351, 1994

20. Borkowsky W, et al: Cell-mediated and humoral immune responses in children infected with human immunodeficiency virus during the first four years of life. J Pediatr 120:371–375, 1992

21. Brichacek B, et al: Increases in HIV-1 replication following vaccination against opportunistic infections. In 24th Annual Keystone Symposium: HIV Pathogenesis. Keystone, CO, Wiley-Liss, 1995

22. Buehler J, Petersen L, Jaffe H: Current trends in the epidemiology of HIV/AIDS. In The Medical Management of AIDS. Sande A, Volberding P, eds. Philadelphia, WB Saunders Co, 1995

23. Bush C, et al: Changes in HIV viral load markers during opportunistic diseases (Abstract). In 35th Interscience Conference on Antimicrobial Agents and Chemotherapy. San Francisco, American Society for Microbiology, 1995

24. Caldwell J, Caldwell P: The African AIDS epidemic. Sci Am 274:62–68, 1996

25. Cameron P, et al: Dendritic cells exposed to human immunodeficiency virus type-1 transmit a vigorous cytopathic infection to CD4 + T cells. Science 257:383–387, 1992

26. Cao J, et al: Molecular determinants of acute single-cell lysis by human immunodeficiency virus type 1. J Virol 70:1340–1354, 1996

27. Capon D, Ward R: The CD4-gp120 interaction in AIDS pathogenesis. Annu Rev Immunol 9:649–678, 1991

28. Chaisson R, Keruly J, Moore R: Race, sex, drug use, and progression of human immunodeficiency virus disease. N Engl J Med 333:751–756, 1995

29. Clerici M, et al: Multiple patterns of alloantigen presenting/stimulating cell dysfunction in patients with AIDS. J Immunol 146:2207–2213, 1991

30. Clerici M, Shearer G: A TH1/TH2 switch is a critical step in the etiology of HIV-1 infection. Immunol today 14:107–111, 1993

31. Cocchi F, et al: Identification of RANTES, MIP-1 alpha, and MIP-1 beta as the major HIV-suppressive factors produced by CD8 + T cells. Science 270:1811–1815, 1995

32. Coffin JM: HIV population dynamics in vivo: Implications for genetic variation, pathogenesis, and therapy. Science 267:483–489, 1995

33. Conner EM, et al: Reduction of maternal-infant transmission of human immunodeficiency virus type 1 with zidovudine treatment. N Engl J Med 331:1173–1180, 1994

34. Connor R, et al: Increased viral burden and cytopathicity correlate temporally with CD4 + T-lymphocyte decline and clinical progression in human immunodeficiency virus type 1-infected individuals. J Virol 67:1772–1777, 1993

35. Courgnaud V, et al: Frequent and early in utero HIV-1 infection. AIDS Res Hum Retroviruses 7:337–341, 1991

36. Crise B, Rose J: Human immunodeficiency virus type 1 glycoprotein precursor retains a CD4-p56lck complex in the endoplasmic reticulum. J Virol 66:2296–2301, 1992

37. Daniel M, et al: Protective effects of a live attenuated SIV vaccine with a deletion in the nef gene. Science 258:1938–1941, 1992

38. Davis B, et al: Absent or rare human immunodeficiency virus infection of bone marrow stem/progenitor cells in vivo. J Virol 65:1985–1990, 1991

39. Deacon N, et al: Genomic structure of an attenuated quasi species of HIV-1 from a blood transfusion donor and recipients. Science 270:988–991, 1995

40. Denis M, Ghadirian E: *Mycobacterium avium* infection in HIV-1-infected subjects increases monokine secretion and is associated with enhanced viral load and diminished immune response to viral antigens. Clin Exp Immunol 97:76–82, 1994

41. Desrosiers R: The simian immunodeficiency viruses. Annu Rev Immunol 8:557–578, 1990

42. deVincenzi I: A longitudinal study of human immunodeficiency virus transmission by heterosexual partners: European Study Group on Heterosexual Transmission of HIV. N Engl J Med 331:341, 1994

43. DiMarzio P, et al: Mutational analysis of cell cycle arrest, nuclear localization, and virion packaging of human immunodeficiency virus type 1 vpr. J Virol 69:7909–7916, 1995

44. Dobrescu D, et al: Enhanced HIV-1 replication in V beta 12 cells due to human cytomegalovirus in monocytes: Evidence for a putative herpesvirus superantigen. Cell 82:753–763, 1995

45. Du Z, et al: Identification of a nef allele that causes lymphocyte activation and acute disease in monkeys. Cell 82:665–674, 1995

46. Duliege A, et al: Natural history of human immunodeficiency virus type 1 infection in children: Prognostic value of laboratory tests on the bimodal progression of disease. Pediatr Infect Dis J 11:630, 1992

47. Embretson J, et al: Massive covert infection of helper T lymphocytes during the incubation period of AIDS. Nature 362:359–362, 1993

48. Emilie D, et al: Cytokines from lymphoid organs of HIV-infected patients: Production and role in the immune disequilibrium of the disease and in the development of B lymphomas. Immunol Rev 140:803–824, 1995

49. Emilie D, et al: Production of interleukins in human immunodeficiency virus-1-replicating lymph nodes. J Clin Invest 86:148–159, 1990

50. European CS: Children born to women with HIV-1 infection: Natural history and risk of transmission. Lancet 337:253, 1991

51. Fang G, et al: Maternal plasma human immunodeficiency virus type 1 RNA level: A determinant and projected threshold for mother-to-child transmission. Proc Natl Acad Sci U S A 92:12100–12104, 1995

52. Feinberg M, Greene W: Molecular insights into human immunodeficiency virus type 1 pathogenesis. Curr Opin Immunol 4:466–474, 1992

53. Feng Y, et al: HIV-1 entry cofactor: Functional cDNA cloning of a seven-transmembrane G protein-coupled receptor. Science 272:872–877, 1996

54. Finkel T, et al: Apoptosis occurs predominantly in bystander cells and not in productively infected cells of HIV- and SIV-infected lymph nodes. Nat Med 1:129–134, 1995

55. Fouchier R, et al: Phenotype-associated sequence variation in the third variable domain of the

human immunodeficiency virus type 1 gp120 molecule. J Virol 66:3183–3187, 1992

56. Frankel S, et al: Replication of HIV-1 in dendritic cell-derived syncytia at the mucosal surface of the adenoid. Science 272:115–117, 1996

57. Garcia J, Alfano J, Miller A: The negative effect of human immunodeficiency virus type 1 Nef on cell surface expression is not species-specific and requires the cytoplasmic domain of CD4. J Virol 67:1511–1516, 1993

58. Gibbs J, et al: Progression to AIDS in the absence of a gene for vpr or vpx. J Virol 69:2378–2383, 1995

59. Giorgi J, et al: Elevated levels of CD38+ T cells in HIV infection add to the prognostic value of low CD4+ T cell levels: Results of 6 years of follow-up. J Acquir Immune Defic Syndr 6:904–912, 1993

60. Goedert J, et al: High risk of HIV-1 infection for first-born twins: The International Registry of HIV-Exposed Twins. Lancet 338:1471, 1991

61. Goldsmith M, et al: Dissociation of the CD4 downregulation and viral infectivity enhancement functions of human immunodeficiency virus type 1 nef. J Virol 69:4112–4121, 1995

62. Golovkina T, et al: Transgenic mouse mammary tumor virus superantigen expression prevents viral expression. Cell 69:637–645, 1992

63. Grant RM, Feinberg MB: HIV replication and pathogenesis Curr Opin Infect Dis 9:7–13, 1996

64. Graziosi C, et al: Lack of evidence for the dichotomy of TH1 and TH2 predominance in HIV-infected individuals. Science 265:248–252, 1994

65. Greene W: Predicting progression to AIDS (Editorial). Ann Intern Med 9:726–727, 1995

66. Groenink M, et al: Phenotype-associated env gene variation among eight related human immunodeficiency virus type 1 clones: Evidence for in vivo recombination and determinants of cytotropism outside the V3 domain. J Virol 66:6175–6180, 1992

67. Groux H, et al: Activation-induced death by apoptosis in CD4+ T cells from human immunodeficiency virus-infected asymptomatic individuals. J Exp Med 175:331–340, 1992

68. Grunfeld C, Feingold K: The metabolic effects of tumor necrosis factor and other cytokines. Biotherapy 3:143–158, 1991

69. Hattori N, et al: The human immunodeficiency virus type 2 vpr gene is essential for productive infection of human macrophages. Proc Natl Acad Sci USA 87:8080–8084, 1990

70. Haynes BF, Pantaleo G, Fauci AS: Toward an understanding of the correlates of protective immunity to HIV infection. Science 271:324–328, 1996

71. Henrard D, et al: Virologic and immunologic characterization of symptomatic and asymptomatic primary HIV-1 infection. J Acquir Immune Defic Syndr 9:305–310, 1995

72. Henrad DR, et al: Natural history of HIV-1 cell-free viremia. JAMA 274:554–558, 1995

73. Herman A, et al: Superantigens: Mechanism of T cell stimulation and role in immune responses. Annu Rev Immunol 9:745–772, 1991

74. Ho D: HIV-1 viremia and influenza. Lancet 339:1549, 1992

75. Ho DD: Time to hit HIV early and hard. N Engl J Med 333:450–451, 1995

76. Ho DD, et al: Rapid turnover of plasma virions and CD4 lymphocytes in HIV-1 infection. Nature 373:123–126, 1995

77. Hoch J, et al: vpr deletion mutant of simian immunodeficiency virus induces AIDS in rhesus monkeys. J Virol 69:4807–4813, 1995

78. Hogarvorst E, et al: Predictors for non- and slow progression in human immunodeficiency virus (HIV) type 1 infection: Low viral RNA copy numbers in serum and maintenance of high HIV-1 p24-specific but not V3-specific antibody levels. J Infect Dis 171:811–821, 1995

79. Huang Y, Zhang L, Ho DD: Biological characterization of nef in long-term survivors of human immunodeficiency virus type 1 infection. J Virol 69:8142–8146, 1995

80. Hugin A, Vacchio M, Morse H: A virus-encoded "superantigen" in a retrovirus-induced immunodeficiency syndrome of mice. Science 252:424–427, 1991

81. Hwang S, et al: Identification of the envelope V3 loop as the primary determinant of cell tropism in HIV-1. Science 253:71–74, 1991

82. Jacquez JA, et al: Role of the primary infection in the epidemics of HIV infection in gay cohorts. J AIDS 7:1169–1184, 1994

83. Jurrians S, et al: The natural history of HIV-1 infection: Virus load and virus phenotype independent determinants of clinical course? Virology 204:223–233, 1994

84. Kaslow R, et al: Influence of combinations of human major histocompatibility complex genes on the course of HIV-1 infection. Nat Med 2:405–411, 1996

85. Kaye J, Ellenberger D: Differentiation of an immature T cell line: A model of thymic positive selection. Cell 71:423–435, 1992

86. Keet I, et al: Predictors of rapid progression to AIDS in HIV-1 seroconverters. AIDS 7:51–57, 1993

87. Kestler H, et al: Importance of the nef gene for maintenance of high virus loads and for development of AIDS. Cell 65:651–662, 1991

88. Kinloch-deLoes S, et al: A controlled trial of zidovudine in primary human immunodeficiency virus infection. N Engl J Med 333:408–413, 1995

89. Kirchhoff F, et al: Brief report: Absence of intact nef sequences in a long-term survivor with nonprogressive HIV-1 infection. N Engl J Med 332:228–232, 1995

90. Koopman G, Pals S: Cellular interactions in the germinal center: Role of adhesion receptors and significance for the pathogenesis of AIDS and malignant lymphoma. Immunol Rev 126:21–45, 1992

91. Koot M, et al: Prognostic value of HIV-1 syncytium-inducing phenotype for rate of CD4+ cell depletion and progression to AIDS. Ann Intern Med 118:681–688, 1993

92. Korostoff J, et al: Neonatal exposure to thymotropic Gross murine leukemia virus induces virus-specific immunologic nonresponsiveness. J Exp Med 172:1765–1775, 1990

93. Koup RA, et al: Temporal association of cellular immune responses with the initial control of viremia in primary human immunodeficiency virus type 1 syndrome. J Virol 68:4650–4655, 1994

94. Kuiken C, et al: Evolution of the V3 envelope domain in proviral sequences and isolates of human immunodeficiency virus type 1 during transition of the viral biological phenotype. J Virol 66:4622–4627, 1992

95. Kunanusont C, et al: HIV-1 subtypes and male-to-fe-

male transmission in Thailand. Lancet 345: 1078–1083, 1995

96. Lang S, et al: Importance of vpr for infection of rhesus monkeys with simian immunodeficiency virus. J Virol 67:902–912, 1993

97. Levy J: Pathogenesis of human immunodeficiency virus infection. Microbiol Rev 57:183–289, 1993

98. Lifson A, et al: Long-term human immunodeficiency virus infection in asymptomatic homosexual and bisexual men with normal CD4+ lymphocyte counts: Immunologic and virologic characteristics. J Infect Dis 163:959–965, 1991

99. Luria S, et al: Expression of the type 1 human immunodeficiency virus Nef protein in T cells prevents antigen-receptor-mediated induction of interleukin 2 mRNA. Proc Natl Acad Sci U S A 88: 5326–5330, 1991

100. Luzuriaga K, et al: Deficient human immunodeficiency virus type 1-specific cytotoxic T cell responses in vertically infected children. J Pediatr 119:230–236, 1991

101. Mackall CL, et al: Age, thymopoiesis, and CD4+ T-lymphocyte regeneration after intensive chemotherapy. N Engl J Med 332:143–149, 1995

102. Mackewicz C, Levy J: CD8+ cell anti-HIV activity: Non-lytic suppression of virus replication. AIDS Res Hum Retroviruses 8:1039–1050, 1992

103. Margolick JB, et al: Failure of T-cell homeostasis preceding AIDS in HIV-1 infection. Nat Med 1: 674–680, 1995

104. Marx P, et al (unpublished) cited in Cohen J: Monkey study prompts high-level public health response (News and Comment). Science 272:805, 1996.

105. Matsuyama T, Kobayashi N, Yamamoto N: Cytokines and HIV-1 infection: Is AIDS a tumor necrosis factor disease? AIDS 5:1405–1417, 1991

106. McCune J: HIV-1: The infective process in vivo. Cell 64:351–363, 1991

107. McKinney R, Wilfert C: Lymphocyte subsets in children younger than 2 years old: Normal values in a population at risk for human immunodeficiency virus infection and diagnostic and prognostic application to infected children. Pediatr Infect Dis J 11:639–644, 1992

108. Meier U-C, et al: Cytotoxic T lymphocyte lysis inhibited by viable HIV mutants. Science 270: 1360–1362, 1995

109. Mellors J, et al: Prognosis in HIV-1 infection predicted by the quantity of virus in plasma. Science 272:1167–1170, 1996.

110. Mellors JW, et al: Quantitation of HIV-1 RNA in plasma predicts outcome after seroconversion. Ann Intern Med 122:573–579, 1995

111. Meltzer M, Gendelman H: Mononuclear phagocytes as targets, tissue reservoirs, and immunoregulatory cells in human immunodeficiency virus disease. Curr Top Microbiol Immunol 181:239–263, 1992

112. Mermin J, et al: Detection of human immunodeficiency virus DNA and RNA in semen by the polymerase chain reaction. J Infect Dis 164:769–772, 1991

113. Meyaard I, et al: Programmed death of T cells in HIV-1 infection. Science 257:217–219, 1992

114. Michael N, et al: Comparison of HIV-1 viral load between HIV-infected patients with and without tuberculosis (Abstract). Third Conference on Retroviruses and Opportunistic Infections. Washington, DC, 1996

115. Miles S, et al: Rapid serologic testing with immune complex-dissociated HIV-1 p24 antigen for early detection of HIV-1 infection in neonates. Southern California Pediatric AIDS Consortium. N Engl J Med 328:297–302, 1993

116. Miller C, et al: Localization of SIV in the genital tract of chronically infected female rhesus macaques. Am J Pathol 141:655–660, 1992

117. Miller M, et al: The HIV-1 nef gene product: A positive factor for viral infection and replication in primary lymphocytes and macrophages. J Exp Med 179:101–113, 1994

118. Miller MD, Feinberg MB, Greene WC: The HIV-1 nef gene acts as a positive viral infectivity factor. Trends Microbiol 2:294–297, 1994

119. Moore J, et al: Development of the anti-gp120 antibody response during seroconversion to human immunodeficiency virus type 1. J Virol 68: 5142–5155, 1994

120. Moskophidis D, et al: Virus persistence in acutely infected immunocompetent mice by exhaustion of antiviral cytotoxic effector T cells. Nature 362: 758–761, 1993

121. Newell ML, Gibb DM: A risk-benefit assessment of zidovudine in the prevention of perinatal HIV transmission. Drug Safety 12:274–282, 1995

122. Nowak M, Anderson R, McLean A: Antigenic diversity thresholds and the development of AIDS. Science 254:963–969, 1991

123. O'Brien T, Shaffer N, Jaffe H: Acquisition and transmission of HIV-1. In Sande M, Volberding P, eds. The Medical Management of AIDS, Philadelphia, WB Saunders Co, 1992, pp 3–17

124. O'Brien W, et al: Changes in plasma HIV-1 RNA and CD4+ lymphocyte counts and the risk of progression to AIDS. N Engl J Med 334:426–431, 1996

125. O'Brien WA, et al: Human immunodeficiency virus-type 1 replication can be increased in peripheral blood of seropositive patients after influenza vaccination. Blood 86:1082, 1995

126. Ohmen J, et al: Evidence for a superantigen in human tuberculosis. Immunity 1:35–43, 1994

127. Oldstone M: Molecular anatomy of viral persistence. J Virol 65:6381–6386, 1991

128. Osborn JE: HIV: The more things change, the more they stay the same (Commentary). Nat Med 1: 991–993, 1995

129. Pantaleo G, et al: Major expansion of CD8+ T cells with a predominant V beta usage during the primary immune response to HIV. Nature 370: 463–467, 1994

130. Pantaleo G, Fauci A: New concepts in the immunopathogenesis of HIV infection. Annu Rev Immunol 13:487–512, 1995

131. Pantaleo G, et al: HIV-1 infection is active and progressive in lymphoid tissue during the clinically latent stage of disease. Nature 362:355–358, 1993

132. Pantaleo G, Graziosi C, Fauci A: New concepts in the immunopathogenesis of human immunodeficiency virus infection. N Engl J Med 328:327, 1993

133. Pantaleo G, Graziosi C, Fauci A: New concepts in the immunopathogenesis of human immunodeficiency virus infection. N Engl J Med 328:327, 1993

134. Pape J, et al: Effect of isoniazid prophylaxis on incidence of active tuberculosis and progression of HIV infection. Lancet 342:268–272, 1993

135. Papiernik M, et al: Thymic abnormalities in fetuses aborted from human immunodeficiency virus type 1 seropositive women. Pediatrics 89:297–301, 1992

136. Parslow T: Post-transcriptional regulation of human retroviral gene transcription. In Human Retroviruses. New York, Oxford University Press, 1993, pp 101–126

137. Paul WE: Can the immune response control HIV infection? Cell 82:177–182, 1995

138. Paxton W, et al: Relative resistence to HIV-1 infection of CD4 lymphocytes from persons who remain uninfected despite multiple high-risk sexual exposure. Nat Med 2:412–417, 1996

139. Perelson A, et al: HIV-1 dynamics in vivo: Virion clearance rate, infected cell life-span, and viral generation time. Science 271:1582–1586, 1996

140. Phair J: Keynote address: Variations in the natural history of HIV infection. Aids Res Hum Retroviruses 10:883–885, 1994

141. Phillips A: Reduction of HIV concentration during acute infection: Independence from a specific immune response. Science 271:497–499, 1996

142. Piatak M, et al: High levels of HIV-1 in plasma during all stages of infection determined by competitive PCR. Science 259:1749–1754, 1993

143. Pizzo P, Butler K: In the vertical transmission of HIV-1, timing may be everything. N Engl J Med 325:652–654, 1991

144. Planelles V, et al: Vpr-induced cell cycle arrest is conserved among primate lentiviruses. J Virol 70:2516–2524, 1996

145. Poli G, Fauci A: Cytokine modulation of HIV expression. Semin Immunol 5:165–173, 1993

146. Pope M, et al: Conjugates of dendritic cells and memory T lymphocytes from skin facilitate productive infection with HIV-1. Cell 78:389–398, 1994

147. Pope M, et al: Low levels of HIV-1 infection in cutaneous dendritic cells promote extensive viral replication upon binding to memory CD4 + T cells. J Exp Med 182:2045–2056, 1995

148. Quinn T: Population migration and the spread of types 1 and 2 human immunodeficiency viruses. Proc Natl Acad Sci U S A 91:2407, 1994

149. Razvi E, et al: Lymphocyte apoptosis during the silencing of the immune response to acute viral infections in normal, lpr, and Bcl-2-transgenic mice. Am J Pathol 147:79–91, 1995

150. Rich E, et al: Increased susceptibility of differentiated mononuclear phagocytes to productive infection with human immunodeficiency virus-1 (HIV-1). J Clin Invest 89:176–183, 1992

151. Rogel ME, Wu LI, Emerman M: The human immunodeficiency virus type 1 vpr gene prevents cell proliferation during chronic infection. J Virol 69:882–888, 1995

152. Rogers M, Jaffe H: Reducing the risk of maternal-infant transmission of HIV: A door is opened. N Engl J Med 331:1222, 1994

153. Roos M, et al: Viral phenotype and immune response in primary human immunodeficiency virus type 1 infection. J Infect Dis 165:427–432, 1992

154. Rowland-Jones S, McMichael A: Immune responses in HIV-exposed seronegatives: have they repelled the virus? Curr Opin Immunol 7:448–455, 1995

155. Saag M, et al: High-level viremia in adults and children infected with human immunodeficiency virus: Relation to disease stage and CD4 + lymphocyte levels. J Infect Dis 164:72–80, 1991

156. Safrit J, Koup R: The immunology of primary HIV infection: Which immune responses control HIV replication? Curr Opin Immunol 7:456–461, 1995

157. Saksela K, et al: Human immunodeficiency virus type 1 mRNA expression in peripheral blood cells predicts disease progression independently of the number of CD4 + lymphocytes. Proc Natl Acad Sci U S A 91:1104–1108, 1994

158. Saksela K, et al: HIV-1 messenger RNA in peripheral blood mononuclear cells as an early marker of risk for progression to AIDS. Ann Intern Med 123:641–648, 1995

159. Schnittman S, et al: Evidence for susceptibility of intrathymic T cell precursors and their progeny carrying T cell antigen receptor phenotypes TCR alpha beta + and TCR gamma delta + to human immunodeficiency virus infection: A mechanism for CD4 + (T4) lymphocyte depletion. Proc Natl Acad Sci U S A 87:7727–7731, 1990

160. Schnittmann S, et al: Preferential infection of CD4 + memory T cells by human immunodeficiency virus type 1: Evidence for a role in the selective T-cell functional defects observed in infected individuals. Proc Natl acad Sci U S A 87:6058–6062, 1990

161. Schubert U, et al: The two biological activities of human immunodeficiency virus type 1 vpu protein involve two separable structural domains. J Virol 70:809–819, 1996

162. Schuitemaker H, et al: Biological phenotype of human immunodeficiency virus type 1 clones at different stages of infection: Progression of disease is associated with a shift from monocyptropic to T cell-tropic virus population. J Virol 66:1354–1360, 1992

163. Schuurman H, et al: The thymus in acquired immune deficiency syndrome. Am J Pathol 134:1329–1338, 1989

164. Scott G, et al: Survival in children with perinatally acquired human immunodeficiency virus type 1 infection. N Engl J Med 321:1791, 1989

165. Shacker T, et al: Reactivation of HSV-2 in HIV infected persons is associated with increased levels of plasma HIV RNA. In Program and Abstracts of the 35th International Conference on Antimicrobial Agents and Chemotherapy, 1995

166. Shearer G, Clerici M: Early T-helper cell defects in HIV infection. AIDS 5:245–253, 1991

167. Shearer GM, Clerici M: Protective immunity against HIV infection: Has nature done the experiment for us? Immunol Today 17:21–24, 1996

168. Simmonds P, et al: Discontinuous sequence change of human immunodeficiency virus (HIV-1) type 1 env sequences in plasma viral and lymphocyte-associated proviral populations in vivo: Implications for models of HIV-1 pathogenesis. J Virol 65:6266–6276, 1991

169. Skowronski J, et al: Altered T cell activation and development in transgenic mice expressing the HIV-1 nef gene. EMBO J 12:703–713, 1993

170. Soto-Ramirez L, et al: HIV-1 Langerhans' cell tropism associated with heterosexual transmission of HIV. Science 271:1291–1293, 1996

171. Spira A, et al: Cellular targets of infection and route of viral dissemination after an intravaginal inoculation of simian immunodeficiency virus into rhesus macaques. J Exp Med 183:215, 1996

172. Stanley S, et al: Human immunodeficiency virus infection of the human thymus and disruption of

the thymic microenvironment. J Exp Med 178: 1151–1163, 1993

173. Stanley S, et al: Effect of immunization with a common recall antigen on viral expression in patients infected with human immunodeficiency virus type 1. N Engl J Med 334:1222–1230, 1996

174. Staprans S, et al: Activation of virus replication after vaccination of HIV-1-infected individuals. J Exp Med 182:1727–1737, 1995

175. Stein D, et al: The effect of the interaction of acyclovir with zidovudine on progression to AIDS and survival. Analysis of data in the Multicenter AIDS Cohort Study. Ann Intern Med 121:100–108, 1994

176. Steinmann G: Changes in the human thymus during aging. In Muller-Hermelink H, ed. The Human Thymus: Histophysiology and Pathology. Berlin, Springer-Verlag, 1986, pp 43–88

177. StLouis M, Kamenga M, Brown C. Risk for perinatal HIV-1 transmission according to maternal immunologic, virologic, and placental factors. JAMA 269:2853, 1993

178. Tenner R, et al: HTLV-III/LAV viral antigens in lymph nodes of homosexual men with persistent generalized lymphadenopathy and AIDS. Am J Pathol 123:9–15, 1986

179. Tersmette M, et al: Evidence for a role of virulent human immunodeficiency virus (HIV-1) variants in the pathogenesis of acquired immunodeficiency syndrome: Studies on sequential HIV-1 isolates. J Virol 63:2118–2125, 1989

180. Tingley D: Disarming the immune system: HIV-1 uses multiple strategies (Research Brief). J NIH Res 1996, pp 33–37

181. Travers K, et al: Natural protection against HIV-1 infection provided by HIV-2. Science 268: 1612–1615, 1995

182. Trono D: HIV accessory proteins: Leading roles for the supporting cast. Cell 82:189–192, 1995

183. Tsai C-C, et al: Prevention of SIV infection in macaques by (R)-9-(2-phosphonylmethoxypropyl)adenine. Science 270:1197–1199, 1995

184. Ward J, et al: The natural history of transfusion-associated infection with human immunodeficiency virus: Factors influencing the rate of progression to disease. N Engl J Med 321:947–952, 1989

185. Wei X, et al: Viral dynamics in human immunodeficiency virus type 1 infection. Nature 373:117–122, 1995

186. Weiser B, et al: Quantitation of human immunodeficiency virus type 1 during pregnancy: Relationship of viral titer to mother-to-child transmission and stability of viral load. Proc Natl Acad Sci U S A 91: 8037–8041, 1994

187. Weiss R: How does HIV cause AIDS? Science 260: 1273, 1993

188. Weissman D, Barker T, Fauci A: The efficiency of acute infection of CD4 + T cells is markedly enhanced in the setting of antigen-specific immune activation. J Exp Med 183:687–692, 1996

189. Willey R, et al: Human immunodeficiency virus type 1 Vpu protein induces rapid degradation of CD4. J Virol 66:7193–7200, 1992

190. Zhang L, et al: Selection for specific sequences in the external envelope protein of human immunodeficiency virus type 1 upon primary infection. J Virol 67:3345–3356, 1993

191. Zhu T, et al: Genotypic and phenotypic characterization of HIV-1 in patients with primary infection. Science 261:1179–1181, 1993

Quantitation of HIV Viral Load: A Tool for Clinical Practice?

MICHAEL S. SAAG

When considering what is the optimum "acquired immunodeficiency syndrome (AIDS) test," AIDS testing must be placed into appropriate historical context. AIDS was first described as a syndrome, a collection of clinical features that were the result of a weakened immune system. It was not until the causative agent of AIDS, human immunodeficiency virus type 1 (HIV-1), was discovered in 1984 that "tests for AIDS" became available. However, since AIDS is a clinical syndrome, there is no such thing as a laboratory test for AIDS per se. Rather, all "AIDS tests" are designed to detect, either directly or indirectly, the presence of underlying HIV-1 infection.

The first test developed to detect HIV-1 infection was isolation of the virus through tissue culture. This was the technique used originally to establish HIV-1 as the causative agent of AIDS. Unfortunately, although sensitive for viral isolation, the tissue culture procedure is expensive, time consuming, and labor intensive. As a result, soon after the initial discovery of HIV-1, several tests were developed using protein products of the newly discovered virus to detect antibodies produced by the infected host. Through these newer techniques, the immunologic "foot-prints" (i.e., antibodies) to the viral infection are detected rather than the virus itself.

The two antibody tests used most commonly are the enzyme-linked immunosorbent assay (ELISA) and the Western blot. In addition to being less expensive, faster, and easier to perform than viral culture, the ELISA and the Western blot test do not require working with live virus and, therefore, are safer. Nonetheless, no test is perfect, and the HIV-1 antibody tests are limited by their reliance on the production of antibody by the host and the absence of cross-reacting antibodies.

Over the last 5 to 6 years, several novel techniques have been developed that directly detect viral protein products or amplify minute fragments of viral RNA and DNA to avoid the pitfalls of antibody testing and the dangers and expense of live virus culture.[25,83] Yet these tests have their own limitations, not the least of which is the interpretation of the results by the clinician ordering the test.

The best way to minimize errors in interpretation of laboratory findings is to understand the methodology of the test, the advantages and limitations of the testing technology, and the application of the test in the context of what is known about the epidemiology and pathogenesis of the underlying disease. This chapter reviews the methodologies of currently available tests for HIV-1, examines their appropriate use and limitations, and discusses the role of each test in the context of diagnosis and as measurements of response to antiretroviral therapy.

METHODOLOGIES

HIV-1 tests can be divided into several groups: virus culture techniques, antibody detection tests, antigen detection tests, viral genome amplification tests, and immune function tests.

This work was supported in part by the University of Alabama at Birmingham General Clinical Research Center (RR00032) and the University of Alabama at Birmingham AIDS Center (AI27767).

Virus Culture Techniques

Peripheral Blood Mononuclear Cell Coculture for HIV-1 Isolation

This technique was used initially to establish HIV-1 as the causative agent of AIDS.[7,72] Viable peripheral blood mononuclear cells (PBMCs) from HIV-1–infected patients are obtained via centrifugation of anticoagulated whole blood (collected in either acid citrate dextran [ACD] tubes or syringes containing preservative-free heparin) over ficoll-hypaque lymphocyte separation medium. Infected PBMCs then are cocultured with PBMCs derived from an uninfected human donor that have been stimulated previously for 24 to 48 hours with phytohemagglutinin (PHA). Growth of the cells in tissue culture is supported by special media (RPMI-1640) that has been supplemented with L-glutamine, fetal bovine serum, gentamicin, and interleukin-2 (to stimulate expression of CD4 receptors for enhanced viral replication and proliferation of lymphocytes). The cultures are observed for evidence of syncytial formation (i.e., multinucleated giant cell formation) as a sign of viral infection in vitro and for the presence of either HIV-1 reverse transcriptase (RT) activity or HIV-1 p24 antigen production in the culture supernatant. Cultures are declared "positive" when at least two consecutive assays detect the presence of RT or p24 antigen in increasing magnitude above a predetermined cutoff value. When performed properly, HIV-1 isolation by PBMC coculture is positive in 95% to 99% of HIV-1–infected patients.[25,83]

Quantitative Cell Culture

Quantitative cell culture is a technique that measures the relative amount of viral load within cells. The cell culture technique is the same as described previously. However, in addition to cocultivating 10^6 patient cells with 10^6 donor cells, serial dilutions of patient cells are also set in culture in decreasing amounts (e.g., 10^6, 10^5, 10^4, 10^3) with 10^6 donor cells[42] (Fig. 4–1A). In this way fewer patient cells are introduced into the coculture system, thereby allowing measurement of relative viral burden. The last positive culture with the fewest number of patient cells represents the end-point. The reciprocal of the end-point dilution indicates the relative number of infected cells in the patient. For example, if the last positive titer is 1×10^4 (10,000), the relative burden signifies 1 of every 10,000 patient cells is infected. If the end-point titer is 1×10^3 (1000), approximately 1 of 1000 cells is infected. This procedure can be improved further by using serial dilutions on a 1:3 basis rather than a 1:10 basis.

Quantitative Plasma Culture

Another means of measuring viral load is through the measurement of free infectious virus in the plasma.[18,20,42,79] This is accomplished through quantitative plasma culture techniques (Fig. 4–1B). Serial dilutions of plasma are prepared by mixing 0.6 ml of plasma with 2.4 ml of culture medium consisting of RPMI-1640, supplemented with L-glutamine, gentamicin, fetal bovine serum, and interleukin-2. One milliliter of each of the dilutions is added to 2×10^6 PHA-stimulated PBMC from an uninfected donor in a microtiter, 96-well tissue culture plate. Culture supernatants are monitored for viral replication at days 7 and 14 after cultivation by an HIV-1 p24 antigen test. The end-point dilution is defined as the smallest volume of plasma that yields a positive culture result. The reciprocal of the smallest volume of plasma indicates the titer expressed as the tissue culture infectious doses per milliliter of plasma. As shown in Fig. 4–1B, a positive dilution of 1:3125 implies that there are more than 3000 free infectious virions per milliliter of plasma in that patient. To ensure accuracy, these tests usually are performed in duplicate and, under special circumstances, in quadruplicate.

HIV Antibody Tests

ELISA

The technology to perform the ELISA was available before the discovery of HIV in 1983 and 1984. This technology was applied rapidly for use as an HIV-1 diagnostic test and was in widespread use by the summer of 1985.[16] As shown in Fig. 4–2, this test uses HIV antigens (proteins) produced in a tissue culture system or through recombinant molecular technology. After the virus has been grown to high titers, the cell culture is lysed. The soluble antigens are then coated onto the wells of a microtiter plate. The test is initiated by adding patient serum to the antigen-coated wells. Anti–HIV-1–specific antibody present in the patient's serum will bind very tightly and specifically with the HIV-1 antigens in the plate. After a washing procedure to remove unbound materials, the

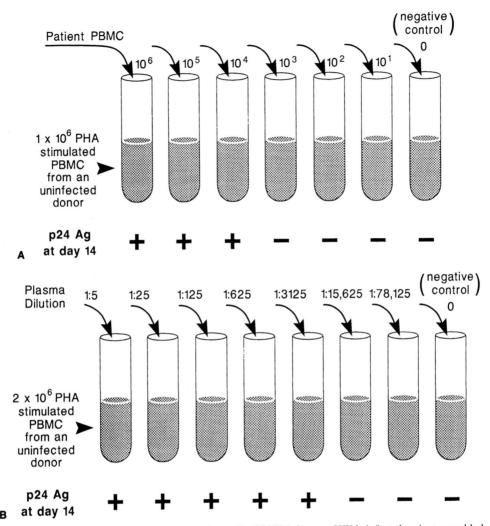

FIGURE 4–1.   *A,* Peripheral blood mononuclear cells (PBMCs) from an HIV-1–infected patient are added in tenfold serial dilutions to a standard amount (e.g., 1×10^6) of phyto-hemagglutin (PHA) -stimulated PBMC from an uninfected donor. The lowest dilution yielding a positive result, as determined by p24 antigen (p24 Ag) positivity in the culture supernatant, represents the end-point. In this example, the end-point dilution is 1×10^4 cells/mm³. *B,* Serial fivefold dilutions of plasma from an HIV-1–infected patient are cocultivated with a standard amount (e.g., 2×10^6) of peripheral blood mononuclear cells from an uninfected donor. As in the quantitative cell dilution assay, the least amount of plasma required to yield a positive culture result represents the end-point. In the example above, the end-point titer is 1:3125.

specific anti–HIV-1 antibodies that have bound to the coated antigen are detected through the addition of a goat antihuman antibody that binds very tightly and specifically to any anti–HIV-1 human antibody bound to HIV-1 antigens on the plate. The goat antihuman antibody has been conjugated to an enzyme that specifically cleaves a colorless substrate and into a product with color (usually yellow). After a washing procedure, the substrate for the enzyme is added. The amount of color present in the well is proportional to the amount of conjugated enzyme bound to the human antibody present. By spectrophotometrically measuring the optical density in the sample well versus that in the negative control well, the amount of HIV-1 antibody can be determined quantitatively.

Through examination of large panels of known HIV-positive sera and comparison of their optical densities with those of known seronegative controls, a cutoff optical density measurement can be determined that distinguishes between a positive and negative result. To make

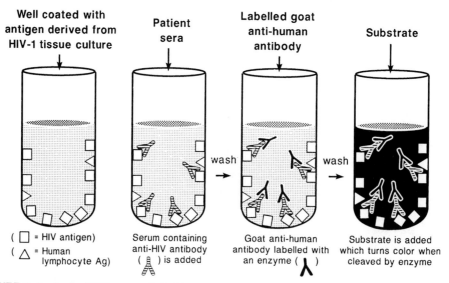

FIGURE 4–2. In the HIV-1 enzyme-linked immunosorbent assay (ELISA) patient serum is added to a microwell plate that has been coated with antigens derived from an HIV-1 tissue culture lysate. Bound anti-HIV antibody from the infected patient is detected via a goat antihuman antibody that has been labeled with an enzyme designed to react with a specific substrate. The cleaved substrate product yields a color that can be measured photometrically. Because the HIV-1 antigens are derived from tissue culture, some human lymphocyte antigens (Ag) may also be present in the well, potentially yielding a false-positive test result (see text for details).

the test more sensitive, the optical density cutoff is established at a lower value. Conversely, to improve specificity, the cutoff can be established at a higher value.

Western Blot Test

The Western blot test is also designed to detect the presence of anti–HIV-1 antibodies. However, in addition to identifying the presence of such antibodies, the Western blot test allows determination of the specific antigen against which the antibody is directed. As shown in Fig. 4–3A, HIV-1 antigens are prepared from a lysate of HIV-1–infected cells and are separated electrophoretically in a polyacrylamide gel. The electrophoretic procedure separates the antigens according to their size: the larger fragments remain toward the top of the gel, and the smaller fragments migrate further down the gel, thereby creating a gradient of antigen by size within the gel. The proteins within the gel are then transferred (blotted) onto nitrocellulose filter paper, which holds the antigens in place for further testing. The nitrocellulose filter is cut into strips that can be incubated with the patient's serum. Anti–HIV-1 antibodies present in this serum bind tightly and specifically to the antigens on the nitrocellulose paper at the point where the antigens migrated. The anti–HIV-1 antibodies can then be detected by

goat antihuman antibody, which is conjugated to either an enzyme or a radioactive probe. Once processed, bands appear at the location where the antibody has bound to antigen. Through the use of reference bands produced as a positive control, the reactivity of the antibodies against specific antigens can be determined (Fig. 4–3B).

The precise criteria for what constitutes a positive Western blot test remain controversial.[6,15,19,65] In general, positive bands from two of the three major antigen groups, the Gag, Pol, and Env regions of the virus, are required for a positive test. The Gag proteins consist of p55, p24, and p18 proteins (p stands for protein), the Pol region codes for reverse transcriptase (p66 and p51) and an endonuclease (p31), and the Env region codes for the envelope glycoprotein gp160 (the precursor product) and its two major subunits, gp120 and gp41 (gp stands for glycoprotein). Recent analyses suggest the use of criteria developed by the Centers for Disease Control and the Association of State, Territorial, and Public Health Laboratory Directors (CDC/ASTPHLD) as the most appropriate for judging results of the Western blot tests.[92] The CDC/ASTPHLD criteria require the presence of at least two of the following bands—p24, gp41, or gp160/120—for a positive result, the presence of no bands for a negative result, and

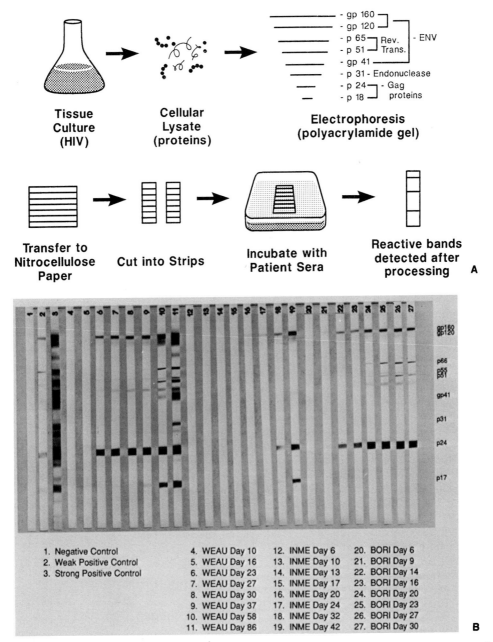

FIGURE 4–3. *A*, Western blot test is performed by separating tissue culture-derived HIV-1 proteins (p) and glycoproteins (gp) via polyacrylamide gel electrophoresis, transferring (blotting) the separated proteins onto nitrocellulose paper, incubating the cut strips of nitrocellulose paper with patient serum, and detecting anti-HIV antibodies that have bound to the HIV-1–associated proteins at the precise point at which they migrated in the gel. Through this procedure, the antibody reactivity against specific antigens can be determined (e.g., anti-Gag, anti-Env, or anti-endonuclease antibodies). *B*, Examples of Western blot tests from three patients (WEAU, BORI, and INME) identified at the time of acute HIV-1 infection (seroconversion). Each lane represents a time point (in days) from the time of presentation with symptomatic acute HIV-1 disease or a positive or negative control (lanes 1 to 3).

the presence of any HIV-1–related (or non–HIV-1–related) band(s) not meeting the criteria for a positive result as an indeterminate result.[65]

Radioimmunoprecipitation Assay

The radioimmunoprecipitation assay (RIPA) is a more time-consuming and labor-intensive test than the Western blot, yet it provides much finer resolution of the high-molecular-weight envelope proteins than the Western blot test.[13] The RIPA requires ongoing cell culture of HIV-1 to provide the appropriate substrate for the assay. HIV-1 replication in lymphocytic cell lines occurs in the presence of radiolabeled amino acids (e.g., ^{35}S-methionine or ^{35}S-cysteine). The radiolabeled amino acids are incorporated into viral proteins during viral replication. A cell lysate is prepared via homogenization of infected cells, and the lysate is then incubated in the presence of patient serum. Anti–HIV-1 antibodies present in the serum react with the radiolabeled antigens and form immune complexes. These complexes are removed by incubating the reaction mixture with protein A-coated Sepharose beads, which bind the Fc portion of immunoglobulin molecules. The beads are separated from the reaction mixture through centrifugation, and the antibody–antigen complexes are eluted from the separated beads by adding a detergent and heating. The immunoprecipitants are then run through an electrophoretic gel, which separates them according to their molecular weight (as in the Western blot procedure). An audioradiograph of the gel yields a banding pattern very similar to that of the Western blot test.

The RIPA is considered more sensitive and specific than the Western blot test.[13,17,34,39] However, the time, expense, and need for active cell lines and radioactive materials make the RIPA a poor choice for routine testing in commercial laboratories. Rather, its use is best reserved for difficult-to-diagnose cases.

Indirect Immunofluorescence Assay

Like the RIPA, the indirect immunofluorescence assay (IFA) requires preparation of HIV-1 antigens that are expressed on infected cells and are stained subsequently.[25] Infected cells are placed on glass slides in a fixed monolayer and are incubated with patient serum. Anti–HIV-1 antibodies present within the serum bind to antigens expressed on the surface of cells, and these bound antibodies are then detected with antihuman antibody that

has been labeled with fluorescein isothiocyanate (FITC), an ultraviolet-activated dye compound. After appropriate processing, the slide is viewed under a fluorescent microscope, and the number of cells, the intensity of staining, and the staining pattern are assessed. IFA can detect the earliest serologic response against the virus (IgM antibodies) during acute infection.[23] However, the time, expense, and expertise required for the IFA procedure make its routine use in a commercial laboratory impractical.

Other Anti–HIV-1 Antibody Tests

A number of rapid screening tests have been developed that may be useful in evaluation of field isolates when large numbers of samples must be screened. The rapid latex agglutination assay uses polystyrene beads that have been coated with recombinant HIV-1 proteins.[77] In the presence of antibodies against these proteins, the beads agglutinate. This test apparently is quite accurate when used by experienced personnel in areas where HIV infection is endemic.[25,75] However, further testing is required to establish its usefulness among populations with lower rates of infection.

An autologous red cell agglutination assay has been developed.[48] In this test a mouse monoclonal antibody directed against human red cells is conjugated with synthetic gp41 envelope protein from HIV. When added to whole blood from the patient, the antibody–gp41 complex binds to the human red cells, and if anti-gp41 antibodies are present in the plasma, agglutination of the red cells occurs rapidly (within a few minutes). Further testing is required to establish the sensitivity and specificity of this assay in large populations.

p24 Antigen Assays

HIV p24 Antigen Test

This assay measures the amount of free viral protein (p24) present in the plasma or tissue culture supernatant.[2] Although this protein may be present in the plasma of patients at all stages of HIV infection, p24 antigenemia is most prevalent during the time of initial seroconversion and again later in the course of more advanced HIV disease.[3,18,36,68,79] The test uses an ELISA sandwich technique in which antibodies to p24 are bound to the bottom of a microtiter well or onto polystyrene beads (Fig.

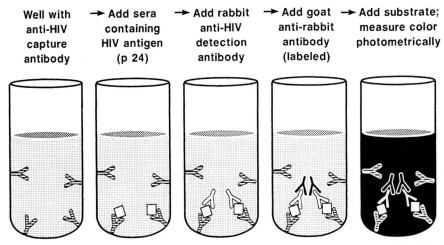

Well with → **Add sera** → **Add rabbit** → **Add goat** → **Add substrate;**
anti-HIV   **containing**   **anti-HIV**   **anti-rabbit**   **measure color**
capture   **HIV antigen**   **detection**   **antibody**   **photometrically**
antibody   **(p 24)**   **antibody**   **(labeled)**

FIGURE 4–4. HIV-1 antigen capture assay is an ELISA-based test that detects the presence of free HIV-1 p24 antigen in patient serum. Free antigen is bound (captured) by specific anti-p24 capture antibodies that have been coated onto a microwell. Bound antigen is detected by specially designed rabbit anti-HIV p24 (detection antibodies), which, in turn, are detected by goat antirabbit antibodies. The goat antibodies have been conjugated with an enzyme that cleaves a specific substrate, yielding a colored product. By photometrically measuring the degree of color in the well, the amount of HIV-1 p24 antigen can be determined quantitatively.

4–4). The bound antibodies are incubated with patient serum or plasma. If free p24 antigen is present in the serum, the antigen is bound tightly and specifically to the capture anti-p24 antibody. After a washing procedure, a second detector anti-p24 antibody is added, followed by addition of an enzyme-linked immunoglobulin, which is directed against the second p24 antibody. With the addition of substrate, the conjugated enzyme cleaves the substrate into a color-generating product that can be measured spectrophotometrically (as in the ELISA anti-HIV antibody procedure). This test was originally developed with the second anti-p24 antibody's having a polyclonal nature. More recently, the use of monoclonal anti-p24 antibodies has increased the sensitivity of the assay substantially. With the more advanced test, p24 antigen levels as low as 7 to 10 pg/ml can be detected reliable.

Acidified p24 Antigen Procedure

A modification of the p24 antigen test was introduced that further increases the test's sensitivity. This modification is based on the concept that p24 antigen, when produced in the presence of significant amounts of anti-p24 antibody, forms antigen–antibody complexes that bind free antigen and prevent detection. Through acidification of plasma, the antigen–antibody complexes can be disrupted, releasing free antigen for detection by the antigen assay.[49,63,73]

The procedure is performed by pretreating patient plasma (or serum) with glycine and incubating it for 1 hour at 37°C. After stabilization of the plasma, the plasma is analyzed for the presence of p24 antigen as described previously. Studies are underway to assess the degree of increased sensitivity by using this technique. Preliminary results indicate that it may be especially helpful in detecting p24 antigen in HIV-1–infected infants in the perinatal period. The acidified p24 antigen assay also may be useful in following patient responses to antiretroviral therapy in clinical trials, although more recent data indicate that regular p24 antigen testing may yield more information.

Polyethylene Glycol Precipitation

Another approach to enhancing p24 antigen sensitivity is through polyethylene glycol precipitation of antibody–antigen complexes before p24 antigen testing. In one study, the sensitivity increased from 38% to 59% after polyethylene glycol precipitation of the complexes.[31] This technique is still under investigation.

Polymerase Chain Reaction Technique

The polymerase chain reaction (PCR) technique, introduced in the late 1980s, represents a major advance in the diagnosis of many disor-

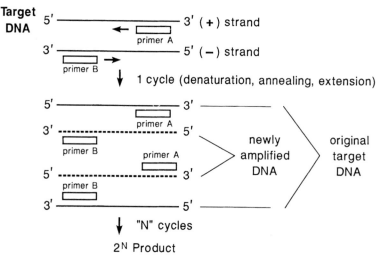

FIGURE 4–5. In the polymerase chain reaction (PCR) technique, target DNA is amplified through a series of cycles, each consisting of (1) denaturation of the double-stranded target DNA, (2) annealing of specially designed complementary primers (A and B) to the target DNA, and (3) extension of the primers into complementary new strands of DNA through the use of a unique heat-stable DNA polymerase (Taq polymerase). By repeating the cycles N times, the amount of original target DNA is amplified exponentially, 2^N (see text for details).

ders, including HIV infection.[68,81] This powerful technique can amplify target DNA existing in very small quantities (as few as 1 copy of HIV per 100,000 cells) through a series of binary replicative cycles (Fig. 4–5).[68,81] Oligonucleotide primers, approximately 25 to 30 bp in length, are carefully designed to bind to a known sequence of the target DNA. These complementary primers bind to highly conserved regions of the genome, usually spaced 150 to 600 bp apart.

Each PCR cycle consists of a period of denaturation (during which the temperatures reach 95°C), followed by an annealing period during which the primers bind to the target DNA (typically with temperatures of 55°C to 60°C) and finally by an extension period during which complementary sequences are generated (temperature, 72°C). The key to the entire reaction is the Taq polymerase, a unique DNA polymerase derived from the bacterium *Thermus aquaticus,* which maintains its activity at high temperatures (72°C). In addition to the Taq polymerase enzyme and primers, the reaction mixture contains the necessary phosphorylated nucleotide products (dATP, dGTP, dCTP, and dTTP), appropriate concentrations of divalent cations (e.g., magnesium), buffers, and the target DNA to allow optimum amplification to occur.

The duration of each portion of the cycle is generally 1 to 3 minutes. At the end of each completed cycle, the amount of DNA in the region of interest is doubled. After a total of a specified number (N) of cycles, the amplified region of DNA exists at 2^N power (usually 20 to 30 cycles are used). Therefore, even if the target DNA initially exists in only a small copy number, the PCR reaction magnifies it several hundred millionfold (e.g., 2^{30} after 30 cycles). The amount of amplified product is easily detected on agarose gel electrophoresis.

The PCR procedure can also be applied to RNA.[38,40,43] In such an instance, RNA is reversed transcribed into cDNA with an animal retrovirus reverse transcriptase (e.g., murine leukemia virus RT), and the cDNA product is then amplified as described previously. In the case of HIV, proviral HIV-1 DNA, genomic RNA, and mRNA have all been amplified successfully.

The major problem with PCR amplification, ironically, is also its greatest strength, (i.e., its incredible sensitivity). When performed properly, there is probably no more powerful molecular biologic technique. Unfortunately, inadvertent contamination of reagents or target DNA or both can lead to false-positive results even in laboratories with the most experienced personnel.[55] The problem with contamination is the limiting obstacle to the widespread use of the PCR technique in clinical practice. Nonetheless, when used properly in laboratories with experienced personnel, this technique allows early detection of infection before the development of a serologic response.[24,92]

Quantitative PCR

Several laboratories have developed techniques to quantitate the amount of HIV proviral DNA and genomic RNA as relative measures of viral load.[1,8,24,26,43,44,66,70] Previously, serial dilutions of target DNA (or cDNA) were PCR-amplified, and the relative intensities of the PCR products were compared to a standard curve. Even with coamplification of highly conserved cellular products (such as the β-globin gene) as positive controls, a high degree of variability was observed. Inefficient RNA extraction, RNAse or DNAse contamination, and variability in PCR efficiency all have contributed to the unreliability of early quantitative PCR techniques.

More recently, several new approaches have been developed that circumvent many of the previously identified obstacles. Competitive PCR techniques, which use an internal standard consisting of known RNA or DNA template matched to the target sequence of interest, have shown more promise in initial studies. One such technique, quantitative competitive PCR (QC-PCR), recently has been applied to a cohort of 66 patients that covers the spectrum of HIV infection.[70] The dynamic range of this assay was from 100 copies per milliliter of plasma to over 21,000,000 copies per milliliter and varied with stage of disease. The mean plasma HIV-1 RNA value for patients with early asymptomatic disease was 78,200 copies per milliliter, with symptomatic disease (ARC) 352,100 copies per milliliter, with advanced disease (AIDS) 2,448,000 copies per milliliter; the highest value, 5,178,000 copies per milliliter, was observed in patients with acute seroconversion syndrome (formerly CDC stage I). Of special interest, the QC-PCR assay was applied to a small number of patients who had been treated with antiretroviral therapy (Table 4–1). Treatment with zidovudine resulted in an 80% to 95% reduction in viral burden as measured by QC-PCR, which was readily reversible within 1 week after cessation of therapy. These data demonstrate both the potential use of more sophisticated viral markers in future clinical studies and the dynamic nature of HIV replication in vivo.

Several other PCR techniques are being developed by a number of investigators.[43,44] These include the Amplicor PCR technique (Roch-Molecular Systems) and the nucleic acid sequence-based amplification (NASBA) technique.[50,61] In addition, a novel non–PCR-based technique has been developed by investigators at Chiron. The so-called branched-chain DNA

TABLE 4–1. VIROLOGIC EFFECT OF ZIDOVUDINE THERAPY OVER 6 WEEKS AS MEASURED BY QC-PCR AND p24 ANTIGEN TECHNIQUES

| Patient ID | HIV RNA (copies per milliliter) | HIV p24 Ag | | Zidovudine (AZT)* | Time on Treatment |
		ICD (pg/ml)	Reg (pg/ml)		
SLMI 0843	84,900	0	0	−	Week 0*
	18,000	0	0	+	Week 1
	33,500	0	0	+	Week 2
	28,100	0	0	+	Week 6
	72,700	0	0	−	Week 7
ARLA 0846	49,100	0	0	−	Week 0
	7300	0	0	+	Week 1
	6500	0	0	+	Week 2
	11,200	0	0	+	Week 6
	58,400	0	0	−	Week 7
MIWI 1278	173,600	79	0	−	Week 0
	21,900	28	0	+	Week 1
	10,900	24	0	+	Week 2
	9200	31	0	+	Week 6
	136,300	47	0	−	Week 7

* For kinetic analysis of viral load over a 6-week period of treatment with zidovudine, patients were studied before initiation of treatment (week 0), after 1, 2, 6 weeks of treatment, and 1 week after temporary discontinuation of treatment (week 7).

Adapted from Pistak M Jr, Saag MS, Yang LC, et al: High levels of HIV-1 in plasma during all stages of infection determined by competitive PCR. Science 259:1749–1754, 1993. Copyright 1993 by the AAAS.

amplification (bDNA) technique is an ELISA-like assay that amplifies signal from target HIV RNA or DNA. The original bDNA assay is less sensitive than PCR assays (cut-off of 10,000 Eq/ml); however, a new, more sensitive assay (second-generation bDNA) can accurately detect down to 500 copies/ml. In general, the bDNA assay is easier to perform and is associated with a low intra-assay variability rate. Despite obvious differences in technique, a remarkable correlation exists between values obtained via quantitative PCR versus bDNA ($r = 0.89$, $p < 0.001$)[12] (see Fig. 4–6).

Based on currently available data viral burden measurements should be used routinely in clinical practice.[80] In recently reported studies, quantitative PCA and bDNA have demonstrated *independent* predictive value in determining the relative risk of clinical progression and/or survival when compared to other markers, including CD4 lymphoma counts.[21,37,57,64,80] In these studies, viral burden measures were better predictors of clinical outcome than other markers, whether using either baseline values or change in the marker in response to antiviral therapy. As all of the viral burden assays become more standardized and more readily available, clinicians will be able to make decisions regarding the effectiveness of antiretroviral therapy based on measurements of viral burden rather than indirect assessments of antiretroviral therapy effects, such as CD4 counts.

EVALUATION OF IMMUNOLOGIC STATUS

CD4 Cell Count

Human lymphocytes possess specific glycoproteins on their surface that play an important role in cell activity and function. Although many surface glycoproteins have been identified, the CD3, CD4, and CD8 cell-surface markers are used most often in the context of HIV infection.[53] The CD3 (T3) cell marker is present on all adult human lymphocytes. The CD8 (T8) cell marker is present on the subset of suppressor or cytotoxic lymphocytes that control or suppress specific ongoing immunologic activity. In contrast, the lymphocytes bearing the CD4 (T4) cell surface marker help or induce immunologic reactions.

CD4 cells respond to the class II major histocompatibility complex (MHC) antigens and release cytokines that activate and augment the immunologic response. CD4+ lymphocytes are the primary targets of HIV infection, and the CD4 receptor is the primary binding site of HIV-1. Throughout the course of chronic HIV-1 infection, the number of CD4 lymphocytes is depleted, and the loss of these cells is associated with development of the characteristic opportunistic infections and malignancies of AIDS.[25,28,29,35,60,71,76,85] Thus the measurement of CD4+ lymphocytes is one of the most impor-

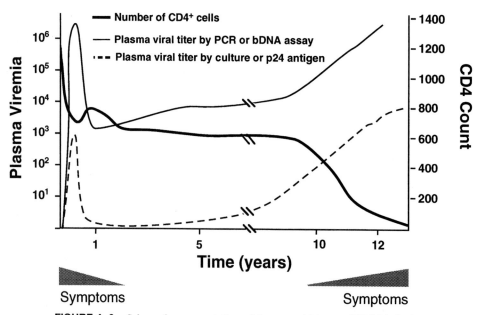

FIGURE 4–6. Schematic representation of the natural history of HIV-1 infection.

tant determinants for clinically staging the disease status of HIV-1–infected patients.

The numbers of CD4 and CD8 cells are measured through the use of specific monoclonal antibodies directed against the surface glycoprotein. These monoclonals are labeled with fluorescent markers, which can be detected when light is passed through the sample. Specialized fluorescent antibody cell sorting (FACS) machines have been developed that automatically count the number of cells labeled with the monoclonal antibody. Using this flow cytometric technique, the percentage of cells bearing the CD4 or CD8 cell-surface markers can be determined.

The FACS analysis yields the percentage of cells carrying a certain surface marker. The absolute CD4 count cannot be measured directly but is calculated by the following formula:

Absolute CD4 count

$$= \text{total white blood count}$$
$$\times \text{percent lymphocytes}$$
$$\times \text{percent CD4 cells.}$$

Clinical staging can be based on either the CD4 percent or the absolute CD4 count. However, most clinical studies have used the absolute CD4 count, even though the percentage value is less subject to fluctuations.[56,87]

Variability in the CD4 percent and the absolute CD4 cell count can be a significant problem both over time and with repeated determinations. CD4 counts normally undergo diurnal variation, with fluctuations of as much as a 150 to 300/mm^3 difference between morning and evening values in normal hosts.[56] Additionally, the longer samples set before processing, the more likely CD4 count values will be artificially elevated. Refrigeration also dramatically increases CD4 cell count values. Such variation has posed difficulties both in clinically staging patients and in following response to therapy in clinical trials.

Another means of clinically following patients is to use the CD4/CD8 ratio.[87] It is determined by dividing the number of CD4 cells by the number of CD8 cells. In uninfected controls, normal values for the CD4/CD8 ratio are 0.5 to 2.0. Normal values for CD4 percent are 40% to 70%, and CD4 counts are generally 500 to 1600/mm^3 in adults.

β_2-Microglobulin

β_2-Microglobulin is a protein present on the surface of all nucleated cells and serves as the light chain of the class T MHC complex.[25] Measurable levels of β_2-microglobulin are increased whenever mononuclear cell activation or cell destruction occurs, as is the case with HIV-1 infection. Serum levels of β_2-microglobulin are determined through radioimmunoassay determination or through an enzyme immunoassay. Several clinical studies have shown that levels >3 mg/liter are associated with increased risk of progression to AIDS among HIV-infected patients.[11,51,54,86] When levels are >5 mg/liter, the likelihood of occurrence of new opportunistic diseases or death increases further.[5,59] Unfortunately, β_2-microglobulin levels are too nonspecific and not sufficiently predictive of clinical outcome to be of value in clinical practice.

Serum Neopterin

Neopterin is produced during guanosine triphosphate metabolism and is increased during periods of cellular activation. The primary source of neopterin apparently is cells of the monocyte-macrophage lineage that release increased amounts of neopterin after stimulation with interferon-γ. Neopterin levels can be determined through high-pressure liquid chromatography or by competitive radioimmunoassay and can be detected in both serum and urine.

Like β_2-microglobulin, elevated levels of neopterin have been correlated to advancing clinical HIV disease.[30,32,33] Levels >15 ng/ml are noted in patients with AIDS as compared to levels in the 3- to 5-ng/ml range for asymptomatic seropositive patients.[75] Like β_2-microglobulin, neopterin levels are not sufficiently predictive of clinical events to be of use in clinical practice.

TEST INTERPRETATION

To interpret results of any HIV-related test appropriately, the natural history of HIV infection and the host immune response must be understood. After initial primary infection with HIV, there is an immunologically silent-window period before the development of detectable antibody (Fig. 4–6). The median time from initial infection to the development of detectable antibody is 2.1 months, with 95% of individuals developing antibody within 5.8 months of initial infection.[45] Although the majority of individuals notice very few, if any, symptoms associated with seroconversion, an estimated 40% to

60% of individuals will develop symptoms of an acute mononucleosis-like syndrome, consisting of sore throat, headache, fever, myalgias, lymphadenopathy, and skin rash.[18,22,46,88,89] When such symptomatic patients have been studied carefully, virus replication is typically quite high, as demonstrated by high levels of plasma HIV RNA, infections free-virus in plasma, and plasma p24 antigen levels.[18,24,61,70] (Fig. 4–7). Within 14 to 21 days after the onset of symptoms, anti–HIV-1 antibodies become detectable, and titers rise very rapidly against both the envelope glycoproteins and p24. Once a patient

develops a mature antibody response, it usually remains detectable for life. The rise in detectable antibody response is associated with a rapid decline in both the p24 antigenemia and plasma viremia (culturable virus), usually to undetectable levels within weeks. The p24 antigenemia and plasma viremia generally return to detectable levels as the patient approaches more advanced disease.[20,42,79] However, viral burden as measured by quantitative PCR remains detectable throughout the course of the disease.[70] Indeed, recent studies demonstrate continued, ongoing, viral replication through-

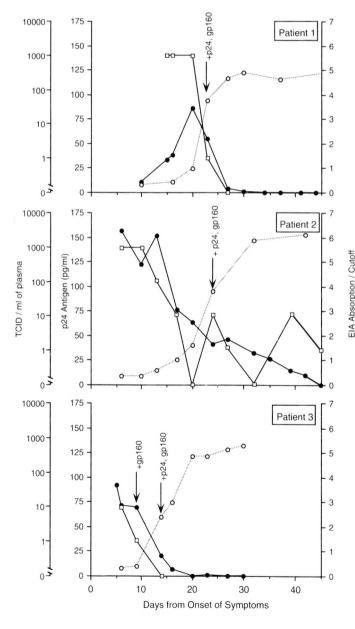

FIGURE 4–7. Detailed analysis of plasma viremia titers (*open squares*), HIV-1 p24 antigen levels (*closed circles*), and anti-p24 antibody levels (*open circles*) in three patients with acute primary HIV-1 infection. The *arrows* indicate the time of first detection of both gp160 and p24 antibodies by Western blot technique (see Fig. 4–3*B*). (From Clark SJ, Saag MS, Decker WD, et al: High titers of cytopathic virus in plasma of patients with symptomatic primary HIV-1 infection. N Engl J Med 324[14]:956, 1991, with permission.)

out *all* stages of HIV infection with extraordinarily high rates of viral replication (~1 billion virions provided daily with a half-life of 1.2 days).

The CD4 count generally decreases during the acute viral-like illness of acute seroconversion (as CD4 counts do with most acute viral syndromes) but usually returns toward normal levels as a healthy immune response is established. Over a period of many years, the CD4 count declines.[85] As the cell count drops below 500/mm^3, antiretroviral therapy usually is initiated.[62] The risk of serious opportunistic infections and death increases substantially as CD4 counts drop below 200/mm^3.[28,29,35,71,76] Prophylactic therapy against the development of *Pneumocystis carinii* pneumonia is indicated when the CD4 cell count approaches 200/mm^3.[62] Much controversy still exists about routine prophylaxis of other opportunistic diseases when CD4 counts drop below 50/mm^3, although current data suggest initiation of routine preventative therapy against *Mycobacterium Avium* complex disease (Chapter 21).

SENSITIVITY, SPECIFICITY, AND MISLEADING TEST RESULTS

Any discussion of HIV testing must address the questions of sensitivity, specificity, positive predictive value, and negative predictive value (Table 4–2). By definition, sensitivity refers to the ability to detect accurately an individual with a particular disorder among those individuals who truly have the disorder. In contrast, specificity is the ability to identify accurately all those individuals who truly do not have the disorder out of all of those individuals within a

population who are unaffected. The sensitivity and specificity of a given test are test specific and are not dependent on the population being tested. Positive and negative predictive values, on the other hand, refer to the test's ability to predict accurately who does or does not have a particular disorder and are critically related to the prevalence of the disorder within the population being tested.

False-negative antibody test results can occur any time an individual is within that 1- to 3-month seronegative window period between the time of initial infection and the development of a detectable immune response. Fortunately, this time period is short, and based on bloodbank transfusion data, the number of false-negative results among low-risk populations is approximately 1 in 40,000 to 1 in 150,000.[90] Other causes of false-negative ELISA reactions to HIV-1 include replacement transfusions, bone marrow transplantation, and commercially available test kits that detect antibody to p24 only (e.g., the ELISA test using recombinant p24 antigen).

False-positive ELISA reactions generally result from crossreacting antibodies, such as those against class II human leukocyte antigens (HLA-DR-4 and DQw-3).[4,10,52] Such antibodies are most often observed in multiparous women and in individuals who have received multiple transfused units of blood. Other autoantibodies (e.g., those against smooth muscle or parietal cells, antimitochondrial antibodies, antinuclear antibodies, and anti–T-cell antibodies) can lead to false-positive results.[9,78,82,84]

A common misconception is that a false-positive ELISA will always be corrected by the confirmatory Western blot test. In fact, false-positive Western blot results do occur, although the frequency of false-positive Western blot results is generally less common than with ELISA results.[82] Antibodies against HLA class I antigens may lead to false-positive gp41 bands, whereas antibodies to class II HLA antigens cause false-positive bands at p31. Other autoantibodies (e.g., antimitochondrial, antinuclear, anti–T-cell, and antileukocyte antibodies) that react with proteins present in the T-lymphocyte cell line that propagated the virus used in the Western blot test also may lead to false-positive test results.[78,82]

The most important parameter when interpreting HIV tests is the positive predictive value. The probability of a positive test result occurring in a truly infected individual is critically dependent on the prevalence of HIV infection of the population tested.[58] As an example, as-

TABLE 4–2. HIV TESTING RESULTS

Test Result	HIV Infection	
	Present	Absent
Positive	True-positive (A)	False-positive (B)
Negative	False-negative (C)	True-negative (D)

Sensitivity (%) $= \dfrac{A}{A + C}$ ($\times$ 100).

Positive predictive value (%) $= \dfrac{A}{A + B}$ ($\times$ 100).

Specificity (%) $= \dfrac{D}{D + B}$ ($\times$ 100).

Negative predictive value (%) $= \dfrac{D}{D + C}$ ($\times$ 100).

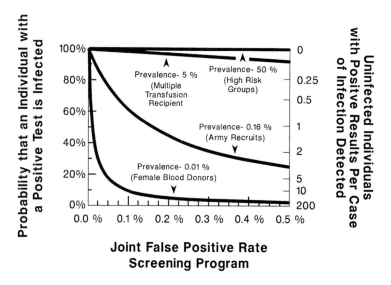

Probability that an Individual with a Positive Test is Infected

Uninfected Individuals with Positive Results Per Case of Infection Detected

Joint False Positive Rate
Screening Program

FIGURE 4–8. Interpretation of a positive HIV antibody test result. The joint false-positive rate from the ELISA and Western blot tests is shown on the *horizontal axis*. The *left vertical axis* demonstrates the probability that a person with a positive test result is truly infected with HIV. The *right vertical scale* shows the number of uninfected individuals falsely identified as infected for every infected person correctly identified. The *four bold lines* represent four populations that might be screened (high-risk groups, transfusion recipients, army recruits, and female blood donors), each of which has a different prevalence of HIV infection (listed accordingly). (From Meyer KB, Pauker SG: Sounding board. Screening for HIV: Can we afford the false positive rate? N Engl J Med 317[4]:240, 1987, with permission.)

suming tests (ELISA and Western blot) of 100% sensitivity and a joint false-positive rate of 0.01%, the rates of truly infected patients among those with positive ELISA and Western blot results vary dramatically, depending on who is tested. In testing intravenous drug users from a major U.S. metropolitan center in which the seroprevalence is 50%, the positive predictive value would approach 100%. Conversely, in screening female school teachers from a rural area in the United States where the prevalence of HIV infection is 0.01%, 50% of the women testing positive would have false-positive test results. If the joint false-positive rate increases to 0.1%, 90% of the women with positive ELISA and Western blot results would be falsely labeled as HIV infected[58] (Fig. 4–8).

Although test specificity has improved over the last 3 to 5 years, the specificities do not equal 100% and in some instances, depending on the experience of the laboratory personnel, may be 99.9% (false-positive rate, 0.1%). For most other tests, this is an acceptable false-positive rate; however, when considering the difficulties in counseling an individual who has a low risk of HIV infection who has just been diagnosed as HIV positive, it becomes quite difficult to know what precisely to tell the patient. In such instances in which the test result does not match the clinical presentation, it is best initially to repeat both the ELISA and the Western blot test at a different laboratory. If the results do not change or are indeterminate, testing at specialized laboratories using either RIPA, IFA,

HIV-1 isolation by cell culture, or, preferably, PCR techniques may be of benefit.

Another difficult problem in antibody test interpretation is how to deal with an indeterminate Western blot result. As described earlier, this situation is created when bands are present on the Western blot that do not meet criteria of a definitively positive test. Several algorithms have been proposed in the literature for dealing with indeterminate Western blots. However, the applied concepts of assessing the risk to the patient combined with repeat testing in another laboratory are a common theme with all these algorithms.[14,27] When retesting a patient who has had an indeterminate result at more than one laboratory, it is recommended that the individual be retested at 3 and 6 months to determine whether he or she was in the process of seroconverting at the original time of testing.

Use of Markers in Clinical Trials and Clinical Practice

Since the discovery of zidovudine as an effective antiretroviral agent (Table 4–1), it is no longer ethically appropriate to have untreated placebo groups in patients with advanced HIV infection. Neither is it appropriate to rely on gross measurements of antiviral efficacy, such as advancing morbidity or mortality, as a means of assessing relative antiviral activity of one compound versus another. As a result, markers of viral replication, such as p24 antigenemia,

TABLE 4–3. SUMMARY OF INTERIM RECOMMENDATIONS

Parameter	Recommendation
Plasma HIV RNA level that suggests initiation of treatment	More than 5000–10,000 copies/ml and a CD4+ count/clinical status suggestive of progression; >30,000–50,000 regardless of laboratory/clinical status
Target level of HIV RNA after initiation of treatment	Undetectable; <5000 copies/ml is an acceptable target
Minimal decrease in HIV RNA indicative of antiviral activity	>0.5 log decrease
Change in HIV RNA that suggests drug treatment failure	Return toward (within 0.3–0.5 log of) pretreatment value
Suggested frequency of HIV RNA measurement	At baseline: 2 measurements, 2–4 weeks apart Every 3–4 months or in conjunction with CD4+ counts Shorter intervals as critical decision points are neared 3–4 weeks after initiating/changing therapy

plasma viremia, quantitative cell culture, quantitative PCR along with indirect markers such as CD4 cell count are being used in various combinations to assess the relative antiretroviral activity of one compound versus another (Table 4–1). Although the definitions of how to use each test most appropriately are still being clarified, viral load measurements, via quantitative PCR or bDNA, are the best measures of antiretroviral activity and can demonstrate the relative antiviral effect of a given regimen within 2 weeks. The long-term clinical benefit of a short-term virologic assessment is still under investigation; however, viral load changes at 8 weeks of therapy have been associated with clinical benefit over time.[21,37]

From a clinical standpoint, however, it is important to separate the goals of experimental therapeutics and the goals of optimum patient care. The goal of antiretroviral therapy is to keep the viral load as low as possible for as long as possible. Based on the predictive nature of viral load and its rapid response to changes in antiretroviral regimens, measurement of viral load in clinical practice should be performed on a routine basis.[80] Table 4–3 summarizes how the measures might be used to initiate antiret-roviral therapy, monitor the response to therapy, and determine when a given regimen may be failing. Plasma HIV RNA levels should be obtained every 3 to 4 months, preferably in conjunction with CD4 cell counts or at shorter intervals as critical decision points are neared. Proper specimen handling is essential for ensuring accurate RNA values, including use of plasma (as opposed to serum), use of EDTA or ACD (rather than heparin) as an anticoagulant, prompt specimen processing (within 2 to 4 hours of phlebotomy), and, ideally, consistent use of the same type of assay (bDNA or quantitative PCR). Plasma HIV RNA assays substantially improve the ability to determine when an antiretroviral regimen is no longer active and, therefore, are likely to reduce the overall cost of care by minimizing continued use of ineffective and expensive treatment regimens.

ACKNOWLEDGMENT

Thanks to Ms. Jane Garrison for her assistance in the preparation of this manuscript, to Katharine Coleman for preparation of the figures, and to Dr. Victoria Johnson for her critical review.

REFERENCES

1. Abbott MA, Poiesz BJ, Byrne BC, et al: Enzymatic gene amplification: Qualitative and quantitative methods for detecting proviral DNA amplified in vitro. J Infect Dis 158(6):1158–1169, 1988
2. Allain J-P, Laurian Y, Paul DA, et al: Long-term evaluation of HIV antigen and antibodies to p24 and gp41 in patients with hemophilia. N Engl J Med 317:1114–1121, 1987
3. Allain J-P, Laurian Y, Paul DA, et al: Serological markers in early stages of human immunodeficiency virus infection in hemophiliacs. Lancet 2:1233–1236, 1986
4. Ameglio F, Dolei A, Benedetto A, et al: Antibodies reactive with nonpolymorphic epitopes on HLA molecules interfere in screening tests for the human immunodeficiency virus. J Infect Dis 156(6):1034–1035, 1987
5. Anderson RE, Lang W, Shiboski S, et al: Use of β_2-

microglobulin level and CD4 lymphocyte count to predict development of acquired immunodeficiency syndrome in persons with human immunodeficiency virus infection. Arch Intern Med 150: 73–77, 1990

6. Barnes DM: New questions about AIDS test accuracy. Science 238:884–885, 1987

7. Barre-Sinoussi F, Chermann JC, Rey F, et al: Isolation of a T-lymphotropic retrovirus from a patient at risk for acquired immune deficiency syndrome (AIDS). Science 220:868–871, 1983

8. Becker-Andre M, Hahlbrock K: Absolute mRNA quantification using the polymerase chain reaction (PCR). A novel approach by a PCR aided transcript titration assay (PATTY). Nucleic Acids Res 17: 9437–9446, 1989

9. Biberfeld G, Bredberg-Raden U, Bottinger B, et al: Blood donor sera with false-positive Western blot reactions to human immunodeficiency virus. Lancet 2:289–290, 1986

10. Blanton M, Balakrishnan K, Dumaswala U, et al: HLA antibodies in blood donors with reactive screening tests for antibody to the immunodeficiency virus. Transfusion 27:118, 1987

11. Calabrese LH, Proffitt MR, Gupta MK, et al: Serum β_2-microglobulin and interferon in homosexual males: Relationship to clinical findings and serologic status to the human T lymphotropic virus (HTLV-III). AIDS Res 1:423–438, 1984

12. Cao Y, Ho DD, Todd J, et al: Clinical evaluation of branched DNA signal amplification for quantifying HIV type-1 in human plasma. AIDS Res Hum Retroviruses 11:353–361, 1995

13. Carlson JR, Yee J, Hinrichs SH, et al: Comparison of indirect immunofluorescence and Western blot for detection of antihuman immunodeficiency virus antibodies. J Clin Microbiol 25:494–497, 1987

14. Celum CL, Coombs RW, Lafferty W, et al: Indeterminate human immunodeficiency virus type 1 Western blots: Seroconversion risk, specificity of supplemental tests, and an algorithm for evaluation. J Infect Dis 164:656–664, 1991

15. Centers for Disease Control: Interpretation and use of the Western blot assay for serodiagnosis of human immunodeficiency virus type 1 infections. MMWR 38:1–7, 1989

16. Centers for Disease Control: Update: Serologic testing for antibody to human immunodeficiency virus. MMWR 36:833–840, 1988

17. Chiodi F, Bredberg-Raden U, Biberfeld G, et al: Radioimmunoprecipitation and Western blotting with sera of human immunodeficiency virus infected patients: A comparative study. AIDS Res Hum Retroviruses 3:165–176, 1987

18. Clark SJ, Saag MS, Decker WD, et al: High titers of cytopathic virus in plasma of patients with symptomatic primary HIV-1 infection. N Engl J Med 324: 954–960, 1991

19. Consortium for Retrovirus Serology Standardization: Serological diagnosis of human immunodeficiency virus infection by Western blot testing. JAMA 260: 674–679, 1988

20. Coombs RW, Collier AC, Allain J-P, et al: Plasma viremia in human immunodeficiency virus infection. N Engl J Med 321:1626–1631, 1989

21. Coombs RW, Welles SL, Hooper C, et al: Association of plasma human immunodeficiency virus type-1

RNA level with risk of progression in patients with advanced infection. J Infect Dis (In press) 1996

22. Cooper DA, Gold J, Maclean P, et al: Acute AIDS retrovirus infection. Lancet 1:537–540, 1985

23. Cooper DA, Imrie AA, Penny R: Antibody response to human immunodeficiency virus after primary infection. J Infect Dis 155:1113–1118, 1987

24. Daar ES, Moudgil T, Meyer RD, et al: Transient high levels of viremia in patients with primary immunodeficiency type 1 infection. N Engl J Med 324: 961–964, 1991

25. Davey RT Jr, Lane HC: Laboratory methods in the diagnosis and prognostic staging of infection with human immunodeficiency virus type 1. Rev Infect Dis 12(5):912–930, 1990

26. Dickover RE, Donovan RM, Goldstein E, et al: Quantitation of human immunodeficiency virus DNA by using the polymerase chain reaction. J Clin Microbiol 28:2130–2133, 1990

27. Dock NL, Kleinman SH, Rayfield MA, et al: Human immunodeficiency virus infection and indeterminate Western blot patterns. Arch Intern Med 151: 525–530, 1991

28. El-Sadr W, Marmor M, Zolla-Pazner S, et al: Four year prospective study on homosexual men: Correlation of immunologic abnormalities, clinical status and serology to human immunodeficiency virus. J Infect Dis 155:789–793, 1987

29. Eyster ME, Gail MH, Ballard JO, et al: Natural history of human immunodeficiency virus infection in hemophiliacs: Effects of T-cell subsets, platelet counts, and age. Ann Intern Med 107:1–6, 1987

30. Fahey JL, Taylor JMG, Detels R, et al: The prognostic value of cellular and serologic markers in infection with human immunodeficiency virus type 1. N Engl J Med 322:166–172, 1990

31. Fiscus SA, Wallmark EB, Folds JD, et al: Detection of infectious immune complexes in human immunodeficiency virus type 1 (HIV-1) infections: Correlation with plasma viremia and CD4 cell counts. J Infect Dis 164:765–769, 1991

32. Fuchs D, Hausen A, Reibnegger G, et al: Neopterin as a marker for activated cell-mediated immunity: Application in HIV infection. Immunol Today 9: 150–155, 1988

33. Fuchs D, Spira TJ, Hausen A, et al: Neopterin as a predictive marker for disease progression in human immunodeficiency virus type 1 infection. Clin Chem 35:1746–1749, 1989

34. Gallo D, Diggs JL, Shell GR, et al: Comparison of detection of antibody to the acquired immune deficiency syndrome virus by enzyme immunoassay, immunofluorescence, and Western blot methods. J Clin Microbiol 23:1049–1051, 1986

35. Goedert JJ, Biggar RJ, Melbye M, et al: Effect of T4 count and cofactors on the incidence of AIDS in homosexual men infected with human immunodeficiency virus. JAMA 257:331–334, 1987

36. Goudsmit J, DeWolf F, Paul DA, et al: Expression of human immunodeficiency virus antigen (HIV-Ag) in serum and cerebrospinal fluid during acute and chronic infection. Lancet 2:177–180, 1986

37. Hammer SM, Katzenstein DA, Hughes MD, et al: Virologic markers and outcome in ACTG 175 (Abstract 524). Third Conference on Retroviruses and Opportunistic Infections, Washington, DC, 1996, p 175

38. Hart C, Schochetman G, Spira T, et al: Direct detec-

tion of HIV RNA expression in seropositive subjects. Lancet 2:596–599, 1988

39. Hedenskog M, Dewhurst S, Ludvigsen C, et al: Testing for antibodies to AIDS-associated retrovirus (HLTV-III/LAV) by indirect fixed cell immunofluorescence: Specificity, sensitivity, and applications. J Med Virol 19:325–334, 1986

40. Hewlett IK, Gregg RA, Ou CY, et al: Detection in plasma of HIV-1-specific DNA and RNA by polymerase chain reaction before and after seroconversion. J Clin Immunoassay 11:161–164, 1988

41. Ho DD, Newmann AU, Perelson AS, et al: Rapid turnover of plasma virions and CD4+ lymphocytes in HIV-1 infection. Nature 373:123–126, 1995

42. Ho DH, Moudgil T, Alam M: Quantitation of human immunodeficiency virus type 1 in the blood of infected persons. N Engl J Med 321:1621–1625, 1989

43. Holodniy M, Katzenstein DA, Sengupta S, et al: Detection and quantification of human immunodeficiency virus RNA in patient serum by use of the polymerase chain reaction. J Infect Dis 163:862–866, 1991

44. Holodniy M, Katzenstein D, Winters M, et al: Measurement of HIV virus load and genotypic resistance by gene amplification in asymptomatic subjects treated with combination therapy. J Acquir Immune Defic Syndr 6:366–369, 1993

45. Horsburgh CR Jr, Ou CY, Jason J, et al: Duration of human immunodeficiency virus infection before detection of antibody. Lancet 2:637–639, 1989

46. Isaksson B, Albert J, Chiodi F, et al: AIDS two months after primary human immunodeficiency virus infection. J Infect Dis 158:866–868, 1988

47. Jacobson MA, Abrams DI, Volberding PA, et al: Serum β_2-microglobulin decreases in patients with AIDS or ARC treated with azidothymidine. J Infect Dis 159:1029–1036, 1989

48. Kemp BE, Rylatt DB, Bundesen PG, et al: Autologous red cell agglutination assay for HIV-1 antibodies: Simplified test with whole blood. Science 241:1352–1354, 1988

49. Kestens L, Goofd G, Gigase PL, et al: HIV antigen detection in circulating immune complexes. J Virol Methods 31:67–76, 1991

50. Kievits T, Van Gemen B, van Strijp D, et al: NASBA isothermal enzymatic in vitro nucleic acid amplification optimized for the diagnosis of HIV-1 infection. J Virol Methods 35:273–286, 1991

51. Klein E, Gindi EJ, Brown DK, et al: Cross-sectional study of immunologic abnormalities in intravenous drug abusers on methadone maintenance in New York City. AIDS 3:235–237, 1989

52. Kuhnl P, Seidl S, Holzberger G: HLA DR4 antibodies cause positive HTLV-III antibody ELISA results. Lancet 1:1222–1223, 1985

53. Lane HC, Fauci AS: Immunologic abnormalities in the acquired immunodeficiency syndrome. Annu Rev Immunol 3:477–500, 1985

54. Lazzarin A: Raised serum β_2-microglobulin levels in different stages of human immunodeficiency virus infection. J Clin Lab Immunol 27:133–137, 1988

55. Lifson AR, Stanley M, Pane J, et al: Detection of human immunodeficiency virus DNA using the polymerase chain reaction in a well-characterized group of homosexual and bisexual men. J Infect Dis 161:436–439, 1990

56. Malone JL, Simms TE, Gray GC, et al: Sources of variability in repeated T-helper lymphocyte counts from human immunodeficiency virus type 1-infected patients: Total lymphocyte count fluctuations and diurnal cycle are important. J Acquir Immune Defic Syndr 3:144–151, 1990

57. Mellors JW: Rinaldo, CR, Jr, Gupta P, et al. Prognosis in HIV-1 infection predicted by the quantity of virus in plasma. Science 272:1167–1170, 1996

58. Meyer KB, Pauker SG: Sounding board: Screening for HIV: Can we afford the false positive rate? N Engl J Med 317(4):238–241, 1987

59. Moss AR, Bacchetti P: Natural history of HIV infection. AIDS 3:550–561, 1989

60. Moss AR, Bacchetti P, Osmond D, et al: Seropositivity for HIV and the development of AIDS or AIDS-related condition: Three year follow-up of the San Francisco General Hospital cohort. BMJ 296:745–750, 1988

61. Mulder J, McKinney N, Christopherson C, et al: Rapid and simple PCR assay for quantitation of human immunodeficiency virus type 1 RNA in plasma: Application to acute retroviral infection. J Clin Microbiol 32:292–300, 1994

62. NIH State-of-the-Art Conference: State-of-the-Art conference on azidothymidine therapy for early HIV infection. Am J Med 89:335–344, 1990

63. Nishanian P, Huskins KR, Stehn S, et al: A simple method for improved assay demonstrates that HIV p24 antigen is present as immune complexes in most sera from HIV-infected individuals. J Infect Dis 162:21–28, 1990

64. O'Brien WA, Hartigan PM, Martin D, et al: Changes in plasma HIV-1 RNA and CD4 lymphocyte counts and the risk of progression to AIDS. N Engl J Med 334:426–431, 1996

65. O'Gorman MRG, Weber D, Landis SE, et al: Interpretive criteria of the Western blot assay for serodiagnosis of human immunodeficiency virus type 1 infection. Arch Pathol Lab Med 115:26–30, 1991

66. Oka S, Urayama K, Hirabayashi Y, et al: Quantitative analysis of human immunodeficiency virus type 1 in asymptomatic carriers using the polymerase chain reaction. Biochem Biophys Res Commun 167:1–8, 1990

67. Ou CY, Kwok S, Mitchell SW, et al: DNA amplification for direct detection of HIV-1 DNA of peripheral blood mononuclear cells. Science 239:295–297, 1988

68. Paul DA, Falk LA, Kessler HA, et al: Correlation of serum HIV antigen and antibody with clinical status in HIV-infected patients. J Med Virol 22:257–363, 1987

69. Perelson AS, Neumann AU, Markowitz M, et al: HIV-1 dynamics in vivo: Virion clearance rate, infected cell life-span, and viral generation time. Science 271:1582–1586, 1996

70. Piatak M Jr, Saag MS, Yang LC, et al: High levels of HIV-1 in plasma during all stages of infection determined by competitive PCR. Science 259:1749–1754, 1993

71. Polk BF, Fox R, Brookmeyer R, et al: Predictors of the acquired immunodeficiency syndrome developing in a cohort of seropositive homosexual men. N Engl J Med 316:61–66, 1988

72. Popovic M, Sarngadharan MG, Read E, et al: Detection, isolation, and continuous production of cytopathic retroviruses (HTLV-III) from patients with AIDS and pre-AIDS. Science 224:497–500, 1984

73. Portera M, Vitale F, La Licata R, et al: Free and anti-body-complexed antigen and antibody profile in apparently healthy HIV-seropositive individuals and in AIDS patients. J Med Virol 30:30–35, 1990

74. Quinn TC, Riggin CH, Kline RL, et al: Rapid latex agglutination assay using recombinant envelope polypeptide for the detection of antibody to the HIV. JAMA 260:510–513, 1988

75. Reddy MM, Grieco MH: Neopterin and alpha and beta interleukin 1 levels in sera of patients with human immunodeficiency virus infection. J Clin Microbiol 27:1919–1923, 1989

76. Redfield RR, Wright DC, Tramont EC: The Walter Reed staging classification for HTLV-III/LAV infection. N Engl J Med 314:131–132, 1986

77. Riggin CH, Beltz GA, Hung C-H, et al: Detection of antibodies to human immunodeficiency virus by latex agglutination with recombinant antigen. J Clin Microbiol 25:1772–1773, 1987

78. Saag MS, Britz J: Asymptomatic blood donor with a false positive HTLV-III Western blot. N Engl J Med 314(2):118, 1986

79. Saag MS, Crain MJ, Decker WD, et al: High-level viremia in adults and children infected with human immunodeficiency virus: Relation to disease stage and CD4+ lymphocyte levels. J Infect Dis 164:72–80, 1991

80. Saag MS, Holodniy M, Kuritzkes DR, et al: HIV viral load markers in clinical practice. Nat Med 2:625–629, 1996

81. Saiki RK, Gelfand DH, Stoffel S, et al: Primer-directed enzymatic amplification of DNA with a thermostable DNA polymerase. Science 239:487–491, 1988

82. Schleupner CJ: Diagnostic tests for HIV-1 infection. In Mandell GL, Douglas RG, and Bennet JE, eds: Principles and Practice of Infectious Diseases, Update 1. New York, Churchill Livingstone, 1989, p 3

83. Sloand EM, Pitt E, Chiarello RJ: HIV testing—state of the art. JAMA 266(20):2861–2866, 1991

84. Smith DM, Dewhurst S, Shepherd S, et al: False-positive enzyme-linked immunosorbent assay reactions for antibody to human immunodeficiency virus in a population of Midwestern patients with congenital bleeding disorders. Transfusion 127:112, 1987

85. Stein DS, Korvick JA, Vermund SH: CD4+ lymphocyte cell enumeration for prediction of clinical course of human immunodeficiency virus disease: A review. J Infect Dis 165:352–363, 1992

86. Taylor CR, Krailo MD, Levine AM: Serum beta-2 microglobulin levels in homosexual men with AIDS and with persistent, generalized lymphadenopathy. Cancer 57:2190–2192, 1986

87. Taylor JMG, Fahey JL, Detels R, et al: CD4 percentage, CD4 number, and CD4:CD8 ratio in HIV infection: Which to choose and how to use. J Acquir Immune Defic Syndr 2:114–124, 1989

88. Tindall B, Barker S, Donovan E, et al: Characterization of the acute clinical illness associated with human immunodeficiency virus infection. Arch Intern Med 148:945–949, 1988

89. Ward JW, Bush TJ, Perkins HA, et al: The natural history of transfusion-associated infection with human immunodeficiency virus: Factors influencing the rate of progression to disease. N Engl J Med 321(14):947–952, 1989

90. Ward JW, Holmberg SD, Allen JR, et al: Transmission of human immunodeficiency virus (HIV) by blood transfusions screened as negative for HIV antibody. N Engl J Med 318(8):473–478, 1988

91. Wei X, Ghosh SK, Taylor ME, et al: Viral dynamics in human immunodeficiency virus type 1 infection. Nature 373:117–122, 1995

92. Wolinsky SM, Rinaldo CR, Kwok S, et al: Human immunodeficiency virus type 1 (HIV-1) infection a median of 18 months before a diagnostic Western blot. Ann Intern Med 111:961–972, 1989

Chapter 5

Limiting the Risks of Health Care Workers

JULIE LOUISE GERBERDING

Health care providers exposed to blood and other body fluids risk infection with human immunodeficiency virus (HIV).[2,7,27,28,36,38,41,43,44,57,64,71] Although rare, nosocomial transmission of HIV to patients is also an important issue. Defining the risks of HIV transmission in health care settings and developing policies for protecting health care providers and their patients are important aspects of care delivery in the acquired immunodeficiency syndrome (AIDS) era. This chapter summarizes the current status of occupational and nosocomial HIV exposure risk assessment, prevention, and management.

PATIENT-TO-PROVIDER TRANSMISSION

The risk of occupational HIV transmission has been evaluated in at least 25 prospective studies of exposed health care providers at several medical centers around the world.[2,7,27,28,36,38,41,43,44,57,64,71] In these studies, both the numerator (number of infections) and the denominator (number of HIV exposures) are known and so the probability of transmission through various exposure routes can be estimated. Pooled data indicate that the **average** risk of HIV transmission associated with needle punctures or similar percutaneous injuries is 0.32% (21 infections following 6498 exposures; 95% confidence interval = 0.18 to 0.46).[28] The current estimate of mucocutaneous transmission risk is 0.03% (1 infection following 2885 exposures through mucous membranes or nonintact skin).[28] This mucocutaneous risk estimate may be biased, however, because the single transmission event was actually reported before prospective data were collected from the involved institution.

These risk estimates are useful in evaluating **populations** of exposed persons, but do not necessarily pertain to the probability of infection in **individual** cases. The factors influencing infectivity have not been completely defined. There is evidence that the amount of virus transmitted during the exposure may be a very important predictor of exposure risk. The exposure inoculum, in turn, is dependent on the titer of virus in the source fluid and the volume of that fluid.

The titer of blood can be approximated (albeit imperfectly) by ascertaining the clinical stage of HIV infection in the source patient. In general, circulating titers of infectious HIV are highest at the time of seroconversion and during advanced stages of AIDS.[18,40,64] Recent data from the Centers for Disease Control and Prevention (CDC) suggest that the odds of acquiring infection after percutaneous exposure are six times higher when the source patient has preterminal AIDS (defined by death within 2 months) than when the source has earlier stages of infection (Table 5–1).[11] This may be a consequence of high virus titers in these patients and could also reflect differences in HIV phenotype or genetic subtypes present in late-stage disease.

Deep (intramuscular) penetrations, large-bore hollow needles, and injections of blood are factors associated with most of the reported needlestick accidents causing occupational infections. In a laboratory model of needle injuries, these same factors predicted the amount of blood transferred to the skin.[51] Deep punctures (defined as injuries penetrating the skin and resulting in spontaneous bleeding), injuries caused by devices visibly contaminated with blood before the accident, and injuries caused by devices that had entered an artery or vein prior to the accident, were independently associated with infection risk in the CDC study.

TABLE 5–1. FACTORS INDEPENDENTLY ASSOCIATED WITH PERCUTANEOUS INJURY TRANSMISSION RISK ($p < .05$) BY LOGISTIC REGRESSION ANALYSIS IN A CASE-CONTROL STUDY

Risk Factor	Odds Ratio
Deep (intramuscular) injury	16.1
Visible blood on sharp device	5.2
Device used to enter blood vessel	5.1
Source patient with terminal AIDS	6.4
ZDV prophylaxis used	0.2

From Centers for Disease Control and Prevention: Case-control study of HIV seroconversion in health-care workers after percutaneous exposure to HIV-infected Blood—France, United Kingdom, and United States, January 1988–August 1994. MMWR 44:929–933, 1995.

(Table 5–1).[11] Large volumes of blood, prolonged duration of contact, and a portal of entry are common features in the reported cases of infection through mucosal surfaces or skin, but the number of cases is too small to identify and quantify risk factors for mucocutaneous infection.[28]

The efficiency of occupational transmission could be influenced by other factors. The presence of intracellular (as opposed to cell-free) virus in the inoculum or the genotype or phenotype of the virus strain may be relevant to transcutaneous infectivity. The immunologic response of the recipient health care provider could affect the probability of successful infection. Recent in vitro studies demonstrate that circulating T lymphocytes from uninfected health care providers who were exposed to HIV proliferate in vitro in response to HIV antigens.[16,17] This observation suggests that the cellular immune system may be an important host response, capable of "aborting" transcutaneous HIV infection.

Blood has been implicated as the source of the exposure in all infections occurring in clinicians. Other body fluids, including saliva, tears, and urine, may contain HIV, but the titer of HIV in these fluids is usually much lower than the titer found in blood and semen. While HIV transmission is very unlikely following exposure to most nonbloody body fluids, these fluids could contain other viruses or pathogens, and should be considered potentially infectious when planning infection-control interventions.

Cutaneous exposure involving intact skin has not been linked to HIV infection in any setting. Although Langerhans' cells and other subcutaneous cells possess CD4 receptors, these cells are protected from primary infection by an intact integument. However, transcutaneous inoculation during parenteral needlestick injury, or contamination of skin wounds or lesions, is hypothesized to promote primary infection of subcutaneous target cells. No HIV transmission risk from close personal contact with patients, exposure to airborne droplets, or contact with contaminated environmental surfaces or fomites has been observed.

Aerosols of infected blood or saliva can occur in dental, pathology, laboratory, and surgical environments. Because masks do not prevent exposure to aerosolized particles smaller than the pore diameter of the mask material, concern about the possibility of aerosolized HIV transmission has alarmed some health care providers. Hepatitis B virus, which is present in much higher titers than HIV among infected patients, has not been recovered from aerosols during experiments performed in dental operatories and dialysis units.[58,59] The absence of HIV seroconversion in prospective studies of dentists practicing in areas where HIV is highly prevalent strongly suggests that aerosol transmission is unlikely to confer a measurable occupational hazard. In fact, aerosols have not been associated with HIV infection in any setting to date.

The cumulative professional risk from repeated exposure to HIV has not been completely determined. The overall risk to a given health care provider depends on the risk from discreet exposure events, the frequency of such events, and the prevalence of HIV in the workplace. Nurses, dentists, surgeons, emergency care providers, and labor and delivery personnel are at highest risk for acquiring hepatitis E (HBV) and also may be at higher risk for HIV infection over a lifetime of practice, especially when practicing in areas where HIV is common (Table 5–2).[27] One prevalence study of more than 3400 orthopedic surgeons documented two cases of nonoccupational infection, but no cases attributable to occupational exposure.[68] Large prospective studies of individuals at risk will be necessary to define the infection rate among health care professionals.

By the end of 1995, 46 cases of documented occupational HIV transmission among health care providers in the United States were reported to the CDC.[7,11,28,38] Occupational transmission was proven by demonstrating HIV antibody seroconversion temporally related to a discreet accidental HIV exposure event. Needlestick exposures or lacerations contami-

TABLE 5–2. BLOODBORNE PATHOGEN PREVALENCE (Prev)* AND INCIDENCE DENSITIES (ID)† AMONG SAN FRANCISCO GENERAL HOSPITAL HEALTH CARE PROVIDERS ENROLLED IN A PROSPECTIVE COHORT STUDY OF OCCUPATIONAL INFECTIONS (1984–1993)

Occupation	HBV‡ Prev	HCV Prev	HIV Prev	HBV ID	HCV§ ID	HIV ID
Physicians	20%	0.6%	0%	1.0	0	0
Dentists	28%	0%	0%	8.4	0	0
Nurses	22%	2.9%	0%	3.7	0.24	0.6
Laboratorians	19%	2.8%	0%	1.7	0	0
Technicians	25%	0%	0%	3.7	0	0
Paramedics	17%	0.4%	0%	0	0	0

* Prevalence = number of persons infected/number of persons at risk × 100%.

† Incidence density = number of infected persons/1000 at-risk person-years of follow-up.

‡ Includes only subjects with no history of prior HBV immunization.

§ Includes only those susceptible individuals not immunized during follow-up.

From Gerberding JL: Incidence and prevalence of human immunodeficiency virus, hepatitis B virus, hepatitis C virus, and cytomegalovirus among health care personnel at risk for blood exposure: Final report from a longitudinal study. J Infect Dis 170:1410–1417, 1994, with permission.

nated by infected blood produced infection in the majority. Inapparent parenteral exposure to blood through breaks in the skin or mucous membrane inoculation with blood was the most likely route of transmission in at least three cases. In addition, 97 health care providers with possible occupational infection were reported to the CDC.[38] These health care providers provided no history of nonoccupational exposure risks and all recalled contact with blood or body fluids. However, the relationship between exposure and infection could not be proven because a baseline HIV test at the time of exposure was not performed.

The infections reported to the CDC almost certainly do not include all cases of occupational infection. In many states, HIV is not a reportable condition until AIDS develops, and some occupational infections may not yet be recognized or reported. Most experts agree that the CDC data do include a large majority of the occupational infections. Efforts to improve surveillance and reporting of cases are in progress. In the future, a more complete assessment of the frequency of such events may be possible. Success will depend, at least in part, on the willingness of exposed health care providers to undergo HIV testing and disclose their serostatus to public health agencies. Concerns about employment, loss of insurance, and stigmatization are strong disincentives for participating in a voluntary HIV reporting system, and must be addressed before reliable surveillance can be accomplished.

PROVIDER-TO-PATIENT TRANSMISSION

Transmission of HIV to patients could occur by direct inoculation of blood or other infected body fluids or through use of contaminated materials or equipment. Direct inoculation is possible when an infected health care provider is injured and then bleeds into the patient; when the contaminated instrument or object causing injury recontacts the patient's tissue; or when the provider is injured by bone, hardware, or other sharp fixed in the patient.[5,62,67] The frequency of injuries severe enough to cause bleeding into the wounds or tissues of patients undergoing invasive procedures is unknown but likely to be low. Recontact exposures, when an instrument that injured a provider then passes through the tissue of the patient, are more common. "Shear injuries" (trauma to the hand while manually tightening sutures) have been proposed as a related mechanism of exposure.[29,35]

The HIV transmission risk associated with recontact exposures is unknown. To date, no HIV infections have been attributed to recontacts during surgical procedures.[8,10,29] However, intraoperative transmission of hepatitis C virus (HCV) and HBV from infected surgeons to their patients has been reported.[5,21,29,35] High circulating titers of virus have been observed in all cases of provider-to-patient HCV and HBV transmission. That most HIV-infected persons well enough to work are likely to have lower titers of infection may be one reason why intraoperative HIV transmission has not been observed.

As of April 1996, the only cases of probable provider-to-patient HIV transmission have been attributed to a single cluster involving a Florida dentist with AIDS.[15] Six patients in this practice were shown to be infected with virus strains that were genetically similar to the dentist's isolates. The exact mechanism by which the patients were infected has not been established. Speculations about the routes of infection include direct inoculation of blood or recontact with a contaminated instrument following sharps injuries to the provider (though no injuries were recalled), cross-contamination via handpieces or instruments that were used on the provider and then subsequently reused without proper disinfection, and intentional exposure. Insufficient evidence is available to identify which, if any, of these potential exposure routes played a role in the transmission events in this practice.

It is probable that additional cases of provider-to-patient HIV transmission will eventually emerge. Even so, these events must be extremely rare. From the public health perspective, nosocomial transmission does not contribute to the AIDS epidemic, and special policies to restrict the practice of infected health care providers will have little if any measurable impact on the spread of the infection.[29] On the other hand, implementing safer surgical techniques that prevent provider injuries and recontacts could be very effective in preventing the growing list of bloodborne pathogens that pose a risk to providers and (albeit rarely) their patients.[25]

PATIENT-TO-PATIENT TRANSMISSION

Instruments contaminated with blood from infected patients could transmit HIV to other patients when proper disinfection procedures are not followed.[9] Even though HIV is a relatively fragile virus, survival in clots of blood or tissue (especially in a warm or moist environment) is possible. If disinfection protocols are not rigorously followed, then nosocomial transmission from one patient to another is potentially a much more common event than is transmission from an infected provider to a patient. The practice of obtaining medication from a vial contaminated by a needle used on a previous patient is contraindicated, but does occasionally occur.[1,56] Although HIV transmission through this route has not been proven, HBV transmission has been associated with multiple-use medication vials. Needle reuse has also been associated with nosocomial infections, including a number of cases of HIV transmission to children.[39]

Accidental infusion of radiolabeled blood products from HIV-infected products for nuclear medicine studies into the wrong patient has resulted in patient infections.[6] A cluster of outpatient surgical patients who received care on the same day as an infected patient has also been reported, but the route of cross-contami-

nation has not been determined.[55] Although rare, these anecdotes clearly illustrate the potential for patient infection when safety protocols and disinfection techniques are not followed.

ALLAYING FEARS OF TRANSMISSION

Fear of AIDS may be masked by denial. Beliefs that HIV-infected patients are not present in the health care environment, that infected patients can be identified and avoided, or that transmission is impossible are often perpetuated, until a case of nosocomial or occupational transmission is reported. The first experience with exposure or infection may precipitate a crisis. Intense anger, depression, surprise, and aggressiveness are reactions frequently described in this setting. Although creating a "zero risk" of infection is not a realistic possibility, a demand for excessive or unreasonable infection control measures often follows the initial crisis. Recognition that some degree of risk is unavoidable and that all are at some risk should be made. Providers should be reminded that the vast majority (99.7%) of occupational exposures to HIV do not result in infection.

Fear of acquiring HIV among clinicians who recognize their risk for exposure is not irrational when the degree of fear is commensurate with the degree of risk. Lack of knowledge about the magnitude of risk or routes of transmission can amplify the perceived risk and should be addressed. More importantly, the anxiety aroused by confronting the complex psychological issues related to homosexuality, morality, and mortality evoked by AIDS patients may be experienced or communicated as fear of infection. For some health care professionals, it is easier to avoid the AIDS patient altogether than to deal with the emotional conflicts encountered while providing care. Fear of contagion provides a convenient and more publicly acceptable excuse. Constructive methods to openly acknowledge the stresses inherent in dealing with HIV should be included in clinical training curricula and staff development programs.

RISK REDUCTION: INFECTION CONTROL

Avoiding contact with potentially infected body fluids and tissues is an essential component of risk reduction for health care providers. Preventing needlestick injuries and other parenteral exposures is likely to have the biggest impact on reducing HIV transmission in most health care settings. Although blood is the only body fluid associated with occupational transmission to date, common sense and concern for preventing transmission of other nosocomial pathogens would dictate that other body fluids also should be considered potentially infectious.

Universal precautions were recommended by the CDC for all patients, regardless of diagnosis, for preventing transmission of bloodborne pathogens.[3,4,19] These precautions include the use of gloves for procedures where contact with blood, bloody body fluids, and certain other fluids (amniotic fluid, semen, vaginal fluid, cerebrospinal fluid, serial transudates/exudates, and inflammatory exudates) might occur; the use of masks and protective eyewear when splatter of such body fluids is anticipated; and the use of gowns or other protective garments when clothing is likely to be soiled.

Body substance isolation (BSI), is an alternative system of infection control practiced by many institutions.[30,34,50] A single standard of precautions, based on the anticipated degree of exposure with *all* body fluids and tissues, regardless of the infectious disease diagnosed or suspected, is implemented at the moment of initial contact with the patient. The main difference between these two infection-control systems is that the CDC isolation system considers the type of infection suspected, while BSI is based on the degree of contact anticipated. However, both universal precautions and BSI emphasize prevention of needlestick injury and use of barrier protection for avoiding exposure to potentially infectious materials, and neither requires the use of labeling of patients or specimens for implementation.

The CDC has recently developed a new isolation system for hospitalized patients.[24] In this new system, components of universal precautions and BSI are merged into "standard precautions." Standard precautions apply to all patients and require the use of gloves, protective clothing, and other barriers as needed to prevent direct contact with all body fluids (except sweat).

All isolation systems include precautions to prevent needle injuries. Safer needle devices, which are engineered to retract, cover, or blunt the needle after use, are gaining acceptance. These new devices may contribute to a reduc-

tion in the frequency of postuse injuries, provided that training is adequate to ensure their proper use, but they are less likely to have an impact on during-use injury rates.[14,42] Techniques involving needles and other sharps during invasive procedures are undergoing scrutiny to prevent injuries that could expose the provider (and then the patient).[25] Using the index finger of the nondominant hand to retract tissue or to palpate the needle tip during suturing accounts for a large proportion of intraoperative injuries. Substituting instruments for manual manipulations or use of special protective coverings is advocated to ameliorate this problem. Gloves constructed of monofilament polymers resistant to tears have become available for use when manipulation of bone fragments or suture wires is needed, but use is not widespread because of the associated decrease in tactile sensation. The benefit of double-gloving, glove-reinforcement, and new glove materials in preventing tissue trauma during suture manipulations has not been evaluated.[33] Efforts are underway to identify other changes that may have a favorable impact on injury risks during invasive procedures.

MANAGING EXPOSURES TO HIV

Determining whether or not exposure has actually occurred is not always simple. Health care workers may not report exposures for a variety of reasons, and may under- or overestimate the severity of the exposure. A careful history will usually permit categorization of the exposure route into one of the following broad categories: (1) needle puncture, (2) injury by non-needle sharp (or similar injury resulting in direct transcutaneous exposure), (3) mucous membrane inoculation, (4) contamination of open skin wound or lesion, (5) contamination of nonintact skin, or (6) a bite.

Needlesticks and other percutaneous accidents should be further characterized to help assess the exposure severity. The presence of factors known or suspected to affect the virus inoculum (virus titer in the source material and exposure volume) should be documented. These include variables associated with transmission in the CDC case-control study (deep punctures, visible bloody device, device used in an artery or vein, and blood from a source patient with preterminal AIDS) (Table 5–1).[11] In addition, the size and type of needle or instrument involved (suture needle, hollow-bore needle, scalpel, etc.), volume of blood actually injected (if any), location of the injury, wound appearance, amount of bleeding (spontaneous or induced), method and timing of decontamination, and duration of time that the contaminating fluid was ex vivo before the exposure occurred all should be established.[28] Similarly, the type, volume, and duration of contact should be estimated for fluids implicated in mucous membrane and skin wound contacts.

Establishing the presence of HIV infection in the source patient can be difficult. HIV exposure can be assumed when patients are diagnosed with AIDS or are known to be HIV-infected. Institutions vary in guidelines for testing source patients whose HIV status is unclear. In most, the probability of HIV infection is assessed by clinical and epidemiologic criteria. Patients perceived to be at risk are then counseled and asked to consent to testing. Routine testing of all source patients is gaining acceptance, especially where legislation has guaranteed access to this information.

The exposed health care worker should be encouraged to have an HIV test or serum banked as soon as possible after exposure has occurred (baseline).[28,31,60] Without a negative baseline HIV test, proving that infection was temporally related to the exposure event is extremely difficult. In rare cases, demonstrating close genetic similarity in virus sequences obtained from the source patient and the infected health care provider can confirm the source of exposure, but these studies are expensive, difficult to obtain, and sometimes difficult to interpret. Subsequent HIV testing, usually performed 6 weeks, 3 months, and 6 months after exposure, is recommended when HIV is present or potentially present in the exposure source. Sequential testing is extremely useful in allaying fears, documenting seronegativity, and rarely, in diagnosing HIV infection. HIV seroconversion occurs within 3 months of exposure in more than half of occupational infections, and is expected within 6 months in virtually all. Most cases of occupational infection documented more than 6 months after exposure did not have a 6-month test, so the time of seroconversion could not be ascertained.

Because symptoms of acute retroviral infection (fever, lymphadenopathy, rash, headache, profound fatigue) are associated with approximately 80% of reported occupational infections, persons sustaining exposures should be advised to return for evaluation if a compatible illness occurs. Enzyme-linked immunosorbent assay (ELISA) HIV antibody tests may be nega-

tive or indeterminate during the early phases of seroconversion illness. Immunoblot, gene amplification, virus cultures, or HIV p24 antigen tests may be more sensitive methods for detecting early infection. The value of gene amplification (polymerase chain reaction [PCR]) in identifying infection in seronegative health care workers remains unproved, but data suggest that latent infections detected by PCR rarely, if ever, are detected in seronegative health care workers.[27] In at least one case of seroconversion, HIV antibody was detected before the PCR test was positive.[36]

Postexposure counseling by experienced care providers familiar with the special medical and psychological needs of exposed health care providers is essential.[20] Counseling should provide information about the degree of risk present, options for follow-up, a description of the confidentiality procedures in place, and infection-control procedures to prevent similar occurrences in the future. Counselors should be alert to the concerns of the sexual partners, coworkers, family, and friends of the exposed worker. Referral for ongoing supportive therapy during the follow-up interval is helpful for the minority of exposed persons who experience difficulty in adjusting to the stress inherent in waiting the 6 months for testing to be complete.

The CDC recommends "safer" sexual practices and other behavior changes to minimize the potential for transmission until infection has been ruled out by a negative antibody test 6 months after the exposure.[60] Unfortunately, this advice frequently produces confusion and anxiety in the exposed person. Counselors are faced with the difficult task of communicating a "mixed message" about the risk of infection: reassurance that occupational transmission is statistically unlikely, and on the other hand, advocacy of behaviors to prevent exchange of body fluids, to avoid pregnancy, and to defer blood donation until infection has been ruled out.

In some centers, advice is individualized to the specific situation. For example, persons sustaining trivial punctures with small-bore non-hollow needles minimally contaminated by blood from a low-risk untested source patient may decide to return for follow-up HIV testing for 6 months, but to comply with safer sex guidelines for a shorter interval of time. Likewise, recipients of deep intramuscular injections of infected blood may be cautioned to compulsively follow all guidelines for preventing transmission.

Patients exposed to provider's blood should be managed with the same standard of care applied to occupational exposures. A system for confidential reporting of such exposures should be developed and communicated to hospital staff. It is the ethical and professional responsibility of the involved provider to undergo testing for bloodborne pathogens and to communicate test results to the clinician responsible for the patient's postexposure care.

POSTEXPOSURE PROPHYLAXIS

Interest in postexposure chemoprophylaxis for occupationally exposed health care workers has increased since zidovudine (ZDV, AZT) was licensed for palliating HIV infection in persons with advanced disease.[26,28,37,45,46,60] Zidovudine or other antiretroviral drugs could prevent or help abort HIV infection when administered soon after exposure by preventing HIV replication in the initial target cells and allowing the antigen-independent or antigen-dependent host defenses to clear the exposure inoculum.

The relevance of animal models of retrovirus infection to human infection with HIV is not established. Experiments using murine, feline, and human retroviruses in animals inoculated with high titers of virus indicate that zidovudine can prevent viremia and illness under some conditions.[23,32,49,52–54,63,65,66,70] Protection is most apparent when treatment is started within 24 hours of exposure. However, the efficacy of postexposure zidovudine in preventing the establishment of asymptomatic latent infection has not been proven in any primate models.

Failure of zidovudine prophylaxis has been documented in at least 11 health care providers who were treated after occupational exposures.[47,48] These cases indicate that zidovudine treatment is not always successful, but in the absence of a controlled trial, the efficacy of postexposure treatment cannot be established. Conduct of such a study is difficult, given the relatively low rate of seroconversion that necessitates evaluation of an extremely large sample of exposed persons to measure efficacy. In the absence of clinical data, interim approaches to the use of zidovudine were adopted.[22,26,37,60,61] In the past few years, about 45% to 50% of persons occupationally exposed to HIV have elected to take zidovudine.[69]

The outcome of two studies has prompted renewed enthusiasm for postexposure treatment. First, data from the AIDS Clinical Trial Group (ACTG) protocol 076 demonstrated that zidovudine treatment could reduce the risk of perinatal HIV transmission by more than 60%.[13,22] This study included only women who had never received zidovudine before, and involved treatment of the infected mothers during the last two trimesters and of the newborns for 6 weeks. Although this experience cannot be generalized to transcutaneous exposures experienced by health care providers, it does demonstrate the prophylactic efficacy of antiretroviral treatment under some clinical circumstances.

The second study, the CDC's case control study of occupational HIV infections, is directly relevant to health care providers.[11] In this study, those who received zidovudine treatment after exposure were 79% less likely (odds ratio = 0.21) to acquire infection than those who did not get treated (Table 5–1), independent of the other variables affecting the probability of transmission. Cases and controls had equal access to treatment. The study's retrospective design precluded determination of the dosing regimen or treatment duration most likely to be effective. Based on this study, the USPHS changed its postexposure treatment guidelines, and is now recommending prophylactic antiviral treatment for percutaneous exposures, especially when other risks for infection are present.[13a]

The frequency of zidovudine resistance among source patients undergoing treatment increases with the duration of therapy. In addition, transmission of zidovudine-resistant virus has been documented. Zidovudine prophylaxis is unlikely to be effective when the exposure involves resistant virus. New postexposure treatment guidelines recommend combination therapy with zidovudine *and* lamivudine (3TC) for serious occupational exposures.[28] A protease inhibitor, usually indinavir (IND), is recommended in addition to the nucleoside analogues when the exposure is especially high risk and/or the source patient has recently taken both zidovudine and lamivudine.

Most parenteral exposures to HIV (99.7%) do not transmit HIV infection. Antiretroviral chemoprophylaxis is a promising but unproved prevention strategy that appears to be protective in select cases. While it is hoped that the incidence of serious adverse events associated with combination treatment will be low, experience with the new agents alone or in combination with zidovudine is extremely limited.[22]

**TABLE 5–3. CURRENT POSTEXPOSURE PROPHYLAXIS (PEP) PROTOCOL
AT SAN FRANCISCO GENERAL HOSPITAL**

Initiation:	ASAP after known or potential exposure to HIV
Duration:	4 weeks
AZT dose:	200 mg PO tid
3TC dose:	150 mg PO bid

May also add a protease inhibitor (e.g., indinavir 800 mg PO tid) if the source patient is AZT/3TC "experienced" and for high-risk exposures

Toxicity monitoring:	Symptoms/focused exam
	Complete blood count/chemistry panel/amylase/urinalysis every 2 weeks while on treatment and at 6 weeks, 3 months, 6 months, 12 months
HIV monitoring:	HIV antibody test at baseline and 6 months (required)
	HIV antibody test at 6 weeks and 3 months (optional)
	HIV PCR ± HIV antigen ± culture if symptoms of acute retrovirus illness occur in a seronegative health care provider

When used, close monitoring for known and potential adverse effects must be included in the follow-up protocol. In the author's view, prophylactic treatment is still experimental therapy, despite the USPHS endorsement. Health care workers electing treatment should carefully consider the potential risks as well as benefits associated with treatment and provide written consent (or perhaps declension) to document their decision about treatment.

Most experts believe that prophylactic treatment should be started as soon as possible (within hours) after the exposure to maximize the chance of efficacy. The optimal dose and duration of treatment has not been established. Treatment is usually recommended for 4 to 6

**TABLE 5–4. POSTEXPOSURE PROPHYLAXIS TREATMENT ADVICE
AT SAN FRANCISCO GENERAL HOSPITAL**

	Source Status		
Exposure Level	**Asymptomatic; Known Low Titer**	**AIDS; Symptomatic Infection**	**Preterminal AIDS; Acute Seroconversion**
A. Percutaneous Injuries			
Superficial injury	Offer	Recommend	Strongly encourage
Visibly bloody device Used in artery or vein	Recommend	Recommend	Strongly encourage
Deep / IM Actual injection	Strongly encourage	Strongly encourage	Strongly encourage
B. Mucosal Exposures			
Small volume and brief contact	Offer	Offer	Offer
Large volume or prolonged contact	Recommend	Recommend	Recommend
Large volume and prolonged contact	Recommend	Recommend	Strongly encourage
C. Cutaneous Exposures			
Small volume and brief contact (e.g., few drops)	Offer only if portal of entry	Offer only if portal of entry	Offer only if portal of entry
Large volume or prolonged contact (e.g., aphoresis machine back-up) (e.g., 20-minute contact)	Offer; recommend if portal of entry	Offer; recommend if portal of entry	Offer; recommend if portal of entry
Large volume and prolonged contact (e.g., paramedic bloodbath)	Offer; recommend if portal of entry	Offer; recommend if portal of entry	Offer; recommend if portal of entry

weeks. Treatment of pregnant women or persons not practicing effective contraception is discouraged. Close monitoring for hematologic, hepatic, pancreatic, renal, and neuralgic dysfunction is essential. Adverse reactions should be reported to the Food and Drug Administration and to the drug manufacturer(s).

At San Francisco General Hospital, a new treatment protocol for postexposure prophylaxis was implemented in April 1996. In collaboration with Dr. David Henderson and colleagues at the National Institutes of Health (NIH), the toxicity of the treatment protocol will be evaluated in a prospective multicenter study (Table 5–3). An interim guide to exposure risk assessment has been prepared to assist persons facing the decision about treatment (Table 5–4). The risk assessment scheme is intended to provide general guidance, and is not an absolute measure of exposure risk.

REFERENCES

1. Alter MJ, Ahtone J, Maynard JE: Hepatitis B transmission associated with a multiple-dose vial in a hemodialysis unit. Ann Intern Med 99:330–333, 1983
2. Cavalcante NJF, Abreu ES, Fernandes ME, et al: Risk of health care professionals acquiring HIV infection in Latin America. AIDS Care 3:311–316, 1991
3. Centers for Disease Control: Recommendations for prevention of HIV transmission in health-care settings. MMWR 36(Suppl 2S):1S–18S, 1987
4. Centers for Disease Control: Update: Universal precautions for prevention of transmission of human immunodeficiency virus, hepatitis B virus, and other bloodborne pathogens in health care settings. MMWR 37:377–382, 387–388, 1988
5. Centers for Disease Control: Recommendations for preventing transmission of human immunodeficiency virus and hepatitis B virus infection to patients during exposure-prone invasive procedures. MMWR 40:1–9, 1991
6. Centers for Disease Control: Patient exposures to HIV during nuclear medicine procedures. MMWR 41:575–578, 1992
7. Centers for Disease Control: Surveillance for occupationally acquired HIV infection—United States, 1981–1992. MMWR 41:823–825, 1992
8. Centers for Disease Control: Update: Investigations of patients who have been treated by HIV-infected health-care workers. MMWR 41:344–346, 1992
9. Centers for Disease Control: Improper infection-control procedures during employee vaccination programs—District of Columbia and Pennsylvania. MMWR 42:969–971, 1993
10. Centers for Disease Control: Update: Investigations of persons treated by HIV-infected health-care workers—United States. MMWR 42:329–331, 337, 1993
11. Centers for Disease Control and Prevention: Case-control study of HIV seroconversion in health-care workers after percutaneous exposure to HIV-infected Blood—France, United Kingdom, and United States, January 1988–August 1994. MMWR 44:929–933, 1995
12. Centers for Disease Control and Prevention: Recommendations of the U S Public Health Service task force on the use of zidovudine to reduce perinatal transmission of HIV. MMWR 43(RR-11):1–20, 1994
13. Centers for Disease Control and Prevention: Zidovudine for the prevention of HIV transmission from mother to infant. MMWR 43:285–288, 1994
13a. Centers for Disease Control: Update: Provisional public health service guidelines for chemoprophylaxis after occupational exposure to HIV. MMWR 45:468–472, 1996
14. Chamberland M, Short LJ, Srivastava P, et al: Efficacy and compliance with use of safety devices to reduce percutaneous injuries during phlebotomy. Second National Conference on Human Retroviruses and Related Infections. Washington, DC, January, 1995
15. Ciesielski C, Marianos D, Ou CY, et al: Transmission of human immunodeficiency virus in a dental practice. Ann Intern Med 116:798–805, 1992
16. Clerici M, Berzofsky JA, Shearer GM, Tacket CO: Exposure to HIV-1 indicated by HIV-specific T helper cell responses before detection of infection by polymerase chain reaction and serum antibodies. J Infect Dis 165:1012–1019, 1992
17. Clerici M, Levin JM, Kessler HA, et al: HIV-specific T-helper activity in seronegative health care workers exposed to contaminated blood. JAMA 271:42–46, 1994
18. Daar ES, Moudgil T, Meyer RD, Ho DD: Transient high levels of viremia in patients with primary human immunodeficiency virus type 1 infection. N Engl J Med 325:733–735, 1991
19. Department of Labor Occupational Safety and Health Administration: Occupational exposure to bloodborne pathogens: Final rule. Fed Register 56:64004–64182, 1991
20. Dilley JW: Counseling health care workers after accidental exposures. Focus 5:3–4, 1990
21. Esteban JI, Gomez J, Martell M, et al: Transmission of hepatitis C virus by a cardiac surgeon. N Engl J Med 334:555–560, 1996
22. Fahrner R, Beekmann SE, Koziol DE, et al: Safety of zidovudine (ZDV) administered as post-exposure prophylaxis to health care workers (HCW) sustaining HIV-related occupational exposures (OE). In Program and Abstracts of the 34th Interscience Conference on Antimicrobial Agents and Chemotherapy, Orlando, October 4–7, 1994. Washington, DC, American Society for Microbiology, 1994, p 133
23. Fazely F, Haseltine WA, Rodger RF, Ruprecht RM: Post-exposure chemoprophylaxis with ZDV or ZDV combined with interferon-alfa: Failure after inoculating rhesus monkeys with high dose of SIV. J Acquir Immune Defic Syndr 4:1093–1097, 1991
24. Garner JL: Guidelines for isolation precautions in hospitals. Infect Control Hosp Epidemiol 17:54–80, 1996
25. Gerberding JL: Procedure-specific infection control

for preventing intraoperative blood exposures. Am J Infect Control 21:364–367, 1992

26. Gerberding JL: Is antiretroviral treatment after percutaneous HIV exposure justified? Ann Intern Med 118:979–980, 1993

27. Gerberding JL: Incidence and prevalence of human immunodeficiency virus, hepatitis B virus, hepatitis C virus, and cytomegalovirus among health care personnel at risk for blood exposure: Final report from a longitudinal study. J Infect Dis 170:1410–1417, 1994

28. Gerberding JL: Management of occupational exposures to blood-borne viruses. N Engl J Med 332:444–451, 1995

29. Gerberding JL: The infected health care provider. N Engl J Med 334:594–595, 1996

30. Gerberding JL, Henderson DK: Design of rational infection control guidelines for human immunodeficiency virus infection. J Infect Dis 156:861–864, 1987

31. Gerberding JL, Henderson DK: Management of occupational exposures to bloodborne pathogens: Hepatitis B virus, hepatitis C virus, and human immunodeficiency virus. Clin Infect Dis 14:1179–1185, 1992

32. Gerberding JL, Marx P, Gould R, et al: Simian model of retrovirus chemoprophylaxis with constant infusion zidovudine with or without interferon-alpha. In Program and Abstracts of the 31st Interscience Conference on Antimicrobial Agents and Chemotherapy. Washington, DC, American Society for Microbiology, 1991

33. Gerberding JL, Quebbeman EJ, Rhodes RS: Hand Protection. In Rhodes RS, Bell DM, eds. The Surgical Clinics of North America: Prevention of Bloodborne Pathogens, vol 75. Philadelphia, WB Saunders Co, 1995, pp 1133–1139

34. Gerberding JL, and the University of California, San Francisco Task Force on AIDS: Recommended infection-control policies for patients with human immunodeficiency virus infection: An update. N Engl J Med 315:1562–1564, 1986

35. Harpaz R, Von Seidlein L, Averhoff FM, et al: Transmission of hepatitis B virus to multiple patients from a surgeon without evidence of inadequate infection control. N Engl J Med 334:549–554, 1996

36. Henderson DK, Fahey BJ, Willy M, et al: Risk for occupational transmission of human immunodeficiency virus type-1 (HIV-1) associated with clinical exposures. A prospective evaluation. Ann Intern Med 113:47–56, 1990

37. Henderson DH, Gerberding JL: Post-exposure zidovudine chemoprophylaxis for health care workers occupationally exposed to the human immunodeficiency virus: An interim analysis. J Infec Dis 160:321–327, 1989

38. Heptonstall J, Porter K, Gill ON: Occupational HIV: Summary of published reports. Public Health Laboratory Services Communicable Disease Surveillance Centre, London, December 1995

39. Hersh BS, Popovici F, Apertrei RC, et al: Acquired immunodeficiency syndrome in Rumania. Lancet 338:645–649, 1991

40. Ho DD, Moudgil T, Alam M: Quantitation of human immunodeficiency virus type 1 in the blood of infected persons. N Engl J Med 321:1622–1625, 1989

41. Ippolito G, Puro V, DeCarlt G, and the Italian Study Group on Occupational Risk of HIV Infection: Arch Intern Med 153:1431–1438, 1993

42. Jagger J, Hunt EH, Bland-Elnaggar J, Pearson RD: Rates of needlestick injury caused by various devices in a university hospital. N Engl J Med 319:284–288, 1988

43. Josephson A, Bottone M, Gerber M, Oppermann N: Blood and body fluid exposure followup in the AIDS era: A two year experience. Am J Infect Control 18:136, 1990

44. Kuhls TL, Viker S, Parris NB, et al: Occupational risk of HIV, HBV and HSV-2 in health care personnel caring for AIDS patients. Am J Public Health 77:1306–1309, 1987

45. LaFon SW, Lehrman SN, Barry DW: Prophylactically administered Retrovir in health care workers potentially exposed to the human immunodeficiency virus. J Infect Dis 158:503, 1988

46. LaFon SW, Mooney BD, McMullen JP, et al: A double-blind, placebo-controlled study of the safety and efficacy of Retrovir (zidovudine, ZDV) as a chemoprophylactic agent in health care workers (Abstract 489). In Program and Abstracts of the 30th Interscience Conference on Antimicrobial Agents and Chemotherapy. Washington, DC, American Society for Microbiology, 1990

47. Lange JMA, Boucher CAB, Hollak CEM, et al: Failure of zidovudine prophylaxis after accidental exposure to HIV-1. N Engl J Med 322:1375–1377, 1990

48. Looke DFM, Grove DI: Failed prophylactic zidovudine after needlestick injury. Lancet 335:1280, 1990

49. Lundgren B, Bottinger D, Ljungdahl-Stahle E, et al: Antiviral effects of 3′-fluorothymidine and 3′-azidothymidine in cynomologous monkeys infected with simian immunodeficiency virus. J Acquir Immune Defic Syndr 4:489–498, 1991

50. Lynch P, Jackson MM, Cummings MJ, Stamm WE: Rethinking the role of isolation practices in the prevention of nosocomial infections. Ann Intern Med 107:243–246, 1987

51. Mast S, Woolwine J, Gerberding JL: Efficacy of gloves in reducing blood volumes transferred during simulated needlestick injury. J Infect Dis 168:1589–1592, 1993

52. Mathes LE, Polas PJ, Hayes KA, et al: Pre- and postexposure chemoprophylaxis: Evidence that 3′-azido-3′-dideoxythymidine inhibits feline leukemia virus disease by a drug-induced vaccine response. Antimicrob Agents Chemother 36:2715–2721, 1992

53. McClure HM, Anderson DC, Ansari AA, et al: Nonhuman primate models for evaluation of AIDS therapy. Ann N Y Acad Sci 616:287–298, 1990

54. McCune JM, Namikawa R, Shih CC, et al: 3′azido-3′-deoxythymidine suppresses HIV infection in SCID-hu mouse. Science 247:564–560, 1990

55. Ragg M: Medically acquired HIV. Lancet 343:47, 1994

56. Oren I, Hershow RC, Ben-Porath E, et al: A common-source outbreak of fulminant hepatitis B in a hospital. Ann Intern Med 110:691–698, 1989

57. Pereira LIA, Souza LCS, Souza MA, et al: Acidentes profissionais com material biologico de paclantes com sindrome da immunodeficiencia adquirida-accompanhamento clinico-serologico. Rev Soc Bras Med Trop 24:169, 1991

58. Petersen NJ: An assessment of the airborne route in hepatitis B transmission. Ann N Y Acad Sci 253:157–166, 1980

59. Petersen NJ, Bond WW, Favero MS: Air sampling technique for hepatitis B surface antigen in a dental operatory. J Am Dent Assoc 99:465–467, 1979

60. Public health service statement on management of occupational exposure to human immunodeficiency virus, including considerations regarding zidovudine postexposure use. MMWR 39:1–14, 1990
61. Puro V, Ippolito G, Guzzanti E, et al: Zidovudine prophylaxis after accidental exposure to HIV: The Italian experience. The Italian Study Group on Occupational Risk of HIV Infection. AIDS 6:963–969, 1992
62. Rose DA, Ramiro N, Perlman J, et al: Usage rates and perforation patterns of 6306 gloves from intra-operative procedures at San Francisco General Hospital. Infect Control Hosp Epidemiol 15:349, 1994
63. Ruprecht RM, et al: Suppression of mouse viraemia and retroviral disease by 3'-azido-3'-deoxythymidine. Nature 323:467–469, 1986
64. Saag MS, Crain MJ, Decker WD, et al: High-level viremia in adults and children infected with human immunodeficiency virus: Relation to disease stage and CD4+ lymphocyte levels. J Infect Dis 164:72–80, 1991
65. Shih CC, Kaneshima H, Rabin L, et al: Post-exposure prophylaxis with zidovudine suppresses human immunodeficiency virus type 1 infection in SCID-hu mice in a time-dependent manner. J Infect Dis 163:625–627, 1991
66. Tavares L, et al: 3'-azido-3'-deoxythymidine in feline leukemic virus-infected cats: A model for therapy and prophylaxis of AIDS. Cancer Res 47:3190–3194, 1987
67. Tokars JI, Bell DM, Culver D, et al: Percutaneous injuries during surgical procedures. JAMA 267:2899–2904, 1992
68. Tokars JI, Chamberland ME, Schable CA, et al: A survey of occupational blood contact and HIV infection among orthopedic surgeons. JAMA 268:489–494, 1992
69. Tokars JI, Marcus R, Culver DH, et al: Surveillance of human immunodeficiency virus infection and zidovudine use among health care workers after occupational exposure to HIV-infected blood: The CDC Cooperative Needlestick Group. Ann Intern Med 118:913–919, 1993
70. Van Rompay KKA, Marthas ML, Ramos RA, et al: Simian immunodeficiency virus (SIV) infection of infant rhesus macaques as a model to test antiretroviral drug prophylaxis and therapy: Oral 3'-azido-3'-deoxythymidine prevents SIV infection. Antimicrob Agents Chemother 36:2381–2386, 1992
71. Wormser GP, Joline C, Sivak S, Arlin ZA: Human immunodeficiency virus infection: Considerations for health care workers. Bull N Y Acad Med 64:203–215, 1988

Section II

MANAGEMENT OF HIV INFECTIONS AND THEIR COMPLICATIONS

Chapter 6

Primary HIV Infection

ANDREW CARR AND DAVID A. COOPER

The first encounter of the human immunodeficiency virus type 1 (HIV-1) with the human immune system provides valuable insights into the immunopathogenesis of HIV-1 infection and the host response to HIV-1. The increasing recognition of this early stage of infection has allowed the definition and investigation of its characteristic clinical, serologic, and immunologic features.[154] Information about these early events could suggest approaches to arresting initial viral infection and spread. Moreover, the identification of patients at this stage of infection affords a rare opportunity to institute counselling to avoid further dissemination of HIV-1 infection in the community.

EPIDEMIOLOGY

Transmission Category

Symptomatic primary HIV-1 infection has been reported in persons from each of the major groups affected by HIV-1 infection: homosexual men and women; injecting drug users; recipients of contaminated blood, blood components, or organs; and health care workers in association with occupational exposure.

It is not yet clear whether the risk of developing symptomatic primary HIV-1 infection after inoculation is greater in any of these groups. If differences do exist, they might be attributable to factors such as differences in the dose of inoculum, the various transmission routes, the antecedent immunocompetence of the various groups, or the concurrent transmission of other organisms.

Prevalence

An acute clinical illness associated with seroconversion for HIV-1 has been reported in 53% to 93% of cases.[53,111,151] In a prospectively studied group of homosexual men, primary HIV-1 infection was the second most common cause (after influenza) of an acute febrile illness lasting more than 3 days.[50] Although asymptomatic seroconversion does occur, a high index of clinical suspicion and prior experience with primary HIV-1 infection greatly increase the recognition rate.

Early recognition of this phase of infection in countries such as Australia was related to several factors including a lower burden of advanced disease, a national health care system that enabled multiple visits and tests over a short period of time without cost implications for the patient, and an excellent level of awareness of community practitioners and the homosexual male community following the first report of primary HIV-1 infection.[40] It is now our experience that many patients present because they believe that they may have primary HIV-1 infection. Similarly, the apparent higher incidence of primary HIV-1 infection among health care workers who acquire HIV occupationally may merely reflect closer monitoring of such subjects by their physicians.

Incubation Period and Duration

The time from infection with HIV-1 until the onset of the acute clinical illness is typically 2 to 4 weeks,[35,44,53,120,160] although incubation periods of 6 days to 6 weeks have been reported. The clinical illness is generally acute in onset[21,42,53,67,78,160] and lasts from 1 to 2 weeks.[21,44,67,78,140,160] In a series of 46 subjects, the median duration was 16 days (range 4 to 56 days)[111] and in a series of 20 subjects, the mean duration was 12.7 days (range 5 to 44 days) with 45% of subjects having an illness that lasted from to 5 to 7 days.[156] The illness can be associated with an appreciable degree of morbidity, and patients may require hospitalization.[35,53,64,160] Most of the clinical manifestations of primary HIV-1 infection are self-limited, although in a few cases mild to moderate symptoms may persist (e.g., fatigue, adenopathy). However, in the majority of cases primary HIV-1 infection is followed by an asymptomatic phase that lasts months to years.

CLINICAL PRESENTATION

The main clinical features of primary HIV-1 infection reflect the broad cellular tropism of HIV-1 during this period (Table 6–1). In a review of 139 cases of primary HIV-1 infection, Clark et al[35] found that the most common physical signs and symptoms were fever (97%), adenopathy (77%), pharyngitis (73%), rash (70%), and myalgia or arthralgia (58%). Meningoencephalitis and diarrhea may also occur. Symptomatic primary HIV-1 infection has been reported only once in a pediatric setting.[39]

Although cases of symptomatic primary HIV-1 infection are more likely to come to the attention of clinicians, asymptomatic infection may also occur.[53,154] It is not clear what factors influence the development or lack of symptoms during primary infection, although a lack of symptoms appears to correlate with a more favorable long-term outcome. Possible viral factors include the inoculum, tropism, and virulence of the infecting HIV strain. Ward et al[166] found that symptomatic primary HIV-1 infection was more common in those infected by persons with late-stage disease than those infected by persons at an earlier disease stage.

General Features

Fever is a consistent sign in patients with symptomatic primary HIV-1 infection and may or may not be associated with night sweats. Myalgia is also common[11,29,35,44,64,67,78,141] and may be associated with muscle weakness and an increased level of serum creatine kinase. Arthralgia may also occur.[35,67,78,146] Lethargy and malaise are frequent, often severe, and may persist for several months after resolution of the other clinical manifestations of primary HIV-1 infection.

Lymphocytopathic Features

Lymphadenopathy develops in approximately 70% of persons, generally in the second week of the illness and usually concomitant with the development of peripheral lymphocytosis, although it is not clear whether the two are related.[152] The lymphadenopathy may be generalized, but the axillary, occipital, and cervical nodes are most commonly involved. Lymphadenopathy may persist after the acute illness but tends to decrease with time. Splenomegaly has also been reported.[28,35,56,118,120,121,134,141,170]

Dermatologic Features

The most frequently reported dermatologic evidence of primary HIV-1 infection is an erythematous, nonpruritic, maculopapular rash (Color Plate IA).[6,11,15,21,25,40,56,67,69,78,101,119,120,133,146] This rash is generally symmetric, with lesions 5 to 10 mm in diameter, and affects the face or trunk, but it can also affect the extremities, including the palms and soles,[21,44] or can be generalized.

Other skin lesions noted during primary HIV-1 infection include a roseola-like rash,[110]

TABLE 6–1. CLINICAL MANIFESTATIONS OF PRIMARY HIV-1 INFECTION

General
Fever
Pharyngitis
Lymphadenopathy
Arthralgia
Myalgia
Lethargy/malaise
Anorexia/weight loss

Neuropathic
Headache/retroorbital pain
Meningoencephalitis
Peripheral neuropathy
Radiculopathy
Brachial neuritis
Guillain-Barré syndrome
Cognitive/affective impairment

Dermatologic
Erythematous maculopapular rash
Roseola-like rash
Diffuse urticaria
Desquamation
Alopecia
Mucocutaneous ulceration

Gastrointestinal
Oral/oropharyngeal candidiasis
Nausea/vomiting
Diarrhea

Respiratory
Cough

diffuse urticaria,[67] a vesicular, pustular exanthem and enanthem,[25] desquamation of the palms and soles,[40,103] alopecia,[29,78] and erythema multiforme.[87] Desquamation and alopecia typically occur in the second month following onset of primary HIV-1 infection, after resolution of other symptoms.

Mucocutaneous Ulceration

Mucocutaneous ulceration is a distinctive feature of primary HIV-1 infection. Ulcers have been reported on the buccal mucosa, gingiva, palate,[15,35,46,56,69,101,120,170] esophagus,[56,69,78,120] anus,[56] and penis.[15,56,69] They are generally round or oval and sharply demarcated, with surrounding mucosa that appears normal.

In one series, 7 (35%) of 20 subjects had mucocutaneous ulceration at the time of presentation, and an additional 5 presented with retrosternal pain on swallowing thought likely to have been caused by esophageal ulceration.[56] In another series, 50% of subjects who presented with odynophagia during primary HIV-1 infection had virus particles that morphologically resembled human retroviruses in esophageal ulcer tissue examined by electron microscopy.[120] Bartelsman et al[12] obtained specimens from small shallow esophageal ulcers from one such patient; histopathology showed only partial desquamation of the squamous epithelium with severe granulocyte infiltration.

Neurologic Features

The isolation of HIV-1 from cerebrospinal fluid (CSF) during primary HIV-1 infection[46,134] indicates that infection of the central nervous system (CNS) can occur soon after exposure (see Chapter 13). Elevated neopterin and β_2-microglobulin levels have also been found in CSF during primary HIV-1 infection, both in individuals with and without clinical meningitis,[145] suggesting that the cellular immune system in the CNS may be activated during this stage in the absence of overt neurologic symptoms or signs.

The most common neurologic symptoms are headaches,[11,28,29,35,64,120] retroorbital pain (particularly exacerbated by eye movements),[120] and photophobia,[67,120] which may reflect an underlying aseptic meningitis.[26,64,67]

Acute encephalitis during primary HIV-1 infection has rarely been reported.[15,26,64,66,67]

Depression, irritability, and mood changes[26,151] suggest that early CNS involvement may also manifest as cognitive or affective impairment. These changes may last weeks to months following resolution of other symptoms.[14]

Other neurologic conditions that may be associated with primary HIV-1 infection include myelopathy,[48] peripheral neuropathy,[118] meningoradiculitis,[108] brachial neuritis,[22,25] facial palsy,[103,118,170] cauda equina syndrome, and Guillain-Barré syndrome.[63] The neurologic manifestations of primary HIV-1 infection are generally self-limited, but persistent neurologic deficit has been reported.[25]

It is not yet clear what factors determine whether neurologic involvement will occur during primary HIV-1 infection. It may be that strains of HIV-1 that are particularly neurotropic or monocytotropic have a high propensity to cause such involvement.

Gastrointestinal Features

Sore throat and pharyngeal edema, with or without exudate, are common during primary HIV-1 infection.[15,21,35,160] Anorexia, nausea, vomiting, and diarrhea have also been reported.[15,29,35,44,141] Oral candidiasis may occur during primary HIV-1 infection, and several cases of esophageal candidiasis have also been reported.[37,110,119,157] In the latter cases, there was an appreciable decline in the absolute number of peripheral CD4+ cells, reflecting that the development of this acquired immunodeficiency syndrome (AIDS)–defining condition occurred in the setting of transient but severe immunodeficiency.[157]

Respiratory Features

Respiratory presentations are not common, although some patients may have a dry cough. Several cases of acute pneumonitis with bilateral diffuse interstitial abnormalities revealed by chest roentgenogram and nonspecific inflammation revealed by fiberoptic bronchoscopy have been reported.[28,56] Primary HIV-1 infection among injecting drug users is associated with a higher prevalence of respiratory symptoms. In one study, 30% of primary HIV-1 infection in such patients was associated with bacterial pneumonia.[104] This may be related to a higher background incidence of bacterial pneumonia in this group[94] exacerbated by the transient immunodeficiency associated with primary HIV-1 infection. *Pneumocystis carinii* pneumonia (PCP) was reported in association with primary HIV-1 infection in three subjects, each of whom had severe CD4+ lymphocytopenia (nadir range 62 to 91/mm^3).[162]

Primary HIV-2 Infection

Two cases of symptomatic primary HIV-2 infection have been reported. In the first case a 19-year-old woman developed an acute clinical illness 3 weeks after her first sexual relationship,[13] that was characterized by painful cervical nodes, fevers, fatigue, and a maculopapular rash on the face and thorax. In the second case a 50-year-old French male resident of the Ivory Coast presented with polyneuritis in association with seroconversion to HIV-2.[127]

LABORATORY FINDINGS

Hematology

Following an initial and transient lymphopenia, lymphocytosis comprised mainly of CD8+ lymphocytes develops (generally in the second to third weeks of infection). The appearance of atypical lymphocytes concomitant with this CD8+ lymphocytosis has been noted in several case reports,[89,146] although it appears to occur in fewer than 50% of patients overall.[56]

There is an increase in the proportion of banded neutrophils during the first week of illness and subsequent decrease in segmented neutrophils in weeks 3 and 4.[56] Mild thrombocytopenia is a common finding in the first 2 weeks of illness,[25,28,29,40,46,56,67,110,160,170] but is rarely of clinical significance. Antiplatelet antibodies and reduced numbers of megakaryocytes on bone marrow examination have been demonstrated,[89] suggesting that both viral-mediated or immune-mediated mechanisms are responsible for the thrombocytopenia. The presence of other autoantibodies has not been documented during primary HIV-1 infection. The erythrocyte sedimentation rate may be increased and C-reactive protein is raised in approximately 50% of patients.[25,29,56,67] No characteristic alterations in hemoglobin levels have been reported.

Liver Function Tests

Elevated serum levels of hepatic transaminases have been noted[15,26,47,56,118,121,146] that are infrequently associated with clinical hepatitis.[141] These generally return to normal within 3 months of presentation.

T-Lymphocyte Subset Enumeration

Primary HIV-1 infection is characterized by rapid changes in peripheral T-cell subsets[46,58,109,129]; therefore, the values obtained at enumeration depend on the time after infection. During the first 1 to 2 weeks after onset of primary HIV-1 infection characteristically there is lymphopenia that affects both CD4+ and CD8+ subsets. It may be profound, and the level of CD4+ cells may be as low as that of patients with advanced HIV-1 disease. The nadir of total, CD4+, and CD8+, lymphocytes occurs a median of 9 days following onset of illness,[42] concurrent with an increase in antibody titres to CD4.[76] This transient lymphopenia is followed 3 to 4 weeks after infection by peripheral lymphocytosis. Although both CD4+ and CD8+ cells contribute to this lymphocytosis, the increase in CD8+ cells is relatively greater, leading to an inversion of the CD4+ :CD8+ ratio. The level of CD8+ cells typically remains higher than that of the CD4+ cells, and there is sustained inversion of the CD4+ :CD8+ ratio. This is similar to data on primary cytomegalovirus (CMV) and Epstein-Barr virus (EBV) infections.[27,47]

Zaunders et al,[173] in a study of T-cell subsets in primary HIV-1 infection, found that the decrease in CD4+ lymphocyte numbers was accounted for mostly by a decline in those expressing CD45RA (i.e., "naive" T lymphocytes). The increased numbers of CD8+ lymphocytes also expressed HLA-DR, CD38, and CD11a/CD18, suggesting that these cells have an activated phenotype. Lastly, the inverted CD4:CD8 ratio was found to have possible diagnostic value for primary HIV infection, as an inverted ratio was not seen in those with other acute viral illnesses (with the exception of acute EBV infection) and was seen in a few patients who were not HIV-1 p24 antigenemic before HIV-specific antibodies were detectable. The most marked increase in the absolute number of CD8+ lymphocytes (and activated CD8+ lymphocytes) was observed in individuals with the most pronounced clinical signs of primary HIV-1 infection.[129]

Immune Function Studies

Severe lymphocytic proliferative hyporesponsiveness to both mitogens and antigens occurs during primary HIV-1 infection[44,109,148] and persists after resolution of the acute illness. Pedersen et al[109] found that pokeweed mitogen (PWM) responses were depressed in each patient at some point in the acute illness, but in most patients reached the lowest level at 6 to 8 weeks after onset of illness. Responses subsequently improved but remained subnormal at 1-year follow-up. Phytohemagglutinin (PHA) responses showed a similar pattern, but were less affected. Rapid and persistent impairment of B-cell function follows primary HIV-1 infection.[148,149] Terpstra et al[149] found that inducible in vitro B-cell activity is impaired soon after seroconversion and remains impaired throughout the first year of infection.

Antibodies to Structural Proteins

Primary HIV-1 infection is confirmed serologically by the appearance of HIV-specific serum antibodies directed against the specific internal and surface proteins that form HIV-1 (see Chapter 3)[4,82] including *gag* (p55, p24, p18), *pol* (p68, p53, p34), and *env* (gp160, gp120, gp41).

In persons with symptomatic primary HIV-1 infection, specific HIV-1 antibodies are usually detectable within the first few weeks of onset of the acute illness.[41,57] Antibodies are generally detected first by enzyme-linked immunosorbent assay (ELISA) for IgM antibody. IgG antibody is then detected, usually 2 to 6 weeks after the onset of illness.[41,57] Differences in the length of the window period according to the type of the ELISA screening tests emphasize the need for consistent use of sensitive screening tests. However, the 3- to 6-month window period commonly cited is conservative, particularly if other tests are used in conjunction.

Immunoblotting usually first shows antibody to p24 or gp41.[41,57] Gaines et al[57] found that all serum samples obtained 2 weeks or more after onset of symptomatic primary HIV-1 infection in 20 patients were seropositive by immunoblotting.

Antibodies to Regulatory Proteins

Antibodies to regulatory proteins (including those produced from the *rev, tat, nef, vpu,* and *vpr* genes) are not used for routine diagnostic tests, but develop early in infection, generally concomitant with, but in some cases prior to, core and envelope seroconversion.[5,33,48,124–126] The significance of the presence of antibodies to regulatory proteins months before *gag* and *env* seroconversion is not clear. The demonstration of anti-*nef* antibodies in HIV-1–seronegative patients without risk factors for HIV-1 infection[122] suggests that there may be an immunologic cross-reaction between *nef* and some cellular protein.

IgM Antibody

The detection of HIV-specific IgM antibodies is a sign of recent infection. IgM antibodies to HIV-1 appear within 2 weeks of infection, precede the IgG response, reach peak titers at 2 to 5 weeks, and then decline to undetectable levels within approximately 3 months.[41,55,57] The first IgM antibodies to appear are directed against *gag* or *env* proteins.[55] However, IgM antibody is not always detected within the first few weeks of infection, and a negative result therefore is not conclusive.[83] Furthermore, technical difficulties with IgM assays, including lack of specificity, reproducibility, and standardization, indicate a need for care in the interpretation of IgM results. In our experience, IgM testing does not provide useful diagnostic information beyond that which can be obtained through Western blotting and assays for serum HIV-1 p24 antigen or DNA and so is not used routinely.

Seronegative HIV-1 Infection and Molecular Diagnosis

Much controversy has surrounded the occurrence and prevalence of "silent" HIV-1 infection among persons who test negative for HIV-1–specific serum antibodies. The potential for silent HIV-1 infection has profound implications for the public health and also for understanding of HIV-1 immunopathogenesis.

Ranki et al[123] first reported the detection of low titer antibodies to recombinant structural or accessory proteins or free HIV-1 antigen in serum from homosexual men 6 to 14 months before ELISA seroconversion. A subsequent study found an appreciable rate of HIV-1 isolation from homosexual men who remained seronegative for a long period.[70] However, results from other cohort studies did not support these findings,[68,88] and it was suggested that the use of relatively insensitive ELISAs in the first studies may have been responsible for misclassification of patients as HIV-1–seronegative in at least some instances.[135] Several investigators have examined the prevalence of silent infection in high-risk seronegative persons further by using the polymerase chain reaction (PCR) method, viral isolation, and in situ hybridization. The results of these studies have been conflicting.[3,36,51,70,74,84,85,87,92,97,114,115,171,172]

In some studies, intermittent positive and low-intensity PCR readouts may lead to false-positive findings.[136,169] Sheppard et al have reported that a major weakness of many studies is that they fail to report the rate of positive PCR results in low-risk individuals.[138] They found an identical frequency and distribution of equivocal PCR reactions in homosexual men who had been at risk for HIV-1 infection and in heterosexual men with presumed low levels of risk, suggesting that latent HIV-1 infection in seronegative homosexual men, if it occurred at all, was a rare phenomenon.

Of those studies that have reported patients with seronegative infection, none have determined the infectious potential of such patients. In our experience, testing of the index cases from whom patients have acquired primary HIV-1 infection has always revealed positive ELISA and Western blot HIV serological results. However, transmission of HIV-1 from infected persons who are themselves in the process of seroconverting has been reported,[31,167] emphasizing that a negative serologic result must always be interpreted in the context of the clinical presentation and the case history.

HIV-1 p24 Antigen

Assay for serum p24 antigen is important if the differential diagnosis includes primary HIV-1 infection. p24 antigen can be detected in serum and CSF in the period before *gag* and *env* seroconversion[4,25,54,72,78,97,147,164] and has been detected in serum as early as 24 hours after the onset of acute illness.[78,163] In one series, p24 antigen was detected in all of 13 patients for whom serum samples were available during the first 18 days after the onset of illness.[163]

False-positive p24 antigen results can occur

and the sensitivity and specificity for diagnosing acute HIV infection is not clear. Whether p24 detection using acid-dissociation pretreatment methods will improve sensitivity is unknown, although this would appear very unlikely during seroconversion prior to the development of p24 antibodies.

The level of serum p24 antigen typically decreases as immune complexes develop,[141,163] the level of serum HIV-1 antibodies increases,[61,72,78,163] and viral load declines. Persistent antigenemia or the reappearance of antigenemia at a later time is associated with an increased risk for the development of severe HIV-1 disease.[50,112]

The isolation of HIV-1 from a range of host cells and tissues during primary HIV-1 infection indicates that the antigenemia of the acute period reflects a true viremia and that patients are potentially highly infectious during the period of primary HIV-1 infection.[73]

Viral Quantitation

Although not useful as a routine diagnostic investigation, the isolation of HIV-1 from a range of host cells and tissues reflects its rapid dissemination throughout the body within days of infection. At the time of presentation, subjects have very high levels of viremia, with peak titres in one study of 1000 to 10,000 tissue-culture–infective doses per milliliter of plasma and 100 to 10,000 infective doses per million of peripheral blood mononuclear cells (PBMC).[44] Quantitative RNA assays show that viral load is about 10^6 copies/ml plasma at this time. Viral RNA can on average be detected 2 days prior to HIV-1 p24 antigen and 9 days prior to HIV-specific antibodies.[24] High viral load in both plasma and PBMC decrease precipitously by about 100-fold within 10 days of presentation.

HIV-1 has been isolated from PBMC,[2,57,67,72,120,134] cell-free plasma,[2,54,57] CSF,[46,134] bone marrow cells,[134] and seminal fluid[155,176] during primary HIV-1 infection.

Histopathology

Lymph node biopsies typically show a reduction of extrafollicular B cells, CD8 + cell follicular infiltration, and only little activation and proliferation of the germinal center cells.[141] The *env* proteins gp120 and gp160 have been found in interfollicular and follicular lymphocytes, endothelial cells, and interdigitating and dendritic reticulum cells.[141] The relative normality of the structure of the germinal centers during primary HIV-1 infection contrasts with the follicular hyperplasia associated with established HIV-1 infection.

Immunohistologic features of the typical erythematous rash generally reveal a normal epidermis and a sparse dermal, mainly perivascular, lymphocytic, and histiocytic infiltrate around vessels of the superficial plexus.[11,21,101] One report noted the infiltrate around the superficial vessels was composed of predominantly CD4+ cells and p24 antigen was detected in occasional cells (possibly Langerhans' cells) of the infiltrate.[101] These findings suggest that the rash of primary HIV-1 infection may be T-cell mediated and directed against HIV-infected Langerhans' cells.

DIFFERENTIAL DIAGNOSIS

Although originally described as "mononucleosis-like"[40] and still described as such in the Centers for Disease Control and Prevention (CDC) classification system of HIV-1 disease,[30] symptomatic primary HIV-1 infection is a distinct and recognizable clinical syndrome. The diagnosis of primary HIV-1 infection should be considered in any person with known possible recent exposure to HIV-1 and who has a febrile illness of acute onset (Table 6–2). The major symptoms and signs that strengthen this diagnosis include mucocutaneous ulceration, maculopapular rash, lymphadenopathy, and nonsuppurative pharyngitis.

The skin rash associated with primary HIV-1 infection is a valuable diagnostic aid. Skin eruptions are rare in patients with EBV or CMV infections (unless antibiotics have been given) or toxoplasmosis, and do not affect the palms

TABLE 6–2. MAJOR DIFFERENTIAL DIAGNOSES

Primary HIV-1 infection
Epstein-Barr virus mononucleosis
Cytomegalovirus mononucleosis
Toxoplasmosis
Rubella
Viral hepatitis
Secondary syphilis
Disseminated gonococcal infection
Primary herpes simplex virus infection
Other viral infection
Drug reaction

TABLE 6–3. CLINICAL FACTORS DIFFERENTIATING EPSTEIN-BARR VIRUS (EBV) MONONUCLEOSIS FROM PRIMARY HIV-1 INFECTION

Primary HIV-1 Infection	EBV Mononucleosis
Acute onset	Insidious onset
Little or no tonsillar hypertrophy	Marked tonsillar hypertrophy
Enanthema on hard palate	Enanthema on border of both hard and soft palates
Exudative pharyngitis uncommon	Exudative pharyngitis common
Mucocutaneous ulcers common	No mucocutaneous ulcers
Rash common	Rash rare (in absence of ampicillin)
Jaundice rare	Jaundice (8%)
Diarrhea possible	No diarrhea

From Gaines H, von Sydow M, Pehrson PO, Lundbergh P: Clinical picture of primary HIV infection presenting as a glandular-fever-like illness. Br Med J 297:1363–1368, 1988, with permission.

and soles in patients with rubella. The rash of pityriasis rosea is typically scaly and may be pruritic; both these features are not found in the rash of a patient with primary HIV-1 infection. Furthermore, constitutional symptoms are generally mild or absent in persons with pityriasis rosea. Histologically, epidermal changes are absent with primary HIV-1 infection, excluding pityriasis rosea as the diagnosis. Mucocutaneous ulceration is a fairly distinctive finding because it is unusual in most of the other differential diagnoses.

The major differences between primary HIV-1 infection and EBV mononucleosis have been detailed by Gaines et al[56] and are summarized in Table 6–3. Although serologic testing for HIV-1 and EBV usually provides the definitive diagnosis, clinicians should be aware that false-positive tests for heterophil antibodies may occur during primary HIV-1 infection. Because HIV-1 remains predominantly a sexually transmitted disease (STD) and because the incubation period of primary HIV-1 infection is comparable to that of most common STDs, primary care physicians managing other STDs should be particularly alert to the clinical manifestations of primary HIV-1 infection and include this in their differential diagnosis.

In patients with meningoencephalitis, other causes of aseptic meningoencephalitis should be excluded.

PROGNOSIS

After resolution of the acute clinical illness, most patients enter a stage of asymptomatic infection that lasts from many months to years. The development of severe HIV-1–related disease within the first 2 years after infection is unusual, although such cases have been reported.[72]

Other viral models have shown that the nature of the acute clinical response may have a role in subsequent disease progression. For example, in hepatitis B virus infection the person with sudden-onset and deep jaundice usually recovers completely, and survivors of fulminant viral hepatitis rarely develop progressive disease. In such patients the severe acute clinical illness reflects an effective cytotoxic immunologic response.

Several reports have suggested that clinical or laboratory-based factors at the time of primary HIV-1 infection may be useful in predicting the subsequent course of disease (Table 6–4). Pedersen et al[111] found that the 3-year progression rate to CDC group IV HIV-1 disease was eight times higher among patients who had a primary illness lasting longer than 14 days than in those with illnesses of shorter duration. Furthermore, each of six patients who developed AIDS during this period had long-lasting illnesses. The 3-year progression rates to CD4+ cell counts $<500/mm^3$ and to recurrence of HIV-1 antigen-

TABLE 6–4. ADVERSE PROGNOSTIC VARIABLES AT THE TIME OF OR IMMEDIATELY AFTER PRIMARY HIV INFECTION

Clinical
  Symptomatic
  Duration >14 days
  Neurologic involvement
  Acquisition of HIV from an index case with late-stage HIV-1 disease

Virologic
  Infection with SI viral strain
  Persistent p24 antigenemia
  Higher HIV RNA viremia following seroconversion

Immunologic
  Low p24 antibody titres
  High gp120 antibody titres
  Level of total plasma IgM before the appearance of specific antibodies
  Presence of specific anti–HIV-1 IgM and IgA after infection
  Immunodeficiency at time of infection
  Persistent low CD4+ lymphocyte count
  High CD38 expression on CD8+ lymphocytes
  Oligoclonal T cell response

emia were also significantly higher for those patients who had long-lasting primary HIV-1 infection. A longer term study by Lindback et al[90] also found that presence and duration of the seroconversion closely correlated with the risk of progression to AIDS, and was 28% at 5 years in those with no illness and 58% in those with an illness. These findings suggest that a severe primary illness could be related to an early and extensive spread of HIV-1 caused by a defective host immune response that could, in turn, adversely influence long-term prognosis.[111] Anecdotal case reports of fatal primary HIV-1 infection in immunosuppressed persons[7,134] and of rapid progression to AIDS in a person treated with prednisolone[113] support this notion. Similarly, Sinicco et al[142] found that 23 patients with symptomatic primary HIV-1 infection had a significantly higher risk of developing AIDS than "asymptomatic" seroconverters (68% at 56 months versus 20% at 66 months). Lastly, Boufassa et al[20] found that neurologic symptoms and signs during primary infection were associated with an even greater risk of disease progression.

Persons with low p24 antibody titers and high gp120 antibody titers at seroconversion developed severe HIV-1 disease more rapidly than did those with high p24 and low gp120 antibody titers and were more likely to have developed p24 antigenemia.[34] Possibly higher quantities of infecting virus may lead to more rapid progression of disease and suppress production of p24 antibody by interfering with the cooperation of T cells with B cells to produce antibodies.[105] In a cohort of 18 hemophiliacs who seroconverted for HIV-1, the level of total plasma IgM before the appearance of specific antibodies and the presence of specific anti–HIV-1 IgM and IgA after infection were predictive of rapid disease progression.[140] The investigators suggested that both these findings probably reflected a general tendency in these patients to mount a prolonged and intense immunoglobulin response.

There is limited evidence that persons who acquire HIV-1 infection from an index case with late-stage HIV-1 disease may have a higher incidence of symptomatic primary HIV-1 infection and subsequent accelerated development of severe disease than those who acquire infection from an index case with asymptomatic disease.[77,161,166] This may be due to a greater virus load in those with advanced HIV disease[65] or the more frequent occurrence of syncytium-inducing (SI) viral strains at this stage of disease.[150,151] Roos et al[129] found that the number of CD4 + cells remained relatively stable in subjects with primary HIV-1 infection who were infected with non–syncytium-inducing (NSI) variants, but declined more rapidly in individuals infected with SI strains. Nielsen et al[107] reported that, in a group of 17 patients, the ability to isolate SI variants during primary infection (from six patients) was associated with a steeper rate of decline of CD4+ cells and clinical progression. Keet et al[77] found that the combination of fever and skin rash, absence of anti–HIV-1 core antibody, and presence of p24 antigen were independent markers of progression to AIDS.

Mellors et al found that HIV RNA load at the first presentation after resolution of HIV seroconversion illness was strongly and independently predictive for HIV disease progression.[102]

An increase in CD38 expression on CD8+ lymphocytes is associated with a poor prognosis, and is independent of changes in both CD4+ lymphocyte count and HIV viral load.[59,60]

Lastly, Imrie et al found that infection with zidovudine-resistant HIV-1 (i.e., HIV with an IC_{90} of greater than 1 μM) did not affect the clinical or CD4+ lymphocyte outcome at 1 year after documented seroconversion.[71]

Although these studies require validation, they suggest that there may be subgroups of patients who should be monitored more intensively and targeted for early intervention.

PREDISPOSING FACTORS

The factors that determine whether an infected person develops symptomatic primary HIV-1 infection have not been elucidated fully. However, several factors seem at least theoretically plausible.

Susceptibility

HIV-1 itself may be an opportunistic infection in an immunocompromised host. In a group of persons with hemophilia, HIV-1 seroconversion after administration of HIV-infected factor VIII preparation was more likely in those who had a preexisting low CD4+ cell count or CD4+ :CD8+ ratio.[95] However, in a large group of homosexual men no difference was found between the antecedent T-cell profiles of 45 seroconverters and 90 matched seronegative

controls.[152] A further study supported these findings but found that anergy to dinitrochlorobenzene (DNCB), a neoantigen, was predictive of subsequent seroconversion and suggested that individuals who could not mount an adequate primary immune response to DNCB (or other novel antigens) were at increased risk of HIV-1 seroconversion.[96] In contrast, anergy to three recall antigens was not predictive of seroconversion.

Source of Infection

There is limited evidence that persons who acquire HIV-1 infection from an index case who has late-stage HIV-1 disease may have a higher incidence of symptomatic primary HIV-1 infection than those who acquire infection from an index case who is at an earlier stage of infection. Ward et al[166] found that symptomatic primary HIV-1 infection was more frequent in 31 patients who were infected by donors in whom AIDS developed within 29 months from the date of donation than in 31 subjects who were infected by donors who developed AIDS more than 29 months after donation (58% versus 23%). Individuals from the first group were also more likely to have developed AIDS 4 years after infection (49% versus 4%). Similarly, van Griensven et al[161] have reported that history of sex with someone with AIDS is a risk factor for accelerated development of severe disease.

Although these studies have not been further substantiated, they suggest that either the nature of the virus in persons with late-stage disease or the greater viral load in such persons may affect the expression of primary HIV-1 infection in the recipient. Ho, Moudgill, and Alam[65] have shown that titers of infectious virus are increased in persons with AIDS and infection from such persons with advanced disease may therefore contain a larger viral inoculum. Tersmette et al[150,151] have shown that persons with severe HIV-1 disease have high replicating and SI HIV-1 variants, which apparently are more virulent in vitro. Roos et al[128] examined the virus phenotype in 19 patients with primary HIV-1 infection who were reviewed for 1 year after infection. They found that the number of CD4+ cells remained relatively stable in 15 of 16 patients with primary HIV-1 infection who were infected with NSI variants but declined rapidly in each of three individuals infected with SI variants.

Concurrent Viral Infections

The host's clinical and immunologic response to primary HIV-1 infection may, in theory, be influenced by concurrent infection with other potentially immunodepressive viruses. If so, this may be particularly relevant in groups of persons such as homosexual men and blood component recipients with a high prevalence of infection with such viruses, including EBV and CMV.

Coinfection of T-cell or monocyte cell lines with CMV and HIV-1 has resulted in enhanced in vitro replication of HIV-1 as measured in a virus-yield assay or by radioimmunoassay for p24 antigen.[144] Furthermore on the molecular level, products of genes of CMV and other herpes viruses are able to *trans*-activate the long terminal repeat of HIV-1 in the presence of the *tat* gene.[106] There are few clinical data on these factors. Three cases of simultaneous infection with CMV and HIV-1 have been reported. In two of them the severity of the acute clinical illness was reported as more severe and of greater duration than that which the authors had generally encountered in either infection alone.[17] In the third case, p24 antigenemia and low absolute numbers of CD4+ cells developed within 18 months of primary HIV-1 infection, suggesting that simultaneous primary infection with CMV may have accelerated expression of HIV-1.[121]

PATHOGENESIS AND VIRAL CLEARANCE

Viral Burden During Primary HIV-1 Infection

The heterogeneous and widespread clinical manifestations of primary HIV-1 infection apparently are based on an immunologic response to rapid and widespread dissemination of HIV-1 after infection.

Primary HIV-1 infection is characterized by high levels of infectious HIV-1 in plasma and PBMC during the first few weeks of infection.[35,44] Titres tend to fall by 4 weeks of onset of illness, concurrently with resolution of symptoms and appearance of anti–HIV-1 antibodies. Sequential isolates of virus from plasma or PBMC obtained throughout primary HIV-1 infection were highly cytopathic for normal donor PBMC and immortalized T lymphocytes. A study of three seroconverting subjects suggests that higher levels of circulating HIV-1 and

failure to effectively control virus replication after initial infection as reflected by continuing high viral titre in plasma may be associated with a poor long-term prognosis.[117] However, in addition to viral quantitative load, other virologic or immunologic factors, including viral phenotype, are likely to contribute to variable rates of CD4+ lymphocyte decline and clinical outcome.

The short and intense period of viral replication[35,44] is followed in the ensuing weeks by a rapid decline in viral load and resolution of the acute illness. Subjects then enter a clinical state of symptomless infection that may last from many months to years. However, during this period of relative clinical latency, HIV-1 accumulates in lymphoid tissue and replicates despite a low viral burden in PBMC.

The viral clearance during primary HIV-1 infection is likely to be due to the emergence of an effective host immune response, although one alternative is the depletion of host target cells.[116] The mechanisms of viral clearance during primary HIV-1 infection have not yet been fully delineated but it appears that humoral, cellular, and cytokine responses each play a role.

It is not yet clear whether a clinical illness is necessarily related to a greater viral burden (or antigenemia). Lindhardt et al[90] found that p24 antigenemia was significantly more common in seroconverters with symptomatic primary HIV-1 infection than in those who seroconverted asymptomatically (56% versus 19%). However, patients who were p24 antigenemic may have been more severely ill and therefore more likely to present clinically. Pedersen et al[111] found no significant difference in the proportion of patients with a long-lasting illness and those without a long-lasting illness who were p24 antigenemic (50% and 41%, respectively).

Strain Selection During Transmission

Studies of HIV seroconverters have found that a single strain of HIV is transmitted in general, although coinfection has been described in one case of homosexual and one case of transfusional transmission (Table 6–5).[24,177] These strains tend to have an NSI phenotype[71,137] but may not be the most common strain in the blood or semen of the source subject,[175,176] suggesting that one or more structural, viral, or immunologic features may influ-

TABLE 6–5. CHARACTERISTICS OF TRANSMITTED HIV STRAINS

Molecular homogeneity (coinfection documented twice only)
NSI more common than SI strains
Not a dominant strain in male genital secretions
About 10% zidovudine resistant in countries where antiretroviral therapy is widespread

ence strain transmission. As discussed below, in countries where antiretroviral therapy is widely used, about 10% of recently transmitted isolates show evidence of zidovudine resistance.[71,99]

Humoral Immune Responses

Neutralizing antibodies may contribute to viral clearance,[1,9,19,158] although a direct correlation between decline in viral load and development of neutralizing antibody has not been demonstrated. Limited data suggest that serum-neutralizing antibodies are not present when viral load falls.[80,158] Antibodies that inhibit syncytium formation and antibodies that mediate antibody-dependent cellular cytotoxicity (ADCC) against virally infected cells also develop soon after infection.[16] HIV-1 immune complexes appear in the blood during the period of declining concentrations of p24 antigen and increasing concentration of IgM and IgG antibodies[163] and may be detected before overt seroconversion.

Cellular Immune Responses

An appreciable CD8+ lymphocytosis has been reported in patients with primary HIV-1 infection,[40,42,58,109,173] generally beginning in the second week after onset of illness. A CD8+ lymphocytosis also occurs in other primary viral infections, such as CMV and EBV, and controls these infections through cytotoxic or suppressor mechanisms. In CMV infection it has been shown that failure to generate a virus-specific cytotoxic T-cell response was associated with severe disease manifestations and persistence of viral infection.[128]

The increase in the number of CD8+ cells during primary HIV-1 infection occurs concomitant with resolution of clinical symptoms and a decrease in the detectable levels of serum p24 antigen,[42] suggesting that the CD8+ cell response to primary HIV-1 infection has a role in

controlling viral replication in vivo as it has been shown to have in vitro.[165]

Roos et al[129] reported that activated CD8+ cells (as identified by expression of HLA-DR and CD38 antigens) were found in all patients with primary HIV-1 infection but were only transiently elevated in those patients with infection with SI variants of HIV. They hypothesized that, after primary HIV-1 infection, SI variants may be selectively cleared by the host immune response and that the isolation of SI variants from these patients may reflect the failure of the CD8+ response to clear the SI variants.

More recently, HIV-specific, CD8+ lymphocyte-mediated, HLA-restricted cytotoxic activity appeared early in HIV seroconversion at a time when HIV-specific neutralizing antibody activity could not be detected.[7,9,80] These cells appear to present with relatively high precursor frequency (0.1% to 1%).[159] Analysis of V-beta T-cell receptor gene usage in these CD8+ lymphocytes has demonstrated different responses between individuals. The V-beta response may be monoclonal, oligoclonal, or polyclonal, with patients generating a polyclonal response appearing to have the best CD4+ count outcome over the medium term.[45]

Another mechanism demonstrable in vitro has been proposed as a means by which CD8+ T lymphocytes suppress HIV replication following primary HIV infection. CD8+ lymphocytes may act by secretion of one or more soluble noncytolytic factors such as RANTES, MIP-1α, MIP-1β, and IL-16, which inhibit HIV replication.[10,38] This soluble suppressor activity has been observed in a small number of HIV seroconverters.[168] However, this activity was also observed in some individuals months prior to seroconversion, suggesting that this activity is not sufficient to prevent infection.

Cytokines

Increased levels of interferon-alpha (IFN-α), tumor necrosis factor-alpha (TNF-α), neopterin, and β2-microglobulin have been detected in blood and CSF during primary HIV-1 infection,[58,98,145,164] reflecting activation of the cellular immune system. High circulating levels of these cytokines are also presumably responsible for the pathogenesis of some of the major clinical manifestations of primary HIV-1 infection (e.g., the symptoms of primary HIV-1 infection such as fevers, chills, myalgia, headache, fatigue, leukopenia, and weight loss are very similar to those found in people receiving exogenous IFN-α).

Primary HIV-1 infection is associated with an early, transient rise in IFN-α and TNF-α in some individuals. Von Sydow et al[164] found that the IFN-α response was sufficiently high to induce suppression of HIV-1 replication. In accordance with this, it was found that p24 antigen levels rapidly declined following the IFN-α peak response that in turn occurred before the development of HIV-specific antibodies and before the rise in CD8+ cells, suggesting that it is a first line of defense against HIV-1 infection, a finding that has some support in a murine model.[131]

The order of appearance of these markers in relation to HIV-1 seroconversion in humans remains unclear.

MANAGEMENT

The mainstays of treatment of primary HIV-1 infection are early recognition and symptomatic treatment. Recognition and early diagnosis of HIV-1 infection are important in order to institute appropriate counseling and prevent further spread of the virus. Moreover, early diagnosis obviates the need for further investigations or empiric therapy, which may not be appropriate. This is especially important in those cases in which neurologic signs are present.

Zidovudine

Although not yet proved, it is possible that antiretroviral intervention during primary HIV-1 infection could prevent persistent HIV-1 infection or lessen the initial viral load and subsequently improve long-term prognosis. In some animal retroviral models, zidovudine has prevented persistent infection or significantly altered disease progression if it was given soon after inoculation.[100,132,133]

These studies have not, however, been uniformly successful. Although the direct applicability of these animal studies to humans is tenuous, zidovudine has subsequently been used by several investigators in the postexposure prophylaxis of HIV-1 in humans. If zidovudine is to have any role in the postexposure prophylaxis of HIV-1 infection, it would be most efficacious if it were administered prior to the initial replicative cycle. Of note, cases have been reported in which zidovudine clearly failed to prevent persistent HIV-1 infection even when administered within 1 hour following inoculation.[7,75,81,93] Nevertheless, zidovudine is clearly effective in preventing perinatal transmission of HIV.[23] Combination antiretroviral therapy might be more effective in preventing transmission.

By the time symptomatic primary HIV-1 infection develops, widespread viral dissemination has already occurred and it is unlikely that treatment at this stage would prevent the establishment of persistent HIV-1 infection.

There are two reports of the effect of treatment with zidovudine during symptomatic primary HIV-1 infection. In a joint Australian-Swedish study, 11 patients with symptomatic primary HIV-1 infection were treated with 1 g of zidovudine daily for a median period of 56 days.[156] Compared with a group of historical controls, no clear evidence of any clinical benefit in terms of resolution of the clinical illness and no indication that the intervention would prevent development of persistent infection emerged. Subjects treated with zidovudine also had a significantly lower CD8+ response in the second month than did a series of untreated, historical controls.[153] It is not clear whether this was due to decreased viral replication and therefore decreased stimulus for CD8+ cell proliferation, or whether zidovudine may have dampened the normal, and presumably protective, CD8+ cell response.[165]

A subsequent double-blind, placebo-controlled trial of zidovudine 250 mg bid for 6 months found that zidovudine was safe but did not shorten the duration of seroconversion illness. After 6 months of therapy, patients receiving zidovudine had higher CD4+ lymphocyte counts (about 140 cells/μl), lower HIV RNA loads (about 0.5 log), and a significant reduction in the number of HIV-related minor opportunistic infections during 18 months of follow-up.[79]

Several cases of primary infection with a zidovudine-resistant strain of HIV-1 have been reported, indicating that horizontal transmission of such strains is possible.[52,71,99] Given the increasing number of persons in the community who are being treated with nucleoside antiretroviral therapy, the possibility of such transmission in cases of primary HIV infection may need to be considered and investigated in individual cases. Preliminary data suggest that zidovudine-resistant transmission occurs in about 10% of seroconverters, but that such transmission is not associated with an adverse outcome at 1 year.[71] There is little information regarding the use of other antiretroviral agents (licensed or investigational) during primary HIV infection[130]; the presence of a zidovudine-resistant isolate in a seroconvertor should make such alternatives more attractive.

Counseling

A diagnosis of HIV infection is likely to be associated with profound psychosocial consequences. Specific factors that must be considered in counseling persons with primary HIV-1 infection include the acute physical distress that many persons experience, the tentative nature of the diagnosis before seroconversion occurs, self-reproach resulting from recent risk behavior, and the potential development of mood disorders. The identification of a patient with primary HIV-1 infection necessarily implies the existence of a source case of infection.

When possible, contact tracing should be implemented to identify this source case. If he or she is identified, counseling for the source person is also indicated. Such persons may be unaware of their infection, may be in the process of seroconverting themselves, or may be unaware of what constitutes safe sex or safe injecting practices. Counseling of such patients also must address their emotional reactions to having infected another individual.

Prevention

Prevention of primary HIV-1 infection remains the only proven intervention strategy. Most cases of primary HIV-1 infection occur as the result of intimate, consensual human activity, and spread of HIV-1 through these modes is totally preventable. The significant changes in sexual practices among homosexual men in urban areas demonstrate that sustained behavior change can be achieved.

REFERENCES

1. Albert J, Abrahamsson B, Nagy K, et al: Rapid development of isolate-specific neutralizing antibodies after primary HIV-1 infection and consequent emergence of virus variants which resist neutralization by autologous sera. AIDS 4:107–112, 1990
2. Albert J, Gaines H, Sonnetborg A, et al: Isolation of human immunodeficiency virus (HIV) from plasma during primary HIV infection. J Med Virol 23:67–73, 1987
3. Albert J, Pehrson PO, Schulman S, et al: HIV isolation and antigen detection in infected individuals and their seronegative sexual partners. AIDS 2:107–111, 1988
4. Alain J-P, Laurian Y, Paul DA, et al: Serological markers in early stages of human immunodeficiency virus infection in haemophiliacs. Lancet 2:1233–1236, 1986
5. Ameisen J-C, Guy B, Chamaret S, et al: Antibodies to the *nef* protein and to *nef* peptides in HIV-1-infected seronegative individuals. AIDS Res Hum Retroviruses 5:279–291, 1989
6. Anonymous: Needlestick transmission of HTLV-III from a patient infected in Africa. Lancet 2:1376–1377, 1984
7. Anonymous: HIV seroconversion after occupational exposure despite early prophylactic zidovudine. Lancet 341:1077–1078, 1993
8. Apperley JF, Rice SJ, Hewitt P, et al: HIV infection due to a platelet transfusion after allogeneic bone marrow transplantation. Eur J Haematol 39:185–189, 1987
9. Ariyoshi K, Harwood E, Chiengsong-Popov R, Weber J: Is clearance of HIV-1 at seroconversion mediated by neutralising antibodies? Lancet 340:1257–1258, 1992
10. Baier M, Werner A, Bannert N, et al: HIV suppression by interleukin-16. Nature 378:563, 1995
11. Balslev E, Thomsen HK, Weismann K: Histopathology of acute human immunodeficiency virus exanthema. J Clin Pathol 43:201–202, 1990
12. Bartelsman JFWM, Lange JMA, van Leeuwen R, et al: Acute primary HIV oesophagitis. Endoscopy 22:184–185, 1990
13. Besnier J-M, Barin F, Baillou A, et al: Symptomatic HIV-2 primary infection. Lancet 335:798, 1990
14. Biggs B, Newton-John HF: Acute HTLV-III infection: A case followed from outset to seroconversion. Med J Aust 144:545–547, 1986
15. Biggar RJ, Johnson BK, Musoke SS, et al: Severe illness associated with appearance of antibody to human immunodeficiency virus in an African. Br Med J 293:1210–1211, 1986
16. Bolognesi DP: Prospects for prevention of and early intervention against HIV. JAMA 261:3007–3013, 1989
17. Bonnetti A, Weber R, Vogt MW, et al: Co-infection with human immunodeficiency virus-type 1 (HIV-1) and cytomegalovirus in two intravenous drug users. Ann Intern Med 111:293–296, 1989
18. Borrow P, Lewicki H, Hahn BH, et al: Virus-specific CD8+ cytotoxic T-lymphocyte activity associated with control of viraemia in primary human immunodificiency virus type 1 infection. J Virol 68:6103–6110, 1994
19. Boucher CAB, de Wolf F, Houweling JTM, et al: Antibody response to a synthetic peptide covering a LAV-I/HTLV-IIIB neutralization epitope and disease progression. AIDS 3:71–76, 1989
20. Boufassa F, Bachmeyer N, Deveau CC, et al: Influence of neurologic manifestations of primary

human immunodeficiency virus infection on disease progression. J Infect Dis 171:1190–1195, 1995

21. Brehmer-Andersson E, Torssander J: The exanthema of acute (primary) HIV infection. Identification of a characteristic histopathological picture? Acta Derm Venereol (Stockh) 70:85–87, 1990

22. Brew BJ, Perdices M, Darveniza P, et al: The neurological features of early and "latent" human immunodeficiency virus. Aust N Z J Med 19:700–705, 1989

23. Bryson YJ, Pang S, Wei LS, et al: Clearance of HIV infection in a perinatally infected infant. N Engl J Med 332:833–838, 1995

24. Busch MP, Herman SA, Henrard DR, et al: Time course and kinetics of HIV viremia during primary infection (Abstract 38). Third National Conference of Human Retroviruses and Related Infections, Washington, DC, January 1996

25. Calabresse LH, Proffitt MR, Levin KH, et al: Acute infection with the human immunodeficiency virus (HIV) associated with acute brachial neuritis and exanthematous rash. Ann Intern Med 107:849–851, 1987

26. Came CA, Tedder RS, Smith A, et al: Acute encephalopathy coincident with seroconversion for anti-HTLV-III. Lancet 2:1206–1208, 1985

27. Carney WP, Rubin RH, Hoffman RA, et al: Analysis of T lymphocyte subsets in cytomegalovirus mononucleosis. J Immunol 126:2114–2116, 1981

28. Casalino E, Bouvet E, Bedos J-P, et al: Acute HIV seroconversion and pneumonitis. AIDS 5:1143–1144, 1991

29. Case records of the Massachusetts General Hospital: Case 33-1989. N Engl J Med 321:454–463, 1989

30. Centers for Disease Control: CDC classification system for human T-lymphotropic virus type III/lymphadenopathy-associated virus infections. MMWR 35:334–339, 1986

31. Centers for Disease Control: Transfusion associated human T-lymphotropic virus type III/lymphadenopathy associated virus infection from a seronegative donor—Colorado. MMWR 35:389–391, 1986

32. Chaix ML, Burgard M, Saragosti S, et al: Sequence analysis revealed divergence of the V3 loop in an infected HIV-1 patient nine months after seroconversion (Abstract 237). Third National Conference of Human Retroviruses and Related Infections, Washington, DC, January 1996

33. Cheingsong-Popov R, Panagiotidi C, Ali M, et al: Antibodies to HIV-1 nef(p27): Prevalence, significance and relationship to seroconversion. AIDS Res Hum Retroviruses 6:1099–1105, 1990

34. Cheingsong-Popov R, Panagiotidi C, Bowcock S, et al: Relation between humoral responses to HIV gag and env proteins at seroconversion and clinical outcome of HIV infection. Br Med J 302:23–26, 1991

35. Clark SJ, Saag MS, Decker WD, et al: High titers of cytopathic virus in plasma of patients with symptomatic primary HIV-1 infection. N Engl J Med 324:954–960, 1991

36. Clerici M, Berzofsky JA, Shearer GM, Tacket CO: Exposure to human immunodeficiency virus type 1—specific T helper cell responses before detection of infection by polymerase chain reaction and serum antibodies. J Infect Dis 164:178–182, 1991

37. Clotet B, Romeu J, Casals A, et al: Spontaneous reso-

lution of Candida esophagitis in a seroconverting patient for HIV antibodies. Am J Gastroenterol 83:1433, 1988

38. Cocchi F, de Vico AL, Garzino-Demo A, et al: Identification of RANTES, MIP-1α and MIP-1β as the major HIV-suppressive factors produced by CD8 + T cells. Science 270:1811–1816, 1995

39. Colebunders R, Greenberg AE, Francis H, et al: Acute HIV illness following blood transfusion in three African children. AIDS 2:125–127, 1988

40. Cooper DA, Gold J, Maclean P, et al: Acute AIDS retrovirus infection. Definition of a clinical illness associated with seroconversion. Lancet 1:537–540, 1985

41. Cooper DA, Imrie AA, Penny R: Antibody response to human immunodeficiency virus following primary infection. J Infect Dis 155:1113–1118, 1987

42. Cooper DA, Tindall B, Wilson EJ, et al: Characterization of T lymphocyte responses during primary HIV infection. J Infect Dis 157:889–896, 1988

43. Cossarizza A, Ortolani C, Mussini C, et al: Lack of selective Vβ deletion in CD4 + or CD8 + lymphocytes and functional integrity of T-cell repertoire during acute HIV syndrome. AIDS 11:547–553, 1995

44. Daar ES, Moudgil T, Meyer RD, Ho DD: Transient high levels of viremia in patients with primary human immunodeficiency virus type I infection. N Engl J Med 324:961–964, 1991

45. Demarest JF, Daucher M, Vaccarezza M, et al: Qualitative differences in the primary immune response to HIV infection may be predictive of subsequent clinical outcome (Abstract 420). Third National Conference of Human Retroviruses and Related Infections, Washington, DC, January 1996

46. Denning DW, Anderson J, Rudge P, et al: Acute myelopathy associated with primary infection with human immunodeficiency virus. Br Med J 294:143–144, 1987

47. de Waele M, Thielmans C, Van Camp BKG: Characterization of immunoregulatory T cells in EBV-induced infectious mononucleosis by monoclonal antibodies. N Engl J Med 304:460–462, 1981

48. de Ronde A, Reiss P, Dekker J, et al: Seroconversion to HIV-1 negative regulation factor. Lancet 2:574, 1988

49. de Wolf F, Goudsmit J, Paul DA, et al: Risk of AIDS related complex and AIDS in homosexual men with persistent antigenaemia. Br Med J 295:569–572, 1987

50. de Wolf F, Lange JMA, Bakker M, et al: Influenza-like syndrome in homosexual men: A prospective diagnostic study. J R Coll Gen Pract 38:443–446, 1988

51. Ensoli F, Fiorelli V, Mezzaroma I, et al: Plasma viraemia in seronegative HIV-1-infected individuals. AIDS 5:1195–1199, 1991

52. Erice A, Mayers DL, Strike DG, et al: Primary infection with zidovudine-resistant human immunodeficiency virus type 1. N Engl J Med 328:1163–1165, 1993

53. Fox R, Eldred LJ, Fuchs EJ, et al: Clinical manifestations of acute infection with human immunodeficiency virus in a cohort of gay men. AIDS 1:35–38, 1987

54. Gaines H, Albert J, von Sydow M, et al: HIV antigenaemia and virus isolation from plasma during primary HIV infection. Lancet 1:1317–1318, 1987

55. Gaines H, von Sydow M, Parry JV, et al: Detection of immunoglobulin M antibody in primary human immunodeficiency virus infection. AIDS 2:11–15, 1988

56. Gaines H, von Sydow M, Pehrson PO, Lundbergh P: Clinical picture of primary HIV infection presenting as a glandular-fever-like illness. Br Med J 297:1363–1368, 1988

57. Gaines H, von Sydow M, Sonnetborg A, et al: Antibody response in primary human immunodeficiency virus infection. Lancet 1:1249–1253, 1987

58. Gaines H, von Sydow MAE, von Stedingk LV, et al: Immunological changes in primary HIV infection. AIDS 4:995–999, 1990

59. Giorgi JV, Ho HN, Hirji K, et al: CD8+ lymphocyte activation of human immunodeficiency virus type 1 serconversion: Development of HLA-DR+ CD38-CD8+ cells is associated with subsequent stable CD4+ cell levels. J Infect Dis 170:775–781, 1994

60. Giorgi JV: HIV pathogenesis and prognostic markers of disease progression: Update from the Multicenter AIDS Cohort Study (Abstract 541). Third National Conference of Human Retroviruses and Related Infections, Washington, DC, January 1996

61. Goudsmit J, de Wolf F, Paul DA, et al: Expression of human immunodeficiency antigen (HIV-Ag) in serum and cerebrospinal fluid during acute and chronic infection. Lancet 2:177–180, 1986

62. Graziosi C, Gantt K, Wilbon G, et al: Oligoclonal expansions of CD8+ T lymphocytes and high levels of expression of pro-inflammatory cytokines are major components of the primary immune response to HIV and EBV infection (Abstract 422). Third National Conference of Human Retroviruses and Related Infections, Washington, DC, January 1996

63. Hagberg L, Maimvail B-E, Svennerholm L, et al: Guillan-Barre syndrome as an early manifestation of HIV central nervous system infection. Scand J Infect Dis 18:591–592, 1986

64. Hardy WD, Daar ES, Sokolov RT Jr, Ho DD: Acute neurologic deterioration in a young man. Rev Infect Dis 13:745–750, 1991

65. Ho DD, Moudgil T, Alam M: Quantification of human immunodeficiency virus type 1 in the blood of infected persons. N Engl J Med 321:1621–1625, 1989

66. Ho DD, Rota TR, Schooley RT, et al: Isolation of HTLV-III from cerebrospinal fluid and neural tissues of patients with neurologic syndromes related to the acquired immunodeficiency syndrome. N Engl J Med 313:1493–1497, 1985

67. Ho DD, Sarngadharan MG, Resnick L, et al: Primary human T-lymphoptropic virus type III infection. Ann Intern Med 103:880–883, 1985

68. Horsburgh CR Jr, Ou C-Y, Holmberg SD, et al: Human immunodeficiency virus type 1 infection in homosexual men who remain seronegative for prolonged periods. N Engl J Med 321:1679–1680, 1989

69. Hulsebosch HJ, Claessen FAP, van Ginkel CJW, et al: Human immunodeficiency virus exanthem. J Am Acad Dermatol 23:483–486, 1990

70. Imagawa DT, Lee MH, Wolinsky SM, et al: Human immunodeficiency virus type 1 infection in homosexual men who remain seronegative for prolonged periods. N Engl J Med 320:1458–1462, 1989

71. Imrie A, Carr A, Duncombe C, et al: Primary infection with zidovudine-resistant HIV-1 does not adversely affect outcome at 1 year. J Infect Dis 1996 (In press)

72. Isaksson B, Albert J, Chiodi F, et al: AIDS two months after primary human immunodeficiency virus infection. J Infect Dis 158:866–868, 1988

73. Jacquez JA, Koopman JS, Simon CP, Longing IM: Role of the primary infection in epidemics of HIV infection in gay cohorts. J Acquir Immune Defic Syndr 7:1169–1184, 1994

74. Jason J, Ou C-Y, Moore JL, et al: Prevalence of human immunodeficiency virus type 1 in hemophiliac men and their sexual partners. J Infect Dis 160:789–794, 1989

75. Jones PD: HIV transmission by stabbing despite zidovudine prophylaxis. Lancet 338:884, 1991

76. Keay S, Wecksler W, Wasserman SS, et al: Association between anti-CD4 antibodies and a decline in CD4+ lymphocytes in human immunodeficiency virus type 1 seroconverters. J Infect Dis 171:312–319, 1995

77. Keet IPM, Krijnen P, Koot M, et al: Predictors of rapid progression to AIDS in HIV-1 seroconvertors. AIDS 7:51–57, 1993

78. Kessler HA, Blaauw B, Spear J, et al: Diagnosis of human immunodeficiency virus infection in seronegative homosexuals presenting with an acute viral syndrome. JAMA 258:1196–1199, 1987

79. Kinloch-Löes S, Hirschel BJ, Hoen B, et al: A controlled trial of zidovudine in primary HIV infection. N Engl J Med 333:408–413, 1995

80. Koup RA, Safrit JT, Cao Y, et al: Temporal association of cellular immune responses with the initial control of viremia in primary human immunodeficiency virus type 1 infection. J Virol 68:4650–4655, 1994

81. Lange JMA, Boucher CAB, Hollak CEM, et al: Failure of zidovudine prophylaxis after accidental exposure to HIV-1. N Engl J Med 322:1375–1377, 1990

82. Lange JMA, Paul DA, de Wolf F, et al: Viral gene expression, antibody production and immune complex formation in human immunodeficiency virus infection. AIDS 1:15–20, 1987

83. Lange JMA, Parry JV, de Wolf F, et al: Diagnostic value of specific IgM antibodies in primary HIV infection. Br Med J 293:1459–1462, 1986

84. Lee T-H, El-Amad Z, Reis M, et al: Absence of HIV-1 DNA in high-risk seronegative individuals using high-input polymerase chain reaction. AIDS 5:1201–1207, 1991

85. Lefrere JJ, Mariotti M, Courouce A-M, et al: Polymerase chain reaction testing of HIV-1 seronegative at-risk individuals. Lancet 335:1400–1401, 1990

86. Legrand E, Neau PD, Masqelier B, et al: HIV-1 specific cytotoxic T-lymphocyte activity after primary infection (Abstract 433). Third National Conference of Human Retroviruses and Related Infections, Washington, DC, January 1996

87. Lewis DA, Brook MG: Erythema multiforme as a presentation of human immunodeficiency virus seroconversion illness. Int J STD AIDS 3:56–57, 1992

88. Lifson AR, Stanley M, Pane J, et al: Detection of human immunodeficiency virus DNA using the polymerase chain reaction in a well characterized

group of homosexual and bisexual men. J Infect Dis 161:436–439, 1990

89. Lima J, Ribera A, Garcia-Bragado F, et al: Antiplatelet antibodies in primary infection by human immunodeficiency virus. Ann Intern Med 106:333, 1987

90. Lindback S, Brostrom C, Karlsson A, Gaines H: Does symptomatic primary HIV-1 infection accelerate progression to CDC stage IV disease, CD4 count below 200 × 10⁶/1, AIDS, and death from AIDS? Br Med J 309:1535–1537, 1994

91. Lindhardt BO, Lauritzen E, Ulrich K, et al: Serological markers of primary HIV infection. Scand J Infect Dis 21:491–496, 1989

92. Loche M, Mach B: Identification of HIV-infected seronegative individuals by a direct diagnostic test based on hybridisation to amplified viral DNA. Lancet 2:418–421, 1988

93. Looke DFM, Grove DI: Failed prophylactic zidovudine after needlestick injury. Lancet 335:1280, 1990

94. Louria DB, Hensle T, Rose J: The major medical consequences of heroin addiction. Ann Intern Med 67:1–22, 1967

95. Ludlam CA, Tucker J, Steel CM, et al: Human T-lymphotropic virus type III (HTLV-III) infection in seronegative haemophiliacs after transfusion of factor VIII. Lancet 2:233–236, 1985

96. Marion SA, Schechter MT, Weaver MS, et al: Evidence that prior immune dysfunction predisposes to human immunodeficiency virus infection in homosexual men. J Acquir Immune Defic Syndr 2:178–186, 1989

97. Mariotti M, Leftere J-J, Noel B, et al: DNA amplification of HIV-1 in seropositive individuals and in seronegative at-risk individuals. AIDS 4:633–637, 1990

98. Martin DH, Pearson JE, Kumar P, et al: Sequential measurement of beta-2-microglobulin levels, p24 antigen levels, and antibody titers following transplantation of a human immunodeficiency virus-infected kidney allograft. J Acquir Immune Defic Syndr 4:1118–1121, 1991

99. Mayers D: Transmission of ZDV-resistant HIV-1. Programme and Abstracts of the Third International Workshop on HIV Drug Resistance. Kauai, HA, August 2–5, 1994

100. McCune JM, Namikawa R, Shih C-C, et al: Suppression of HIV infection in AZT-treated SCIDhu mice. Science 247:564–566, 1990

101. McMillan A, Bishop PE, Aw D, Peutherer JF: Immunohistology of the skin rash associated with acute HIV infection. AIDS 3:309–312, 1989

102. Mellors JW, Kingsley LA, Rinaldo CR, et al: Quantitation of HIV-1 RNA in plasma predicts outcome after seroconversion. Ann Intern Med 122:573–579, 1995

103. Mercey DE, Loveday C, Miller RF: Sclerosing cholangitis rapidly following anti-HIV-1 seroconversion. Genitourin Med 67:239–243, 1991

104. Mientjes GHC, van Ameijden EJC, Weigel HM, et al: Clinical symptoms associated with seroconversion for HIV-1 among misusers of intravenous drugs: Comparison with homosexual seroconvertors and infected and non-infected drug misusers. Br Med J 306:371–373, 1993

105. Mittler R, Hoffman M: Synergism between HIV gp120 and gp120 specific antibody in blocking human T cell activation. Science 245:1380–1382, 1989

106. Mosca JD, Bednarik DP, Raj NBK, et al: Herpes simplex virus type-1 can reactivate transcription of latent human immunodeficiency virus. Nature 325:67–70, 1987

107. Nielsen C, Pedersen C, Lundgren JD, Gerstoft J: Biological properties of HIV isolates in primary HIV-1 infection: Consequences for the subsequent course of infection. AIDS 7:1035–1040, 1993

108. Paton P, Poly H, Gonnaud P-M, et al: Acute meningoradiculitis concomitant with seroconversion to human immunodeficiency virus type 1. Res Virol 141:427–433, 1990

109. Pedersen C, Dickmeiss E, Gaub J, et al: T-cell subset alterations and lymphocyte responsiveness to mitogens and antigen during severe primary infection with HIV: A case series of seven consecutive HIV seroconverters. AIDS 4:523–526, 1990

110. Pedersen C, Getstoft J, Lindhardt BO, Sindrup J: *Candida* esophagitis associated with acute human immunodeficiency virus infection. J Infect Dis 156:529–530, 1987

111. Pedersen C, Lindhardt BO, Jensen BL, et al: Clinical course of primary HIV infection: Consequences for subsequent course of infection. Br Med J 299:154–157, 1989

112. Pedersen C, Nielsen CM, Vestergaard BF, et al: Temporal relation of antigenaemia and loss of antibodies to core antigens to development of clinical disease in HIV infection. Br Med J 295:567–569, 1987

113. Pedersen C, Nielsen JO, Dickmeiss E, Jordal R: Early progression to AIDS following primary HIV infection. AIDS 3:45–47, 1989

114. Pezzella M, Mannella E, Mirolo M, et al: HIV genome in peripheral blood mononuclear cells of seronegative regular sexual partners of HIV-infected subjects. J Med Virol 28:209–214, 1989

115. Pezzella M, Rossi P, Lombardi V, et al: HIV viral sequences in seronegative people at risk detected by in situ hybridisation and polymerase chain reaction. Br Med J 298:713–716, 1989

116. Phillips AN: Is the reduction in high virus level due to the HIV-specific immune response? (Abstract 455) Third National Conference of Human Retroviruses and Related Infections, Washington, DC, January 1996

117. Piatak M Jr, Saag MS, Yang LC, et al: High levels of HIV-1 in plasma during all stages of infection determined by competitive PCR. Science 259:1749–1754, 1993

118. Piette AM, Tusseau F, Vignon D, et al: Acute neuropathy coincident with seroconversion for anti-LAV/HTLV-III. Lancet 1:852, 1986

119. Podzamczer D, Casanova A, Santamaria P, et al: Esophageal candidiasis in the diagnosis of HIV-infected patients. JAMA 259:1328–1329, 1988

120. Rabeneck L, Popovic M, Gartner S, et al: Acute HIV infection presenting with painful swallowing and esophageal ulcers. JAMA 263:2318–2322, 1990

121. Raffi F, Boudart D, Billaudel S: Acute co-infection with human immunodeficiency virus (HIV) and cytomegalovirus. Ann Intern Med 112:234–235, 1990

122. Ranki A, Jarvinen K, Valle S-L, et al: Antibodies to recombinant HIV-1 *nef* protein detected in HIV-1 infection as well as in non risk individuals. J Acquir Immune Defic Syndr 3:348–355, 1990

123. Ranki A, Valle S-L, Krohn M, et al: Long latency period precedes overt seroconversion in sexually

transmitted human immunodeficiency virus infection. Lancet 2:589–593, 1987

124. Reiss P, de Ronde A, Dekker J, et al: Seroconversion to HIV-1 *rev-* and *tat-*gene-encoded proteins. AIDS 3:105–106, 1989

125. Reiss P, de Ronde A, Lange JMA, et al: Antibody response to the viral negative factor (*nef*) in HIV-1 infection: A correlate of levels of HIV-1 expression. AIDS 3:227–233, 1989

126. Reiss P, Lange JMA, de Ronde A, et al: Antibody response to viral proteins U (*vpu*) and R (*vpr*) in HIV-1 infected individuals. J Acquir Immune Defic Syndr 3:115–122, 1990

127. Ritter J, Chevallier P, Peyramond D, Sepetjan M: Serological markers during an acute HIV-2 infection. Vox Sang 59:244–245, 1990

128. Rook AH: Interactions of cytomegalovirus with the human immune system. Rev Infect Dis 10(Suppl 3):460–467, 1988

129. Roos MTL, Lange JMA, Goede REY, et al: Virus phenotype and immune response in primary human immunodeficiency virus type 1 (HIV-1) infection. J Infect Dis 165:427–432, 1992

130. Rouleau D, Conway B, Patenaude P, et al: Combination antiretroviral therapy for the treatment of acute HIV infection (Abstract 287). Third National Conference of Human Retroviruses and Related Infections, Washington, DC, January 1996

131. Ruprecht RM, Chou T-C, Chipty F, et al: Interferon-alpha and 3′-azido-3′-deoxythymidine are highly synergistic in mice and prevent viremia after acute retrovirus exposure. J Acquir Immune Defic Syndr 3:591–600, 1990

132. Ruprecht RM, O'Brien LG, Rossoni LD, et al: Suppression of mouse viraemia and retroviral disease by 3′-azido-3′-deoxythymidine. Nature 323:467–469, 1986

133. Rustin MHA, Ridely CM, Smith MD, et al: The acute exanthem associated with seroconversion to human T-cell lymphotropic virus III in a homosexual man. J Infect 12:161–163, 1986

134. Ruutu P, Suni J, Oksanen K, Ruutu T: Primary infection with HIV in a severely immunosuppressed patient with acute leukemia. Scand J Infect Dis 19:369–372, 1987

135. Saab AJ: Latency preceding seroconversion in sexually transmitted HIV infection. Lancet 2:1402, 1987

136. Sabino EC, Delwart E, Lee TZ, et al: Identification of low-level contamination of blood as basis for detection of human immunodeficiency virus (HIV) DNA in anti-HIV-negative specimens. J Acquir Immune Defic Syndr 7:853–859, 1994

137. Schacker TW, Hughes J, Shea T, Corey L: Virologic course of primary HIV infection (Abstract 480). Third National Conference of Human Retroviruses and Related Infections, Washington, DC, January 1996

138. Sheppard HW, Dondero D, Aron J, Winkelstein W Jr: An evaluation of the polymerase chain reaction in HIV-1 seronegative men. J Acquir Immune Defic Syndr 4:819–823, 1991

139. Sherman MP, Dock NL, Ehrlich GD, et al: Evaluation of HIV type 1 Western blot–indeterminate blood donors for the presence of human or bovine retroviruses. AIDS Res Hum Retrovirus 11:409–414, 1995

140. Simmonds P, Beatson D, Cuthbert RJG, et al: Deter-

minants of HIV disease progression: Six year longtitudinal study in the Edinburgh haemophilia/HIV cohort. Lancet 1:1159–1163, 1991

141. Sinicco A, Palestro G, Caramello P, et al: Acute HIV-1 infection: Clinical and biological study of 12 patients. J Acquir Immune Defic Syndr 3:260–265, 1990

142. Sinicco A, Fora R, Sciandra M, et al: Risk of developing AIDS after primary acute HIV-1 infection. J Acquir Immune Defic Syndr 6:575–581, 1993

143. Sinicco A, Biglino A, Sciandra M, et al: Cytokine network and acute HIV-1 infection. AIDS 7:625–631, 1993

144. Skolnik PR, Kosloff BR, Hirsch MS: Bidirectional interaction between human immunodeficiency virus type 1 and cytomegalovirus. J Infect Dis 157:508–514, 1988

145. Sonnerborg AB, von Stedingk L-V, Hansson L-O, Strannegard OO: Elevated neopterin and beta$_2$-microglobulin levels in blood and cerebrospinal fluid occur early in HIV-1 infection. AIDS 3:277–283, 1989

146. Steeper TA, Horwitz CA, Hanson M, et al: Heterophil-negative mononucleosis-like illnesses with atypical lymphocytosis in patients undergoing seroconversions to the human immunodeficiency virus. Am J Clin Pathol 89:169–174, 1988

147. Stramer SL, Heller JS, Coombs RW, et al: Markers of HIV infection prior to IgG antibody seropositivity. JAMA 262:64–67, 1989

148. Teeuwsen VJP, Siebelink KHJ, de Wolf F, et al: Impairment of in vitro immune responses occurs within 3 months after HIV-1 seroconversion. AIDS 4:77–81, 1990

149. Terpstra FG, Al BJ, Roos MTL, et al: Longitudinal study of leukocyte function in homosexual men seroconverted for HIV: Rapid and persistent loss of B cell function after HIV infection. Eur J Immunol 19:667–673, 1989

150. Tersmette M, Gruters RA, de Wolf F, et al: Evidence for a role of virulent HIV variants in the pathogenesis of AIDS obtained from studies on a panel of sequential HIV isolates. J Virol 63:2118–2125, 1989

151. Tersmette M, Lange JMA, de Goede REY, et al: Association between biological properties of human immunodeficiency virus variants and risk for AIDS and AIDS mortality. Lancet 1:983–985, 1989

152. Tindall B, Barker S, Donovan B, et al: Characterization of the acute clinical illness associated with human immunodeficiency virus infection. Arch Intern Med 148:945–949, 1988

153. Tindall B, Carr A, Goldstein D, Cooper DA: Administration of zidovudine during primary HIV-1 infection may be associated with a less vigorous response. AIDS 7:127–128, 1993

154. Tindall B, Cooper DA: Primary HIV infection. Host responses and intervention strategies. AIDS 5:1–14, 1991

155. Tindall B, Evans LA, Cunningham P, et al: Identification of HIV-1 in semen following primary HIV-1 infection. AIDS 6:949–952, 1992

156. Tindall B, Gaines H, Imrie A, et al: Zidovudine in the management of primary HIV infection. AIDS 5:477–484, 1991

157. Tindall B, Hing M, Edwards P, et al: Severe clinical manifestations of primary HIV infection. AIDS 3:747–749, 1989

158. Tsang MI, Evans LA, McQueen P, et al: Neutralizing antibodies against sequential autologous human immunodeficiency virus type 1 isolates after seroconversion. J Infect Dis 170:1141–1147, 1994

159. Vaccarezza M, Demarest JF, Daucher M, et al: Kinetics of HIV-specific cytotoxic activity during primary HIV infection (Abstract 421). Third National Conference of Human Retroviruses and Related Infections, Washington, DC, January 1996

160. Valle S-L: Febrile pharyngitis as the primary sign of HIV infection in a cluster of cases linked by sexual contact. Scand J Infect Dis 19:13–17, 1987

161. Van Griensven GJP, de Vroome EMM, de Wolf F, et al: Risk factors for progression of human immunodeficiency virus (HIV) infection among seroconverted and seropositive homosexual men. Am J Epidemiol 132:203–210, 1990

162. Vento S, Di Perri G, Garofano T, et al: *Pneumocystis carinii* pneumonia during primary HIV-1 infection. Lancet 342:24–25, 1993

163. von Sydow M, Gaines H, Sonnerborg A, et al: Antigen detection in primary HIV infection. Br Med J 296:238–240, 1988

164. von Sydow M, Sonnerborg A, Gaines H, Strannegard O: Interferon-alpha and tumor necrosis factor in serum of patients in varying stages of HIV infection. AIDS Res Hum Retroviruses 7:375–380, 1991

165. Walker CM, Moody DJ, Stites DP, Levy JA: CD8 + lymphocytes can control infection *in vitro* by suppressing virus replication. Science 234:1563–1566, 1986

166. Ward JW, Bush TJ, Perkins HA, et al: The natural history of transfusion-associated HIV infection: Factors influencing progression to disease. N Engl J Med 321:947–952, 1989

167. Ward JW, Holmberg SD, Allen JR, et al: Transmission of human immunodeficiency virus (HIV) by blood transfusion screened as negative for HIV antibody. N Engl J Med 318:473–478, 1988

168. Weissman D, Barker T, Daucher J, et al: Identification of multiple and distinct CD8 positive T cell suppressor activities (Abstract 423). Third National Conference of Human Retroviruses and Related Infections, Washington, DC, January 1996

169. Winkelstein W Jr, Royce RA: Median incubation time for human immunodeficiency virus (HIV). Ann Intern Med 112:797, 1990

170. Wiselka MJ, Nicholson KG, Ward SC, Flower AJE: Acute infection with human immunodeficiency virus associated with facial nerve palsy and neuralgia. J Infect 15:189–194, 1987

171. Wolinsky SM, Rinaldo CR, Kwok S, et al: Human immunodeficiency virus type 1 (HIV-1) infection a median of 18 months before a diagnostic Western blot. Evidence from a cohort of homosexual men. Ann Intern Med 111:961–972, 1989

172. Yagi MJ, Joesten ME, Wallace J, et al: Human immunodeficiency virus type I (HIV-1) genomic sequences and distinct changes in CD8 + lymphocytes precede detectable levels of HIV-1 antibodies in high-risk individuals. J Infect Dis 164:183–188, 1991

173. Zaunders J, Carr A, McNally L, et al: Effects of primary HIV-1 infection on subsets of CD4 + and CD8 + T lymphocytes. AIDS 9:561–566, 1995

174. Zhang LQ, Diaz RS, Mosley J, et al: Host-specific divergence of HIV-1 in patients infected from the same blood donor source (Abstract 235). Third National Conference of Human Retroviruses and Related Infections, Washington, DC, January 1996

175. Zhu T, Mo H, Wang N, et al: Genotypic and phenotypic characterization of HIV-1 in patients with primary infection. Science 261:1179–1181, 1993

176. Zhu T, Wang N, Carr A, et al: Genetic characterization of human immunodeficiency virus type 1 in blood and genital secretions: Evidence for viral compartmentalization and selection during sexual transmission. J Virol 70:3098–3107, 1996

177. Zhu T, Wang N, Carr A, et al: Evidence for coinfection by multiple strains of human immunodeficiency virus type 1 infection subtype B in an acute seroconvertor. J Virol 69:1324–1327, 1995

Chapter 7

Initiating Routine Care for the HIV-Infected Adult

HARRY HOLLANDER

While there has been tremendous excitement generated by gains in the understanding of the biology of the human immunodeficiency virus (HIV) and how these might be applied to definitive antiviral treatment approaches, more rudimentary elements of medical care remain an important part of the overall therapeutic approach of the HIV-infected adult. As one study suggested, the mortality benefit of *Pneumocystis* prophylaxis and treatment outweighed the benefit of zidovudine monotherapy during the mid-1980s.[27] With this in mind, the United States Public Health Service formulated guidelines for the routine care and follow-up of HIV-infected patients that emphasize prevention against and screening for opportunistic infections rather than the nuances of current antiretroviral therapy.[38] This chapter provides an overview of HIV natural history from a clinical perspective, makes recommendations for the health care maintenance of infected individuals, and reviews the available data about the efficacy of such interventions. A detailed discussion of the issues of timing and choice of antiretroviral therapy is contained in Chapter 8.

CLINICAL HISTORY OF HIV INFECTION

Provision of timely, rational preventive therapy depends upon a detailed understanding of the relationship of clinical events and the degree of immunosuppression. This natural history is now well understood, having been studied in homosexual and bisexual men, intravenous drug users, transfusion recipients, and vertically infected children.[1,8,14,20,33,39] The cumulative risks of the development of acquired immunodeficiency syndrome (AIDS) in these studies differ. In the San Francisco City Clinic cohort, 54% of patients progressed to an AIDS diagnosis 11 years after seroconversion.[33] In transfusion recipients, 49% develop AIDS after 7 years,[39] and 25% of hemophiliacs develop AIDS 9 years after seroconversion.[14] In one study of 32 vertically infected children, 6 (20%) died within 18 months after birth.[1] The European Collaborative Study[8] of 600 children born to HIV-infected mothers showed that 13% were vertically infected. AIDS developed in 26% of infected children by 1 year, and 17% had died. The differences in progression rates may reflect variations in inoculum size, immunologic state of the individual, or other as yet unidentified cofactors for progression. However, all these studies suggest a progressively increasing risk with time. There has been intense interest recently in the small minority of individuals who are long-term nonprogressors clinically and immunologically, but unfortunately, these individuals are the exception in clinical practice.

Multiple possible predictors of HIV disease progression have been studied. One Italian study found that individuals who were symptomatic with the acute retroviral syndrome were more likely to have rapid progression of disease than asymptomatic seroconverters. The most reliable clinical factors are the development of thrush, persistent fever, unexplained diarrhea, and involuntary weight loss.[17,20,23,30] Oral hairy leukoplakia and cutaneous herpes zoster also are important clues to disease progression.[1,30] The presence of generalized lymphadenopathy has not been independently associated with a more rapid disease progression. However, the rapid involution of previously persistently enlarged lymph nodes is a poor prognostic sign.[20] Age greater than 35 years is also associated with a worse prognosis.[17] An interesting recent observation is that individuals who smoke have a more rapid development of *Pneumocystis carinii* pneumonia (PCP) than do nonsmokers.[25] Two studies came to opposite conclusions about the influence of depression on the rate of CD4 decline.[3,21]

Laboratory markers for disease progression include anemia, neutropenia, CD4+ cell counts, low CD4+ percent, CD4+/CD8+ ratios, elevated β_2-microglobulin, elevated serum neopterin levels, and p24 antigenemia.[9,13,17,22,24,30,31,37,40] The CD4+ cell count (expressed as the absolute number, percent of CD4+, or CD4+/CD8+ ratio) has emerged as the best immunologic predictor of HIV disease progression (see Chapter 4 for a discussion of the prognostic utility of viral load measurements). A number of recent studies have correlated CD4 count with risk of opportunistic infection and death.

Data from the multicenter AIDS cohort study of 1665 seropositive persons without AIDS at the time of enrollment in the study found the highest risk of progressing to PCP in patients with a CD4+ cell count <200/mm^3. Compared to patients with a CD4+ cell count >200/mm^3, the relative risk was 4.9. For those with a CD4+ cell count <200/mm^3, the presence of thrush, fever, unintentional weight loss, or persistent fatigue increased the risk of developing PCP.[30] Although combining p24 antigen data with CD4 count does not improve the ability to prognosticate progression, combining β_2-microglobulin levels with CD4 count does.[10,11,27]

An Australian study stratified the risk of specific opportunistic infections according to CD4+ cell count. Candidiasis and tuberculosis occurred with CD4+ cell counts of 250 to 500; Kaposi's sarcoma, lymphoma, and cryptosporidiosis, with 150 to 200; PCP, *Mycobacterium avium* complex, herpes simplex virus, toxoplasmosis, cryptococcosis, and esophageal candidiasis with 75 to 125; and cytomegalovirus retinitis with <50.[6] Importantly, there is great geographic variability in opportunistic infection incidence and prevalence. As the HIV epidemic becomes entrenched in parts of the world with other endemic infections, these infections may become frequent opportunistic complications in HIV-seropositive people; an example of this is histoplasmosis in the midwestern United States.

A study from the National Cancer Institute retrospectively looked at the risk of death as a function of CD4+ cell counts in 55 patients. Of 41 deaths, all but 1 occurred in patients with CD4+ cell counts less than 50/mm^3. The median survival time of patients whose CD4+ count had fallen below 50/mm^3 was 1 year.[40]

HIV infection alters the natural history of some common infections, most notably syphilis and hepatitis B. Syphilis is discussed in Chapter 27. HIV-induced suppression of cell-mediated immunity resulted in the development of the chronic carrier state of hepatitis B in 23% of HIV-infected persons compared to 4.3% in non–HIV-infected controls in a study from Australia.[2] Patients with depressed CD4 cell counts were more likely to develop chronic HBV infection and less likely to develop clinical icterus than non–HIV-infected persons.

STAGING OF HIV INFECTION

Determining the stage of HIV disease has several important implications. From an epidemiologic and surveillance point of view, accurate reporting of individuals with advanced HIV disease allows the tracking of changing trends within the epidemic. More importantly for the individual with HIV infection, accurate staging helps both provider and patient formulate an overall prognosis and therapeutic strategy. Accurate staging is also crucial to individuals trying to obtain medical and other benefits as a result of their HIV disease. In the initial evaluation of an individual with known HIV infection, a complete baseline physical examination should be done. Repeated routine physical examinations have proved unhelpful in a variety of medical screening settings. Similarly, it is difficult to justify the time and expense of repeated full examinations in infected persons. Nevertheless, a focused examination may uncover important new data. The pertinent pieces of the examination with potential findings are listed in Table 7–1. A recent study that examined the ability of primary care physicians to diagnose common HIV-related physical findings was somewhat discouraging. The majority of physicians overlooked generalized lymphadenopathy, and only 25% were able to correctly identify hairy leukoplakia or Kaposi's sarcoma. Diagnostic acumen correlated with the amount of prior HIV experience.[28]

As noted, many laboratory markers of disease progression have been identified (Table 7–2). Early in the epidemic, there was a greater degree of enthusiasm for measuring many of these markers, but experience has demonstrated little incremental predictive value when any of these tests are added to the measurement of the

TABLE 7–1. IMPORTANT PHYSICAL EXAMINATION FINDINGS

General
  Weight loss
Skin
  Seborrheic dermatitis
  Folliculitis
  Dermatophytosis
  Kaposi's sarcoma
  Bacillary angiomatosis
Mouth
  Candidiasis (pseudomembranous and erythematous)
  Hairy leukoplakia
  Aphthous ulcers
  Periodontal disease
Lymphatic System
  Localized lymphadenopathy*
  Splenomegaly
Neuropsychiatric
  Mood or affect disorders
  Psychomotor slowing
  Eye movement abnormalities
  Hyperreflexia (if feasible, simple motor tests, such as timed gait, and quantifiable neuropsychiatric tests, such as digit symbol substitution, are more sensitive to early neurologic disease than is bedside examination)

*Generalized lymphadenopathy does not correlate with increased disease progression.

CD4 lymphocyte count and percentage. Thus, despite some limitations in the utility of CD4 counts (such as decreased prognostic value once antiretroviral therapy has been started[5]), this remains the most important laboratory value in the staging of and therapeutic planning for an infected individual. Currently, there is debate about the appropriate routine use of markers of viral load in evaluating patients and making decisions about therapy. While it is

TABLE 7–2. LABORATORY MARKERS OF HIV DISEASE PROGRESSION

Nonspecific Markers
  Decreased hematocrit value
  Decreased albumin
  Elevated erythrocyte sedimentation rate
Immunologic Markers
  Decreased CD4 lymphocytes
  Decreased CD4/CD8 lymphocyte ratio
  Elevated serum β_2-microglobulin
  Elevated serum neopterin
  Elevated serum acid labile interferon
  Absent or decreased levels of anti-p24 antibody
HIV-Specific Markers
  p24 antigenemia
  Positive serum HIV culture
  Quantitative polymerase chain reaction (PCR) of proviral DNA in cells or RNA in serum
  Syncytium-inducing strains of HIV

clear that viral load measurements can provide predictive information independent of CD4 count and indicate early antiretroviral activity (see Chapters 3 and 8), it has not yet been established that application of this new, relatively expensive technology improves the clinical decision making or outcome for individual patients. When considering the use of any surrogate marker test, it is imperative to recall that results must be interpreted in the context of laboratory variation as well as simple historical and examination findings, which themselves may provide powerful prognostic information that should drive clinical decision making.

After the initial visit, both clinical and laboratory reassessment are important. One approach is to stratify asymptomatic individuals on the basis of complete blood count and CD4 studies. For those with normal results, an initial follow-up frequency of 3 to 6 months is adequate. In contrast, individuals with low, intermediate, or rapidly declining CD4 values might be seen every 2 to 3 months, with a shorter follow-up period if symptoms are present. Once the decision is made to embark on medical therapy, follow-up recommendations intensify accordingly.

The basic approach to the practical management of HIV-related health care by stage of disease is illustrated in Table 7–3.

PROPHYLAXIS OF OPPORTUNISTIC INFECTIONS

Experience with *P. carinii* has reinforced the principle that, when possible, prophylaxis of opportunistic infection should be attempted in patients with HIV infection (Chapter 20). Table 7–4 lists issues to consider when planning prophylactic therapy. Several uncertainties are identified in the table. First, data to allow prediction of a given infection in HIV-infected individuals are limited.[6,30] Thus, improved diagnosis and staging are fundamental in the planning of rational prophylaxis. Second, efficacy or lack thereof in other treatment settings does not necessarily predict the outcome of prophylaxis. An example is the trend toward decreased CMV infection in renal transplant recipients receiving high doses of acyclovir. Third, prophylaxis may lead to undesirable therapeutic trade-offs. For example, use of a highly effective antimicrobial that has synergistic toxicity with an antiretroviral could, on balance, be detrimental. Fourth, the past several years have demonstrated the clinical signifi-

TABLE 7–3. APPROACH BY STAGE OF INFECTION

At Time of First Contact
  Baseline history and examination
  Hematology and CD4 count
  Screen for syphilis (RPR), tuberculosis (PPD and chest x-ray), toxoplasmosis (IgG)
  Cervical Pap smear
  Update vaccinations (Pneumovax, (?) *Haemophilus* B, (?) hepatitis B)
  Assess need for formal counseling and other support services
Early-Stage Disease (CD4 count >500/mm³)
  Monitor clinical status, CD4 count every 3–6 mo
  Continue routine health care maintenance
Middle-Stage Disease (CD4 count of 200–500/mm³)
  Continue to monitor clinical status, CD4 count every 3–4 mo
  Consider PCP prophylaxis as CD4 approaches lower end of range (Chapter 20)
  See Chapter 8 for recommendations regarding antiretroviral therapy
  Continue health care maintenance measures
Late-Stage Disease (CD4 count <200/mm³)
  Consider yearly ophthalmologic examinations
  PCP prophylaxis
  Consider other opportunistic infection prophylaxis (Chapters 21 to 24 and 26)
  See Chapter 8 for recommendations regarding antiretroviral therapy

cance of antimicrobial resistance in this population. Whether the use of prophylactic therapy merits risking the development of resistance that could render later therapy useless must be considered. This is particularly germane for infections treatable with only one or a few efficacious agents. Finally, cost of therapy is a major consideration. Given these competing issues, it should not be surprising that, at present, there are few ideal prophylactic agents. A travel history should always be obtained to identify people at risk for geographically limited infections, such as coccidioidomycosis.

In light of the practical difficulties with antimicrobial prophylaxis, strategies aimed at avoidance of acquisition of pathogens are highly desirable. The 1995 USPHS guidelines

TABLE 7–4. CRITICAL ISSUES IN OPPORTUNISTIC INFECTION PROPHYLAXIS

Geographic and other risk factors for specific infections
Likelihood of reactivation of the infection
Availability of effective, bioavailable antimicrobials
Acceptable long-term toxicity profile
Compatibility with other therapies, particularly antiretrovirals
Development of drug resistance
Cost of therapy

emphasize the discussion of behavioral risk factors that place people at risk for becoming infected with a variety of potential opportunists.[38] For example, individuals with pets should be given guidance to reduce exposure to organisms as diverse as enteric bacterial pathogens, *Bartonella henselae,* and *Toxoplasma gondii.* Similarly, advice regarding safer sexual practices, handling of drinking water, travel, and, where applicable, occupational exposures can theoretically reduce the risk of other opportunistic infections, some of which are not effectively treated with available antimicrobial regimens.

VACCINATION

Several infections may be preventable by vaccination. Clinical efficacy data are not available, but the majority of people with early HIV disease (CD4+ cell count > 500/mm³) will mount an appropriate antibody response to some serotypes represented in pneumococcal vaccine.[16] Since the incidence of adverse effects is no higher in this population, polyvalent pneumococcal vaccine should be administered to each HIV-infected person at the time of first contact. The need for a booster is unknown. HIV-infected individuals are also susceptible to *Haemophilus influenzae* type B disease.[4] As with pneumococcal vaccine, it has been found that higher antibody responses to *H. influenzae* vaccine are found in those individuals with earlier HIV disease and higher CD4 counts.[36] Because this is a less common complication in adults than pneumococcal disease, routine vaccination is not yet recommended.

Seasonal influenza vaccination is still advocated, but the wisdom of this recommendation is questionable for the following reasons. First, there is no evidence that influenza causes more severe disease in an HIV-infected population. Second, antibody response to immunization is generally poor, even in individuals with preserved CD4 counts.[24] Finally, influenza vaccination has been shown to lead to short-term increase of HIV burden.[26] Although the ultimate significance of this burst of replication is unknown, this observation raises concerns about the risk/benefit ratio of vaccination in general, and suggests a conservative approach that targets only high-morbidity complications as candidates for vaccination.

OTHER HEALTH CARE MAINTENANCE

Guidelines for general preventive health care in adults should be followed in HIV-infected adults. Gynecologic cancer screening is particularly important in women, given the high incidence of cervical cancer if there is concurrent papillomavirus infection (Chapter 28). Similar risks of squamous carcinoma exist in men with anal papillomavirus infection. In addition, several preventive interventions deserve special attention. Routine dental care is desirable, since oral lesions are common, prognostic, and often treatable (Chapter 12). Regular eye examinations should be considered, especially when the CD4 count drops to a level below $100/mm^3$.

Identifying individuals with preexisting or current psychologic or psychiatric problems is crucial for establishing adequate counseling and mental health care and for palliating associated symptoms. Nutritional intervention is not routinely indicated but should be considered in instances where there is significant weight loss, anorexia, or diarrhea (Chapter 13).

DOES THE CURRENT HEALTH CARE MAINTENANCE STRATEGY WORK?

Despite perceptions of practitioners that the type of comprehensive intervention described above is the correct approach, there are few data directly addressing this issue. One very optimistic study was carried out in an urban population in Boston.[12] It prospectively evaluated newly diagnosed HIV-seropositive patients with a standardized protocol structured similarly to the one described above. The initial charges were slightly more than $400 per person. For the population screened, the yield was impressive, with the need for tuberculosis prophylaxis identified in about 25% and *Pneumocystis* prophylaxis in 35%. While these results might not be entirely applicable to other demographic settings, they do suggest that the application of a standardized battery of screening examinations to HIV-infected adults may find a significant number of individuals who may immediately benefit from currently available treatments.

In contrast, a Seattle study was more sobering.[7] When evaluating a standardized patient, less than a third of primary care physicians performed recommended screenings and pneumococcal vaccination. Furthermore, only half of the physicians would have prescribed *Pneumocystis* and tuberculosis prophylaxis according to published guidelines. One strategy for improving physician adherence to practice guidelines may be the incorporation of more sophisticated medical information systems that can actively prompt providers when an intervention or measurement is indicated.[34]

SUMMARY

Comprehensive care of HIV-infected adults remains a complex mix of the art and science of medicine. Clinicians struggle to keep up with advances in molecular virology and try simultaneously to counsel, educate, and comfort patients. There is now evidence that simple interventions that can be carried out by *any* practitioner can improve length, and undoubtedly, quality of life for infected people. Although some data point to less than optimal delivery of these health care maintenance measures, the overall message is positive as long as providers are willing to take the time to speak with patients and balance basics of care with more cutting-edge issues.

REFERENCES

1. Blanche S, Rouzioux C, Moscata M-L, et al: A prospective study of infants born to women seropositive for human immunodeficiency virus type 1. N Engl J Med 320:1643–1648, 1989
2. Bosworth NJ, Cooper DA, Donovan B: The influence of human immunodeficiency virus type I infection on the development of the hepatitis B virus carrier state. J Infect Dis 163:1138–1140, 1991
3. Burack JH, Barrett DC, Stall RD, et al: Depressive symptoms and CD4 lymphocyte decline among HIV-infected men. JAMA 270:2568–2573, 1993
4. Casadevall A, Dobroszycki J, Small C, et al: *Haemophilus influenzae* type B bacteremia in adults with AIDS and at risk for AIDS. Am J Med 92:587–590, 1992
5. Choi S, Lagakos SW, Schooley RT, et al: CD4 and lymphocytes are an incomplete surrogate marker for clinical progression in persons with asymptomatic HIV infection taking zidovudine. Ann Intern Med 118:674–680, 1993
6. Crowe SM, Carlin JB, Stewart KI, et al: Predictive value of CD4 lymphocyte numbers for the development of opportunistic infections and malignancies in HIV-infected persons. J AIDS 4:770–776, 1991
7. Curtis JR, Paauw DS, Wenrich MD, et al: Physicians'

ability to provide initial primary care to an HIV-infected patient. Arch Intern Med 155:1613–1618, 1995

8. European Collaborative Study: Children born to women with HIV-1 infection: Natural history and risk of transmission. Lancet 337:253–260, 1991

9. Eyster ME, Ballard JO, Gail MH, et al: Predictive markers for the acquired immunodeficiency syndrome (AIDS) in hemophiliacs: Persistence of p24 antigen and low T4 cell count. Ann Intern Med 110:963–969, 1989

10. Fahey JL, Taylor JMG, Detels R, et al: The prognostic value of cellular and serologic markers in infection with human immunodeficiency virus type 1. N Engl J Med 332:166–172, 1990

11. Farzadegan H, Chmiel J, Odaka N, et al: Association of antibody to human immunodeficiency virus type 1 core protein (p24), CD4 lymphocyte number and AIDS-free time. J Infect Dis 166:1217–1222, 1993

12. Freedberg KA, Malaban A, Samet JH, Libman H: Initial assessment of patients infected with human immunodeficiency virus: The yield and cost of laboratory testing. J Acquir Immune Defic Syndr 7:1134–1140, 1994

13. Goedert JJ, Biggar RJ, Melbye M, et al: Effect of T4 count and cofactors on the incidence of AIDS in homosexual men infected with the human immunodeficiency virus. JAMA 257:331–334, 1987

14. Goedert JJ, Kessler CM, Aledort LM, et al: A prospective study of human immunodeficiency virus type 1 infection and the development of AIDS in subjects with hemophilia. N Engl J Med 321:1141–1148, 1989

15. Greenspan D, Greenspan JS, Hearst NG, et al: Relation of oral hairy leukoplakia to infection with the human immunodeficiency virus and risk of developing AIDS. J Infect Dis 155:475–481, 1987

16. Juan K-L, Ruben FL, Rinaldo CR, et al: Antibody responses after influenza and pneumococcal immunization in HIV-infected men. JAMA 257:2047–2050, 1987

17. Kaslow RA, Phair JP, Friedman HB: Infection with the human immunodeficiency virus: Clinical manifestations and their relationship to immune deficiency—a report from the multicenter AIDS cohort study. Ann Intern Med 107:474–480, 1987

18. Lange JM, Paul DA, Huisman HG, et al: Persistent HIV antigenemia and decline of HIV core antibodies associated with transition to AIDS. Br Med J 293:1459–1462, 1986

19. Larder BA, Darby G, Richman DD: HIV with reduced sensitivity to zidovudine (AZT) isolated during prolonged therapy. Science 243:1731–1734, 1989

20. Lifson AR, Rutherford GW, Jaffe HW: The natural history of human immunodeficiency virus infection. J Infect Dis 158:1360–1367, 1988

21. Lyketsos CG, Hoover DR, Guccione M, et al: Depressive symptoms as predictors of medical outcomes in HIV infection. JAMA 270:2563–2567, 1993

22. McHugh TM, Sites DP, Busch MP, et al: Relationship of circulating levels of HIV antigen, anti-p24 antibody and HIV containing immune complexes in patients infected with HIV. J Infect Dis 158:1088–1091, 1988

23. Melbye R, Biggar R, Ebbesen P, et al: Long-term seropositivity for human T-lymphotrophic virus type III in homosexual men without the acquired immunodeficiency syndrome: Development of immuno-logic and clinical abnormalities. Ann Intern Med 104:496–500, 1986

24. Nelson KE, Clements ML, Miotti P, et al: The influence of human immunodeficiency virus (HIV) infection on antibody responses to influenza vaccines. Ann Intern Med 109:383–388, 1988

25. Nieman RB, Fleming J, Coker RJ, et al: The effect of cigarette smoking on the development of AIDS in HIV-1-seropositive individuals. AIDS 7:705–710, 1993

26. O'Brien WA, Grovit-Ferbas K, Namazi A, et al: Human immunodeficiency virus-type 1 replication can be increased peripheral blood of seropositive patients after influenza vaccination. Blood 86:1082–1089, 1995

27. Osmond D, Charlebois E, Lang W, et al: Changes in AIDS survival time in two San Francisco cohorts of homosexual men, 1983 to 1993. JAMA 271:1083–1087, 1994

28. Paauw DS, Wenrich MD, Curtis JR, et al: Ability of primary care physicians to recognize physical findings associated with HIV infection. JAMA 274:1380–1382, 1995

29. Phair JP: Estimating prognosis in HIV-infection. Ann Intern Med 118:742–744, 1993

30. Phair J, Munoz A, Detels R, et al: The risk of *Pneumocystis carinii* pneumonia among men infected with human immunodeficiency virus type 1. N Engl J Med 322:161–165, 1990

31. Polk BF, Fox R, Brookmeyer R, et al: Predictors of the acquired immunodeficiency syndrome developing in a cohort of seropositive homosexual men. N Engl J Med 316:61–66, 1987

32. Richman DD, Grimes JM, Lagakos SW: Effect of stage of disease and drug dose on zidovudine susceptibilities of isolates of human immunodeficiency virus. J AIDS 3:743–746, 1990

33. Rutherford GW, Lifson AR, Hessol NA, et al: Course of HIV-1 infection in a cohort of homosexual and bisexual men: An 11 year follow-up study. Br Med J 301:1183–1188, 1990

34. Safran C, Rind DM, Davis RB, et al: Guidelines for management of HIV infection with computer-based patient's record. Lancet 346:341–346, 1995

35. Sinicco A, Fora R, Sciandra M, et al: Risk of developing AIDS after primary acute HIV-1 infection. J Acquir Immune Defic Syndr 6:575–581, 1993

36. Steinhoff MC, Auerbach BS, Nelson KE, et al: Antibody responses to *Haemophilus influenzae* type B vaccines in men with human immunodeficiency virus infection. N Engl J Med 325:1837–1842, 1991

37. Taylor JMG, Fahey JL, Detels R, Giorgi JV: CD4 percentage, CD4 number, and CD4/CD8 ratio in HIV infection: Which to choose and how to use. J AIDS 2:114–124, 1989

38. United States Public Health Service/Infectious Disease Society of America: Prevention of opportunistic infections in persons infected with human immunodeficiency virus. Clin Infect Dis 21:S1–141, 1995

39. Ward JW, Bush TJ, Perkins HA, et al: The natural history of transfusion-associated infection with human immunodeficiency virus. Factors influencing the rate of progression to disease. N Engl J Med 321:947–957, 1989

40. Yarchoan R, Venzon DJ, Pluda JM, et al: CD4 count and the risk for death in patients infected with HIV receiving antiretroviral therapy. Ann Intern Med 115:184–189, 1991

Chapter 8

Antiretroviral Therapy

PAUL A. VOLBERDING

Antiretroviral therapy is a key element of the overall management of human immunodeficiency virus (HIV)–infected persons. When properly used, antiretroviral therapy can delay the onset of acquired immunodeficiency syndrome (AIDS), prolong survival, and interrupt transmission. Despite these advantages, however, antiretroviral drugs have clear limitations. They do not usually completely inhibit viral replication and the disease eventually continues to progress despite their use. Also, antiretroviral treatment can be expensive, inconvenient, and has side effects in many patients. It must also be acknowledged that antiretroviral therapy, while important, is only part of a comprehensive treatment program for HIV disease and that opportunistic disease recognition, prophylaxis, and management, and attention to the many psychosocial and financial difficulties caused by HIV disease are also crucial. Nevertheless, it is critical that antiretroviral therapy be used and that decisions regarding its use be based on the most current information.

As has been true of AIDS care in general, optimism regarding the effects of antiretroviral therapy has varied during the epidemic. Recently, however, important clinical trial results have stimulated this field. These, combined with new insights from basic pathogenesis investigations, make it clear that aggressive HIV therapy can be made more clinically effective without a concomitant increase in drug toxicity. Both in HIV therapy and in our understanding of HIV pathogenesis, the tool of HIV RNA quantitation provides important new insights and has rapidly been incorporated into clinical investigations and clinical practice.

While substantial optimism arises from the development and clinical testing of potent new drugs and drug combinations, recent trials continue to highlight the benefits of those antiretroviral drugs that in this very new field, are considered to be "old". Zidovudine monotherapy, for example, has, in recent trials, been shown to be effective in reducing vertical transmission of the virus from HIV-infected pregnant women,[6] in treating those recently infected with HIV,[27] and in preventing infection in health care workers accidentally sustaining puncture wounds from sharp objects contaminated with HIV-infected blood.[43] Finally, optimism arises from trials in patients with established infection of potent new therapies that are rapidly becoming available for prescription use. Particularly as these new therapies are optimally monitored and their use adjusted with HIV RNA quantitation, it is reasonable to expect continued progress and longer survival.

This review will begin by considering the background of HIV quantitation, particularly the insight this assay can provide regarding the tests of newer drugs. Recent clinical trial results, especially those involving these new drugs or new applications of previous drugs, will be summarized. The review will finish by proposing personal guidelines for clinical use of antiretroviral treatment strategies and HIV RNA quantitation.

HIV RNA QUANTITATION

Direct quantitative measurement of HIV has become practical for clinical use. Still, these assays are not yet uniformly available and some questions remain regarding their application. The number of HIV RNA molecules in the plasma provides a direct measurement of the titer of HIV virions. Plasma HIV RNA can be measured using either of two general techniques. Because the absolute concentration of RNA is so minute even with very high virus loads, one method of measurement requires that the RNA first be amplified through polymerase chain reaction (PCR) techniques.[37,38] Quantitative PCR is thus often referred to as *target amplification*. In the second approach, the amount of target HIV RNA is not amplified, but rather the sensitivity of its detection is increased by amplifying the signal the RNA generates in the assay system. This approach is referred to as *signal amplification* and is the method used by the branched-chain DNA (bDNA).[9] Here, HIV RNA is attached to the bottom of an assay plate and then a complex, multiply-branched DNA molecule is attached to it. Indicator compounds on the ends of the branches of DNA are excited in the assay system, generating light. The amount of light is then used to quantify the amount of starting HIV RNA in the patient's specimen.

Direct HIV quantitation using either assay is rapidly proving clinically useful. The baseline HIV RNA titer is an important predictor of disease,[33,34] stronger than CD4, in fact, and higher levels have, at least in some studies, also been associated with a greater risk of vertical transmission.[1–3] HIV quantitation is almost certainly of value in optimizing antiretroviral therapy. Changes in HIV RNA titer occur rapidly with the introduction of antiretroviral drugs,[24,49] with reductions ranging from approximately 3-fold with monotherapy zidovudine to as much as 1000 or more fold with current combinations employing nucleoside analogs and protease inhibitors. HIV RNA titer also has been shown to rise with some drugs at the time of the onset of phenotypic drug resistance.[40] These observations suggest that serial HIV RNA determinations be obtained as antiretroviral therapy is initiated and these results be used to estimate the magnitude and duration of therapeutic benefit. In this way, more effective control of HIV replication might be maintained and inappropriate and expensive drugs more rapidly discontinued. This monitoring may reduce the confusion generated by the proliferation of agents in combinations and the growing impossibility of comparing all possible treatment strategies directly in prospective clinical trials. In general, the lower the HIV RNA following therapy (in comparable populations) the more potent that therapy is assumed to be.

Guidelines for the use of HIV RNA testing in managing individual patients on antiretroviral therapy will be offered in this review after first examining some details of the drug regimens in common use.

KEY CLINICAL QUESTIONS IN HIV THERAPY

Several common and practical questions in HIV therapy must be addressed. A considera-

tion of the answers forms the main body of this review.

Should Antiretroviral Drugs Be Used Routinely?

This basic question has generated a surprising amount of controversy. More recently, however, a consensus has grown given newer clinical trial results that show substantial benefit. Treatment with effective antiretroviral agents reduces plasma HIV RNA levels and increases CD4 cell counts. This has been seen in many clinical trials, although the magnitude and duration of benefit vary by the drug regimen, disease stage, and prior treatment history. Treatment also delays the time to symptomatic disease or AIDS. Again, this has been seen in multiple clinical trials and the degree of this benefit varies. The most stringent evidence of antiretroviral benefit is longer survival. This was seen in the original zidovudine phase III trial[16] and since then in multiple epidemiologic cohorts. Until recently, however, there was little evidence that initiating therapy before the onset of symptoms prolonged survival more than when this therapy was used after the patient became symptomatic. As will be discussed, however, data from several clinical trials have now shown this benefit when more potent therapies (typically with antiretroviral combinations) are used. Therefore, antiretroviral therapy at some point during HIV infection should be considered essential and it is expected that the magnitude of benefit will be even further enhanced with the use of increasingly potent drugs and combinations optimized by the use of HIV RNA monitoring.

Growing consensus favors treatment with antiretroviral drugs because:
- HIV RNA titers fall.
- CD4 cell counts rise.
- Time until HIV-related symptoms begin is prolonged.
- Survival is improved with more aggressive therapy.

When Should Antiretroviral Drug Therapy Be Initiated?

The ideal trial to answer the question of when to best initiate antiretroviral therapy cannot be performed. It would require a placebo-controlled randomization to a wide variety of drugs and combinations and would require a huge number of previously untreated patients with various predefined disease stages probably followed until mortality differences could be recorded. Instead, we must consider, with all limitations, an examination of completed trials, few of which are now placebo controlled and many of which use laboratory rather than clinical end-points. The most important group of patients, in practice, are those with established infection, but this review will first consider several somewhat unique groups where initial therapy might be employed. In each of these groups, there is a growing consensus favoring therapy.

Postexposure Prophylaxis

The risk of unintended HIV exposure varies widely. While the vast majority (>90%) of recipients of HIV-infected blood transfusions become infected, the risk of a single unprotected sexual exposure is estimated at 1 in approximately 500 or less[35] and the risk of HIV infection from an accidental needlestick injury ranges from 1 in 200 to 1 in 400.[22] Because of the low absolute risk of isolated sexual and occupational exposure, prospective controlled trials of prophylaxis have not been conducted, but recently the Centers for Disease Control and Prevention (CDC) released results from an important retrospective, case-controlled evaluation of zidovudine monotherapy of occupational exposures to health care workers.[43] After adjusting for the estimated magnitude of risk, depth of puncture, type of needle, etc., those health care workers who received zidovudine in various doses and durations following exposure had a significant (>75%) reduction in the frequency of subsequent HIV infection. Based on this, such early prophylaxis can be recommended. The optimum drug or combination, dose, and treatment duration is not known but many currently favor aggressive use of two or three drugs, perhaps for as little as 2 weeks, to attempt to block initial viral spread. Because of concern about exposure to zidovudine-resistant strains, zidovudine should only be used in combination with another nucleoside analog and, perhaps, with a potent protease inhibitor as well. Standard doses of all drugs should be used.

Primary Infection

Evidence is accumulating that the initial spread of HIV within the lymphatic system and the success of host control of replication, whether through immunologic or other mechanisms, are important factors in determining the later rate of disease progression.[4,33] Thus, attempts to inhibit HIV replication in those with recent infection are interesting. Despite fear that antiviral therapy of primary HIV infection may prove detrimental by reducing the vigor of the host response, this was not seen in one prospective placebo-controlled trial of zidovudine in this setting. In this small European trial, a group of mostly symptomatic recently infected persons was found to benefit from zidovudine given as standard dosage for 6 months.[27] After therapy, a sustained benefit was detected in HIV titer and CD4 cell count and in a reduction in the subsequent rate of minor clinical infections. Given these data, many would recommend treating recently acquired HIV infection, probably for at least 6 months. The prevalence of zidovudine-resistant mutations in primary infection is 5% to 15%. This, and the greater activity of zidovudine when used along with another reverse transcriptase inhibitor or with both a reverse transcriptase and protease inhibitor, make such combinations worth considering in cases of primary infection as well as in established disease.

Pregnant HIV-Infected Women

Numerous studies have identified a risk of vertical transmission from an HIV-infected pregnant woman to her newborn child.[1,14,15] The degree of risk varies but in the United States is approximately 25%. An extremely important trial, ACTG 076, found that treatment of the woman with zidovudine in the third trimester and peripartum and of the newborn after delivery decreased vertical transmission to approximately 8.4%.[6] Recent work suggests that this effect of zidovudine was independent of the mother's HIV RNA titer and may have represented prophylaxis of the newborn.[42] At any rate, the data are similarly striking and make it imperative that all pregnant women have access to HIV testing and that such testing be particularly recommended in women at higher estimated HIV risk. All pregnant HIV-infected women should be treated with indicated antiretrovirals for their own health and all women should have such therapy recommended in the later stages of pregnancy to decrease the rates of transmission. The best drug(s) for the prevention of vertical transmission is not known but, again, may well involve several agents given simultaneously.

Established HIV Infection

Within approximately 6 months of the initial HIV infection, the virus has spread widely in the body and the HIV titer has stabilized at a level, termed the HIV "set-point," which is held relatively constant until advanced stages of HIV disease.[33] After infection is established, therapy is aimed at achieving a durable reduction in HIV replication of sufficient magnitude to slow clinical progression and prolong survival. Recent trials have demonstrated important benefits of antiretroviral treatment across a wide spectrum of established HIV infection, particularly when the CD4 cell count is 500/mm³ or below, in both symptomatic and asymptomatic states. Although zidovudine monotherapy has a laboratory and clinical benefit in this population, other therapies, especially those in which a second drug is added to zidovudine, are even more beneficial; survival may be prolonged beyond that achieved with zidovudine monotherapy.

Arriving at a consensus on the optimum time to initiate antiretroviral treatments has been complicated by clinical trials of modestly effective therapy with seemingly disappointing or conflicting results. Whereas, zidovudine was shown to delay the onset of AIDS in one placebo-controlled trial of asymptomatic patients with CD4 cell counts below 500/mm,[3,47] a simultaneous companion trial found no such benefit in an asymptomatic population with CD4 cell counts above that threshold.[46] In neither study was survival additionally prolonged by earlier as opposed to somewhat delayed drug use, even though the loss of CD4 cells was slowed by zidovudine therapy. In a 3-year trial in those with CD4 cell counts above or below 500/mm³, no reduction of clinical progression was seen with zidovudine monotherapy despite a CD4 cell benefit.[5] Another trial in a comparable population (asymptomatic, CD4 cell counts 400 to 750/mm³) found a zidovudine benefit in reducing progression to mild symptoms, but lacked the statistical power to detect an effect, if any, on mortality or progression to overt AIDS.[7]

As a group, these trials strongly suggest that zidovudine monotherapy is of real benefit in asymptomatic HIV infection, but that its effect is modest, limiting the detection of benefit in those with very early disease stages. Thus, these results lead to the recommendation to use zidovudine monotherapy in those with CD4 cell counts below 500/mm³ but not when the CD4 cell count was higher than 500/mm³.[41] Even among those asymptomatic HIV-infected patients with CD4 counts below 500/mm³, however, real enthusiasm for zidovudine therapy was often limited. Many clinicians elected to defer zidovudine use until further CD4 cell loss or until the onset of symptoms.

Countering this, in the end, pessimistic view of antiretroviral therapy are the positive results of recent clinical trials in both previously treated or untreated populations using more potent strategies. The trials ACTG 175 in the United States[20] and Delta in Europe[18] explored the initial use of zidovudine in combination with didanosine or zalcitabine or didanosine by itself (in ACTG 175 only) while other trials studied combinations of zidovudine and lamivudine. Another group of trials have begun to examine stavudine as monotherapy or in combination with didanosine or lamivudine, and almost any combination of nucleoside reverse transcriptase inhibitors with nonnucleoside inhibitors or, in particular, with the protease inhibitors. In some trials clinical endpoints are being used, whereas others have relied primarily on changes in RNA or CD4 levels to evaluate response.

No clinical trial or even group of trials can tell us with precision or permanence when antiretroviral therapy should commence. It is even difficult to compare separate clinical trials to say which of the many possible treatments are superior. Also, concepts of HIV pathogenesis and natural history change as new laboratory assays come into use; opinions on the efficacy of therapy rise or fall with the latest results, and new drugs and combinations make even recently completed trials seem dated.

Most clinical trials of antiretroviral therapy have been designed around arbitrary CD4 cell thresholds (e.g., 500/mm³). This has made some sense, as CD4 cell counts remain predictive, especially at very low levels, of disease progression and mortality. In addition, CD4 cells accurately predict the risk for certain preventable opportunistic infections, especially *Pneumocystis carinii* pneumonia. Several prospective trials support the use of antiretroviral therapy when the CD4 cell count is below 500/mm³ even in the absence of symptoms. The most recent of these confirm that therapy can not only delay symptomatic progression, but also can prolong survival.

HIV RNA titer is another marker to consider in initiating antiretroviral therapy. Data are rapidly emerging that show a closer correlation between baseline HIV RNA titer or a subsequent therapy-induced change in this titer and survival and disease progression than is seen with CD4 cell counts.[20,33] In two separate studies, values above 30,000 to 50,000 copies/mm³ were associated with much more rapid progression and death—65% mortality in 3 to 5 years in one study compared to a 0% mortality in those in the lowest HIV RNA quartile (approximately 5000 copies/mm³ or below).[33] The two intermediate HIV RNA quartiles had correspondingly intermediate progression risks. Moreover, HIV RNA titers were a more accurate and stable predictor of this risk than either baseline or change in the CD4 cell count. Even for those with higher CD4 cell counts, progression and death were common when the HIV RNA levels were in the upper range. While it may be premature to make definite recommendations regarding the specific HIV RNA titer at which to initiate antiretroviral therapy, it would appear prudent to strongly consider such therapy, particularly in those above the lowest quartile. As intercurrent infections or other sources of antigenic stimulation (e.g., influenza vaccinations) can temporarily raise HIV RNA titer, the test should not be done within several weeks of such events.

Reasonable, if temporary, guidelines may, thus, be possible regarding the initial use of antiretroviral therapy.

- Treat if possible before the onset of HIV-related symptoms.
- In general treat when the CD4 cell count falls to or below 500/mm³.
- Consider treatment if the HIV RNA titer is above 5000 copies/mm³ in those whose CD4 cell count is above 500/mm³, and recommend treatment if the HIV RNA is greater than 30,000 to 50,000 copies/ml, or if the CD4 cell count is rapidly declining.
- Treat HIV-infected pregnant women and those with recent unintended HIV exposures.
- Consider therapy for primary HIV infection.

Choice of Initial Antiretroviral Treatment

For established HIV infection, a number of single-agent combination therapy trials have been reported—many of the latter still in preliminary fashion. As reviewed briefly above, these results, often quite promising, are useful in deciding whether or not to use *any* antiretroviral therapy and in estimating when this treatment should commence. It is more difficult to know with any certainty which of these drugs or combinations is best or whether one specific treatment is best used before another. It is tempting to assume that one should first

use that treatment which most completely suppresses HIV replication as reflected in HIV RNA titers but this has not been proven. Current data suggest that this treatment would involve a combination of two nucleoside analogs and a potent protease inhibitor. In a second approach,[42] one would begin with two nucleoside drugs, adding a protease inhibitor at a later time. Alternatively, one might use the combination of nucleosides with protease inhibitors as initial therapy but restrict it for those patients who, at baseline, have a higher progression risk as estimated by their HIV RNA titer, rate of CD4 fall, or some combination of those. Clearly, these are very different approaches to initial therapy, and the choice among them must be made in the absence of firm data. To some degree this will reflect the treatment philosophy of the physician and patient. Fortunately, viral load monitoring allows adjustments if therapy is not optimal.

Before proposing guidelines for the choice of initial HIV therapy, one might review selected drugs (Tables 8–1 and 8–2) and clinical trials using these agents in previously untreated HIV-infected persons. Here, key variables in design and analysis should be examined, as a direct comparison of treatments under exactly comparable conditions is rarely possible.

The specific choice of the best initial antiretroviral treatment should be based on an assessment of the potency, expected duration of benefit, resistance, toxicity, potential interactions with other medications, ease of use, and cost. This assessment is somewhat subjective and the information is rapidly changing as more trials are conducted. Nevertheless, some recommendations have emerged. Initial therapy should include, at a minimum, two nucleoside analogs. Most data and experience support the inclusion of zidovudine as one of these drugs. The second drug can be didanosine, zalcitabine, or lamivudine (listed in order of their development). Of these, clinical endpoint data are strongest for didanosine or zalcitabine, which emerged in the ACTG 175[20] and Delta[18] trials as more effective when combined with zidovudine than zidovudine used alone with respect to both laboratory and clinical outcomes. Lamivudine with zidovudine may be somewhat more durably potent than these drugs, but the combination has been tested less using clinical end-points.[13] Certainly lamivudine is less toxic and more convenient than didanosine or zalcitabine. Resistance studies suggest a possible benefit from using

TABLE 8–1. CLINICAL GLOSSARY OF ANTIRETROVIRAL DRUGS

	Drug	Proprietary Name	Dose/ Frequency	Toxicity	Comments
Nucleoside Analog Reverse Transcriptase Inhibitors	Zidovudine (ZDV, AZT)[46,50]	Retrovir	200 mg tid	Anemia, neutropenia, nausea, vomiting	Resistance relatively common, may be reduced when used with potent combinations
	Didanosine (ddI)[23,30]	Videx	200 mg bid	GI disturbances, pancreatitis, peripheral neuropathy	Less neurotoxic than zalcitabine; requires gastric neutralization with antacids which can interfere with absorption of other drugs; avoid use in patients with high potential for pancreatitis (drugs, alcohol, prior history)
	Zalcitabine (ddC)[23,30]	HIVID	0.75 mg tid	Rash, oral ulcers, peripheral neuropathy	No significant pancreatic toxicity; most effective in previously untreated patients, especially with higher CD4 cell counts
	Stavudine (d4T)[25,39]	Zerit	40 mg bid	Peripheral neuropathy	Less neurotoxic than didanosine or zalcitabine
	Lamivudine (3TC)[29,44]	Epivir	150 mg bid	None significant	Resistance develops rapidly but restores zidovudine sensitivity
Protease Inhibitor	Saquinavir[28]	Invirase	600 mg tid	None significant	Metabolized by cytochrome P-450. May interact with other drugs (e.g., ketoconazole, ritonavir)
	Indinavir[19]	Crixivan	800 mg tid	Nephrolithiasis, hyperbilirubinemia	Elevated bilirium is benign; frequency of renal stones 2% to 3%; more rapid resistence in noncompliant patients
	Ritonavir[8,31]	Norvir	600 mg bid	Circumoral paresthesias, nausea, headache	Cross-resists with indinavir
	Agouron AG 1343[48]	Nelfinavir Viracept	None decided	None significant	
Nonnucleoside Reverse Transcriptase Inhibitor	Delavirdine[36]		None decided	Rash	Rapid resistance, effect more durable when used in combination
	Nevirapine[21]		None decided	Rash	Rapid resistance; less compromise in efficacy with high doses

didanosine or zalcitabine first, as the dominant resistance mutation of lamivudine (codon 184) may reduce the later effectiveness of these two other drugs. This, however, has not been established in vivo.

For patients who cannot tolerate a regimen that includes zidovudine or who prefer another drug, stavudine-based regiments are a reasonable alternative. Again, most would use this drug at full dose in combination, although the data are far less developed than those with zidovudine. Stavudine combined with didanosine was tested in one trial and found to be active with respect to laboratory variables and surprisingly well tolerated.[39] Only one case of peripheral neuropathy was reported in the 76 patients evaluated. The combination of stavudine with lamivudine is under investigation but has been popular, as both drugs are well tolerated and can be taken twice daily.

In general, data support combination therapy, but monotherapy may be an option for some patients. Data from ACTG 175 show substantial benefit with didanosine monotherapy and preliminary data with stavudine monotherapy show antiviral activity.

The use of nonnucleoside reverse transcriptase inhibitors with any of these other regimens is also of growing interest. Preliminary studies of nevirapine or delavirdine[17] suggest

TABLE 8–2. KEY TRIALS OF SELECTED DRUGS OR COMBINATIONS IN INITIAL HIV THERAPY

Selected Drug or Drug Combination	Trial	Population	CD4 Benefit	RNA Benefit*	Clinical Benefit	Comments
ZDV	BW 02[16]	Advanced disease	Yes	NA	Yes, survival	Short trial; significant survival difference
	ACTG 019[47] in those with baseline CD4 counts <500/mm^3	Asymptomatic, 1500 subjects followed median 12 mo	Yes	NA	Yes; reduced progression to AIDS, ARC	No additional survival benefit compared to later use
	ACTG 019[46] with CD4 counts >500/mm^3	1600 patients, all asymptomatic	Yes; Longer time to reach 500 cells/mm^3	NA	No; same time to AIDS or death	
	Concorde[5]	1700 asymptomatic subjects with any CD4 cell count at entry; 40% >500/mm^3	Yes	NA	No	Reanalysis suggested measurable benefit if baseline CD4 <500/mm^3
ddI	ACTG 116a[10]	Most asymptomatic; no or less than 16 wk prior ZDV therapy	Not compared to ZDV	NA	Not compared to ZDV	Needs to be compared with ACTG 175, Delta
	ACTG 175[20]	One arm with ddI; most asymptomatic; CD4 <500/mm^3; 40% of overall group ZDV naive	Yes	Yes (2+)	Yes	Progression to AIDS, death or CD4 loss decreased significantly with ddI
d4T	Katlama[25]	Asymptomatic; CD4 cell count 400–750/mm^3	Yes	Yes (2+)	?	Minimal neuropathy
3TC	Monotherapy arm of NUCA 3001[12]		Yes	Yes (1+)	?	Surprising degree and duration of effect especially considering rapid onset of drug resistance
ZDV + ddI	ACTG 175[20]	As above	Yes	Yes (2+)	Yes	Best arm overall; significant survival advantage compared with ZDV
	Delta[18]	More advanced than ACTG 175	Yes	Yes (2+)	Yes	Best arm for naive patients
ZDV + ddC	ACTG 175[20]	As above	Yes	Yes (2+)	Yes	Best arm for naive patients; significant survival advantage
	Delta[18]	As above	Yes	Yes (2+)	Yes	Somewhat inferior to ZDV + ddI
ZDV + 3TC	NUCA 3001[12]	Moderate disease	Yes	Yes (2–3+)	?	Trend to fewer symptomatic progressions; durable response (past 76 weeks)
d4T + ddI	Pollard[39]	Early to moderate disease	Yes	Yes (2–3+)	?	Essentially no peripheral neuropathy
ZDV + 3TC + indinavir	Merck[32]	Moderate disease; mean CD4 142/mm^3	Yes	Yes (4+)	?	Small trial; only toxicity that of ZDV; 85% patients had nondetectable HIV RNA at 24 wk
ZDV + ddC + saquinavir	ACTG 229†	Moderate–advanced disease	Yes	Yes (2–3+)	?	Modest benefit; minimal toxicity
ZDV + ddI + indinavir	Merck[32]	Moderate disease mean CD4 = 150 naive	Yes	Yes (3–4+)	?	Minimal peripheral neuropathy but GI intolerance of ddI or even ddI buffer in placebo relatively common
ZDV + ddC + ritonavir	Abbott	CD4 50–250 (mm^3)	Yes	Yes (3+)	?	Open label

* Estimate of potency.
† From Collier A, Coombs RW, Schoenfeld DA, et al: Treatment of human immunodeficiency virus infection with saquinavir, zidovudine, and zalcitabine. N Engl J Med 334:1011–1017, 1996, with permission.

durable activity in higher doses in at least some patients. Such combinations should not be recommended as initial therapy, however, until more clinical data become available.

The most current pressing concern regards the role of protease inhibitors as a part of an initial treatment regimen for established HIV infection. Such combinations may be the most potent as measured by HIV RNA effects (2 to 3-log reductions)[11] but have not been fully tested with clinical end-points. Saquinavir is well tolerated but expensive and of limited potency because of the low bioavailability (about 4%) of its current formulation. Indinavir and ritonavir share resistance mutations and are thus likely to be cross-resistant in vivo, whereas saquinavir may develop resistance through separate pathways that do not fully overlap those of indinavir and ritonavir. It is thus possible that initial use of saquinavir will not impair later response to indinavir or ritonavir, but this has yet to be shown in vivo. Data with indinavir show that previous low-dose therapy compromises later effectiveness, raising the concern that similar consequences might follow prior therapy with lower potency compounds. Because ritonavir blocks the hepatic metabolism of saquinavir,[26] combinations of these agents should be avoided until drug level monitoring is available. Also, *many* drugs have an altered metabolism when combined with ritonavir, and the clinician prescribing ritonavir should review all available information regarding these interactions.

Interim treatment recommendations include the following:

• Start patients on a two-drug combination of a nucleoside analog and reverse transcriptase inhibitor. Zidovudine and either didanosine, zalcitabine, or lamivudine can be recommended.
• For zidovudine-intolerant individuals, the combination of stavudine with didanosine is a reasonable alternative.
• For patients with more advanced or rapidly progressing HIV disease or with a higher HIV RNA load (e.g., >30,000 to 50,000/mm^3) initial therapy might include a protease inhibitor added to the combinations already discussed.
• An alternative recommendation is to begin all therapy with the most potent combination available, typically two nucleoside drugs and one protease inhibitor.

TABLE 8–3. GUIDELINES FOR HIV RNA USE*

Select assay (RT-PCR, bDNA) and use same assay for serial determinations in any patient
Follow lab directions closely regarding specimen processing
Avoid testing shortly after vaccination or opportunistic infection
Obtain baseline HIV RNA in all patients
Obtain duplicate value prior to initiating antiretroviral therapy
Perform HIV RNA titer within 2–4 wk of starting new therapy and expect >8-fold reduction from baseline; If see <8-fold reduction, alter therapy

* Repeat assay every 3–4 mo and change therapy if value approaches baseline after initial suppression.

How Should Patients Be Monitored for Continuing Benefit?

Despite ready agreement that, to date, antiretroviral therapy is of declining benefit over time, there is little consensus on the best practical means for deciding when to change to a second and potentially better drug or combination. If a patient experiences serious new clinical problems while still on initial therapy, one has probably waited too long, but it is possible that minor clinical problems may be useful in deciding when to change treatments. Also, CD4 cell counts are used by many clinicians and, if changes are substantial, may be useful. It is clear that in groups of patients in clinical trials, CD4 cell count changes correlate with the clinical benefits of therapy, but the wide variance of determination limits its usefulness in individual patient management.

Another test of potential value in making clinical decisions is the HIV RNA titer. The potential utility of HIV quantitation is great and tentative guidelines may be offered.[45] The clinician should be aware that such guidelines are based on preliminary data and might be altered with more experience (Table 8–3). First, as repeated testing is required, a clinician should choose which test, quantitative PCR (RT-PCR) or bDNA, to use for serial comparisons. HIV RNA quantitation should be obtained when the patient is first seen and in duplicate as a baseline when therapy is beginning. The titer should be measured within 4 weeks of initiating or changing antiretroviral therapy. Effective therapy should decrease baseline titer by at least 3-fold. If this degree of suppression is not obtained, therapy should be altered by adding or replacing specific drugs. The lower the maximal suppression titer below the 3-fold threshold, the more potent the therapy is estimated to be. Once therapy is initiated or changed, and after the first repeat titer, follow-up determinations may be obtained at 3 to 4-month intervals and therapy should be discontinued or changed if the viral suppression appears to be waning. As the results are sensitive to improper specimen processing, care should always be taken to follow usage guidelines closely. In most cases, the optimum anticoagulant is ethylenediaminetetraacetic acid (EDTA), and plasma should be promptly separated and frozen or refrigerated.

What Therapies Should Be Used Next?

The primary overall goal of antiretroviral therapy is to maintain viral suppression for as long as possible. Unfortunately, all antiretroviral treatments will, over time, lose activity, making secondary alternatives necessary. Although a simple algorithm is not possible given the number of potential combinations and pa-

tient variables, some principles can be offered (Table 8–4). The optimum choice of secondary (and tertiary) treatment is likely to be complicated by many factors. For example, what was the prior therapy, how long was it used, was the drug (or drugs) tolerated? Even though many would like to have a set of simple guidelines for these common clinical questions, such a scheme would be hazardous, and would be increasingly so as new drugs are rapidly approved and become available.

If a patient becomes intolerant to a given drug, it should be replaced in that combination with another drug or drugs. Zidovudine intolerance may require replacement with stavudine, for example, for which at least some data exist supporting its use in combination with didanosine or lamivudine.[39] Intolerance to didanosine due to pancreatitis may require a change to lamivudine or zalcitabine. Even when few clinical data exist, various combinations may be attempted using HIV RNA titers to evaluate short-term treatment success.

TABLE 8–4.   GUIDELINES FOR SECONDARY HIV THERAPY*

Existing Therapy	Failure Due to Toxicity	Failure Due to Loss of Activity

Zidovudine	Switch to:
	    Didanosine
	    Stavudine
	    Didanosine or zalcitabine + protease
	       inhibitor
	    Stavudine + protease inhibitor
		Add:
		    Didanosine
		    Lamivudine
		    Zalcitabine
		    Add/switch to didanosine or
		       zalcitabine + protease inhibitor
		Switch to:
		    Stavudine + protease inhibitor

Zidovudine + didanosine	Switch to:
	    Zidovudine + lamivudine
	    Stavudine + protease inhibitor
	    Zalcitabine + protease inhibitor
		Switch to:
		    Zidovudine + lamivudine
		    Stavudine + protease inhibitor
		    Didanosine + protease inhibitor

Zidovudine + zalcitabine	Switch to:
	    Zidovudine + lamivudine
	    Didanosine + protease inhibitor
	    Stavudine + lamivudine
		Zidovudine + lamivudine
		Stavudine + protease inhibitor
		Didanosine + protease inhibitor
		Stavudine + lamivudine

Zidovudine + lamivudine	Switch to:
	    Didanosine + zalcitabine + protease
	       inhibitor
	    Stavudine + protease inhibitor
		Didanosine or zalcitabine + protease
		    inhibitor
		Stavudine + protease inhibitor

Didanosine	Switch to:
	    Zidovudine + lamivudine
	    Stavudine + lamivudine
		Zidovudine + lamivudine
		Stavudine + protease inhibitor

didanosine or zalcitabine + protease inhibitor	Switch to:
	    Zalcitabine or didanosine + protease
	       inhibitor 1
	    Didanosine or zalcitabine + protease
	       inhibitor 2
		Zalcitabine or didanosine + protease
		    inhibitor 2

Zidovudine + didanosine or zalcitabine + protease inhibitor	Switch to:
	    Zalcitabine or didanosine + protease
	       inhibitor 2
		Zalcitabine or didanosine + protease
		    inhibitor 2

* The role of nonnucleoside transcriptase is to be established.

When Should HIV Therapy Be Stopped?

Many patients with extensive prior HIV therapy and advanced debilitating disease request that antiretroviral drugs be discontinued. In general, this request can be honored, as the clinical benefits of such therapy may be limited. Also, after extensive prior therapy, many patients will no longer have an RNA or CD4 effect, even with otherwise potent combinations. Here too, discontinuation may be reasonable.

The one disadvantage to discontinuing therapy, though, centers on the potential continuing value of antiretroviral drugs with respect to central nervous system (CNS) disease. Recent data suggest that HIV found in the CNS may retain drug sensitivity even when this has been lost in the periphery. As some drugs, especially lamivudine, are so well tolerated, continuing therapy as long as the drug is tolerated may be considered.

DIRECTIONS IN HIV THERAPY

It seems clear that antiretroviral therapy of increasing efficacy and tolerability is available and that monitoring with HIV RNA assays will help in determining the optimum use of these new drugs. In this way, it is expected that survival can be prolonged and that symptomatic disease can be substantially delayed. Therapy can prevent transmission following occupational exposures and can prevent vertical transmission in pregnancy. Finally, therapy in very early infection may also prove of significant value.

REFERENCES

1. Boyer PJ, Dillon M, Navaie M, et al: Factors predictive of maternal-fetal transmission of HIV-1: Preliminary analysis of zidovudine given during pregnancy and/or delivery. JAMA 271(24):1925–1930, 1994
2. Bryson YJ: The role of plasma RNA as a determinant of risk maternal-fetal HIV transmission and early progression of disease in perinatally-infected infants (Abstract). Third Conference on Retroviruses and Opportunistic Infections, Washington, DC, 1996, p 17
3. Burchett SK, Kornegay J, Pitt J, et al: Assessment of maternal plasma HIV viral load as a correlate of vertical transmission (Abstract). Third Conference on Retroviruses and Opportunistic Infections, Washington, DC, 1996, p 40
4. Coffin JM: Viral/cellular kinetics: Fitness dynamics (Abstract). Third Conference on Retroviruses and Opportunistic Infections, Washington, DC, 1996, p 39
5. Concorde Coordinating Committee: Concorde: MRC/ANRS randomised double-blind controlled trial of immediate and deferred zidovudine in symptom-free HIV infection. Lancet 343:871–881, 1994
6. Connor EM, Sperling RS, Gelber R, et al: Reduction of maternal-infant transmission of human immunodeficiency virus type 1 with zidovudine treatment. N Engl J Med 331:1173–1225, 1994
7. Cooper DA, Gatell JM, Kroon S, et al: Zidovudine in persons with asymptomatic HIV infection and CD4+ cell counts greater than 400 per cubic millimeter. N Engl J Med 329:297–303, 1993
8. Danner SA, Carr A, Leonard JM, et al. A short-term study of the safety, pharmacokinetics, and efficacy of Ritonavir, an inhibitor of HIV-1 protease. N Engl J Med 334:1528–1533, 1995
9. Dewar RL, Highbarger HC, Sarmiento MD, et al: Application of branched DNA signal amplification to monitor human immunodeficiency virus type 1 burden in human plasma. J Infect Dis 170:1172–1179, 1994
10. Dolin R, Amato DA, Fischl MA, et al: Zidovudine compared with didanosine in patients with advanced HIV type 1 infection and little or no previous experience with zidovudine. Arch Intern Med 155:961–974, 1995
11. Emini EA: Protease inhibitors (Abstract). Third Conference on Retroviruses and Opportunistic Infections, Washington, DC, 1996, p 1
12. Eron JJ, Benoit SL, Jemsek J, et al: Treatment with lamivudine, zidovudine, or both in HIV-positive patients with 200 to 500 CD4+ cells per cubic millimeter. N Engl J Med 333:1662–1669, 1995
13. Eron JJ, Quinn JB, Hill-Price S, et al: 52 Week follow-up of NUCA 3001: 3TC, zidovudine or both in the treatment of HIV-positive patients with CD4 cell counts of 200–500 cells/mm^3 (Abstract) Third Conference on Retroviruses and Opportunistic Infections, 1996, Washington, DC, 1996, p 14
14. European Collaborative Study: Children born to women with HIV-1 infection: Natural history and risk of transmission. Lancet 337:253–260, 1991
15. European Collaborative Study: Risk factors for mother-to-child transmission of HIV-1. Lancet 339:1007–1012, 1992
16. Fischl MA, Richman DD, Griego MH, et al: The efficacy of azidothymidine (AZT) in the treatment of patients with AIDS and AIDS-related complex. N Engl J Med 317:185–191, 1987
17. Freimuth WW, Wathen LK, Cox SR, et al: Delavirdine in combination with zidovudine causes sustained antiviral and immunological effects in HIV-1 infected individuals (Abstract). Third Conference on Retroviruses and Opportunistic Infections, Washington, DC, 1996, pp 40–41
18. Gazzard B: Further results from European/Australian Delta Trial (Abstract). Third Conference on Retroviruses and Opportunistic Infections, Washington, DC, 1996, p 40
19. Gulick R, Mellors J, Havlir D, et al: Potent and sustained antiretroviral activity of indinavir (IDV) in combination with zidovudine (ZDV) and lamivud-

ine (3TC) (Abstract). Third Conference on Retroviruses and Opportunistic Infections, Washington, DC, 1996, p 162

20. Hammer S: Virologic markers and outcome in ACTG 175 (Abstract). Third Conference on Retroviruses and Opportunistic Infections, Washington, DC, 1996, p 17

21. Havlir D, Cheeseman SH, McLaughlin M, et al: High-dose nevirapine: Safety, pharmacokinetics, and antiviral effect in patients with human immunodeficiency virus infection. J Infect Dis 171:537–545, 1995

22. Henderson DK, Fahey BJ, Willy M, et al: Risk for occupational transmission of human immunodeficiency virus type 1 (HIV-1) associated with clinical exposures. Ann Intern Med 113:740–746, 1990

23. Hirsch MS, D'Aquila RT: Therapy for human immunodeficiency virus infection. N Engl J Med 328: 1686–1695, 1993

24. Ho DD, Neumann AU, Perelson AS, et al: Rapid turnover of plasma virions and CD4 lymphocytes in HIV-1 infection. Nature 373:123–125, 1995

25. Katlama C, Molina JM, Rozenbaum W, et al: Stravudine in HIV infected patients with CD4 > 350/mm^3. Results of a double-blind randomized placebo controlled study (Abstract). Third Conference on Retroviruses and Opportunistic Infections, Washington, DC, 1996, p 14

26. Kempf D, Marsh K, Denissen J, et al: Coadministration with ritonavir enhances the plasma levels of HIV protease inhibitors by inhibition of cytochrome P450 (Abstract). Third Conference on Retroviruses and Opportunistic Infections, Washington, DC, 1996, p 79

27. Kinloch-De Loes S, Hirschel BJ, Hoen B, et al: A controlled trial of zidovudine in primary human immunodeficiency virus infection. N Engl J Med 333: 408–413, 1995

28. Kitchen VS, Skinner C, Ariyoshi K, et al: Safety and activity of saquinavir in HIV infection. Lancet 345: 952–955, 1995

29. Larder BA, Kemp SD, Harrigan PR: Potential mechanism for sustained antiretroviral efficacy of AZT-3TC combination therapy. Science 269:696–699, 1995

30. Lipsky JJ: Zalcitabine and didanosine. Lancet 341: 30–32, 1993

31. Markowitz M, Saag M, Powderly WG, et al: A preliminary study of ritonavir, an inhibitor of HIV-1 protease, to treat HIV-1 infection. N Engl J Med 334: 1534–1539, 1995

32. Massari F, Conant M, Mellors J, et al: A phase II open-label, randomized study of the triple combination of indinavir, zidovudine and didanosine versus indinavir alone and zidovudine/didanosine in antiretroviral naive patients (Abstract). Third Conference on Retroviruses and Opportunistic Infections, Washington, DC, 1996, p 14

33. Mellors JW: Rinaldo CR Jr, Gupta P, et al: Prognosis in HIV-1 infection predicted by the quantity of virus in plasma. Science 272:1167, 1996

34. Mellors JW, Kingsley LA, Rinaldo CR Jr, et al: Quantitation of HIV-1 RNA in plasma predicts outcome after seroconversion. Ann Intern Med 122:573–579, 1995

35. Padian NS, Shiboski SC, Jewell NP: The effect of number of exposures on the risk of heterosexual HIV transmission. J Infect Dis 161:883–887, 1990

36. Perelson AS, Neumann AU, Markowitz M, et al: HIV-1 dynamics in vivo: Virion clearance rate, infected cell life-span, and viral generation time. Science 271:1582–1586, 1996

37. Piatak M, Saag MS, Yang LC, et al: Determination of plasma viral load in HIV-1 infection by quantitative competitive polymerase chain reaction. AIDS 7: S65–S71, 1993

38. Piatak M, Saag MS, Yang LC, et al: High levels of HIV-1 in plasma during all stages of infection determined by competitive PCR. Science 259: 1749–1754, 1993

39. Pollard R, Peterson D, Hardy D, et al: Antiviral effect and safety of stavudine and didanosine combination therapy in HIV-infected subjects in an ongoing pilot randomized double-blinded trial (Abstract). Third Conference on Retroviruses and Opportunistic Infections, 1996, Washington, DC, 1996, p 14

40. Saag MS, Emini EA, Laskin OL, et al: A short-term clinical evaluation of L-697,661, a non-nucleoside inhibitor of HIV-1 reverse transcriptase. N Engl J Med 329:1065–1072, 1993

41. Sande MA, Carpenter CCJ, Cobbs G, et al: Antiretroviral therapy for adult HIV-infected patients. JAMA 270:2583–2589, 1993

42. Sperling RS, Shapiro EE, Coombs R, et al: Maternal plasma HIV-1 RNA and the success of ZDV in the prevention of mother-child transmission (Abstract). Third Conference on Retroviruses and Opportunistic Infections, 1996, Washington, DC, 1996, p 40

43. State and Territorial Health Departments, CDC Cooperative Needlestick Surveillance Group: Case-control study of HIV seroconversion in health-care workers after percutaneous exposure to HIV-infected blood—France, United Kingdom, and United States, January 1988–August 1994. MMWR 44:929–933, 1995

44. van Leeuwen R, Katlama C, Kitchen V, et al: Evaluation of safety and efficacy of 3TC (lamivudine) in patients with asymptomatic or mildly symptomatic human immunodeficiency virus infection: A phase I/II study. J Infect Dis 171:1166–1171, 1995

45. Volberding PA: HIV quantification: Clinical applications. Lancet 347:71–73, 1996

46. Volberding PA, Lagakos SW, Grimes JM, et al: A comparison of immediate with deferred zidovudine therapy for asymptomatic HIV-infected adults with CD4 cell counts of 500 or more per cubic millimeter. N Engl J Med 333:401–407, 1995

47. Volberding PA, Lagakos SW, Koch MA, et al. Zidovudine in asymptomatic human immunodeficiency virus infection. N Engl J Med 322:941–949, 1990

48. Webber S, Shetty B, Wu E, Zorbas M: *In vitro* and *in vivo* metabolism and cytochrome P450 induction studies with the HIV-1 protease inhibitor, VIRACEPT™ (AG1343) (Abstract) Third Conference on Retroviruses and Opportunistic Infections, Washington, DC, 1996, p 79

49. Wei X, Ghosh SK, Taylor ME, et al: Viral dynamics in human immunodeficiency virus type 1 infection. Nature 373:117–122, 1995

50. Wilde MI, Langtry HD: Zidovudine. An update of its pharmacodynamic and pharmacokinetic properties, and therapeutic efficacy. Drugs 46:515–578, 1993

51. Collier AC, Coombs RW, Schoenfeld DA, et al: Treatment of human immunodeficiency virus infection with saquinavir, zidovudine, and zalcitabine. N Engl J Med 334:1011–1017, 1996

Drug Interactions and Toxicities in Patients with AIDS

BELLE L. LEE

The potential for drug interactions leading to adverse reactions is great in patients with the acquired immunodeficiency syndrome (AIDS), since multiple drugs are commonly prescribed to these patients. In addition, patients with AIDS have a higher incidence of adverse reactions to drugs that are commonly used in the treatment of opportunistic infections than non-AIDS patients have. As a result of the high rate of adverse reactions, use of available drugs often is limited. An appreciation of the potential drug interactions and knowledge of the most frequently occurring adverse reactions can increase the chance of a successful therapeutic response.

DRUGS USED TO TREAT *PNEUMOCYSTIS CARINII* PNEUMONIA (Chapter 20)

Trimethoprim-Sulfamethoxazole

Trimethoprim-sulfamethoxazole therapy has been associated with adverse effects in up to 100% of patients with AIDS.[33,52,103] These adverse reactions occur more often in white patients with human immunodeficiency virus (HIV) infection and AIDS than in HIV-seronegative patients. Many of these adverse reactions are thought to be mediated by a toxic metabolite of sulfamethoxazole, hydroxylamine. Anaphylaxis and fatal blistering skin

eruptions, such as erythema multiforme or Stevens-Johnson syndrome, can occur but are rare, especially in patients with HIV infection.[70] Medina et al[72] reported that 57% of patients with AIDS receiving trimethoprim-sulfamethoxazole developed major toxicity requiring a change of therapy to pentamidine as compared to 30% of those receiving trimethoprim-dapsone. The incidence of minor toxicities was equal in both groups, with 2.7 reactions occurring per patient, but mild elevation of alanine aminotransferase or aspartate aminotransferase levels (to five times normal) or neutropenia (<50% baseline value) was more common in the group assigned to trimethoprim-sulfamethoxazole.

Drug interactions reported with use of trimethoprim-sulfamethoxazole include warfarin (increased prothrombin time),[83] procainamide (decreased clearance of procainamide),[51] and phenytoin (increased half-life of phenytoin).[104] The prothrombin time or the concentrations of these drugs should be monitored closely when they are given concurrently with trimethoprim-sulfamethoxazole.

Trimethoprim-Dapsone

The major adverse reactions associated with trimethoprim-dapsone therapy are intolerable rash (10%), nausea and vomiting (7%), neutropenia (3%), elevation of aminotransferase concentrations (3%), thrombocytopenia (3%), and severe methemoglobinemia (3%) (Table 9–1).[72] Hyperkalemia has been associated with both trimethoprim-sulfamethoxazole and trimethoprim-dapsone therapy. In a comparative

Portions of this chapter appeared previously in *Clinical Infectious Diseases*, March 1992, published by The University of Chicago Press, and *Current Opinion in Infectious Diseases*, April 1992, published by Current Science.

TABLE 9–1. *PNEUMOCYSTIS CARINII* PNEUMONIA THERAPY

Drug	Major Adverse Reactions	Interactions
Trimethoprim-sulfamethoxazole	Rash Fever Transaminase elevation Neutropenia Nausea/vomiting Thrombocytopenia Hyperkalemia	Warfarin: increased prothrombin time Procainamide: decreased clearance by trimethoprim Phenytoin: increased half-life of phenytoin Dapsone: increased dapsone levels by trimethoprim
Dapsone	Rash Nausea/vomiting Anemia Methemoglobinemia Transaminase elevation Neutropenia Thrombocytopenia	Trimethoprim: increased trimethoprim levels by dapsone Rifampin: decreased half-life of dapsone ddI: decreased absorption of dapsone
Pentamidine	Nephrotoxicity Hypoglycemia* Hyperglycemia Transaminase elevation Hyperkalemia Neutropenia Thrombocytopenia Pancreatitis* Ventricular arrhythmia*	Foscarnet: severe hypocalcemia, increased risk of nephrotoxicity
Clindamycin	Diarrhea *Clostridium difficile* colitis Rash Transaminase elevation Nausea	Kaolin antidiarrheals: decreased absorption of clindamycin Neuromuscular blocking agents: enhanced neuromuscular blockade
Primaquine	Rash Transaminase elevation Hemolysis Methemoglobinemia	
Atovaquone	Rash Fever Transaminase elevation	Zidovudine: increased levels by atovaquone

* Potentially life threatening.

trial using doses of trimethoprim about 50% higher than currently recommended, hyperkalemia occurred more frequently in patients treated with trimethoprimdapsone (53%) than in patients treated with trimethoprim-sulfamethoxazole (20%).[72]

Concurrent use of dapsone and trimethoprim will increase the plasma concentrations of both drugs, possibly due to decreased renal secretion of these drugs.[62] Rifampin can decrease the half-life of dapsone as a result of enzyme induction, and probenecid can cause a significant reduction in the urinary excretion of dapsone.[110] As the concurrent administration of dapsone and ddI will result in decreased absorption of dapsone because of the buffered vehicle for ddI,[74] dapsone and ddI should be administered at least 2 hours apart (Chapter 8).

Pentamidine

The use of intravenous pentamidine is limited by the high frequency of adverse reactions. Nephrotoxicity can range from mild azotemia to severe tubular necrosis.[55] Both hypoglycemia and hyperglycemia have been associated with pentamidine therapy; the latter often is not reversible. This toxicity probably is caused by a direct cytolytic effect of pentamidine on the beta islet cells of the pancreas. One report found that the risk of hypoglycemia is increased with higher doses of pentamidine, prolonged therapy, or retreatment within 3 months.[102] Other complications include elevation in liver enzymes, hyperkalemia, leukopenia, thrombocytopenia, acute pancreatitis, and ventricular arrhythmias.[87,103] Rapid infusion of pentamidine can result in a precipitous drop in blood pressure.

Deaths from pentamidine administration generally have been attributed to hypotension, ventricular arrythmias, or unrecognized hypoglycemia.

Several drugs are best avoided when administering pentamidine. The combined use of pentamidine and foscarnet can result in severe hypocalcemia and may increase the risk of nephrotoxicity. Drugs that may cause pancreatitis (e.g., ddI) or hypoglycemia (e.g., sulfonylureas) also should be avoided as cotherapy.

Aerosolized pentamidine is generally free of all but local (bronchospastic) complications. However, acute pancreatitis[36] and mild hypoglycemia have been reported in association with this therapy. In addition, an increased risk of spontaneous pneumothorax has occurred.[80]

Clindamycin

Gastrointestinal side effects, particularly diarrhea and nausea, are the most frequent adverse reactions associated with use of clindamycin. In retrospective and prospective studies, the frequency of clindamycin-associated diarrhea has varied from 0.3% to 21% and of pseudomembranous colitis from 1.9% to 10%.[54] Diarrheal side effect is more common with oral than with parenteral therapy. Rash may also occur in association with clindamycin therapy. In clinical trials of the combination of clindamycin with primaquine for the treatment of acute *Pneumocystis carinii* pneumonia, rash was the most common side effect (61%), followed by diarrhea (17%), elevation in serum transaminases, and mild methemoglobinemia.[6,85] In only 2% were these side effects dose limiting. A trial of clindamycin for prophylaxis against *Toxoplasma gondii* infection in 52 HIV-infected patients with a CD4 cell count <200/mm^3 was halted prematurely because of diarrhea (30.8%) and rash (21.2%).[47] Although isolated cases of reversible neutropenia have been reported with use of clindamycin, this drug is generally not myelosuppressive and apparently does not enhance zidovudine hematologic toxicity. Mean half-life, peak concentration, and area under the curve (AUC) of zidovudine are unchanged by clindamycin.[48]

Use of neuromuscular blocking agents in combination with clindamycin may result in skeletal muscle weakness or respiratory depression or both caused by enhancement of neuromuscular blockage.[100] Use of kaolin- or attapulgite-containing antidiarrheals can decrease oral absorption of clindamycin. Any antiperistaltic agent can prolong or worsen pseudomembranous colitis by delaying the elimination of toxin. Erythromycin can displace clindamycin from its ribosomal binding site. Therefore, concurrent use is not recommended.

Primaquine

Hemolysis can occur with administration of primaquine and is particularly severe in patients with substantial deficiency of the glucose-6-phosphate dehydrogenase enzyme. Methemoglobinemia also may result, particularly with the use of high doses of primaquine or in patients with NADH methemoglobin reductase deficiency. More rarely, granulocytopenia or gastrointestinal disturbances occur.[69]

Atovaquone

Atovaquone has been approved for the treatment of mild to moderately severe cases of *P. carinii* pneumonia in patients who are intolerant of trimethoprim-sulfamethoxazole. Adverse reactions have been mild and infrequent and include fever, rash, and increases in serum aminotransferase concentrations. In an open-label trial of 34 patients, 27 (79%) were treated successfully with atovaquone, and all survived. In four (12%) of the patients, atovaquone was discontinued because of possible toxicity (fever and rash).[27] In a large comparative trial of trimethoprim-sulfamethoxazole and atovaquone, atovaquone was found to be less effective than trimethoprim-sulfamethoxazole but had fewer treatment-limiting adverse effects. These adverse effects included rash (4%); liver dysfunction (3%); and vomiting, fever, nausea, and pruritus (1% each).[42]

Atovaquone is highly protein (99.9%) bound in plasma. Therefore, caution should be used when administering atovaquone concurrently with other drugs that are highly bound to plasma proteins, as competition for binding sites may occur. The extent of plasma protein binding of atovaquone in human plasma is not affected by the presence of therapeutic concentrations of phenytoin (15 μg/ml).

Atovaquone can increase the AUC of zidovudine by inhibiting the glucuronidation of zidovudine. In patients who are receiving both atovaquone and zidovudine and are experiencing hematologic adverse effects from zidovud-

TABLE 9–2. ANTIFUNGAL AGENTS

Drug	Major Adverse Reactions	Interactions
Amphotericin B	Hyperkalemia Nephrotoxicity Fever Chills Nausea	Zidovudine: additive bone marrow toxicity Digitalis, carbenicillin, ticarcillin: enhanced hypokalemic effect of amphotericin B Nephrotoxic agents (aminoglycoside): additive nephrotoxicity
Flucytosine (5-FC)	Nausea/vomiting Agranulocytosis Aplastic anemia	Amphotericin B, ganciclovir: additive hematologic toxicity Antacids: decreased 5-FC absorption
Fluconazole	Nausea Headache Skin rash Abdominal pain Vomiting/diarrhea	Cyclosporin A: increased cyclosporin A levels Rifampin: decreased half-life of fluconazole Phenytoin, warfarin: decreased metabolism of phenytoin and warfarin Sulfonylureas: increased hypoglycemia
Ketoconazole	Nausea Vomiting Hepatitis Adrenal suppression Gynecomastia	ddI, cimetidine, antacids: decreased levels of ketoconazole Cyclosporin A: increased cyclosporin A levels Terfenadine: inhibited terfenadine metabolism Phenytoin: inhibited phenytoin metabolism Rifampin: increased ketoconazole metabolism; decreased absorption Isoniazid: decreased itraconazole levels
Itraconazole	Nausea/vomiting Diarrhea Rash Headache Hypertension	Terfenadine: increased terfenadine levels, leading to cardiovascular adverse events Astemizole: inhibits astemizole metabolism Cyclosporin A, digoxin: increased levels of cyclosporin A and digoxin Phenytoin, rifampin, H_2 antagonists: decreased itraconazole levels Coumarin-like drugs: enhanced anticoagulant effect Isoniazid: decreased itraconazole levels Oral hypoglycemic agents: enhanced hypoglycemic effects

ine, doses of zidovudine can be decreased by one third.[66]

DRUGS USED TO TREAT FUNGAL INFECTIONS (Chapter 23)

Amphotericin B

Toxic reactions associated with both amphotericin B and liposomal amphotericin B therapy in humans include fever, chills, nausea, electrolyte imbalance, and renal toxicity (Table 9–2). Liposomal amphotericin B infusion may also lead to cardiopulmonary toxic effects.[68]

Caution must be taken to monitor the serum potassium concentration when digitalis and amphotericin are coadministered. Carbenicillin or ticarcillin given concomitantly with amphotericin B may also exacerbate hypokalemia. Amphotericin B administered with either miconazole or ketoconazole may be less effective than amphotericin B alone.[96] Nephrotoxicity attributed to the concurrent use of gentamicin and amphotericin B has been described in four patients.[95] Both antibiotics are nephrotoxic and may have additive toxic effects when given in combination.

Flucytosine

Nausea and vomiting occur frequently with flucytosine administration. Spacing ingestion in 5- to 10-minute intervals may help alleviate this problem. The hematologic toxicity is believed to be dose related, and excessive serum levels are associated with bone marrow toxicity. Agranulocytosis and aplastic anemia have been reported. Hepatic necrosis has been reported but is rare and is probably dose related.[5]

Fluconazole

Fluconazole given either orally or intravenously is generally well tolerated. In approximately 4000 patients treated with fluconazole, the overall incidence of side effects was 16%.[34] Hepatotoxicity and exfoliative skin disorders are rare occurrences with fluconazole treatment.

There are several potential drug interactions with fluconazole.[61] Coadministration of fluconazole and cyclosporin A may lead to the accumulation of cyclosporin A, and monitoring of cyclosporin A level is recommended.[61] Rifampin decreases the half-life of fluconazole. Thus, increasing the dosage of fluconazole may be necessary when coadministered with rifampin.[17,61] Concomitant administration of fluconazole and phenytoin results in a clinically significant increase in the phenytoin concentrations.[9,61] Serum concentrations of phenytoin, therefore, should be closely monitored, and the necessity of modifying the dosage of phenytoin for patients being treated with fluconazole should be anticipated. Concurrent use of fluconazole with tolbutamide, chlorpropamide, glyburide, and glipizide[34,61] has increased the plasma concentrations of these oral hypoglycemic agents, and hypoglycemia has been noted. Blood glucose concentrations should be monitored, and reduction in the dose of the oral hypoglycemic agents may be necessary. Concurrent use of warfarin with fluconazole may decrease the metabolism of warfarin, resulting in an increase in prothrombin time.[61] Prothrombin time must be monitored carefully in patients receiving warfarin or a coumarin-type anticoagulant.

Ketoconazole

Nausea and vomiting commonly occur with ketoconazole administration. The drug may be given with food, but absorption is reduced. Reversible hepatitis has been observed and does not appear to be dose related. Adrenal suppression and gynecomastia have been reported and probably are due to inhibition of steroid synthesis.[5]

Plasma levels of ketoconazole are markedly reduced when the drug is administered with cimetidine, antacids, or ddI.[8,61] Since bioavailability of oral ketoconazole is already reduced in patients with AIDS, largely as a result of gastric hypochlorhydria,[58] and because the absorption of ketoconazole requires a gastric pH <3–4, ketoconazole should be administered at least 2 hours before antacid administration or in an acidic fluid, such as fruit juice. Coadministration of cyclosporin A and ketoconazole sig-

nificantly increases the serum levels and prolongation of the half-life of cyclosporin A.[61] Coadministration of ketoconazole and phenytoin may alter the disposition of both drugs.[61] As ketoconazole can inhibit the metabolism of terfenadine and torsades de pointes has been reported following coadministration of these two drugs,[78] such combination therapy should be avoided. Because concomitant administration of rifampin and ketoconazole resulted in an 80% decrease in ketoconazole levels,[61] these drugs should not be given together. Isoniazid can accelerate the metabolism of ketoconazole, sometimes requiring increased doses of ketoconazole for optimal therapeutic effect.

Itraconazole

In a number of clinical trials conducted in the United States of patients with systemic fungal disease with itraconazole, treatment was discontinued in 10.5% of a total of 602 patients as a result of adverse reactions. These adverse reactions primarily consisted of nausea (10.6%), vomiting (5.1%), diarrhea (3.3%), rash (8.6%), headache (3.8%), and fatigue (2.8%).

Coadministration of terfenadine with itraconazole is contraindicated. Rare cases of serious cardiovascular adverse events, including death, ventricular tachycardia, and torsades de pointes, have been observed in patients taking these drugs together because itraconazole increased terfenadine concentrations.

Pharmacokinetic data indicate that ketoconazole inhibits the metabolism of astemizole, resulting in elevated plasma levels of astemizole and its active metabolite desmethylastemizole, which may prolong QT intervals. Based on the chemical resemblance of itraconazole and ketoconazole, coadministration of astemizole and itraconazole is contraindicated. Coadministration of itraconazole and cyclosporine or digoxin has led to increased plasma concentrations of the latter two drugs.[53] When digoxin is given concurrently with itraconazole, digoxin concentrations should be monitored, and the dose of digoxin may need to be reduced. Although no studies have been conducted, case reports suggest that the dose of cyclosporine should be reduced by 50% when itraconazole doses greater than 100 mg daily are given. Cyclosporine levels should be monitored frequently, and the dose should be adjusted appropriately.

When itraconazole was coadministered with phenytoin, rifampin, or H_2 antagonists, reduced plasma concentrations of itraconazole were reported.[99] Plasma concentrations of itraconazole should be monitored when any of these drugs is taken concurrently, and the dose of itraconazole should be increased if necessary. Phenytoin can decrease the AUC of itraconazole by 90%.[25] This magnitude of interaction is likely to account for reports of therapeutic failures in patients with fungal infections who are receiving both itraconazole and phenytoin. Because monitoring of itraconazole serum concentrations in patients is not currently routinely available, patients with fungal infections who are receiving phenytoin should be treated with an alternative antifungal agent.

It has been reported that itraconazole enhanced the anticoagulant effect of coumarin-like drugs.[108] Therefore, prothrombin time should be monitored carefully in patients receiving itraconazole and coumarin-like drugs simultaneously. Plasma concentrations of azole antifungal agents are reduced when given concurrently with isoniazid.[7] Itraconazole plasma concentrations should be monitored when itraconazole and isoniazid are coadministered. Severe hypoglycemia has been reported in patients concomitantly receiving azole antifungal agents and oral hypoglycemic agents. Blood glucose concentrations should be monitored carefully when itraconazole and oral hypoglycemic agents are coadministered.

DRUGS USED TO TREAT TOXOPLASMOSIS (Chapter 24)

Pyrimethamine, Sulfadiazine

Treatment with pyrimethamine and sulfadiazine for *Toxoplasma* encephalitis is effective in 80% to 90% of patients.[20,67] Unfortunately, toxicity develops in 60% to 70% of patients and has resulted in the discontinuation of therapy in 30% to 45% of patients.[37,67] Adverse reactions include severe rash, leukopenia, thrombocytopenia, and elevated liver enzyme levels.[37,67] Because therapy for toxoplasmosis in patients with AIDS is lifelong, bone marrow toxicity may also preclude therapy with antiretroviral agents, such as zidovudine. In addition, there is some evidence that zidovudine antagonizes the antitoxoplasma activity of pyrimethamine.[46] Sulfadiazine-induced crystalluria has been described in patients with AIDS.[77]

Serious pancytopenia and megaloblastic anemia have been reported in patients under treatment with pyrimethamine and either trimethoprim-sulfamethoxazole or other sulfonamides.[95] The additive adverse reactions seem to reflect a depression of the normal folate metabolism caused by the combined actions of both drugs. Hematologic variables should be monitored closely if both drugs are given simultaneously.

Clindamycin

See under "Drugs Used to Treat *Pneumocystis carinii* Pneumonia."

DRUGS USED TO TREAT *MYCOBACTERIUM TUBERCULOSIS* INFECTION (Chapter 22)

Isoniazid

Isoniazid frequently causes a rise in serum transaminases, although clinical hepatitis is rare. The frequency of hepatotoxicity rises proportionally with the age of the individual ($\leq 0.3\%$ in persons <35 years of age, $\leq 2.3\%$ in persons >50 years of age). In addition, risk is increased in persons who are slow acetylators of the drug, in those who ingest alcohol daily (Table 9–3),[49] and in those with preexisting liver disease who are taking rifampin concomitantly.

A pyridoxine-responsive peripheral neuropathy may occur, which frequently is greater in persons who acetylate the drug slowly[92] or who are malnourished. Rash and nausea may occur occasionally. Use of aluminum-containing antacids may decrease the absorption of isoniazid. Inhibition of hepatic microsomal enzymes by isoniazid can result in elevation of phenytoin, carbamazepine, coumarin-like anticoagulants, benzodiazepines, and theophylline serum levels.[54,100] Flushing may occur in some patients who ingest certain fish or cheese while receiving isoniazid because of inhibition of histamine metabolism by isoniazid.[54] Isoniazid may cause niacin deficiency by inhibiting niacin incorporation into nicotinamide adenine dinucleotide (NAD).[100] Increased metabolism of

TABLE 9–3. ANTIMYCOBACTERIAL THERAPY

Drug	Major Adverse Reactions	Interactions
Mycobacterium tuberculosis		
Isoniazid	Transaminase elevation Peripheral neuropathy Nausea Rash	Antacids: decreased absorption of isoniazid Carbamazepine, coumarin, benzodiazepines, theophylline, phenytoin: increased levels of these drugs by isoniazid Cycloserine: increased CNS toxicity Ketoconazole: increased ketoconazole metabolism Sulfonylureas: loss of glucose control
Rifampin	Transaminase elevation Orange discoloration of bodily secretions Hypersensitivity syndrome	Oral contraceptives, corticosteroids, cyclosporine, coumarin, methadone, theophylline, digoxin, levothyroxine, quinidine, propranolol, dapsone: increased metabolism of these drugs by rifampin Ketoconazole, fluconazole: decreased levels of ketoconazole and fluconazole Tolbutamide, trimethoprim: decreased half-life of tolbutamide and trimethoprim Aminosalicylates: impair absorption of rifampin
Ethambutol	Retrobulbar neuritis Hyperuricemia	Aluminum salts: decreased ethambutol absorption
Pyrazinamide	Transaminase elevation Hyperuricemia Arthralgia Nausea	Probenecid: increased half-life of probenecid
Mycobacterium avium		
Ciprofloxacin, ofloxacin	Nausea/vomiting Diarrhea Abdominal pain	Theophylline: increased levels of theophylline Antacids: decreased absorption of quinolones ddI: decreased ciprofloxacin bioavailability Sucralfate: decreased levels of ciprofloxacin
Clofazimine	Skin discoloration Nausea Retinal degeneration	Rifampin: decreased absorption of rifampin
Clarithromycin	Nausea Diarrhea Abdominal pain Headache	Theophylline, carbamazepine: increased levels of theophylline and carbamazepine Zidovudine: increased levels of zidovudine
Azithromycin	Diarrhea Abdominal pain Headache Dizziness	Antacids: decreased azithromycin absorption
Rifabutin	Rash Neutropenia Gastrointestinal intolerance Headache Myalgias	Zidovudine: decreased zidovudine levels Drugs (e.g., phenytoin, warfarin) metabolized by cytochrome P-450 enzymes potentially can interact with rifabutin

isoniazid, with resultant decreased effectiveness, may occur with alcohol ingestion or with concurrent use of prednisolone. Because isoniazid may increase the already troublesome CNS toxicity of cycloserine, caution should be used when these two drugs are given together. Since isoniazid can increase the metabolism of ketoconazole, increased doses of ketoconazole may be needed. Blood glucose should be monitored carefully in patients receiving concomitant sulfonylureas, as isoniazid may lead to a loss of glucose control.

Rifampin

Hepatotoxicity caused by rifampin administration is relatively uncommon, occurring in ≤1% of patients.[32] In the early weeks of therapy, interference with excretion by rifampin may cause a transient elevation in serum bilirubin. A hypersensitivity syndrome comprised of flushing, fever, redness of the eyes, and thrombocytopenia may occur, generally within 3 hours of the ingestion of the drug, particularly in patients receiving intermittent therapy.[32] Rifampin causes a reddish discoloration of body fluids, such as urine, tears, and sweat.

Although early reports suggested that antituberculous medications were tolerated as well in HIV-infected patients as in others, recently investigators have reported an increased frequency of adverse effects, particularly in association with rifampin administration. In one study, adverse drug reactions to antituberculous medications occurred more frequently in patients with AIDS than in non-AIDS patients (26% versus 3%).[15] Another study found a frequency of side effects of 39% in HIV-infected patients compared with 22% of seronegative controls. The most frequent side effects were elevation in serum transaminase levels and fever.[93] In a third study, 18% of patients required an alteration in antituberculous therapy because of adverse effects, substantially higher than the 3.7% rate reported from the same clinic in non–HIV-infected patients.[90] Twelve percent of adverse reactions were believed associated with rifampin therapy and consisted primarily of rash and hepatitis. In one patient, life-threatening anaphylaxis was reported in association with ingestion of rifampin.[105] Nearly all major side effects occurred during the first 2 months of therapy.[90]

The AUC of ketoconazole decreases by >80% when administered concurrently with rifampin, and serum levels of ketoconazole decrease,[25] causing the Food and Drug Administration to recommend that the two drugs not be administered together.[61] Concurrent administration of fluconazole with rifampin also results in a decrease in the AUC and half-life of fluconazole.[17] However, the magnitude of change is considerably smaller (~23%). Thus, administering fluconazole together with rifampin is acceptable, although an increase in the dosage of fluconazole may be necessary.[61]

There are many potential drug interactions with rifampin because of its induction of enzymes in the cytochrome P-450 system. The half-life of oral hypoglycemic agents, such as tolbutamide, is shortened with concurrent administration of rifampin.[54] Induction of liver enzymes by rifampin may cause increased metabolism of oral contraceptive agents, corticosteroids, cyclosporine, coumarin-like anticoagulants, methadone, theophylline, levothyroxine, digoxin, quinidine, and propranolol, so that close observation, monitoring of serum levels if possible, and adjustment of dosage of these agents or identification of alternative agents for a given indication may be necessary in the patient receiving rifampin.[54] A similar mechanism of interaction may cause a sevenfold to tenfold decrease in serum levels of dapsone when administered concurrently with rifampin. However, this decrease was not believed to be clinically important when its use was evaluated in patients with leprosy.[84]

Aminosalicylates may impair the absorption of rifampin, resulting in decreased serum concentrations. For this reason, ingestion of the two should be separated by at least 6 hours. Concurrent use of rifampin and trimethoprim may significantly increase the rate of clearance and shorten the elimination half-life of trimethoprim.[95]

Ethambutol

Retrobulbar neuritis is the main complication of ethambutol therapy. Symptoms include central scotomata, red-green color blindness, and blurred vision. This complication is dose related, occurring in ~5% of patients receiving 25 mg/kg/day and rarely if at all in patients receiving 15 mg/kg/day.[91] It apparently is not related to the cumulative dose of drug administered. Hyperuricemia occasionally occurs. Aluminum salts may decrease the absorption of ethambutol, but the reduction in absorption is generally small and variable, and it is doubtful that a significant clinical effect will occur.

Pyrazinamide

The most important side effect associated with pyrazinamide therapy is hepatotoxicity. However, the risk for it is small and is related to administration of large doses of the drug (40 to 50 mg/kg/day) for prolonged periods of time. There is no apparent additive risk for hepatotoxicity when pyrazinamide is administered in combination with isoniazid and rifampin. The other main side effect is arthralgia, associated with the increased serum levels of uric acid due to suppression of urinary secretion and excretion. Acute gouty arthritis, however, is rare. Nausea or vomiting or both may occur, although rarely.[1]

Pyrazinamide causes a prolonged half-life of probenecid, so its suppression of urate excretion may be neutralized. Rifampin may enhance the renal excretion of uric acid, in both the presence and absence of pyrazinamide.[95]

DRUGS USED TO TREAT *MYCOBACTERIUM AVIUM* COMPLEX INFECTION (Chapter 21)

Rifampin

See under "Drugs Used to Treat *Mycobacterium tuberculosis* Infection."

Ethambutol

See under "Drugs Used to Treat *Mycobacterium tuberculosis* Infection."

Quinolones (Ciprofloxacin, Ofloxacin)

The quinolones are generally well tolerated. Gastrointestinal symptoms have been reported most frequently (3% to 6%) and have included nausea, abdominal discomfort, vomiting, and diarrhea.[12,40] Colitis associated with *Clostridium difficile* has been reported infrequently after quinolone therapy.[40] Stimulatory effects on the central nervous system, such as anxiety, nervousness, insomnia, euphoria, and tremor, occur in 1% to 4% of patients. Seizures have been reported with ciprofloxacin, and it should be used with caution in epileptic patients. Hallucinations are reported rarely in patients administered ciprofloxacin.

Theophylline serum levels can markedly increase in some patients with concurrent use of ciprofloxacin.[12] Therefore, theophylline levels should be monitored in patients who receive theophylline and ciprofloxacin concurrently. Simultaneous administration of antacids containing magnesium or aluminum hydroxide or both with the quinolones leads to a reduction in the bioavailability of the latter.[81] It is believed that ciprofloxacin forms insoluble chelates with aluminum and magnesium ions in the gut, reducing absorption. This interaction is of potential concern not only in patients using antacids for gastrointestinal symptoms but also in patients with compromised renal function and on hemodialysis or continuous ambulatory peritoneal dialysis who use antacids as phosphate binders. Similarly, cations in ddI tablets can reduce the bioavailability of ciprofloxacin.[86] Sucralfate can significantly reduce ciprofloxacin concentrations, and the two drugs should not be administered concurrently.[31]

Clofazimine

Clofazimine therapy is generally tolerated well in the doses administered to treat *M. avium* complex infection (50 to 100 mg/day). Adverse reactions include a reversible discoloration of the skin and body fluids, gastrointestinal intolerance, and visceral deposition of crystal.[41] Generalized retinal degeneration believed to be due to clofazimine has been described, so visual acuity should be closely monitored in patients receiving long-term therapy.[19] In six male patients with leprosy who received rifampin in conjunction with clofazimine, a statistically significant reduction in the rate of rifampin absorption and time to reach maximum serum concentration was noted.[30] However, since bioavailability was unaffected, the interaction probably is not clinically significant.

Clarithromycin

Clarithromycin has shown promise in the treatment of disseminated *M. avium* complex infection. It is fairly well tolerated as a standard dose of 1 g given orally twice a day. In a large series of 3437 patients, 18% of the patients developed mild to moderate adverse reactions.[2] The most common adverse reactions were nausea (3%), diarrhea (3%), dyspepsia (2%), abdominal pain (2%), and headache (2%) (Table 9–3). Clarithromycin can inhibit the metabolism of theophylline and carbamazepine and thus increase the serum concentrations of both.[31,96] It can also increase the concentrations of digoxin by altering the flora in the distal portion of the intestine that metabolizes digoxin.[75] Therefore, the concentrations of theophylline, carbamazepine, and digoxin should be monitored closely in patients receiving clarithromycin concomitantly. Clarithromycin may also increase the concentrations of zidovudine, although the clinical significance of this interaction is unclear.

Azithromycin

The safety and tolerance of azithromycin were assessed in approximately 4000 patients. Diarrhea was the most common adverse reaction (3.6%), followed by abdominal pain (2.5%) and other gastrointestinal complaints. Central nervous system effects, predominantly headache and dizziness, occurred in 1.3% of patients.[45]

There are no published prospective drug interaction studies with azithromycin. Until further data are available, caution should be used when administering azithromycin concomitantly with such drugs as theophylline, carbamazepine, phenytoin, and warfarin, all known to interact with erythromycin and clarithromycin (Table 9–3).

Rifabutin

Results of phase III, placebo-controlled studies are conflicting with regard to the toxicity of the rifamycin antibiotic rifabutin. Some investigators have reported no increase in the frequency of adverse reactions, whereas others using the same dosage (300 mg/day) have noted an increased incidence of rash and neutropenia.[11,97] Other potential adverse effects include gastrointestinal intolerance, headache, and myalgias. In studies using doses of up to 2400 mg/day, however, painless discoloration of the urine,[98] flushing erythema of the head and trunk,[98] skin discoloration, hepatitis,[89] and reversible arthralgias or arthritis have been reported. In one study, two of nine patients developing arthritis also had uveitis and stomatitis.[89] The potential drug interactions have been incompletely evaluated to date. However, since induction of the cytochrome P-450 enzyme system occurs in association with rifabutin treatment, certain interactions may be expected with drugs (e.g., warfarin, phenytoin, oral contraceptives, dapsone) that are also metabolized by the cytochrome P-450 system. In addition,

serum concentrations of zidovudine were decreased by about half when rifabutin was administered concomitantly.[75] The clinical significance of this interaction is unknown.

DRUGS USED TO TREAT CYTOMEGALOVIRUS INFECTION
(Chapter 26)

Ganciclovir

The most frequent toxicities occurring with ganciclovir therapy are those involving the hematopoietic system. In particular, neutropenia and thrombocytopenia may occur and are generally reversible with discontinuation of ganciclovir therapy. Although the incidence of lowering of the granulocyte count is approximately 40%, this is a dose-limiting problem in <20% of individuals.[100] Thrombocytopenia may also occur, although less frequently (incidence, ~20%; dose-limiting frequency, 5% to 10%). Other than neutropenia and thrombocytopenia, the most frequent adverse events observed are anemia, fever, rash, and abnormalities of liver function tests (Table 9–4).

In several reports, coadministration of ganciclovir with zidovudine has resulted in additive hematologic toxicity.[39,76] Many patients are unable to tolerate these two drugs in combination. Less frequent drug interactions include the occurrence of generalized seizures in six patients receiving imipenem-cilastatin concurrently with ganciclovir, and a reduction in renal clearance because of inhibition of renal tubular secretion by probenecid.

TABLE 9–4. ANTIVIRAL AGENTS

Drug	Major Adverse Reactions	Interactions
Acyclovir	Nausea Headache Nephrotoxicity Neurologic toxicity	Probenecid: decreased acyclovir clearance
Ganciclovir	Neutropenia Thrombocytopenia Anemia Fever Rash Transaminases elevation	Zidovudine: additive hematologic toxicity Imipenem-cilastatin: increased risk of seizures Amphotericin B, antineoplastic agents, flucytosine: increased bone marrow toxicity
Foscarnet	Nephrotoxicity Hypocalcemia Hypercalcemia Neurologic toxicity	Nephrotoxic agents: additive nephrotoxicity Pentamidine: additive hypocalcemia and nephrotoxicity

Foscarnet

The spectrum of potential toxicities associated with foscarnet therapy is broad (Table 9–4). Impairment in renal function is the most common dose-limiting toxicity, is generally reversible, and is often associated with proteinuria. Postmortem studies of patients with acute renal failure occurring in association with foscarnet therapy have demonstrated acute tubular necrosis or tubular interstitial nephritis.[82] In several patients, crystals have been demonstrated in the glomerular capillaries.[4] Polydipsia and polyuria due to nephrogenic diabetes insipidus also have been described.[28] Investigations have suggested that careful adjustment of dosage according to serial serum creatinine and weight determinations and hydration with normal saline solution as an adjunct to foscarnet infusion may prevent renal toxicity in most patients.[23] In addition, the avoidance of concomitant administration of other drugs with nephrotoxic potential, such as pentamidine, aminoglycosides, and amphotericin B, has been recommended.

As foscarnet is a pyrophosphate analog, its administration might be expected to result in altered calcium or phosphorous metabolism. Serum calcium levels may either increase or decrease during foscarnet administration. Chelation of ionized calcium is believed to occur, especially after larger doses. Concomitant treatment with pentamidine administration in one case series of four patients resulted in severe symptomatic hypocalcemia.[109] Also, hyperphosphatemia is a relatively common occurrence in patients receiving foscarnet (although generally not a cause of adverse symptoms). Possible explanations include the replacement of phosphorous in bone by foscarnet and the inhibition of sodium and phosphate transport across renal tubular membranes.[16]

DRUGS USED TO TREAT HERPES SIMPLEX AND VARICELLA ZOSTER VIRAL INFECTION (Chapter 26)

Acyclovir

Acyclovir is, in general, a remarkably well-tolerated agent. When administered orally (2 to 4 g/day), the most frequent adverse effects are nausea (2% to 8%) and headache (0.6% to 6%). Rarely are side effects dose limiting. High-dose intravenous infusion has been associated

with transient rises in serum creatinine concentration. Dehydration, preexisting renal insufficiency, and high-dose bolus infusion may predispose the patient to precipitation of the drug in the renal tubules, causing a reversible crystalline nephropathy.[24] Gastrointestinal symptoms may be associated with intravenous infusion as well, particularly when peak serum levels of acyclovir exceed 25 μg/ml.[3] Also, encephalopathic and neuropsychiatric changes have been noted sporadically in patients receiving intravenous acyclovir (~1%).[101]

As probenecid can decrease the clearance of acyclovir by 30%, acyclovir dosage may need to be reduced when these two drugs are coadministered if the dose of acyclovir is above 10 mg/kg/day or there is preexisting renal insufficiency.

Foscarnet

See under "Drugs Used to Treat Cytomegalovirus Infection."

ANTIRETROVIRAL AGENTS
(Chapter 8)

Zidovudine

The major toxicities associated with zidovudine are anemia and neutropenia.[29] They are inversely related to the CD4 lymphocyte count, hemoglobin concentration, and granulocyte count and directly related to dosage and duration of therapy.[18] Significant anemia most commonly occurs after 4 to 6 weeks of therapy. Myopathy, nausea, malaise, fatigue, and insomnia also may occur in zidovudine-treated patients (Table 9–5). Zidovudine has been associated with seizures, macular edema, and the Stevens-Johnson syndrome, although the causal relationship is uncertain.[71]

The combination of zidovudine and ganciclovir is poorly tolerated in patients with AIDS and serious cytomegalovirus disease, with 82% developing severe to life-threatening hematologic toxicity.[39] It is thought that the toxicity is not a result of pharmacologic interaction but of a combined myelosuppressive toxicity of the two drugs. Therefore, close monitoring of hematologic characteristics should accompany concurrent administration.

Probenecid inhibits hepatic glucuronidation and secretion of zidovudine through the renal tubules, resulting in increased serum concen-

TABLE 9–5. ANTIRETROVIRAL AGENTS

Drug	Major Adverse Reactions	Interactions
Zidovudine (AZT)	Anemia Neutropenia Myopathy Anorexia Nausea Fatigue Headache Malaise Myalgia Insomnia	Ganciclovir: increased hematologic toxicity Probenecid: increased zidovudine levels Trimethoprim-sulfamethoxazole: increased anemia and neutropenia; trimethoprim increased zidovudine levels Phenytoin: increased or decreased phenytoin levels Methadone: decreased zidovudine metabolism
Dideoxyinosine (ddI)	Pancreatitis Peripheral neuropathy Hyperamylasemia Diarrhea (due to antacid) Hyperuricemia Transaminase elevation	Dapsone, ketoconazole, quinolones, tetracycline: decreased absorption by ddI Sulfadiazine, pyrazinamide: increased urate levels Pentamidine: increased risk of pancreatitis
Zalcitabine (ddC)	Peripheral neuropathy Pancreatitis Vomiting Rash Stomatitis	Drugs that can cause peripheral neuropathy or pancreatitis: additive or synergistic toxicity with ddC
Stavudine (d4T)	Peripheral neuropathy, pancreatitis, arthralgia, hypersensitivity, myalgia, anemia, asthenia, gastrointestinal disturbances, headache, and insomnia	Medications associated with neuropathy should be avoided during stavudine therapy
Lamivudine (3TC)	Pancreatitis, peripheral neuropathy, rash, cough, dizziness, fatigue, gastrointestinal distress, headache, insomnia, and hair loss	Trimethoprim-sulfamethoxazole: increased lamivudine levels Zidovudine: increased zidovudine levels Medications associated with pancreatitis, and peripheral neuropathy should be avoided during lamivudine therapy
Saquinavir	Diarrhea Abdominal discomfort Nausea Asthenia Rash Paresthesia	Rifampin, rifabutin: decreased saquinavir levels Ketoconazole: increased saquinavir levels
Ritonavir	Nausea Vomiting Diarrhea Asthenia Circumoral paresthesia Headache	Clarithromycin: increased clarithromycin levels Ethinyl estradiol: decreased ethinyl estradiol levels Theophylline: decreased theophylline levels Rifabutin: increased rifabutin levels
Indinavir	Nephrolithiasis, asymptomatic hyperbilirubinemia, abdominal pain, asthenia/fatigue, flank pain, malaise, nausea, diarrhea, vomiting, acid regurgitation, anorexia, dry mouth, back pain, headache, insomnia, dizziness, somnolence and taste perversion	Rifabutin: increased in rifabutin levels Ketoconazole: increased in indinavir levels Terfenadine, cisapride, astemizole, triazolam, midazolam, rifampin: potential drug interactions can occur with indinavir, do not recommend co-administration of these drugs with indinavir

trations and a prolonged elimination half-life.[22] These results may increase the risk of toxicity or permit a reduction in daily zidovudine dosage. However, one small trial observed a very high incidence of rash in patients receiving probenecid concurrently with zidovudine.[50]

Anemia and neutropenia are more common when zidovudine and trimethoprim-sulfameth-oxazole are combined. Trimethoprim can decrease the renal clearance of zidovudine and possibly increase the serum concentration of zidovudine.[63]

Zidovudine can either decrease or increase phenytoin concentrations. Therefore, phenytoin concentrations should be monitored in patients receiving both agents. Methadone has been shown to decrease zidovudine metabolism, but no dosage adjustment is currently recommended.

2′,3′-Dideoxyinosine (ddI)

The major clinical toxicities associated with ddI therapy include pancreatitis and peripheral neuropathy. In a phase I study,[60] reversible neuropathy was related to both daily dosage and to total dose of drug administered. The incidence of neuropathy was 34% of all phase I patients treated with doses at or below the currently recommended dose but was 14.2% in controlled trials. In one study, acute pancreatitis occurred in 5 of 37 (13.5%) patients[60] and was not clearly related to the dose of ddI. In the U.S. Expanded Access Program, 13.8% of 166 persons developed pancreatitis, of whom 2 died.[94] However, in randomized controlled trials, frequency of pancreatitis has been lower, approximately 2.3%. Predisposing factors to the development of pancreatitis with administration of ddI include a prior history of pancreatitis, advanced HIV disease, and low CD4 count ($<50/mm^3$). Preliminary reports suggest that concurrent administration of ganciclovir with ddI may increase the frequency of acute pancreatitis, but this has not been well documented. Because both pentamidine and ddI can cause pancreatitis, ddI therapy should be withheld during acute *P. carinii* pneumonia treatment with pentamidine. Since there have been instances of pancreatitis associated with aerosolized pentamidine, cotherapy with ddI should be undertaken with caution.

Drugs that require an acidic environment for absorption (e.g., traconazole ketoconazole, dapsone) should be ingested at least 2 hours before ddI. The buffered vehicle for ddI (i.e., a magnesium-aluminum antacid) produces an acutely alkaline gastric environment that may decrease the absorption of these drugs. ddI should not be ingested concurrently with tetracycline or the quinolone antibiotics because absorption of antimicrobials may be impaired.

Because food reduces the bioavailability of ddI by twofold, it is recommended that ddI be given under fasting conditions.[88]

Optic neuritis[56] and fulminant hepatitis[57] have been associated with ddI therapy. Other dose-limiting toxicities include elevation in liver function tests, diarrhea, and abdominal pain.

Zalcitabine (ddC)

The most common adverse effect reported with ddC is a dose-dependent sensorimotor peripheral neuropathy occurring in 17% to 31% of treated patients (Table 9–5).[73] Other potential adverse effects include esophageal ulceration,[43] congestive cardiomyopathy,[38] arthralgias,[73] and dermatologic eruptions.[10] Rash occurs fairly commonly and develops during the first 4 to 6 weeks of therapy but usually resolves despite continuation of therapy.[10] There are isolated case reports of acute pancreatitis due to ddC, but the incidence appears to be less than 1%. However, caution must be observed in patients with a prior history of pancreatitis and in those with other risk factors for pancreatitis, such as alcohol abuse. One study described a syndrome of rash, fever, stomatitis, and varying other manifestations in patients receiving intravenous doses of ddC ranging from 0.03 mg/kg q8h to 0.25 mg/kg q8h.[107] A single case of anaphylaxis and several cases of urticaria have been reported.

Zalcitabine can decrease the AUC of isoniazid by 40%. The mechanism for this interaction is a chemical binding of the excipient of zalcitabine to isoniazid. Dosing of isoniazid and zalcitabine should be separated by at least 1 hour.[64] Zalcitabine can increase the maximum concentration and time to reach maximum concentration of dapsone. This interaction, however, is probably not clinically significant.[65] Because ddC can cause peripheral neuropathy and pancreatitis (concomitant administration of medications associated with the development of peripheral neuropathy (e.g., isoniazid, vincristine) or with pancreatitis (e.g., parenteral pentamidine) should also be avoided.

Stavudine (d4T)

Stavudine (d4T) is indicated for the treatment of patients with advanced HIV infection who are intolerant of approved therapies. The most frequently reported adverse effect with stavudine is peripheral neuropathy. Peripheral neuropathy occurred in 15 to 21% of patients treated with stavudine. Pancreatitis has been reported less than 1% in patients enrolled in clinical trials. Other adverse effects that have been reported with less frequency include arthralgia, hypersensitivity, myalgia, anemia, asthenia, gastrointestinal disturbances, headache, and insomnia.*

Since stavudine has been shown to cause peripheral neuropathy, medications associated with the development of neuropathy should be avoided during stavudine therapy.

Lamivudine (3TC)

Lamivudine (3TC) is indicated in combination with zidovudine, in the treatment of HIV infection or AIDS. In one study, 14 of 97 pediatric patients (14%) being treated with lamivudine monotherapy developed pancreatitis. Pancreatitis was seen in only 3 of 656 adult patients (<0.5%) who received lamivudine. Paresthesias and peripheral neuropathy are also reported more frequently in children. Other adverse effects that have been reported include rash, cough, dizziness, fatigue, gastrointestinal distress, headache, insomnia and hair loss.**

Concurrent administration of trimethoprim-sulfamethoxazole resulted in a 44% increase in lamivudine AUC and a 30% decrease in lamivudine renal clearance. No adjustment in dose is necessary unless the patient has renal function impairment.

Concurrent administration of lamivudine resulted in a 39% increase in the peak plasma concentration of zidovudine, this increase is not thought to be significant to patient safety.**

Since lamivudine has been shown to cause pancreatitis and peripheral neuropathy, medications associated with the development of pancreatitis and peripheral neuropathy should be avoided during lamivudine therapy.

Saquinavir

Saquinavir in combination with nucleoside analogues is indicated for the treatment of advanced HIV infection. In 688 patients who received saquinavir alone or in combination with zidovudine or zalcitabine, the most frequently reported adverse events were diarrhea, abdominal discomfort, and nausea.[44]

There are no drug interactions reported with saquinavir and the concomitant administration

of zidovudine or zalcitabine. However, the coadministration of saquinavir with rifampin or rifabutin resulted in decreased AUC of saquinavir by 80% and 40%, respectively. Because of this significant interaction, an alternative antimycobacterial agent is recommended for patients who are also receiving saquinavir. Ketoconazole can increase the maximum concentration of saquinavir by threefold; however, the clinical significance of this interaction is unknown.

Ritonavir

The safety profile of ritonavir is similar to saquinavir. Nausea, vomiting, diarrhea, asthenia, circumoral paresthesia, and headache were the adverse events most commonly reported by patients taking ritonavir.[21]

Drug interactions that have been reported with ritonavir that do not require any dosage adjustments include didanosine, fluconazole, sulfamethoxazole, and zidovudine.[13,14] The coadministration of clarithromycin and ritonavir can increase the AUC of clarithromycin by 77%. Dosage adjustment may be required especially in patients with renal dysfunction. Ritonavir can decrease the AUC of ethinyl estradiol by 41%. The dose of ethinyl estradiol needs to be increased or another contraceptive should be given. Ritonavir can also decrease the AUC of theophylline by 45%. An increase in the theophylline dose may be required.

Ritonavir can significantly affect the pharmacokinetics of rifabutin, with increases in mean maximum concentrations and AUC values by approximately 2 and 3.5-fold, respectively. Because of the significant increases, an alternative for antimycobacterial prophylaxis or therapy is recommended for patients taking ritonavir.†

Indinavir

Nephrolithiasis, including flank pain with or without hematuria, has been reported in approximately 4% (79/2205) of patients receiving indinavir in clinical trials. In general, these events were not associated with renal dysfunction and resolved with hydration and temporary

---

* Zerit (Stavudine), Bristol-Myers Squibb, Package Insert, July 1994.

** Epivir (Lamivudine), Glaxo Wellcome, Package Insert, January 1996.

---

† Norvir (Ritonavir), Abbott Laboratories, Ritonavir Formulary Kit, January 1996.

interruption of therapy (e.g., 1–3 days).[‡] Asymptomatic hyperbilirubinemia has occurred in approximately 10% of patients treated with indinavir. In <1% this was associated with elevations in ALT or AST. Hyperbilirubinemia and nephrolithiasis occurred more frequently at doses exceeding 2.4 g/day compared to doses ≤2.4 g/day.[‡]

Drug-related clinical adverse experiences of moderate or severe intensity in ≥2% of patients treated with indinavir include abdominal pain, asthenia/fatigue, flank pain, malaise, nausea, diarrhea, vomiting, acid regurgitation, anorexia, dry mouth, back pain, headache, insomnia, dizziness, somnolence and taste perversion.

The administration of indinavir with rifabutin can result in a 32% decrease in indinavir

---

‡ Crixivan (Indinavir Sulfate), Merck & Co., Inc. Package Insert, March 1996.

AUC and a 204% increase in rifabutin AUC. When indinavir is used concomitantly with rifabutin, the dose of rifabutin should be decreased to half the standard dose.

Ketoconazole can increase the AUC of indinavir by 68%. Dose reduction of indinavir should be considered when administering ketoconazole concurrently.

Drug interactions that have been reported with indinavir, that do not require dose modification include zidovudine, lamivudine, stavudine, ethinyl estradiol, cimetidine, quinidine, grapefruit juice, trimethoprim-sulfamethoxazole, fluconazole, isoniazid, and clarithromycin.

Because of the potential interactions between indinavir and terfenadine, cisapride, astemizole, triazolam, midazolam, and rifampin, the manufacturer recommends that these drugs should not be administered concurrently with indinavir.[‡]

REFERENCES

1. Alford RH: Antimycobacterial agents. In Mandell GL, Douglas RG, Bennett JE, eds. Anti-Infective Therapy. New York, John Wiley & Sons, 1985, p 290
2. Anderson G. Clarithromycin in the treatment of community-acquired lower respiratory tract infections. J Hosp Infect 19(A):21–27, 1991
3. Bean B, Aeppli D: Adverse effects of high-dose intravenous acyclovir in ambulatory patients with acute herpes zoster. J Infect Dis 151:362, 1985
4. Beaufils H, Deray G, Katlana C, et al: Foscarnet and crystals in glomerular capillary lumens (Letter). Lancet 336:755, 1990
5. Bennett JE: Antifungal agents. In Mandell GL, Douglas RG, Bennett JE, eds. Anti-Infective Therapy. New York, John Wiley & Sons, 1985, pp 307–324
6. Black JR, Feinberg J, Murphy RL, et al: Clindamycin and primaquine as primary treatment for mild and moderately severe *Pneumocystis carinii* pneumonia in patients with AIDS. Eur J Clin Microbol Infect Dis 10:204–207, 1991
7. Blomley M, Teare EL, de Belder A, et al: Itraconazole and anti-tuberculosis drugs. Lancet 336:1255, 1990
8. Blum RA, D'Andrea DT, Floentino BM, et al: Increased gastric pH and the bioavailability of fluconazole and ketoconazole. Ann Intern Med 114:755–757, 1991
9. Blum RA, Wilton JH, Hilligoss DM, et al: Effect of fluconazole on the disposition of phenytoin. Clin Pharmacol Ther 49:420–425, 1991
10. Broder S, Yarchoan R: Dideoxycytidine: Current clinical experience and future prospects. Am J Med 88 (Suppl 5B):31S–33S, 1990
11. Cameron W, Sparti P, Pietroski N, et al: Rifabutin prevents *M. avium* complex bacteremia in patients

with AIDS and CD4 ≤ 200 (Abstract 888). 32nd Interscience Conference for Antimicrobial Agents and Chemotherapy, Anaheim CA, 1992
12. Campoli-Richards DM, Monk JP, Price A, et al: Ciprofloxacin. A review of its antibacterial activity, pharmacokinetic properties and therapeutic use. Drugs 35:373–447, 1988
13. Cato A, Hsu A, Granneman R, et al: Assessment of the pharmacokinetic interaction between The HIV-1 protease inhibitor ABT-538 and fluconazole. Program and Abstracts of the 35th Interscience Conference on Antimicrobial Agents and Chemotherapy, San Francisco, California, 1995
14. Cato A, Hsu A, Granneman R, et al: Assessment of the pharmacokinetic interaction between The HIV-1 protease inhibitor ABT-538 and zidovudine. Program and Abstracts of the 35th Interscience Conference on Antimicrobial Agents and Chemotherapy, San Francisco, California, 1995
15. Chaisson RE, Schecter GF, Theuer CP, et al: Tuberculosis in patients with the acquired immunodeficiency syndrome: Clinical features, response to therapy and survival. Am Rev Respir Dis 136:570–574, 1987
16. Chrisp P, Clissold SP: Foscarnet: A review of its antiviral activity, pharmacokinetic properties and therapeutic use in immunocompromised patients with cytomegalovirus retinitis. Drugs 41:104–129, 1991
17. Coker RJ, Tomlinson DR, Parkin J, et al: Interaction between fluconazole and rifampicin. Br Med J 301:818, 1990
18. Collier AC, Bozzette S, Coombs RW, et al: To examine the vivo effect of acyclovir and a range of doses of zidovudine. N Engl J Med 323:1015–1021, 1990
19. Cunningham CA, Friedberg DN, Carr RE: Clofazamine-induced generalized retinal degeneration. Retina 10(2):131–134, 1990

20. Dannenman B, McCutchan JA, Isrealski DM, et al: Treatment of toxoplasmic encephalitis in patients with AIDS. Ann Intern Med 116:33–43, 1992

21. Danner SA, Carr A, Leonard JM, et al: A short-term study of the safety, pharmacokinetics, and efficacy of ritonavir, an inhibitor of HIV-1 protease. N Engl J Med 333:1528–1533, 1995

22. De Miranda P, Good SS, Yarchoan R, et al: Alteration of zidovudine pharmacokinetics by probenecid in patients with AIDS or AIDS-related complex. Clin Pharmacol Ther 46:494–499, 1989

23. Deray G, Katlama C, Dohin E: Prevention of foscarnet nephrotoxicity (Letter). Ann Intern Med 113:332, 1990

24. Dorsky DI, Crumpacker CS: Drugs five years later: Acyclovir. Ann Intern Med 107:859–874, 1987

25. Ducharme MP, Slaughter RL, Warbasse LH, et al: Itraconazole and hydroxyitraconazole serum concentrations are reduced more than tenfold by phenytoin. Clin Pharmacol Ther 58:617–624, 1995

26. Engelhard D, Stutman HR, Marks MI: Interaction of ketoconazole with rifampin and isoniazid. N Engl J Med 311:1681–1683, 1984

27. Falloon J, Kovacs J, Hughes W, et al: A preliminary evaluation of 566C80 for the treatment of *Pneumocystis* pneumonia in patients with the acquired immunodeficiency syndrome. N Engl J Med 325(22):1534–1538, 1991

28. Farese RV Jr, Schambelan M, Hollander H, et al: Nephrogenic diabetes insipidus associated with foscarnet treatment of cytomegalovirus retinitis. Ann Intern Med 112:955–956, 1990

29. Fischl MA, Parker CB, Pettinelli C, et al: A randomized controlled trial of a reduced daily dose of zidovudine in patients with the acquired immunodeficiency syndrome. N Engl J Med 323:1009–1014, 1990

30. Garrelts JC: Clofazamine: A review of its use in leprosy and *Mycobacterium avium* complex infection. DICP 25:525–531, 1991

31. Garrelts JC, Godley PJ, Peterie JD, et al: Sucralfate significantly reduces ciprofloxacin concentrations in serum. Antimicrob Agents Chemother 34:931–933, 1990

32. Girling DJ: Adverse reactions to rifampicin in antituberculosis regimens. J Antimicrob Chemother 3:115, 1977

33. Gordin FM, Simon GL, Wofsy CB, Mills J: Adverse reactions to trimethoprim-sulfamethoxazole in patients with acquired immunodeficiency syndrome. Ann Intern Med 100:495–499, 1984

34. Grant SM, Clissold SP: Fluconazole. A review of its pharmacodynamics and pharmacokinetic properties, and therapeutic potential in superficial and systemic mycoses. Drugs 39(6):877–916, 1990

35. Hardy DJ, Guay DRP, Jones RN: Clarithromycin, a unique macrolide: A pharmacokinetic, microbiological, and clinical overview. Diagn Microbiol Infect Dis 5:931, 1992

36. Hart CC: Aerosolized pentamidine and pancreatitis. Ann Intern Med 111:691, 1989

37. Haverkos HO: Assessment of therapy for toxoplasma encephalitis. The TE Study Group. Am J Med 82:907, 1987

38. Herskowitz A, Willoughby SB, Baughman KL, et al: Cardiomyopathy associated with antiretroviral therapy in patients with human immunodeficiency virus infection: A report of 6 cases. Ann Intern Med 116:311–313, 1992

39. Hochster H, Dieterich D, Bozzette S, et al: Toxicity of combined ganciclovir and zidovudine for cytomegalovirus disease associated with AIDS. Ann Intern Med 113:111–117, 1990

40. Hooper DC, Wolfson JS: Fluoroquinolone antimicrobial agents. N Engl J Med 324:381–394, 1991

41. Hudson V, Cox F, Taylor L, et al: Pulmonary clofazamine crystals in a child with acquired immunodeficiency syndrome and disseminated *Mycobacterium avium-intracellulare* infection. Pediatr Infect Dis J 7(12):880–882, 1988

42. Hughes W, Leoung G, Kramer F, et al: Comparison of atovaquone (566C80) with trimethoprim-sulfamethoxazole to treat *Pneumocystis carinii* pneumonia in patients with AIDS. N Engl J Med 328:1521–1527, 1993

43. Indorf AS, Pegram PS: Esophageal ulceration related to zalcitabine (ddC). Ann Intern Med 117:133–134, 1992

44. Invirase (saquinavir mesylate), Roche Package Insert, December 1995

45. Israel D, Polk RE: Focus on clarithromycin and azithromycin: Two new macrolide antibiotics. Hosp Formul 27:115–134, 1992

46. Israelski DM, Tom C, Remington JS: Zidovudine antagonizes the action of pyrimethamine in experimental infection with *Toxoplasma gondii*. Antimicrob Agents Chemother 33:30–34, 1988

47. Jacobson MA, Besch CL, Child C, et al: Randomized study of clindamycin or pyrimethamine prophylaxis for toxoplasmic encephalitis in patients with advanced HIV disease (Abstract 298). Thirty-first Interscience Conference on Antimicrobial Agents and Chemotherapy, Chicago, 1991

48. Jones DR, Black JR: Evaluation of pharmacokinetic interactions between the combination of primaquine plus clindamycin and zidovudine (Abstract Th.B. 400). Sixth International Conference on AIDS, San Francisco, 1990

49. Kopanoff DE, Snider DE Jr, Caras GJ: Isoniazid-related hepatitis: A U.S. Public Health Service cooperative surveillance study. Am Rev Respir Dis 117:991–1001, 1978

50. Kornhauser DM, Petty BG, Hendrix CW, et al: Probenecid and zidovudine metabolism. Br Med J 2:473–475, 1989

51. Kosoglou T, Rocci ML Jr, Vlasses PH: Trimethoprim alters the disposition of procainamide and N-acetylprocainamide. Clin Pharmacol Ther 44:467–477, 1988

52. Kovacs JA, Hiemenz JW, Macher AM, et al: *Pneumocystis carinii* pneumonia: A comparison between patients with the acquired immunodeficiency syndrome and patients with other immunodeficiencies. Ann Intern Med 100:663–671, 1984

53. Kramer MR, Marshall SE, Denning DW, et al: Cyclosporine and itraconazole interaction in heart and lung transplant recipients. Ann Intern Med 113:327–329, 1990

54. Kucers A, Bennett N: The Use of Antibiotics. A Comprehensive Review With Clinical Emphasis, ed 4. Philadelphia, JB Lippincott Co, 1987

55. Lachaal M, Venuto RC: Nephrotoxicity and hyperkalemia in patients with acquired immunodeficiency syndrome treated with pentamidine. Am J Med 87:260–263, 1989

56. Lafeuillade A, Aubert L, Chaffanjon P, Quilichini R: Optic neuritis associated with dideoxyinosine. Lancet 337:615–616, 1991

57. Lai KK, Gang DL, Zawacki JK, Cooley TP: Fulminant hepatic failure associated with 2',3'-dideoxyinosine (ddI). Ann Intern Med 115:283–284, 1991

58. Lake-Bakaar G, Tom W, Lake-Bakaar D, et al: Gastropathy and ketoconazole malabsorption in the acquired immunodeficiency syndrome (AIDS). Ann Intern Med 109:471–473, 1988

59. Lalonde RG, Deschenes JG, Seamone C: Zidovudine-induced macular edema. Ann Intern Med 114: 297–298, 1991

60. Lambert JS, Seidlin M, Reichman RC, et al: 2',3'-Dideoxyinosine (ddI) in patients with the acquired immunodeficiency syndrome or AIDS-related complex. N Engl J Med 322:1333–1340, 1990

61. Lazar JD, Wilner KD: Drug interactions with fluconazole. Rev Infect Dis 12:327–333, 1990

62. Lee BL, Medina I, Benowitz NL, et al: Dapsone, trimethoprim and sulfamethoxazole plasma levels during treatment of *Pneumocystis* pneumonia in patients with acquired immunodeficiency syndrome: Evidence of drug interactions. Ann Intern Med 110:606–611, 1989

63. Lee BL, Safrin S, Makrides BS, et al: Trimethoprim decreases the renal clearance of zidovudine. Program and Abstracts of the 93rd Annual Meeting of the American Society for Clinical Pharmacology and Therapeutics. Clin Pharmacol Ther 51:183, 1992

64. Lee BL, Tauber MG, Chambers HF, et al: The effect of zalcitabine on the pharmacokinetics of isoniazid in HIV-infected patients. Program and Abstracts of the 34th Interscience Conference on Antimicrobial Agents and Chemotherapy, Orlando, Florida, 1994

65. Lee BL, Tauber MG, Chambers HF, et al: Zalcitabine and dapsone pharmacokinetic interaction in HIV-infected patients. Program and Abstracts of the 96th Annual meeting of the American Society for Clinical Pharmacology and Therapeutics, San Diego, California, 1995

66. Lee BL, Tauber MG, Chambers HF, et al: Atovaquone inhibits the glucuronidation and increases the plasma concentrations of zidovudine. Program and Abstracts of the 34th Interscience Conference on Antimicrobial Agents and Chemotherapy, Orlando, Florida, 1994

67. Leport C, Raffi F, Matheron S, et al: Treatment of central nervous system toxoplasmosis with pyrimethamine/sulfadiazine combination in 35 patients with the acquired immunodeficiency syndrome. Am J Med 84:94, 1988

68. Levine S, Walsh T, Martinez A, et al: Cardiopulmonary toxicity after liposomal amphotericin B infusion. Ann Intern Med 114:664–666, 1991

69. Marr JJ: Antiparasitic agents. In Mandell GL, Douglas RG, Bennett JE, eds. Anti-Infective Therapy. New York, John Wiley & Sons, 1985, pp 383–384

70. Masur H: Prevention and treatment of *Pneumocystis* pneumonia. N Engl J Med 327:1853–1860, 1992

71. McLeod GX, Hammer SM: Zidovudine: Five years later. Ann Intern Med 117:487–501, 1992

72. Medina I, Mills J, Leoung G, et al: Oral therapy for *Pneumocystis carinii* pneumonia in the acquired immunodeficiency syndrome. A controlled trial of trimethoprim-sulfamethoxazole versus dapsone-trimethoprim. N Engl J Med 323:776–782, 1990

73. Merigan TC, Skowron G, ddC Study Group of the AIDS Clinical Trials Group of the National Institute for Allergy and Infectious Diseases: Safety and tolerance of dideoxycytidine as a single agent. Am J Med 88(Suppl 5B):11S–15S, 1990

74. Metroka CE, McMechan MF, Andrada R, et al: Failure of prophylaxis with dapsone in patients taking dideoxyinosine. N Engl J Med 325:737, 1991

75. Midoneck SR, Etingin OR: Clarithromycin related toxic effects of digoxin. N Engl J Med 333:1505, 1995

76. Millar AB, Miller RF, Patou G, et al: Treatment of cytomegalovirus retinitis with zidovudine and ganciclovir in patients with AIDS: Outcome and toxicity. Genitourin Med 66:156–158, 1990

77. Molina J, Belenfant X, Doco-Lecompte T, et al: Sulfadiazine-induced crystalluria in AIDS patients with toxoplasma encephalitis. AIDS 5:587–589, 1991

78. Monahan BP, Ferguson CL, Killeavy ES, et al: Torsades de pointes occurring in association with terfenadine use. JAMA 264:2788–2790, 1990

79. Narang P, Nightingale S, Manzone C, et al: Does rifabutin affect zidovudine disposition in HIV+ patients? (Abstract PoB 3888). VIII International Conference on AIDS, Amsterdam, The Netherlands, 1992

80. Newsome GS, Ward DJ, Pierce PF: Spontaneous pneumothorax in patients with acquired immunodeficiency syndrome treated with prophylactic aerosolized pentamidine. Arch Intern Med 150: 2167–2168, 1990

81. Nix DE, Watson WA, Lener ME, et al: Effects of aluminum and magnesium antacids and ranitidine on the absorption of ciprofloxacin. Clin Pharmacol Ther 46:700–705, 1989

82. Nyberg G, Blohme I, Persson H, Svalander C: Foscarnet-induced tubulointerstitial nephritis in renal transplant patients. Transplant Proc 22:241, 1990

83. O'Reilly RA, Motley CH: Racemic warfarin and trimethoprim-sulfamethoxazole interaction in humans. Ann Intern Med 91:34–36, 1979

84. Pieters FA, Woonick F, Zuidema J: Influence of once-monthly rifampicin and daily clofazamine on the pharmacokinetics of dapsone. Eur J Clin Pharmacol 34:73–76, 1988

85. Ruf B, Rohde I, Pohle HD: Efficacy of clindamycin/primaquine versus trimethoprim/sulfamethoxazole in primary treatment of *Pneumocystis carinii* pneumonia. Eur J Clin Microbiol Infect Dis 10:207–210, 1991

86. Sahai J, Gallicano K, Oliveras L, et al: Cations in the didanosine tablet reduce ciprofloxacin bioavailability. Clin Pharmacol Ther 53:292–297, 1993

87. Sands M, Kron MA, Brown RB: Pentamidine: A review. Rev Infect Dis 7:625–634, 1985

88. Shyu WC, Knupp CA, Pittman KA, et al: Food-induced reduction in bioavailability of didanosine. Clin Pharmacol Ther 50:503–507, 1991

89. Siegal FP, Eilbott D, Burger H, et al: Dose-limiting toxicity of rifabutin in AIDS-related complex: Syndrome of arthralgia/arthritis. AIDS 4:433–441, 1990

90. Small PM, Schecter GF, Goodman PC, et al: Treatment of tuberculosis in patients with advanced human immunodeficiency virus infection. N Engl J Med 324:289–294, 1991

91. Snider DE Jr: Pyridoxine supplementation during isoniazid therapy. Tubercle 61:191, 1980

92. Snider DE Jr, Long MW, Cross FS, Farer LS: Six-months isoniazid-rifampicin therapy for pulmonary tuberculosis. Report of a United States public health service cooperative trial. Am Rev Respir Dis 129:573, 1984

93. Soriano E, Mallolas J, Gatell JM, et al: Characteristics of tuberculosis in HIV-infected patients: A case control study. AIDS 2:429–432, 1988

94. Steinberg JP, Gunthel CJ, White RL, et al: Outcomes and toxicities on 2′,3′-dideoxyinosine (ddI) in the expanded access program (Abstract 707). Thirty-first Interscience Conference on Antimicrobial Agents and Chemotherapy, Chicago, 1991

95. Stockley IH: Drug Interactions. A Source Book of Drug Interactions, Their Mechanisms, Clinical Importance and Management, ed 2. Oxford, Blackwell Scientific Publications, 1991

96. Sud IJ, Feingold DS: Effect of ketoconazole on the fungicidal action of amphotericin B in *Candida albicans*. Antimicrob Agents Chemother 23:185–187, 1983

97. Sullam P, Burnside A, Dereskini S, et al: Safety profile of rifabutin for the prevention of *M. avium* complex bacteremia in patients with AIDS and CD4 ≤ 200 (Abstract PoB 3265). Several International Conference on AIDS, Amsterdam, The Netherlands, B131, 1992

98. Torseth J, Bhatia G, Harkonen S, et al: Evaluation of the antiviral effect of rifabutin in AIDS-related complex. J Infect Dis 159:1115–1118, 1989

99. Tucker RM, Denning DW, Hanson LH, et al: Interaction of azoles with rifampin, phenytoin, and carbamazepine: In vitro and clinical observations. Clin Infect Dis 14:165–174, 1992

100. USP DI: Drug Information for the Health Care Professional, ed 11, vols 1A and 1B. The United States Pharmacopeial Convention, 1991

101. Wade JC, Meyers JD: Neurologic symptoms associated with parenteral acyclovir treatment after marrow transplantation. Ann Intern Med 98:921, 1983

102. Waskin H, Stehr-Green JK, Helmick CG, Sattler FR: Risk factors for hypoglycemia associated with pentamidine therapy for *Pneumocystis* pneumonia. JAMA 260:345–347, 1988

103. Wharton JM, Coleman DL, Wofsy CT, et al: Trimethoprim-sulfamethoxazole or pentamidine for *Pneumocystis carinii* pneumonia in the acquired immunodeficiency syndrome. Ann Intern Med 105:37–44, 1986

104. Wilcox JB: Phenytoin intoxication and co-trimoxazole (Letter). N Z Med J 94:235–236, 1981

105. Wurtz RM, Abrams D, Becker S, et al: Anaphylactoid drug reactions to ciprofloxacin and rifampicin in HIV-infected patients (Letter). Lancet 1:955–956, 1989

106. Yakatan GJ, Rasmussen CE, Reis PJ, et al: Bioinequivalence of erythromycin ethylsuccinate and enteric-coated erythromycin pellets following multiple oral doses. J Clin Pharmacol 25:36–42, 1985

107. Yarchoan R, Perno CF, Thomas RV, et al: Phase I studies of 2′,3′-dideoxycytidine in severe human immunodeficiency virus infection as a single agent and alternating with zidovudine. Lancet 1:76–78, 1988

108. Yeh J, Soo SC, Summerton C, et al: Potentiation of action of warfarin by itraconazole. Br Med J 301:669, 1990

109. Youle MS, Clarbour J, Gazzard B, Chanas A: Severe hypocalcemia in AIDS patients treated with foscarnet and pentamidine (Letter). Lancet 1:1455–1456, 1988

110. Zuidema J, Hilbers-Modderman ESM, Merkus FWHM: Clinical pharmacokinetics of dapsone. Clin Pharmacokinet 11:299–315, 1936

Chapter *10*

Alternative Therapies for HIV

DONALD I. ABRAMS

Despite more than a decade of progress in understanding the molecular virology and pathophysiology of the human immunodeficiency virus (HIV), the disease caused by infection with this novel retrovirus remains incurable. Baffled by the continued lack of effective therapies, the affected community launched an alternative treatment movement in the early 1980s that has now grown to a point where most practicing providers caring for patients with HIV infection are likely to be interacting with patients who have utilized alternative therapies.

The use of alternative therapies is not unique to patients with HIV disease. Eisenberg et al conducted a telephone interview with 1539 adults in 1990 to determine the prevalence, costs, and patterns of use of unconventional medicine in the United States.[29] Of those surveyed, 34% reported using one or more such therapies in the past year. Although exercise (26%) and prayer (25%) were the two most frequently reported modalities reported, they were excluded from the overall 34% result. Still, relaxation techniques (13%), chiropractic treatment (10%), massage (7%), imagery (4%), and spiritual healing (4%) were all cited more frequently than any interventions requiring ingestion of a substance. Weight loss programs, lifestyle diets, herbal medicine, and megavitamin therapy were only reported by 2% to 4% of the respondents. The highest use of unconventional therapies was reported by non-black persons, age 25 to 49, with higher income and educational levels. Eighty-three per cent of those using alternative therapies for serious medical conditions also sought treatment from a medical doctor. However, nearly three quarters of those using unconventional therapies did not inform their doctor. The authors extrapolate from their findings to estimate that annual visits to providers of unconventional

therapy number 425 million, a figure that exceeds the number of visits to all primary care physicians, at an approximate cost of $13.7 billion. Concluding that the frequency and use of unconventional therapy is higher than previously reported, the authors urge physicians to ask their patients about their use of such treatments whenever they obtain a medical history.

Use of alternative therapies has been studied extensively in patients with malignant diseases. Research has documented that increased use of unorthodox treatments is related to disillusionment with standard medical practice.[17] Higher use of alternative therapies is noted among patients with diseases for which treatment is limited. It is therefore not surprising that people with HIV infection have become frequent users of alternative therapy. Numerous studies have estimated that from 40% to 70% of patients with HIV infection in the United States are utilizing alternative or complementary therapies.[2,8,37,59] Surveys have reported similar percentages of patients with HIV infection in Europe using unconventional therapies.[52,85,86]

As the epidemic expands globally, it is important to note that oftentimes what is considered to be ''alternative'' therapy in one culture is actually ''traditional'' in another. This is highlighted by a small study from Rwanda of traditional versus modern medicine for the acquired immunodeficiency syndrome (AIDS).[49] Factors and perceptions determining choice between traditional and Western medicine were assessed among urban African women confronting AIDS. Forty women and 25 traditional healers (58% males) were interviewed. The majority of the women were using both traditional healers and Western medicine concurrently. The traditional healers were AIDS aware and interested in collaborating with Western trained physicians. All of the women stated that the traditional healers treat certain illnesses better than Western medicine. Western providers were consulted for their perceived appropriateness for specific illnesses and for access to diagnostic medical technology. As the populations affected by HIV infection continue to expand worldwide into diverse ethnic groups and global information exchange becomes more easily accomplished, the blurring of the line separating alternative and orthodox therapies will likely continue to increase.

A BRIEF HISTORY OF ALTERNATIVE THERAPY FOR HIV

The history of the alternative therapy movement is intricately associated with the availability and perceived efficacy of orthodox antiretroviral interventions. At the beginning of the epidemic, before the etiologic agent had been identified, early alternative therapies included high-dose intravenous or oral vitamin C and topical application of the sensitizer dinitrochlorobenzene (see below). As immunomodulators and antivirals such as isoprinosine and ribavirin began early clinical trials as possible orthodox treatments at research centers, they could also be obtained over-the-counter in easily accessed foreign markets. Alternative use and acquisition of therapies filled the gap caused by the absence of a standard treatment during the first 5 years of the epidemic.

Zidovudine was approved in late 1986 for use in patients with symptomatic HIV disease and CD4 cell $<200/mm^3$ (see Chapter 8).[32] This made an orthodox treatment available by prescription to patients for the first time. There was a brief slowdown in interest in alternatives. However, when it became clear that newer and possibly better antiviral agents would not soon be released, the alternative movement surged again from 1987 through 1989. In 1989 results of large clinical trials demonstrated that zidovudine prevented progression to advanced HIV disease in patients treated earlier in their course of infection.[33,88] This led to the approval of the drug for patients with fewer than $500/mm^3$ CD4 cells, allowing increased numbers of individuals to obtain a licensed agent by prescription from their provider. At the same time the expanded-access program for dideoxyinosine (ddI) was initiated, giving patients for whom zidovudine failed or whose disease progressed access to another potentially beneficial

therapeutic agent.[23,53] The strength of the alternative therapies movement and the fact that the treatment activists would likely gain access to ddI in an unmonitored fashion even in the absence of the "parallel track" were probably factors that encouraged expanded-access programs to be initiated for speedier delivery of drugs to interested individuals while they were still in early stages of conventional clinical trials.

Even with antiretroviral therapies available by prescription, individuals with HIV infection continue to use alternative treatments. Some employ these alternatives as "complementary" to their prescribed antiretroviral medication. However, as experience with nucleoside analogues increased over the years, the perceived benefits of these agents became less evident. Some patients opted for a strictly alternative pathway. Mayer et al reported in 1993 that of a group of 232 HIV-positive men with AIDS or CD4 lymphocyte counts $<500/mm^3$, all eligible for treatment under existing guidelines, one third had never taken zidovudine.[59] Forty-six per cent of those who took zidovudine used it in combination with nonconventional therapies. Zidovudine users were more likely to have AIDS and lower CD4 counts, not be treated in a clinic, and have private insurance. Those who reported using complementary therapy in conjunction with their zidovudine were reported to be sicker, but otherwise similar to those who used zidovudine alone.

In 1993 the alternative therapy movement picked up more steam following the preliminary report of the results of the large collaborative Concorde trial, which evaluated early versus deferred zidovudine therapy in patients with asymptomatic HIV infection.[1] The study suggested that although a definite CD4 cell benefit was apparent throughout the trial in the early-treatment group, the previously reported decrease in progression of disease was short-lived and did not extend through the entire 3 years of follow-up. Similarly, although the study was not large enough to have statistical power to use death as an end-point, no survival benefit was seen for those who had early intervention with zidovudine. In fact, there were more deaths in the early-treatment group compared to the deferred cohort; a disturbing, although not statistically significant finding. Wider dissemination of the Concorde results at the 1993 International Conference on AIDS in Berlin, coupled with discouraging news from combination-therapy studies and trials of other agents for which prior expectations had been high, combined to throw a shroud of disenchantment over currently available treatments.[20] Further disillusionment greeted the recommendations from the State-of-the-Art Conference on antiretroviral therapy for adult HIV-infected patients.[73]

We are currently entering a new era in which antiretroviral therapies are again being embraced by patients and providers alike. Surrogate marker information from trials combining zidovudine and lamivudine (3TC), with even more impressive responses when adding a protease inhibitor, have increased enthusiasm for the conventional licensed agents[26,30,40,50,57] (see Chapter 8). The need to fill gaps with alternatives has recently declined again as the market incorporates three new protease inhibitors into the anti-HIV armamentarium. Although agents aimed specifically at the retrovirus are being utilized less frequently, alternatives are still being sought for those manifestations of HIV disease in which orthodox medicine seems to be failing. Immune reconstitution and wasting are the two current areas where the highest interest remains.

Despite possible progress in the fight against the retrovirus, until there is a cure, patients with HIV/AIDS are likely to continue to empower themselves by seeking alternative or complementary interventions. This underscores the importance of providers maintaining a direct line of communication with their patients regarding their use of alternative treatments. Primary providers caring for patients with HIV infection should become cognizant and conversant with the use of potential alternative therapies to better understand symptoms as they relate to side effects of these agents and to be aware of potential interactions with prescribed medications.

CURRENTLY USED ALTERNATIVE THERAPIES

The popularity of a number of the alternative treatments has waxed and waned over the last decade. The rationale behind the use of many of these agents and results from various trials of early popular alternative therapies have been reviewed elsewhere.[2,4,5] A few of the earliest favorites are again being used to an appreciable extent within the community while other new interventions are becoming more widely touted as complementary treatments (Table 10–1). Providers should be aware of these agents, their rationale for use, and their potential toxicities. With increasing frequency, agents initially chosen as alternatives have begun to enter orthodox clinical trials through university centers or the government-sponsored AIDS Clinical Trial Group (ACTG) or the Community Programs for Clinical Research on AIDS (CPCRA) of the National Institutes of Allergy and Infectious Diseases (NIAID).

Vitamin C and Antioxidants

Vitamin C was one of the first interventions proposed as a potential alternative therapy.[5] The rationale was based on anecdotal observations of broad antiviral activity and in vitro activity against a human retrovirus.[11] High doses (up to 50 g/day) were administered by either oral routes or intravenous infusion. Patients were advised to escalate their vitamin C intake to "bowel tolerance"—to ingest as much ascorbate as possible without developing completely intolerable diarrhea. As many of the early advocates of ascorbate therapy died secondary to progression of their AIDS-related illness, enthu-

TABLE 10–1. ALTERNATIVE THERAPIES IN CURRENT USE

Agent	Nature of Agent	Suggested Activity	Potential Side Effects
Antioxidants	Vitamin C Beta-carotene	Antiviral Free radical scavengers	GI distress
Dinitrochlorobenzene	Organic compound used in photographic processing	Enhanced cellular immunity	Contact dermatitis
NAC	Cysteine precursor, mucolytic, acetaminophen antidote	Antiviral via tumor necrosis factor (TNF) inhibition	None reported
Chinese herbs	Traditional herbal mixture	Symptom palliation	Generally none seen, but numerous possible
Tumeric	Curcumin, food spice component	Antiviral via LTR inhibition	Ulcers seen in rats

siasm for further pursuit of this agent waned in the community.

In the ensuing years a resurgence of interest in the potential therapeutic utility of antioxidants in general and vitamin C in particular emerged. At a National Institutes of Health (NIH)–sponsored conference in 1990, the biologic and clinical actions of vitamin C were reviewed.[12] Vitamin C was reported to be the first line of defense against free radical damage. It is postulated that oxidative stress is toxic to lymphocytes, thus potentiating the destructive effect of HIV in infected patients. In addition to this potential role in preserving immune function, recent reports support the notion of in vitro antiretroviral activity. Continuous exposure of HIV-infected cells to noncytotoxic ascorbate concentrations was shown to significantly inhibit viral replication in both chronically and acutely infected cell lines.[41] A subsequent study from the same group of researchers from the Linus Pauling Institute of Science and Medicine suggests that another benefit of vitamin C is its ability to raise intracellular glutathione levels, which leads to synergistic in vitro anti-HIV activity when combined with N-acetylcysteine[47] (see below). This supplementary HIV-specific information, coupled with the general wave of enthusiasm generated by results of large studies of vitamin/antioxidant therapies in non–HIV-related conditions, has spawned a new wave of ascorbate activists, reminiscent of those in the early 1980s. The current proponents of vitamin C treatment for HIV infection are even more convinced that because vitamins are not patentable, they will never be seriously studied in clinical trials because they pose a threat to the pharmaceutical industry and the medical profession. Despite this rhetoric, the CPCRA proposed a vitamin C/beta carotene trial to be conducted through its community-based clinical trials network to attempt finally to generate some clinical information. Rather than embark on a large full-scale efficacy trial initially, it was decided that a dose-escalating pilot study should first be performed to evaluate tolerance as well as antiretroviral activity using HIV RNA viral load determinations.

The impetus to study beta carotene in conjunction with vitamin C comes from preliminary studies involving this carotenoid with provitamin A activity. Deficiency of vitamin A is associated with increased frequency and severity of infections and beta carotene has been reported to have an immunostimulating effect. This information led to a double-blind, placebo-controlled, crossover trial of beta carotene in 21 HIV-infected patients.[22] Participants received either beta carotene 180 mg daily or placebo for 4 weeks, after which they received the alternate intervention for the next 4 weeks. Beta carotene treatment resulted in a statistically significant rise in total white blood cell count and percent change in CD4 count and CD4:CD8 ratios. Although the absolute CD4 count rose on beta carotene and fell during placebo, these changes did not reach statistical significance. The authors concluded that further studies are needed to determine whether beta carotene may have an adjunctive role in the treatment of persons with HIV infection. A recently reported small controlled trial from France suggested that beta carotene was less of an antioxidant and immune modulator than supplemental selenium.[21]

One of the attractions of alternative therapies has always been to obtain potential benefits with less adverse effects than traditional medicine interventions. Vitamins would seem to meet this criteria of minimal expected toxicity. However, several recently completed large trials employing vitamin supplementation for preventive health have shed some concern on the safety of beta carotene. A randomized, double-blind, placebo-controlled trial evaluated the effects of beta carotene and alpha-tocopherol in over 29,000 middle-aged male smokers.[7] The objective was to assess the impact of the supplements on the reduction of lung and other cancers. The cohort was followed for a median of 6.1 years, yielding nearly 170,000 person-years of follow-up. Surprisingly, among beta carotene recipients there was an overall 8% excess mortality compared to nonrecipients, with more deaths due to lung cancer, ischemic heart disease, and ischemic and hemorrhagic stroke. The authors remark that "an adverse effect of beta carotene seems unlikely; in spite of its formal statistical significance; therefore, this finding may well be due to chance." Unfortunately, the attribution of the 8% excess mortality to chance did not hold up as the National Cancer Institute recently confirmed the surprising detrimental effect of supplemental beta carotene from two additional studies.[35] One trial followed over 22,000 physicians who took either 50 mg of beta carotene daily or placebo for 12 years. Another involved over 18,000 smokers, ex-smokers, and asbestos workers. No benefit from beta carotene was discerned and the smokers' trial was halted early because of increased rates of death from cancer and heart disease in beta carotene recipients compared to controls. This large body of evidence calls into question the potential safety of something as seemingly benign as beta carotene. This sobering finding has not yet been incorporated into the collective consciousness of the AIDS alternative treatment community, who also may benefit more from ingesting vitamins directly from natural food sources than from store-bought supplements.

DNCB

Another of the early AIDS alternative treatments that continues to be used, particularly in the San Francisco Bay Area, is the chemical 1-chloro-2,4-dinitrobenzene (DNCB).[80] DNCB is an organic compound used in the processing of color photography. It has a medical application as a topical sensitizer used as an agent for anergy testing. It also has been used successfully in the treatment of common warts and alopecia areata.[79] A community dermatologist in San Francisco reported observing an increase in the CD4 lymphocyte number in patients repeatedly painted with sensitizing quantities of DNCB in a 1% concentration dissolved in acetone while experimenting with the compound as a potential therapy for patients with AIDS-related Kaposi's sarcoma.[62] Word spread throughout the community that the dermatologist was seeing improvement in immune function. Because DNCB was a widely available chemical, a group purchased the compound in kilogram quantities from photographic supply houses and produced the treatment solution in bulk. It was subsequently distributed to individuals interested in DNCB's potential immunomodulating effect and its activity against Kaposi's sarcoma. A network of similar buyers' groups took shape, thereby creating an infrastructure for drug distribution of alternative treatments on a national level. These "guerilla clinics" became the forerunners of the current "buyers' clubs" that continue in the current for-profit distribution of potentially therapeutic agents for patients with HIV infection.

Enthusiasm for DNCB waned when it became apparent that it had no efficacy against lesions of Kaposi's sarcoma, when many of the early users died of progressive HIV infection, and with the availability of nucleoside analogue antiretroviral therapy. A persistent cohort of proponents, however, continued to support weekly "painting" of DNCB onto the skin of patients with HIV infection. Not convinced that HIV is solely responsible for the pathogenesis of AIDS and more supportive of an underlying autoimmune mechanism, staunch DNCB advocates seemed vindicated by news that HIV infects the Langerhans' cells of the skin.[13] A possible theoretical mechanism for DNCB's rationale as a treatment for HIV infection now seemed plausible. The principal antigen-presenting cell for contact sensitization is the Langerhans' cell. It is postulated that DNCB may allow the immune system to rid itself of HIV-infected Langerhans' cells by the cell-mediated immune system response that results from topical application of DNCB. As replacement Langerhans' cells may ultimately become infected as well, treatment with DNCB must be continued indefinitely. This author, in collaboration with DNCB activists and other university researchers, wrote a protocol to study the effects of DNCB application on viral infection of Langerhans' cells that was rejected for funding. Small trials with immunologic and clinical end-points have been conducted by the remaining DNCB enthusiasts. Stricker et al reported on the results of weekly DNCB application in a cohort of 24 HIV-positive gay men with a mean CD4 cell count of 353/mm^3 at study entry. Fourteen of the patients were on no antiretroviral therapy. The mean duration of follow-up was 12 months. CD4 cell counts decreased significantly to a mean of 251/mm^3. The CD8 count also declined during the course of therapy. A significant increase in natural killer cell number from 99 to 162/mm^3 was observed. Two participating patients developed Kaposi's sarcoma. The authors conclude that prolonged use of topical DNCB was associated with a stable clinical course in most patients, despite a significant decrease in CD4 T cells, and that lack of disease progression was associated with a stable CD8 count, and may be related to a persistent increase in natural killer cells—probably due to DNCB-induced delayed-type hypersensitivity that may be beneficial in HIV disease.[81] A study of 19 Brazilian patients treated for 21 months with topical DNCB by Stricker's associates demonstrated CD4 and CD8 cell rises and decreased parasitic infections compared to historical controls.[83]

Topical DNCB application was compared to acetone sham treatment in a 6-month placebo-controlled trial in patients receiving no antiretroviral therapies.[55] The CD4 counts increased slightly in both groups during the course of the study, but the control group demonstrated a greater increase in CD8 lymphocytes. A higher proportion of the DNCB-treated subjects (10 of 15) experienced a net decline in CD4 cells compared to the controls (5 of 13). There were no differences in clinical disease progression in the two cohorts. In a companion report, eight individuals receiving both DNCB and Chinese herbs underwent serial lymph node biopsies and viral load determinations. DNCB application did not affect viral burden or viral replication in peripheral blood or lymphoid tissue over the 6 months of the trial.[19] The DNCB enthusiasts dismiss these findings by suggesting that Chinese herbs are immunosuppressants and that viral load measurements are irrelevant, as the agent is not purported to work via an antiviral mechanism. Although DNCB application is nontoxic aside from the local contact dermatitis reaction that it is expected to produce, recommendations from the staunch advocates that for best results patients discontinue their nucleoside analogues as well as some of their other conventional therapies has troubled some providers monitoring patients on this regimen. The incongruity between the vehemence of DNCB's supporters and the available objective results is certainly perplexing, but not at all unique to this alternative therapy.

Cysteine Precursors and Other Tumor Necrosis Factor Inhibitors

Cysteine, an essential amino acid, is utilized in the biosynthesis of the peptide glutathione. Patients with HIV infection have decreased intracellular glutathione levels.[14,76,77] N-acetylcysteine (NAC) is the N-acetyl derivative of cysteine. It is available in aerosolized form as a mucolytic treatment for bronchitis in Europe and it is administered systemically in the United States for management of acetaminophen overdosage (Mucomyst). It is believed that cysteine precursors may indirectly inhibit HIV replication by raising intracellular glutathione levels.[71] In vitro cysteine and NAC raise intracellular glutathione and inhibit HIV-1 replication in persistently infected cell lines.[48,61] This may occur by blocking the effects of tumor necrosis factor (TNF) in HIV-infected cells.[18] TNF levels are elevated in people with HIV infection and may be associated with accelerated HIV replication.[34,51] A review of the multifactorial nature of the pathogenesis of HIV disease implicates TNF-α as a cytokine that may contribute to symptoms, especially in HIV-related wasting, as

well as up-regulation of HIV infection.[31] Agents that may block TNF-α were recommended for evaluation in clinical trials. A number of agents popular as alternative therapies in addition to NAC have TNF blockade as their presumed mechanism of action (see below). Because of its easy availability from foreign markets, its biochemical rationale, and its lack of significant toxicity (occasional dyspepsia, diarrhea), NAC ranks as one of the biggest selling items in buyers' clubs nationwide.

The NIAID conducted a small study to evaluate the safety, pharmacokinetics, and antiviral activity of NAC administered intravenously and orally.[89] Eligible patients with HIV infection and fewer than 500/mm^3 CD4 lymphocytes received 6 weeks of escalating intravenous NAC thrice weekly. This was followed by 6 weeks of oral administration of doses ranging from 600 to 4800 mg daily. Twenty-two of the 23 patients enrolled with a mean CD4 count of 209/mm^3 were receiving concurrent antiretroviral therapy; 100 mg/kg was the maximum tolerated dose. First-order pharmacokinetics were observed after intravenous treatment with a half-life of 30 minutes. However, Walker et al reported that following oral administration, plasma-free NAC was barely detectable (22 μM). Although the implication was that there was little or no oral bioavailability, NAC supporters countered that it is rapidly converted into cysteine and subsequently glutathione following ingestion and therefore it is not surprising that NAC blood levels should be scant. Similarly, if NAC is not absorbed, how can it be an effective mucolytic or antidote to acetaminophen? The hepatic protection could be conceivably explained by the first-pass phenomenon. The NIAID study, however, showed no significant changes in CD4 cell counts, p24 antigen levels, HIV plasma viremia, or plasma cysteine levels. Advocates were unphased, however, and suggested that the real end-point to be measured is the intracellular glutathione level, which is currently being investigated. Of concern, however, is the recent report of an in vitro evaluation demonstrating that NAC and glutathione enhanced the replication of HIV-1 in macrophages up to 160%, leading the investigators to conclude that "other oxygen radical scavengers than NAC should be considered as therapeutic agents in AIDS."[66]

Thalidomide

Another inhibitor of TNF-α that has become increasingly popular in the HIV alternative therapies community is thalidomide, the infamous sedative associated with birth defects when taken by pregnant women. The drug has continued to be used as a treatment for erythema nodosum leprosum, where it has been demonstrated to decrease TNF production.[71] Thalidomide enhances the degradation of TNF-α messenger RNA.[64] The first clinical application of thalidomide in HIV-infected patients was its use in treating patients with HIV, tuberculosis, and wasting in Thailand. Investigators noted a significantly increased weight gain in patients treated with thalidomide in addition to their antituberculosis therapy compared to those receiving antibiotics alone. Through the down-regulation of TNF-α, thalidomide is also able to reduce the production of HIV-1 in acutely infected human monocytes in vitro.[56,63] As news of these potential beneficial properties of thalidomide spread, alternative therapy activists began to obtain the drug from foreign markets for distribution through the buyers' club network. At the same time, the ACTG was conducting placebo-controlled clinical trials of thalidomide for treatment of idiopathic aphthous stomatitis and esophagitis. The early termination of the oral ulcer trial because of the tremendous benefit of thalidomide treatment increased the community's interest in obtaining wider access to the agent. Simultaneously, however, the U.S. Food and Drug Administration (FDA) was becoming more concerned about the widespread uncontrolled distribution of this emotionally charged drug through the buyer's club mechanism.[24] They demanded that the groups cease sales of thalidomide. The pharmaceutical manufacturer developed a placebo-controlled trial for patients with HIV-related wasting syndrome that had restrictive entry criteria and was slow to accrue. Subsequently, responding to increasing pressure from the activist community, the company and the FDA established a compassionate-use program for individuals with severe HIV-related weight loss. Unfortunately, despite the absence of any efficacy data, the manufacturer is charging "cost recovery" fees that significantly exceed the buyers' club prices.

Ketotifen, an antihistamine available in Europe, is also purported to have anti-TNF activity.[9] A German study in patients with wasting reported patients sustained a 6-pound weight gain in a 12-week trial.[43] This has catapulted ketotifen into the ranks of best-sellers at the New York PWA Health Group buyers' club.

Other Alternative Treatments for Wasting

In addition to TNF inhibitors, other treatments for HIV-associated wasting and weight loss are also being increasingly utilized by the alternative therapies community (Table 10–2). With numerous available licensed antiretroviral therapies, wasting has emerged as a therapeutic target for alternative intervention. No longer troubled by a dearth of antiretroviral agents, treatment activists noted the paucity of effective available therapies for the wasting syndrome. With two appetite stimulants licensed and trials suggesting efficacy of an extremely expensive subcutaneous hormonal intervention, efforts have been directed toward evaluating other potential therapies for wasting.[36,65,67,82,87]

Testosterone and its derivatives have been increasingly utilized in an attempt to increase lean body mass.[10] In addition to testosterone supplementation in the subset of patients with HIV infection who are also hypogonadal, men with testosterone levels within the normal range have also turned to supplemental testosterone to counteract wasting.[27] Intramuscular or transdermal testosterone therapy requires prescription and cooperation of a primary care provider.[70] Individuals seeking a testosterone-like benefit have been turning to dehydroepiandrosterone (DHEA), a naturally occurring adrenal steroid. DHEA was previously studied for possible immunomodulatory or antiretroviral

TABLE 10–2. ALTERNATIVE THERAPIES USED FOR WASTING

Agent	Nature of Agent	Suggested Activity	Potential Side Effects
Thalidomide	Sedative	Decreased TNF-α ? Antiviral	Sedation Teratogenecity
Ketotifen	Antihistamine	Decreased TNF-α	Sedation
Anabolic steroids including DHEA	Hormones	Increased lean body mass	Androgenizing effects
Marijuana	Cannabis	Appetite stimulant	Mental status changes ?Pulmonary effects

activity when AIDS patients were discovered to have depleted stores.[60] In a phase I dose-escalating trial, Dyner et al enrolled 31 subjects onto a 16-week trial.[28] Participants were treated with oral DHEA 250 to 750 mg three times a day with surrogate end-point monitoring. No changes were appreciated in lymphocyte subsets or p24 antigen levels; a transient increase in serum neopterin levels was noted. Although the unimpressive findings from this initial phase I trial may have inhibited further studies, DHEA has become an increasingly popular buyers' club item. Purchased as a "smart drug" by people without HIV infection, DHEA is being utilized by the AIDS community for its possible impact on increasing lean body mass. Injectable anabolic steroids, particularly deca-durabolin usually in conjunction with testosterone, is also becoming an increasingly popular alternative therapy for HIV-related weight loss and wasting. A placebo-controlled trial has been proposed for study in the ACTG.

The active component of marijuana, tetrahydrocannabinol, is one of the licensed therapies for the anorexia associated with HIV-related wasting.[36,82] In some circles, individuals prefer to inhale their cannabinoids rather than ingest them.[38] In San Francisco, a Cannabis Buyers' Club currently serves over 2000 clients with AIDS and other life-threatening conditions. On producing a physician's letter confirming the diagnosis, an individual can select from a variety of different vintages of marijuana to purchase for medical uses. Prompted by the widespread use and availability of inhaled marijuana in the HIV patient population, the Community Consortium, the Bay Area community-based clinical trials organization, set out to conduct a trial to determine the safety and evaluate the possible effectiveness of inhaled marijuana in patients with AIDS-related wasting syndrome.[6,39,78] One of the primary objectives of the proposed trial was to investigate the safety of smoked marijuana by assessing its impact over 12 weeks of the trial on pulmonary function tests, lymphocyte subset analyses, and HIV viral load. In addition, body composition analyses and appetite assessment tools were to be used to obtain an initial assessment of the usefulness of inhaled marijuana as compared to dronabinol in this small pilot study. Three different strengths of marijuana for the trial were to be supplied by a grower in the Netherlands. The pilot study was approved by the FDA, the university's institutional review board, and provisionally by the Research Advisory Panel of California, pending finalization of the source of the marijuana. The Drug Enforcement Administration, however, was reluctant to grant a Schedule I license because of the complex issue of international importation of the marijuana. A domestic source was sought and the FDA recommended approaching the National Institutes on Drug Abuse (NIDA). After 9 months of deliberation without communication, NIDA rejected the request claiming that the trial was scientifically flawed. In the meantime, countless AIDS patients in San Francisco and elsewhere continue to smoke marijuana in hopes that it may ameliorate their weight loss, with little information available on possible detrimental effects. The Community Consortium is determined to pursue all possibilities to be able to conduct the trial to obtain important safety information on the impact of smoking marijuana in this clinical situation.

Chinese Herbs and Acupuncture

A significant number of individuals with HIV infection seek alternative therapies from other than Western health care providers. Specifically in the San Francisco Bay Area, where much traditional Chinese medicine is practiced by the large local Asian community, patients with HIV infection in various stages have taken advantage of the abundance of providers as an alternative to Western medicine. These therapies are generally sought, not specifically as antiretroviral or immunomodulatory interactions, but as treatment for certain clinical or systemic manifestations of HIV disease, including wasting, nausea, sleep disturbances, and pain syndromes. Anecdotal reports of effectiveness of these interventions in patients for whom previous attempts at Western treatments have failed are abundant.

In an effort to obtain pilot information on the efficacy of Chinese herbal therapies in patients with symptomatic HIV infection, a collaborative trial was conducted in the AIDS Clinic at San Francisco General Hospital using treatments prepared by a Doctor of Oriental Medicine.[15] The herbal formulation was a 31-herb combination based on two herbal formulas, Enhance and Clear Heat, which have been used extensively in the treatment of patients with HIV infection. These herbs were selected for their purported antiviral and immunomodulatory properties. Thirty HIV-positive patients with CD4 cell counts between 200 and

$500/mm^3$, without a prior AIDS-defining diagnosis, were enrolled. All patients had to report experiencing at least two HIV-related symptoms to be eligible for the trial. In this randomized, double-blind, placebo-controlled pilot study, participants took 28 pills a day for 12 weeks. Outcome variables evaluated included changes from baseline in overall well-being, physical and social functioning, and symptoms. Changes in weight, CD4 count, hemoglobin, depression, and adherence to the regimen were also measured. Compliance was excellent and the only adverse reaction was the development of diarrhea requiring discontinuation of therapy in one placebo recipient. No significant changes were seen in any of the major outcome variables studied. The number of symptoms was reduced in subjects on herbs but not in those on placebo. Median life satisfaction change was greater in the herbal group. Believing that one was taking the active herb preparation was strongly associated with reporting that the treatment had helped, but not with changes in life satisfaction or symptoms.[16] After presentation of these results at an international AIDS conference, a practitioner from China commented that it is not possible to evaluate Chinese herbal interventions in a placebo-controlled manner and that no one should expect isolated herbal capsule preparations to work in the absence of the entire herb and outside of the context of a regimen including acupuncture. Regardless, we are now proceeding with trials of Chinese herbal preparations for treatment of cryptosporidium-negative diarrhea and for mild anemia funded by the Office of Alternative Medicine of the NIH.[58]

Perhaps the same caution will apply to the interpretation of a multicenter trial of acupuncture for the treatment of HIV-related peripheral neuropathy being conducted by the CPCRA. Cognizant of the wide use of acupuncture for this painful condition which is often refractory to other analgesic interventions, the CPCRA designed a factorial trial of a standard acupuncture regimen and amitriptylene compared with placebo. A target enrollment of 260 patients was sought for this study. Patients were initially randomized to receive one of four treatment arms for 14 weeks. The protocol defined study medication as follows: "Amitriptyline 75 mg/day or placebo, in combination with standardized acupuncture with Spleen 9, 7, 6 (Lower Three Kings) or alternate points acupuncture (Lower Three Jesters). Standardized additional points may be used with the Lower

Three Kings depending on patient symptoms."[25]

Although this certainly sounds quite progressive for a government sponsored protocol, the response from patients has been less than enthusiastic. First, many are not interested in possibly being randomized to an active amitriptylene arm because they aware of all of the associated side effects. Those who may be particularly attracted to the study because of the opportunity to receive acupuncture treatments are disappointed by the 50% chance of having needles inserted in sham points for 14 weeks. Although the exact efficacy of amitriptylene itself for the indication of HIV-related neuropathy has never been formally studied, the known benefit from other neuropathic syndromes has been extrapolated by many providers who are uncomfortable with the prospect of offering a quarter of the randomized patients both placebo drug and alternate-points acupuncture for 14 weeks. To address some of these issues, the original factorial design of the study was modified. Centers can now choose to randomize patients to amitriptylene versus placebo or to the acupuncture versus sham acupuncture arms. It is hoped that the protocol modification will allow the trial to accrue rapidly to shed light on this interesting East-meets-West treatment evaluation.

Curcumin

Alternative treatment activists are extremely adept at keeping up with basic science literature that may suggest any potential therapeutic intervention that has a glimmer of hope for arresting HIV. Harvard researchers described three inhibitors of HIV-1 long terminal repeat (LTR)–directed gene expression and viral replication.[54] The LTR governs activation of latent provirus. The activity of the LTR is determined by a complex interaction of positive and negative transcriptional regulators binding to specific sequences within the LTR. Tumor necrosis factor, for example, is felt to be a potent LTR activator. Compounds that block activation or suppress activity of the HIV-1 LTR could be useful for extending the viral latency period or inhibition of the persistent progressive infection. Curcumin, the major active component of the spice tumeric, has been demonstrated by these investigators to block HIV LTR activity. It was effective in both acute and chronically infected cells. This information generated enthusiasm among activists to call for the initiation of clinical trials investigating the antiretroviral activity of tumeric. An anthropological anecdote describes different rates of progression of HIV disease in Trinidad, speculating on a possible contribution of tumeric: 40% of the population of Trinidad is of Indian descent and another 40% is of African descent. Studies from several years ago in Trinidad suggested that those of African descent were ten times more likely to have the disease than persons of Indian descent.[46] Notwithstanding possible differences in risk behavior, an inference is made suggesting a benefit to eating more curry. Of note, curcumin is not soluble in water and very little has been detected in the bloodstream of animals after feeding. High doses have produced gastric ulceration in rats.

An "accelerated pilot" study of curcumin was conducted by a community-based clinical trial group in Los Angeles. The Search Alliance trial enrolled 19 patients with CD4 cell counts from 50 to 400/mm^3 of whom 50% were positive for HIV p24 antigen at entry. Participants received 2.5 g of encapsulated tumeric (70% curcumin) in three daily divided doses. The trial to assess safety and potential antiretroviral activity was initially scheduled to last 8 weeks, but was extended to 20. Of the initial 19 participants, 4 developed opportunistic infections, 2 withdrew for nonmedical reasons, and 2 withdrew because of nausea and upset stomach, leaving 11 evaluable patients. Among these patients, no significant changes in CD4 cell counts or p24 antigen levels were found. CD8 lymphocyte counts rose slightly. HIV viral load measured by PCR dropped 2.2 logs from week 4 through 12 but was back to baseline by week 20. The investigators concluded that "the initial results of this pilot study indicate that curcumin looks less promising as an antiretroviral agent. Curcumin appears to behave like other new agents (i.e., protease inhibitors), with low bioavailability, transient viral load reduction, and rapid viral resistance emergence."[74] The Community Research Initiative of New England (CRINE), another community-based clinical trial group, recently reported on the results of a 40-patient trial of curcumin.[42] Participants received either high-dose (4.8 g daily) or low-dose (2.7 g daily) of tumeric in an immediate or 8-week deferred initiation of treatment study design. In addition to safety, laboratory, and lymphocyte subset analyses, HIV RNA was assayed using the reverse transcriptase polymerase chain reaction (RT-PCR) technique. In contrast to the Search Alliance trial, the CRINE study reported that neither high- nor low-dose curcumin appeared to significantly decrease HIV RNA copy number or to change CD4+ cell counts. These trials would seem to have closed the book on curcumin as a potential alternative antiretroviral intervention.

SPV-30 Boxwood Evergreen

With enthusiasm waning for curcumin as a possible antiretroviral intervention and with the relative abundance of licensed available nucleoside analogues and protease inhibitors, SPV-30 is one of the few alternative agents being utilized for its purported anti-HIV activity.[75] SPV-30, a boxwood evergreen extract, was found to be virtually nontoxic in an initial phase I trial conducted in France in 1992. In the placebo-controlled pilot study, individuals receiving SPV-30 during the 6-month trial experienced a 100-cell CD4 increase compared to a 50-cell decline in those on placebo. These results reportedly led to the initiation of a larger phase II/III trial in France under the direction of Montagnier. A Boston activist, upon first learning about SPV-30, contacted the French manufacturer and arranged to gain access to the product. What began as an attempt to obtain SPV-30 for himself and some friends has developed into a project supplying 6 months of product to 500 individuals in a "trial-by-mail." Participants receive a free 2-month supply of SPV-30 in return for completing a questionnaire and supplying specified laboratory results, including HIV RNA levels. The study is open label and available to individuals regardless of CD4 cell count as long as they have been on a stable background regimen for at least 60 days prior to commencing the trial. Preliminary results from patients who have participated for 2 to 4 months indicate some increases in CD8 cells and an average viral load drop of 0.5 log at 2 months, and increases in CD4 cells after 4 months. The organizer of the "informal study" is "pleased . . . that we were able to get a promising, apparently non-toxic all natural alternative therapy in the hands of a substantial number of individuals in order to achieve real data as to its effectiveness."[75] Whether any useful information will emerge from this uncontrolled experiment remains to be seen.

ACQUISITION OF ALTERNATIVE THERAPIES

The "mail-order" acquisition of SPV-30 is another example of the organizational underpinnings of the HIV alternative therapies movement. Although many individuals procure alternative therapies on their own, an increasing number are using the services of buyers' clubs. A cottage industry has developed based on importation and resale of desirable alternative treatments. Initially established as centers for sale of vitamins and herbal remedies to patients interested in restoring immune function, buyers' clubs have now moved on to the business of providing patients with a veritable menu of desired alternative regimens and orthodox agents acquired through alternative means. Recently, the FDA has been making an increased effort to keep abreast of what agents require buyers' club distribution in an effort to shepard them more quickly into clinical trials or expanded access in order to lessen the need for buyers' clubs. However, numerous health care providers have taken advantage of the ease of acquisition of agents through the buyers' club mechanism instead of doing the copious amounts of paperwork and monitoring required to obtain similar agents through expanded-access programs. Despite the fact that the drugs available through expanded-access programs are free of charge to the patient, many prefer the ease of obtaining agents through buyers' clubs.

Individuals with HIV infection and their providers obtain information about which alternative treatments are currently being used through a number of regular publications. As an infrastructure for distribution of alternatives was established with an increasing number of complementary treatments from which to choose, a need for information dissemination arose. Organizations and publications devoted entirely to the spread of up-to-date information on available underground treatments began to appear in 1987. Project Inform, a community-based group of AIDS activists, was one of the first organizations established to provide such information. Using a 24-hour hotline and monthly newsletter, Project Inform quickly became one of the major clearinghouses for the alternative treatment movement.[69] They recently published *The HIV Drug Book,* a comprehensive illustrated guide to the most frequently used HIV/AIDS treatments, including some alternatives, in a useful reference format.[68] *AIDS Treatment News,* a biweekly update of AIDS treatment information, was first published in 1987.[44-46] With a current circulation of 5000, the newsletter informs readers of both alternative and experimental treatments. *Treatment Issues, the Gay Men's Health Crisis Newsletter of Experimental AIDS Therapies,* also appeared in 1987.[84] It cautions subscribers that "describing an experimental therapy should not be misconstrued as recommending it. All new treatments should be conducted under a physician's care." Ironically, however, as the availability of these sophisticated publications geared at the consumer population increased, the providing physicians were frequently ignorant of the particular new agent about which their patient was inquiring as a potential therapeutic intervention. Focused at the health care provider in addition to the consumer is the *AIDS/HIV Treatment Directory.*[3] This frequently updated directory reviews both orthodox and unorthodox agents that are currently in early and later stages of clinical development.

Practitioners caring for patients with AIDS have a number of options with regard to their ultimate approach to the use of alternative treatments (Table 10–3). Some providers may remain unaware of the use of alternatives, and some may choose to ignore that their patients are using unprescribed agents. Often patients fear that they cannot be forthcoming with their provider, being concerned about possible condemnation for not being fully content or confident with medications prescribed by their primary care physician. Condemning a patient's use of alternative treatment regimens without trying to understand what motivates the individual to seek these options is counterproductive in establishing and maintaining trust in the doctor–patient relationship.

Physicians should acknowledge the possibility that their patients are using alternative therapies. In taking a history they should stress in a nonjudgmental manner the need to under-

TABLE 10–3. PROVIDERS' ATTITUDES TOWARD ALTERNATIVE THERAPIES IN THEIR HIV PATIENT POPULATION

Remain unaware
Ignore
Condemn
Acknowledge
Monitor
Encourage
Refer

stand all medications and substances their patients are ingesting so they can best be able to evaluate the patient's clinical condition and determine what, in fact, may be the adverse effects of potential treatments. In some situations providers enter into a partnership with the patient and choose to assist in monitoring their use of alternative treatments. Some providers have taken an even more active stance in their approach to the use of alternative treatments by their patients. Often discouraged by the slow pace of drug development for HIV disease and enthusiastic about early in vitro reports of activity, some providers have encouraged the use of unorthodox, unproved treatments by their patients, especially for patients with advanced disease whose life span may not permit them to survive until actual clinical trials of an agent commence or to benefit from the result of such studies. These providers may encourage patients to seek alternative therapies and in fact refer them to a buyers' club to obtain the agents.

with regard to possible interaction of these agents with prescribed medications or over-the-counter therapeutics. If a patient is participating in a clinical trial to investigate another experimental agent and is not fully reporting alternative treatments being ingested, data could be invalidated. Patients, in their desire to obtain a potentially useful intervention, often coupled with desperation resulting from their declining clinical status, may be willing to pay for costly alternative treatment. The financial risk is coupled with the possibility that the agent may have very little chance of producing a positive effect. The dilemma was summarized in describing why a task force to investigate AIDS consumer fraud and quackery was established by the California State Attorney General's Office: "With so much unknown about AIDS, and with existing treatments so unsatisfactory, it will be hard to find consensus on how to distinguish legitimate, unproven and unconventional treatment attempts from unconscionable schemes to exploit people's desperation."[44]

POTENTIAL RISK OF ALTERNATIVE THERAPIES

HIV prefers to target cells of the immune system that are stimulated in some fashion. The effect of many alternative treatments on the status of the immune system remains unknown at this time (Table 10–4). Therefore, care must be taken that agents not activate lymphocytes, thus making them more susceptible to HIV infection. On the other hand, some substances may also suppress cellular or other aspects of the immune system and may ultimately prove detrimental to patients with HIV infection. For this reason it is desirable that individuals be cautioned against taking underground complementary therapies without being monitored by their physician.

A study by Greenblatt et al[37] clearly demonstrates the potential risk of alternative therapies

POTENTIAL BENEFITS OF ALTERNATIVE THERAPIES

Despite significant progress made in the past decade, there still is no cure for HIV infection. Individuals infected with the virus undergo decimation of their cellular immune system and ultimately develop life-threatening opportunistic infections or malignancies. Numerous potential antiretroviral, immunomodulatory, and antibiotic regimens are under study through NIAID's ACTG and CPCRA mechanisms. Other agents are being tested as pilot studies in academic medical centers and AIDS treatment clinics nationwide and throughout the world. However, AIDS is currently the leading cause of death in the United States in men age 25 to 44 and has become the leading cause of death in women in this age group in New York City. Knowing this grave prognosis, individuals in earlier stages of HIV infection and their advocates are anxious to expedite evaluation and approval of potentially efficacious agents.

The alternative therapies movement offers the possibility for evaluating increased numbers of potentially useful drugs. Even in the absence of careful monitoring and protocol analysis, should one of the alternatives turn out to be the "magic bullet," it is likely that this would not go unrecognized. As the alternative treatment movement has matured, however, in-

TABLE 10–4. POTENTIAL RISKS OF ALTERNATIVE THERAPIES

Immune stimulation or suppression
Interaction with prescribed medications
Invalidation of data if enrolled in clinical trial
Prohibition from participation in orthodox clinical trial
Potential strain on patient–provider relationship
Financial considerations
Potential for fraud and quackery

TABLE 10–5. IMPACT OF THE ALTERNATIVE THERAPY MOVEMENT

Importation for personal use allowed
Buyer's club industry established
Parallel track and expanded-access mechanisms created
Protocols for patients with prior drug exposure designed
Accelerated approval modified by FDA
Office of Alternative Medicine established

creased interest in scientific method and clinical trials design has been demonstrated by its advocates. Often these spokespersons for the alternative treatment movement are very helpful in educating their peers and their community about the necessity of following clinical protocols for drug evaluation. Increasing collaboration is being observed between the AIDS treatment activists and the medical establishment. Much of this has been due to the energy of the AIDS Coalition to Unleash Power (ACT UP), a group instrumental in increasing awareness about the sense of urgency to develop and promote expedited drug development for patients with HIV disease.

The impact of the alternative therapy movement can already be appreciated (Table 10–5). The process of drug approval has accelerated markedly and AIDS drugs are reaching the market in record times. The FDA responded to the alternative treatment movement in a number of ways over the past decade. By allowing importation of these agents for personal use, codifying the parallel track expanded-access program, coexisting with the buyers' club industry, and conducting timely reviews for accelerated approval, the FDA has demonstrated that it is not responding to the epidemic in a vacuum. Further evidence that the Public Health Service is listening carefully to the public is seen in the establishment of the Alternative Medicine Office at the National Institutes of Health.[58]

It is hoped that even more effective therapies for HIV infections and their manifestations will emerge in the near future. The alternative therapies movement has encouraged strides in modernizing and accelerating the drug approval process that will benefit patients with AIDS and HIV infection as well as those with other serious and life-threatening diseases. Unfortunately, in the absence of a cure for AIDS, the need for alternatives persists. John James, the editor of *AIDS Treatment News* and an effective treatment activist, poignantly summarizes the quandary: "In the past years, the only way the AIDS community could move a drug forward in the face of institutional neglect was to develop it as an 'alternative' treatment—i.e. let it go into widespread use—in the hope that if there were any substantial value it would be noticed, and if not, the substance would be retired through the usual 'drug of the month' process. Maybe we can do better today."[45]

Providers caring for patients with HIV infection should make every attempt to inform themselves about complementary therapies that may be in use in their community. Establishing trusting and open communication will enable the health professionals to enter a caring partnership with their patients, including those who may be empowering themselves in the presence of this relentless scourge by using alternative treatments.

REFERENCES

1. Aboulker JR, Swart AM: Preliminary analysis of the Concorde trial. Lancet 341:889–890, 1993
2. Abrams D: Dealing with alternative therapies for HIV. In Sande M, Volberding P, eds. The Medical Management of AIDS, ed 4. Philadelphia, WB Saunders Co, 1995, pp 183–207
3. Abrams D, Cotton D, Markowitz M, Mayer K, eds. AIDS/HIV treatment directory. Am Found AIDS Res (AmFAR) 7(1):1993
4. Abrams DI: Alternative therapies. In Repoza NP, ed. HIV Infection and Disease; Monographs for Physicians and Other Health Care Workers. Chicago, AMA Press, 1989, pp 163–175
5. Abrams DI: Alternative therapies in HIV infection. AIDS 4:1179–1187, 1990
6. Abrams DI, Child CC, Mitchell TF: Marijuana, the AIDS wasting syndrome, and the U.S. government (response). N Engl J Med 333:671, 1995
7. Alpha-Tocopherol, Beta Carotene Cancer Prevention Study Group: The effect of vitamin E and beta carotene on the incidence of lung cancer and other cancers in male smokers. N Engl J Med 330:1029–1035, 1994
8. Anderson WH: Patient use and assessment of conventional and alternative therapies for HIV infection and AIDS. AIDS 74:561–564, 1993
9. Ballmaier M, Rohde F, Schedel I, Deicher H: Ketotifen inhibits the production and secretion of TNF-alpha in PBMC cultures of HIV-infected patients (Abstract PuA 1009). Eighth International Conference on AIDS, Amsterdam, 1992
10. Bhasin S, Storer T, Strakova J, et al: Testosterone increases lean body mass, muscle size and strength in hypogonadal men. Clin Res 42:74A, 1991
11. Blakeslee JR, Yamamoto N, Hinuma Y: Human T-cell leukemia virus I induction by 5-iodo-2′-deoxyuri-

dine and N-methyl-N-nitro-N-nitrosoguanidine: Inhibition by retinoids, L-ascorbic acid, and DL-a tocopherol. Cancer Res 45:3471–3476, 1985

12. Block G, Henson DE, Levine M: Vitamin C: A new look. Ann Intern Med 114:909–910, 1991

13. Braathen LR, Ramirez G, Kunze ROF, et al: Latent infection of epidermal Langerhans cells in HIV-positive individuals. Res Virol 142:119–121, 1991

14. Buhl R, Ari Jaffe H, Holroyd KS, et al: Systemic glutathione deficiency in symptom-free HIV-seropositive individuals. Lancet 2:1294–1298, 1989

15. Burack JH, Cohen MR, Abrams DI: Chinese herbal treatment of HIV-associated symptoms (PO-B29-2191). Ninth International Conference on AIDS, Berlin, 1993, p 500

16. Burack JH, Cohen MR, Hahn JA, Abrams DI: A pilot randomized controlled trial of Chinese herbal treatment for HIV-associated symptoms. J Acquir Immune Defic Syndr 1996 (In press)

17. Cassileth BR, Lusk EJ, Strouse TB, et al: Contemporary unorthodox treatments in cancer medicine: A study of patients, treatments and practitioners. Ann Intern Med 101:105–112, 1989

18. Chen P, Schwartz D: Procysteine inhibits TNF-alpha induced HIV production in U1 cells. (PO-A13-0248). Ninth International Conference on AIDS, Berlin, 1993, p 176

19. Cohen O, Pantaleo G, Loveless M, et al: Effects of dinitrochlorobenzene therapy on viral load and cytokine expression in lymphoid tissue of HIV-infected individuals. IDSA 33rd Annual Meeting, San Francisco, 1995, p 135

20. Concorde Coordinating Committee: Concorde: MRC/ANRS randomised double-blind controlled trial of immediate and deferred zidovudine in symptom-free HIV infection. Lancet 343:871–878, 1994

21. Constans J, Pellegrin JL, Delmas MC, et al: One year supplementation of HIV-positive patients with selenium or betacarotene. Third Conference on Retroviruses and Opportunistic Infections, Washington, DC, 1996, p 122

22. Coodley GO, Nelson HD, Loveless MO, et al: Beta carotene in HIV infection. J Acquir Immune Defic Syndr 6:272–276, 1993

23. Cooley TP, Kunches LM, Saunders CA, et al: Once-daily administration of 2,3-dideoxyinosine (ddI) in patients with the acquired immunodeficiency syndrome or AIDS-related complex: Results of a phase I trial. N Engl J Med 322:1340–1345, 1990

24. Cooper S: Thalidomide, gentrified. Notes from the Underground: The PWA Health Group Newsletter 31:1–3, 1996

25. CPCRA 022: The efficacy of a standardized acupuncture regimen and amitriptyline compared with placebo as a treatment for pain caused by peripheral neuropathy in HIV-infected patients, 1993, p iii

26. Danner SA, Carr A, Leonard JM, et al: A short term study of the safety, pharmacokinetics, and efficacy of ritonavir, an inhibitor of HIV-1 protease. N Engl J Med 333:1528–1533, 1995

27. Dobs AS, Dempsey MA, Landenson PW, et al: Endocrine disorders in men infected with HIV. Am J Med 84:611–616, 1988

28. Dyner TS, Lang W, Geaga J, et al: An open-label dose-escalation trial of oral dehydroepiandrosterone tolerance and pharmacokinetics in patients with HIV

disease. J Acquir Immune Defic Syndr 6:459–465, 1993

29. Eisenberg DM, Kessler RC, Foster C, et al: Unconventional medicine in the United States: Prevalence, costs and patterns of use. N Engl J Med 328:246–252, 1993

30. Eron JJ, Benoit SL, Jemsek J, et al: Treatment with lamivudine, zidovudine, or both in HIV-infected patients with 200 to 500 CD4+ cells per cubic millimeter. N Engl J Med 333:1662–1669, 1995

31. Fauci AS: Multifactorial nature of human immunodeficiency virus disease: Implications for therapy. Science 262:1011–1018, 1993

32. Fischl MA, Richman DD, Grieco MH, et al: Azidothymidine (AZT) in the treatment of patients with AIDS and AIDS-related complex. A double-blind, placebo-controlled trial. N Engl J Med 317:185–191, 1987

33. Fischl MA, Richman DD, Hansen N, et al: The safety and efficacy of zidovudine (AZT) in the treatment of subjects with mildly symptomatic human immunodeficiency virus type 1 (HIV) infection. A double-blind, placebo-controlled trial. Ann Intern Med 112:727–737, 1990

34. Folks TM, Clouse KA, Justement J, et al: Tumor necrosis factor alpha induces expression of human immunodeficiency virus in a chronically infected T cell clone. Proc Natl Acad Sci USA 86:2365–2368, 1989

35. Gorman C: Beta no more: A diet supplement taken by millions doesn't work. Time 147(5):66, 1996

36. Gorter R, Seefried M, Volberding P: Dronabinol effects on weight in patients with HIV infection. AIDS 6:127–128, 1992

37. Greenblatt RM, Hollander H, McMaster JR, et al: Polypharmacy among patients attending an AIDS clinic: Utilization of prescribed unorthodox, and investigational treatments. J Acquir Immune Defic Syndr 4:136–143, 1991

38. Grinspoon L, Bakalar JB: Marijuana as medicine: A plea for reconsideration. JAMA 273:1875–1876, 1995

39. Grinspoon L, Bakalar JB, Doblin R: Marijuana, the AIDS wasting syndrome, and the U.S. Government. N Engl J Med 333:670–671, 1995

40. Gulick R, Mellors J, Havlir D, et al: Potent and sustained antiretroviral activity of indinavir in combination with zidovudine and lamivudine. Third Conference of Retroviruses and Opportunistic Infections. Washington, DC, 1996, p 162

41. Harakeh S, Jariwalla RJ, Pauling L: Suppression of human immunodeficiency virus replication by ascorbate in chronically and acutely infected cells. Proc Natl Acad Sci U S A 87:7245–7249, 1990

42. Hellinger JA, Cohen CJ, Dugan ME, et al: Phase I/II randomized, open-label study of oral curcumin safety, and antiviral effects on HIV-RT PCR in HIV+ individuals. Third Conference on Retroviruses and Opportunistic Infections, Washington, DC, 1996, p 78

43. Herbarth L, Suttmann U, Ballmaier M, et al: Effects of ketotifen on HIV infected individuals (PO-B29-2189). Ninth International Conference on AIDS, Berlin, 1993, p 500

44. James JS: AIDS Treatment News No 31, June 5, 1987

45. James JS: New kind of HIV antiviral: Food spice, cancer drug show activity. AIDS Treatment News No 174, May 7, 1993

46. James JS: Curcumin update: Could food spice be low-

cost antiviral? AIDS Treatment News No 176, June 4, 1993

47. Jariwalla RJ, Harakeh S: HIV suppression by ascorbate and its enhancement by glutathione precursor (PO-B-3697). Eighth International Conference on AIDS, Amsterdam, 2:B207, 1992

48. Kalebic T, Kinter A, Poli G, et al: Suppression of human immunodeficiency virus expression in chronically infected monocytic cells by glutathione, glutathione ester and N-acetylcysteine. Proc Natl Acad Sci U S A 88:986–990, 1991

49. King R, Homsy J, Serufilira A, et al: Traditional medicine vs. modern medicine for AIDS (PO-B-3394). Eighth International Conference on AIDS, Amsterdam, 2:B152, 1992

50. Kitchen VS, Skinner C, Ariyoshi K, et al: Safety and efficacy of saquinavir in HIV infection. Lancet 345:952–955, 1995

51. Lahdevirta J, Maury CP, Teppo AM, et al: Elevated levels of circulating cachectin/tumor necrosis factor in patients with acquired immunodeficiency syndrome. Am J Med 85:289–291, 1988

52. Laifer G, Ruettimann S, Langewitz W, et al: Frequent use of alternative therapies and higher subjective benefit compared to traditional medicine in HIV-infected patients (PO-B-3395). Eighth International Conference on AIDS, Amsterdam, 2:B152, 1992

53. Lambert JS, Seidlin N, Reichman RC, et al: 2′,3′-dideoxyinosine (ddI) in patients with the acquired immunodeficiency syndrome or AIDS-related complex: A phase I trial. N Engl J Med 322:1333–1340, 1990

54. Li CJ, Zhang LJ, Dezube BJ, et al: Three inhibitors of type 1 human immunodeficiency virus long terminal repeat-directed gene expression and virus replication. Proc Natl Acad Sci U S A 90:1839–1842, 1993

55. Loveless M, Bradley B, Fields L, Dharmananda S: Effect of dinitrochlorobenzene (DNCB) cutaneous sensitization on HIV disease progression. IDSA 33rd Annual Meeting, San Francisco, 1995, p 134

56. Makonkawkeyoon S, Limson-Probre RNR, Moreira AL, et al: Thalidomide inhibits replication of human immunodeficiency virus type 1. Proc Natl Acad Sci U S A 90:5974–5978, 1993

57. Markowitz M, Saag M, Powderly WG, et al: A preliminary study of ritonavir, an inhibitor of HIV-1 protease, to treat HIV-1 infection. N Engl J Med 333:1534–1539, 1995

58. Marwick C: Alternative medicine office urged to act rapidly. JAMA 270:1409, 1993

59. Mayer K, Seage G, Gross M, et al: Predictors of therapeutic choices among HIV-infected homosexual males (PO-B32-2236). Ninth International Conference on AIDS, Berlin, 1993, p 508

60. Merril CR, Harrington MG: Plasma dehydroepiandrosterone levels in HIV infection. JAMA 261:1149, 1989

61. Mihm S, Ennen J, Pessara U, et al: Inhibition of HIV-1 replication and NF-nB activity by cysteine and cysteine derivatives. AIDS 5:497–503, 1991

62. Mills BL: Stimulation of T-cellular immunity by cutaneous application of dinitrochlorobenzene. J Am Acad Dermatol 6:1089–1090, 1986

63. Moreira AL, Ye W, Shen Z, et al: Thalidomide reduces HIV-1 production in acutely infected human monocytes in vitro. Third Conference on Retroviruses and

64. Moreira AL, Sampaio EP, Zmuidzinas A, et al: Thalidomide exerts its inhibitory action on TNF-alpha by enhancing mRNA degradation. J Exp Med 177:1675, 1993

65. Mulligan K, Grunfeld C, Hellerstein MK, et al: Anabolic effects of recombinant human growth hormone in patients with weight loss associated with HIV infection. J Clin Endocrinol Metab 77:956–962, 1993

66. Nottet HSLM, van Asbeck BS, de Graaf L, et al: Role for oxygen radicals in the self-sustained HIV-1 replication in monocyte-derived macrophages: Enhanced HIV-1 replication by N-acetyl-L-cysteine (PO-A12-0199). Ninth International Conference on AIDS, Berlin, 1993, p 168

67. Oster MH, Enders SH, Samuels ST, et al: Megestrol acetate in patients with AIDS and cachexia. Ann Intern Med 121:400–408, 1994

68. Petrow S, ed: The HIV Drug Book. New York, Pocket Books, 1995

69. PI Perspective. (Quarterly) Project Inform.

70. Place VA, Atkinson L, Prather DA, et al: Transdermal testosterone replacement through genital skin. In Nieschlag E, Behre HM, eds. Testosterone—Action, Deficiency, Substitution. Berlin and Heidelberg, Springer-Verlag, 1990, pp 165–181

71. Roderer M, Stahl FJI, Raju PA, et al: Cytokine-stimulated human immunodeficiency virus replication is inhibited by N-acetyl-L-cysteine. Proc Natl Acad Sci U S A 87:4884–4888, 1990

72. Sampaio EP, Moreira AL, Sarno EN, et al: Prolonged treatment with recombinant interferon-g induces erythema nodosum leprosum in lepromatous leprosy patients. J Exp Med 175:1729, 1992

73. Sande MA, Carpenter CCJ, Cobbs CG, et al: Antiretroviral therapy for adult HIV infected patients: Recommendations from a state-of-the-art conference. JAMA 270:2583–2589, 1993

74. SEARCHLIGHT, Spring 1994

75. SPV-30 study: A one man crusade. Press release, Boston, June 26, 1995

76. Staal FJT, Ela SW, Roederer, et al: Glutathione deficiency and human immunodeficiency virus infection. Lancet 339:909–912, 1992

77. Staal FJT, Roederer M, Anderson MT, et al: Intracellular glutathione deficiency in AIDS: Implications for therapy (PO-A-2400). Eighth International Conference on AIDS, Amsterdam, 2:A69, 1992

78. Steele FR: Keeping a lid on marijuana research. Nat Med 1:853–854, 1995

79. Stricker RB, Elswood BF, Abrams DI: Dendritic cells and dinitrochlorobenzene (DNCB): A new treatment approach to AIDS. Immunol Lett 29:191–196, 1991

80. Stricker RB, Elswood BF. Topical dinitrochlorobenzene in HIV disease. J Am Acad Dermatol 28:796–797, 1993

81. Stricker RB, Elswood BF, Goldberg B, et al: Analysis of lymphocyte subsets in HIV-infected patients treated with topical dinitrochlorobenzene (DNCB) (PO-B28-2140). Ninth International Conference on AIDS, Berlin, 1993, p 492

82. Struwe M, Kaemfper SH, Geiger CF, et al: Effect of dronabinol on nutritional status in HIV infection. Ann Pharmacol 27:827–831, 1993

83. Traub A, Margulis SB: Use of dinitrocholorobenzene

(DNCB) as an immune modulatory in HIV-positive patients: A pilot study from Brazil. Blood 86(10)(S1):935a, 1995

84. Treatment Issues: The GMHC newsletter of experimental AIDS therapies. New York, GMHC.

85. Valentine C, Weston R, Kitchen V, et al: Anonymous questionnaire to assess consumption of prescribed and alternative medication and patterns of recreational drug use in an HIV positive population (TH-B-1508). Eighth International Conference on AIDS, Amsterdam, 1:204, 1992

86. Van Dam F, De Boer J, Cleijne W, et al: The use of remedies and alternative therapies by patients with symptomatic HIV infection (PO-B-3402). Eighth International Conference on AIDS, Amsterdam, 2: B154, 1992

87. Von Roehn JH, Armstrong D, Kotler DP, et al. Megestrol acetate in patients with AIDS related cachexia. Ann Intern Med 121:393–399, 1994

88. Volberding PA, Lagakos SW, Koch MA, et al: Zidovudine in asymptomatic human immunodeficiency virus infection. A controlled trial in persons with fewer than 500 CD4-positive cells per cubic millimeter. N Engl J Med 322:941–949, 1990

89. Walker RE, Lane H, Boenning C, et al: The safety, pharmacokinetics, and antiviral activity of N-acetylcysteine in HIV-infected individuals (MO-B-0022). Eighth International Conference on AIDS, Amsterdam, 1:72, 1992

Chapter 11

Dermatologic Care in the AIDS Patient

TIMOTHY G. BERGER

Skin disease is an extremely common complication of human immunodeficiency virus (HIV) infection, affecting up to 90% of persons.[3] Some of the skin conditions are common ones also seen in uninfected persons (e.g., seborrheic dermatitis), but of increased severity. Other skin diseases are relatively unique to HIV infection (e.g., Kaposi's sarcoma [KS]). The average HIV-infected patient has at least two and often more different skin conditions simultaneously. It is useful to classify the cutaneous disorders seen with HIV disease as either infectious disorders, hypersensitivity disorders and drug reactions, or neoplasms. The treatment of these conditions is summarized in Table 11–1.

The type of skin disease seen in the course of HIV disease relates to the patient's immune status. In general, in persons with early HIV disease (CD4 count >500/mm^3), only skin diseases typical of the risk factors for HIV disease are seen (e.g., genital herpes simplex virus [HSV], genital warts). At this stage, human papilloma virus (HPV) infection (warts) is resistant to therapy. KS may appear at this stage. Less common are thrush, oral hairy leukoplakia, and herpes zoster. During the early symptomatic phase (CD4 count 200 to 500/mm^3), (formerly called ARC), disorders of subtle immune imbalance occur: candidiasis, oral hairy leukoplakia, herpes zoster, psoriasis, seborrheic dermatitis, and atopic dermatitis. Response to treatment is normal. Once the CD4 count is less than 200/mm^3, (acquired immunodeficiency syndrome [AIDS]), skin disease becomes somewhat different. Opportunistic infections such as cryptococcosis and histoplasmosis may occur on the skin, and skin infections become chronic. Chronic herpes simplex is one example. At this stage, HIV-specific inflammatory diseases also appear. Pruritus from any cause is uncommon with a CD4 count >200 to 300/mm^3, and is very common below these CD4 counts. Drug reactions, insect bite hypersensitivity, and itchy folliculitis are all manifestations of the enhanced cutaneous reactivity seen in AIDS. Once the CD4 count is <50/mm^3, bizarre patterns of skin disease occur. Biopsies are frequently required to confirm diagnoses. Treatment failures, drug resistance, and chronicity are the hallmark findings of this stage of HIV disease.

INFECTIOUS CUTANEOUS DISORDERS

Bacterial Infections

Staphylococcus aureus is the most common cutaneous bacterial pathogen.[5] The following patterns of staphylococcal infection may be seen: folliculitis, bullous impetigo, ecthyma, abscesses, hidradenitis suppurativa-like plaques, and cellulitis. Folliculitis is the most common form of staphylococcal infection seen in HIV-infected persons (Fig. 11–1). The central trunk, groin, and face are the most common sites of infection. The primary lesion is a follicular pustule, but lesions may be almost urticarial. Many HIV-infected patients with staphylococcal folliculitis of the trunk have severe pruritus, and this represents one of the more treatable pruritic eruptions seen in HIV disease.[5] Often many of the lesions have been excoriated and the patient must be carefully examined for a primary lesion adequate for culture. Bullous impetigo is quite common in the groin and axillae, presenting as flaccid blisters that quickly rupture leaving small superficial erosions with a peripheral scale. The lesions are usually asymptomatic, and occur more commonly during hot, humid

TABLE 11–1. DIAGNOSIS AND TREATMENT OF SKIN CONDITIONS COMMONLY SEEN WITH HIV INFECTION

Condition	Morphology	Location	Treatment	Duration
Staphylococcal folliculitis	Erythematous follicular pustules or papules; may be pruritic	Face, trunk, groin	Dicloxacillin, 500 mg PO qid, *or* other penicillinase-resistant antistaphylococcal antibiotic Refractory: add rifampin, 600 mg qd to above	7–21 days First 5 days antibiotic therapy with above
Bacillary angiomatosis	Friable, vascular papules, cellulitic plaques, subcutaneous nodules	Skin, bone, liver, spleen, lymph node	Erythromycin, 500 mg qid *or* Doxycycline, 100 mg bid	Skin: 8 weeks Visceral: unknown, but consider 16 weeks
Herpes zoster (shingles)	Grouped vesicles on erythematous bases	Dermatomal distribution; may spill onto adjacent dermatomes	Acute: acyclovir, 800 mg PO 5 times per day Dissemination, severe immunosuppression, or involvement of ophthalmic branch of trigeminal nerve: acyclovir, 10 mg/kg IV q8h (corrected for creatinine clearance)	7–10 days Give IV until no new blisters for 72 h, then finish orally as above
Herpes simplex	Grouped vesicles on erythematous bases, rapidly evolving into superficial mucocutaneous ulcerations or fissures; necrotizing ulcers may be seen when chronic	Face, hand, or anogenital area	Acute: acyclovir, 200–400 mg PO 5 times per day Oral acyclovir failure or dissemination: acyclovir, 5 mg/kg IV q8h (corrected for creatinine clearance) Maintenance: acyclovir, 200 mg PO tid or 400 mg, PO bid Acyclovir resistance: foscarnet	7–10 days or until ulcers healed Indefinitely

Molluscum contagiosum	2- to 5-mm pearly flesh-colored papules, often with central umbilication	Face, anogenital area	Cryotherapy *or* Electrosurgery *or* Curettage	For all treatments: repeat at 2- to 3-week intervals until resolved
Insect bite reactions	Erythematous, urticarial papules	Scabies: axillae, groin, finger webs Fleas: lower legs Mosquitoes: upper and lower extremities	Scabies: lindane 1% lotion for 12 h; permethrin (Elimite) 5% lotion for 12 h Fleas, mosquitoes: 1. Insect repellants 2. Antihistamines 3. Insecticide spray of environment (fleas)	Twice, 1 week apart Constant, regular use
Photosensitivity	Eczematous eruption	Face (tip of nose), extensor forearms, neck	1. Sun protection, sunscreens 2. Discontinuation of photosensitizing medications 3. Topical steroids	Continuous for *1* and *2*; as needed for *3*
Eosinophilic folliculitis	Urticarial follicular papules	Trunk, face	Astemizole, 10 mg qd Itraconazole 200–400 mg daily *and* Topical steroids *or* Ultraviolet light	Constant treatment
Seborrheic dermatitis	Fine, white scaling without erythema (dandruff) to patches and plaques of erythema with indistinct margins and yellowish, greasy scale	Scalp, central face, eyebrows, nasolabial and retroauricular folds, chest, upper back, axillae, groin	Hydrocortisone 2.5% cream and ketoconazole 2% cream applied bid Maintenance: Hydrocortisone 1% cream and ketoconazole 2% cream applied bid	Until lesions resolve Indefinitely
Psoriasis and Reiter's syndrome	Sharply marginated plaques with a silvery scale	Elbows, knees, lumbosacral area	Triamcinolone acetonide 0.1% cream tid	Indefinitely

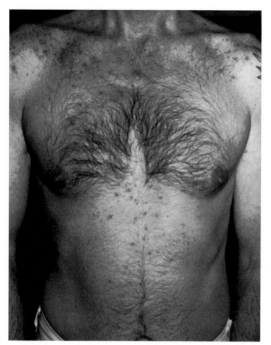

FIGURE 11–1. Pruritic bacterial folliculitis of the trunk. *Staphylococcus aureus* was cultured from a lesion; the condition cleared with oral antibiotics.

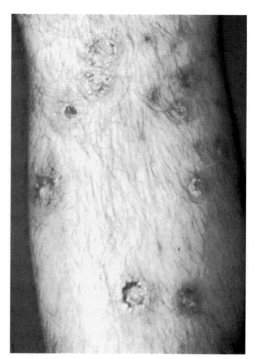

FIGURE 11–2. Ecthyma showing punched-out staphylococcal ulcers of the lower leg.

weather. Ecthyma is a punched-out ulcer with a sharp border. The base may be purulent, or may be covered with a thick, adherent crust (Fig. 11–2). Lesions are most common on the lower legs, commonly overlying a preexisting dermatitis. Violaceous tender cystic plaques and nodules in the axillae and groin may be due to *S. aureus* alone, as are virtually all suppurative abscesses. All of the above patterns may be accompanied by an associated cellulitis (Color Plate II*A*.)

The treatment of cutaneous staphylococcal infections is determined by the severity of the infection and the presence of systemic symptoms. Patients with chills, fever, large abscesses, or cellulitis are usually admitted for intravenous therapy. Abscesses should be incised and drained. Localized infection may be treated on an outpatient basis with oral agents once cultures are taken. Patients are reexamined after 3 to 5 days to ensure improvement and to be sure the appropriate antibiotic was chosen. A penicillinase-resistant penicillin or first-generation cephalosporin is the first choice for therapy. Since nasal carriage approaches 50% in these patients, rifampin 600 mg in a single daily dose for at least 5 days or intranasal mupirocin may be added in refractory or relapsing cases.

Washing with benzoyl peroxide washes or antibacterial soaps may be beneficial to prevent relapse, but should be accompanied by vigorous lubrication, since dry skin is so common.

Viral Infections

The herpes viruses are common cutaneous viral pathogens; herpes simplex (HSV) and varicella zoster viruses frequently cause skin disease. **Herpes zoster** occurs in up to 8% of HIV-infected persons, and the average CD4 count for the initial episode is 315/mm³.[2] Any person, especially under age 65, who develops shingles should be queried about risk factors for HIV infection. Usually the course of herpes zoster is uneventful, although persistent postherpetic neuralgia may occur. In patients with more advanced HIV disease, herpes zoster may be very painful, severe, and prolonged. Dissemination may occur, but is usually limited to skin. Disseminated herpetic lesions are almost always due to varicella zoster; disseminated herpes simplex is rare in HIV disease.

Herpes simplex infections occur in the genital, digital, and orofacial areas. Once the CD4 count is <200/mm³ herpetic lesions present as persistent nonhealing ulcers. It is not unusual for lesions to be secondarily infected, so cultures may yield *S. aureus* or other pathogens. A viral culture or fluorescent antibody examination should be performed. If this is negative, a biopsy of the edge of the ulcer should be considered. It is sometimes impossible clinically to diagnose chronic ulcerations in HIV-infected persons, and multiple cultures and a skin biopsy may be required.

Molluscum contagiosum is extremely common in patients with AIDS. Lesions present as umbilicated, pearly 2- to 5-mm papules on the face, genital area, and scattered on the trunk. There is a particular predilection for lesions to occur on the eyelids. Lesions may number from one to hundreds. Occasional lesions may exceed 1 cm (giant molluscum) (Fig. 11–3). Their pearly border and telangiectasias may lead to the misdiagnosis of basal cell carcinoma. Extensive molluscum of more than one anatomic region (e.g., face and groin), is highly suggestive of a CD4 count <50/mm³. Complete eradication is extremely difficult. Lesions are usually treated with destructive modalities (cryotherapy with liquid nitrogen, light electrocautery, or curettage). Topical retinoic acid (Retin A) applied once nightly to the face may slow down the rate of appearance but, unless applied to the point of severe irritation, does little for established lesions. It cannot be used on the eyelids or genitalia. We and others have seen disseminated cryptococcosis, penicilliosis, and herpetic folliculitis mimic molluscum contagiosum.[4]

Parasitic Infections

Acanthamebiasis is a rare form of encephalitis that may occur in both immunocompetent and immunosuppressed hosts. It may occur in advanced AIDS (CD4) count <50/mm³).[8] In AIDS patients, skin lesions are the most common presentation (75% of cases), and may precede evidence of involvement of other tissues by weeks to months. Lesions occur as deep-seated nodules that suppurate, crust, or weep serosanguinous fluid. They occur most commonly on the extremities, but with time, generalization occurs. Sinusitis is commonly present, and the palate or nasal septum may be perforated. The diagnosis is established by biopsy of an ulcer, which will show suppurative and granulomatous inflammation with vasculitis. The vasculitis is uncommon in other infectious granulomas and should alert the pathologist to search for acanthameba. The organisms are hard to identify on routine histologic material, as they resemble macrophages. Special stains are not very useful; therefore, the clinician must notify the pathologist that acanthameba is a possible diagnosis. The prognosis is dismal, despite multidrug therapy.

HYPERSENSITIVITY DISORDERS

This section contains those disorders that cause the pruritic eruptions so common in AIDS. Many of these disorders are poorly characterized, their pathogenesis is not understood, and the optimal treatments are unknown.[1] Excluding drug reactions, I believe the ability to diagnose three fourths of the pruritic eruptions seen in AIDS is quite good for our current state of knowledge.

Drug Reactions

It has been long recognized that in approximately 50% of persons treated with trimethoprim-sulfamethoxazole (TMP-SMX) for *Pneumocystis* pneumonia, a widespread morbilliform eruption will develop[6] (Color Plate II *B*). The rash may resolve with continued treatment, but often persists or progresses. Therapy may be continued if symptoms are not too severe. Pro-

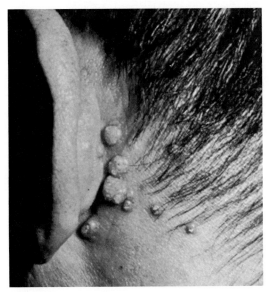

FIGURE 11–3. Extensive molluscum contagiosum of the head and neck, an almost certain indication of advanced HIV disease with a helper T cell count of <200/mm³.

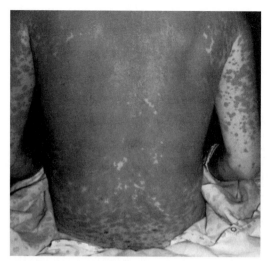

FIGURE 11–4. Drug-induced erythema multiforme major.

ications that have caused these reactions. In some patients, this reaction pattern develops to many chemically unrelated medications. These patients may have increasingly severe reactions with each medication exposure and erythema multiforme major may eventually develop.

In addition to morbilliform reactions, erythema multiforme, and fixed drug eruptions are seen with dramatically increased frequency in HIV-infected individuals. In some patients, the erythema multiforme may be quite severe—appearing as Stevens-Johnson syndrome or toxic epidermal necrolysis (Fig. 11–4). These severe reactions are most commonly due to sulfa drugs and anticonvulsants used to treat central nervous system (CNS) toxoplasmosis or *Pneumocystis* pneumonia.[12] Any HIV-infected person with a widespread eruption should be evaluated for the possibility of its being medication induced.

gression to a life-threatening reaction has not been reported **during that treatment episode.** Similar reactions are seen as a result of virtually all other medications given to HIV-infected patients, but seem to be most common with antibiotics, especially the penicillins and sulfa drugs. Cutaneous reactions are rare with certain frequently used medications, especially acyclovir and the antiretrovirals. It is unknown whether rechallenge at the full dose or desensitization is the best approach for reinstituting needed med-

Insect Bite Reactions

Scabies, flea bites, and mosquito bites may all be extremely florid in patients with HIV disease. These eruptions present as nonfollicular papules to cellulitic plaques with marked pruritus. The nature of the offending arthropod is determined by the distribution of the eruption, and by identification of the biting insects in the pa-

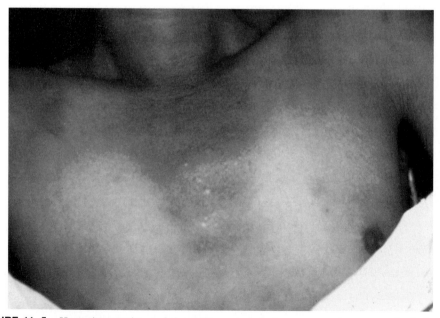

FIGURE 11–5. Hyperpigmentation and dermatitis exclusively in sun-exposed areas may be induced by certain medications (sulfa drugs, NSAIDs) or may be due to HIV infection alone.

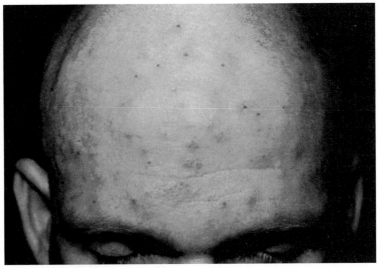

FIGURE 11–6. Eosinophilic folliculitis of the forehead.

tient's environment. In San Francisco, fleas are a common cause of lower leg pruritic papules, nodules, and blisters, whereas in Miami, mosquitoes are the most important cause.[11] In all patients, the fingerwebs, genitalia, axillae, and

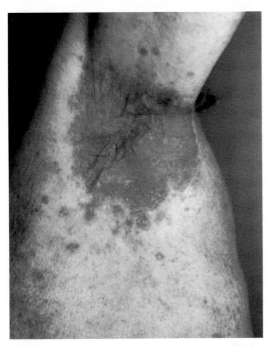

FIGURE 11–7. Seborrheic dermatitis of the axilla in a patient with AIDS. Seborrheic dermatitis commonly is accentuated in the axillae and groin in HIV-infected persons and is distinguished from cutaneous candidiasis by a negative potassium hydroxide scraping. The patient was treated successfully with a mild topical steroid and an imidazole cream mixed together and applied twice daily.

feet should be carefully examined for lesions. When lesions are found in these areas, they should be scraped to search for scabetic mites. Scabies is spread by close personal contact, so the affected person must also be examined for sexually transmitted diseases. Treatment of scabies is with lindane or permethrin applied to the whole body once for 12 hours and repeated 1 week later. Lindane treatment may fail in persons with more advanced HIV infection (with CD4 counts $<150/mm^3$). Five per cent permethrin (Elimite) has been effective in some of these patients. Extensive, crusted scabies (Norwegian scabies) may occur in patients with advanced HIV disease. It is nonpruritic and mimics psoriasis. Daily sequential applications of permethrin, crotamiton (Eurax), or 6% sulfur in petrolatum are recommended (Elimite 1 day, Eurax or sulfur for 6 days comprising 1 week of therapy). This is repeated for several weeks until the patient is cured.

Other insect bite reactions are treated by three steps: (1) *Eliminate the biting insects* from the patient's environment with insecticides, (2) *make the patient less attractive to the insect* with insect repellents (products containing diethyl toluamide [DEET]), and (3) *block the patient's reaction to the bite* with potent antihistamines taken regularly—not as needed. At least a generous nightly dose should be given (e.g., hydroxyzine 50 to 75 mg), with additional doses during the day if this is inadequate. Persistent pruritic papules are treated with medium- to high-potency topical steroids until they resolve.

Photosensitivity

The presence of HIV disease alone, or the medications that HIV-infected patients take, may lead to cutaneous eruptions predominantly in sun-exposed areas; that is, photodermatitis.[10] These eruptions initially may resemble an enhanced sunburn, but may progress or initially appear as pruritic scaly patches. They frequently are excoriated, become thickened, and often cause an increase or loss of skin pigment (Fig. 11–5), especially in persons of color. With time, the eruption may extend to unexposed skin. Short-wave ultraviolet irradiation (UVB) is the usual precipitating spectrum. Photodermatitis is managed by (1) discontinuation of potential photosensitizers (sulfa drugs, nonsteroidal antiinflammatory drugs [NSAIDs]); (2) protecting the patient from the sun with sunscreens, hats and clothing, and sun avoidance; and (3) applying a medium- to high-potency topical steroid to the lesions. In my experience, this is relatively easy to manage if the pattern is recognized. If allowed to persist, the patient may progress to a state of enhanced photosensitivity that will not respond to these simple measures. Black men with a CD4 count $<50/mm^3$ are at particular risk for severe photodermatitis.

Pruritic Folliculitis

Some HIV-infected persons with pruritic folliculitis have *S. aureus* infection.[5] A skin biopsy is required to rule out other infectious processes (systemic fungal infections) and to determine the composition of the inflammatory infiltrate. Eosinophilic folliculitis is the most common nonstaphylococcal folliculitis in HIV-infected persons. It occurs in patients with CD4 counts $\leq 200/mm^3$. Characteristically, it is a chronic, waxing and waning eruption with moderate to severe pruritus.[9,14] The primary lesion is an edematous papule ≤ 1 cm, with a tiny central pustule. The lesions are scattered on the upper trunk, head (especially forehead), neck, and proximal upper extremities (Fig. 11–6); 90% of lesions occur above a line drawn across the nipples. Culture results for bacteria are uniformly negative, and patients do not respond to antibiotics effective against *S. aureus*. Skin biopsy reveals inflammation containing eosinophils surrounding and involving the hair follicle. In my experience, chronic use of antihistamines, especially as-

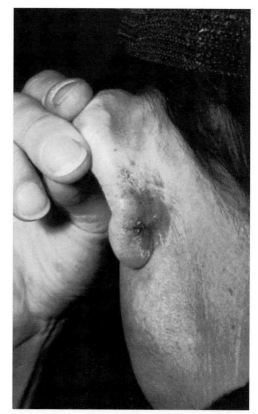

FIGURE 11–8. Seborrheic dermatitis in the retroauricular area. Erosion, weeping, and secondary staphylococcal infection are common in this location.

temizole or loratidine, and potent topical steroids are partially effective. Astemizole may cause cardiac toxicity when given with erythromycin (and related medications) and with imidazole antifungals (ketoconazole, itraconazole, or fluconazole). Phototherapy with UVB or paoralen plus ultraviolet A (PUVA) may be beneficial. Itraconazole in a dose of 200 to 400 mg/day may cause improvement in about 60% of patients with eosinophilic folliculitis. Prolonged (4- to 6-week) topical therapy chronically every other day with 5% permethrin cream or sulfacet R may lead to a more sustained remission. Accutane (isotretinoin) in a dose of about 0.75 to 1.0 mg/kg/day may also be of benefit.[9]

Papulosquamous Disorders

Three dermatologic disorders characterized by scaling patches and plaques are seen commonly in HIV-infected persons—seborrheic dermatitis, psoriasis, and Reiter's syndrome.[3] These papulosquamous disorders form a spectrum from mild and skin only (seborrheic der-

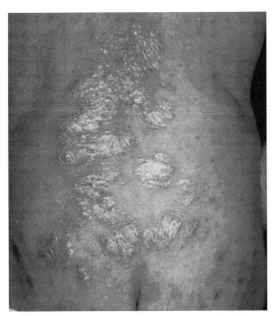

FIGURE 11–9. Typical plaquelike psoriasis that began in the sixth decade in this HIV-infected man. Pruritus was severe.

matitis), to moderate or severe, and skin only (psoriasis), to severe with systemic findings (severe psoriasis or Reiter's syndrome).[13,15] There is considerable overlap and a mild form may progress to a more severe form.

Seborrheic dermatitis is extremely common, affecting to varying degrees most persons with symptomatic HIV disease. Lesions are usually located in the hairy areas of the central face, scalp, chest, back, and groin (Figs. 11–7 and 11–8). The lesions are mildly erythematous with a yellowish greasy scale. When limited to the face, lesions are usually asymptomatic, but scalp and trunk lesions are often pruritic. Therapy for the scalp includes the regular use of a dandruff shampoo containing ketoconazole (Nizoral), selenium sulfide (e.g., Selsun Blue), zinc pyrithione (e.g., Head and Shoulders, Danex, Zincon), or sulfur and salicylic acid (e.g., Van Seb, Sebulex). In addition, a medium-potency steroid solution (triamcinolone 0.1%) may be applied. For facial; trunk, and groin lesions, a topical imidazole cream (ketoconazole 2%, clotrimazole 1%), plus a low-potency topical steroid (hydrocortisone 1% to 21/2) may be applied twice daily. For refractory trunk lesions, the strength of the topical steroid may be increased.

Psoriasis often begins after HIV infection, although preexisting psoriasis may also flare following infection. The initial lesions frequently begin like seborrheic dermatitis, but extend to the axillae and groin, and finally involve the elbows, knees, and lumbosacral areas (Fig. 11–9). The lesions of psoriasis and seborrheic dermatitis in the axillae and groin are identical. When psoriasis involves the trunk, it tends to form more fixed, less easily treatable lesions with a thicker scale. Psoriasis of the palms and soles often begins as superficial pustules that evolve into a hyperkeratotic papules identical to the keratoderma blenorrhagicum of Reiter's syndrome (Fig. 11–10). Arthritis may occur with psoriasis alone or as a part of Reiter's syndrome.

Mild to moderate psoriasis is managed with topical steroids and tar. Patients with severe psoriasis and HIV disease may note a significant

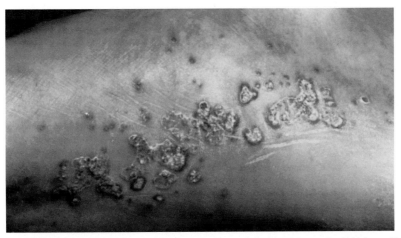

FIGURE 11–10. Pustules evolving into keratotic plaques on the sole. This was the initial manifestation of psoriasis in this HIV-infected person. Although the lesions were identical to those of Reiter's syndrome, this patient had no other characteristic stigmata.

improvement of their skin lesions with zidovudine therapy.[7] This response is dose related, and currently recommended lower doses (1000 mg/day) may have limited benefit. Etretinate, a vitamin A analog, is frequently beneficial, nonimmunosuppressive, and well tolerated in HIV-infected persons. The starting dose is 25 mg/day.

REFERENCES

1. Berger TG: Evaluation and treatment of pruritus in the HIV-infected patient. In Volberding P, Jacobson MA, eds. AIDS Clinical Review 1989. New York, Marcel Dekker, Inc, 1989, pp 205–220
2. Buchbinder SP, Katz MH, Hessol NA, et al: Herpes zoster and human immunodeficiency virus infection. J Infect Dis 166:1153–1156, 1992
3. Coldiron BM, Bergstresser PR: Prevalence and clinical spectrum of skin disease in patients infected with human immunodeficiency virus. Arch Dermatol 125:357–361, 1989
4. Concus AP, Helfand RF, Imber MJ, et al: Cutaneous cryptococcosis mimicking molluscum contagiosum in a patient with AIDS. J Infect Dis 158:897–898, 1988
5. Duvic M: Staphylococcal infections and the pruritus of AIDS-related complex. Arch Dermatol 123:1599, 1987
6. Gordin FM, Simon GL, Wofsy CB, et al: Adverse reactions to trimethoprim-sulfamethoxazole in patients with the acquired immunodeficiency syndrome. Ann Intern Med 100:495–498, 1984
7. Kaplan MH, Sadick NS, Wieder J, et al: Antipsoriatic effects of zidovudine in human immunodeficiency virus-associated psoriasis. J Am Acad Dermatol 20: 76–82, 1989
8. Murakawa GJ, McCalmont T, Altman J, et al: Disseminated acanthamebiasis in patients with AIDS. Arch Dermatol 131:1291–1296, 1995
9. Otley CC, Avram MR, Johnson RA: Isotretinoin treatment of human immunodeficiency virus-associated eosinophilic folliculitis. Results of an open, pilot trial. Arch Dermatol 131(9):1047–1050, 1995
10. Pappert A, Grossman M, DeLeo V: Photosensitivity as the presenting illness in four patients with human immunodeficiency viral infection. Arch Dermatol 130:618–623, 1994
11. Penneys NS, Nayar JK, Bernstein H, et al: Chronic pruritic eruption in patients with acquired immunodeficiency syndrome associated with increased antibody titers of mosquito salivary gland antigens. J Am Acad Dermatol 21:421–425, 1989
12. Porteous DM, Berger TG: Severe cutaneous drug reactions (Stevens-Johnson syndrome and toxic epidermal necrolysis) in human immunodeficiency virus infection. Arch Dermatol 127:740–741, 1991
13. Reveille JD, Conant MA, Duvic M: Human immunodeficiency virus-associated psoriasis, psoriatic arthritis, and Reiter's syndrome: A disease continuum? Arthritis Rheum 33:1574–1578, 1990
14. Rosenthal D, LeBoit PE, Klumpp L, et al: HIV-associated eosinophilic folliculitis: A unique dermatosis associated with advanced HIV infection. Arch Dermatol 127:206–209, 1991
15. Winchester R, Bernstein DH, Fischer HD, et al: The cooccurrence of Reiter's syndrome and acquired immunodeficiency. Ann Intern Med 106:19–26, 1987

Chapter *12*

Oral Complications of HIV Infection

JOHN S. GREENSPAN and DEBORAH GREENSPAN

Oral lesions have been recognized as prominent features of acquired immunodeficiency syndrome (AIDS) and human immunodeficiency virus (HIV) infection since the beginning of the epidemic.[31,46] Some of these changes are reflections of reduced immune function manifested as oral opportunistic conditions, which are often the earliest clinical features of HIV infection. Some, in the presence of known HIV infection, are highly predictive of the ultimate development of the full syndrome, whereas others represent the oral features of AIDS itself. The particular susceptibility of the mouth to HIV disease is a reflection of a wider phenomenon. Oral opportunistic infections occur in a variety of conditions in which the teeming and varied microflora of the mouth take advantage of local and systemic immunologic and metabolic imbalances. They include oral infections in patients with primary immunodeficiency,[74] leukemia,[3] and diabetes,[29] and those resulting from radiation therapy, cancer chemotherapy, and bone marrow suppression.[2,10,17]

Oral lesions seen in association with HIV infection are classified in Table 12–1, and our general approach to the diagnosis and management of oral HIV disease is summarized in Table 12–2. Standardized definitions and diagnostic criteria for these lesions have been proposed.[18,45,95] In the prospective cohorts of HIV-infected homosexual and bisexual men in San Francisco, hairy leukoplakia is the most common oral lesion (20.4%), and pseudomembranous candidiasis is the next most common (5.8%).[23] Others have shown that a simplified staging system for HIV infection, based on CD4 + cell depletion and oral disease, is more effective than the Walter Reed and other staging classifications.[100]

CANDIDIASIS

The pseudomembranous form of oral candidiasis (thrush) was described in the first group of AIDS patients and is a harbinger of the full-blown syndrome in HIV-seropositive individuals.[67,85] We have shown that both oral candidiasis and hairy leukoplakia predict the development of AIDS in HIV-infected patients independently of CD4 counts.[15] However, it is not well recognized that oral candidiasis can take several forms, some of them subtle clinical appearances.[15,42,43,107] The most common form, pseudomembranous candidiasis, appears as removable white plaques on any oral mucosal surface (Fig. 12–1). These plaques may be as small as 1 to 2 mm or may be extensive and widespread. They can be wiped off, leaving an erythematous or even bleeding mucosal surface.

The erythematous form (Fig. 12–2) is seen as smooth red patches on the hard or soft palate, buccal mucosa, or dorsal surface of the tongue. These lesions may seem insignificant and may be missed unless a thorough oral mucosal examination is performed in good light.

Angular cheilitis due to *Candida* infection produces erythema, cracks, and fissures at the corner of the mouth. We have found that erythematous candidiasis is as serious a prognostic indicator of the development of AIDS as pseudomembranous candidiasis.[15]

Diagnosis of oral candidiasis involves potassium hydroxide preparation of a smear from the lesion (Fig. 12–3). Culture provides information about the species involved.

Oral candidiasis in patients with HIV infection usually responds[33] to topical antifungal agents, including nystatin vaginal tablets, 100,000 units tid, dissolved slowly in the mouth; nystatin oral pastilles, 200,000 units,

TABLE 12–1. ORAL LESIONS IN HIV INFECTION

Fungal	Viral
Candidiasis	Herpes simplex
Pseudomembranous	Herpes zoster
Erythematous	Cytomegalovirus ulcers
Angular cheilitis	Hairy leukoplakia
Hyperplastic	Warts
Histoplasmosis	**Neoplastic**
Geotrichosis	Kaposi's sarcoma
Cryptococcosis	Non-Hodgkin's lymphoma
Aspergillosis	Squamous cell carcinoma (?)
Bacterial	**Other**
HIV-associated gingivitis	Recurrent aphthous ulcers
HIV-associated periodontitis	Immune thrombocytopenic purpura
Necrotizing stomatitis	Salivary gland disease
Mycobacterium avium complex	
Klebsiella stomatitis	
Bacillary angiomatosis	

one pastille five times daily; or clotrimazole oral tablets, 10 mg, one tablet five times daily. Oral ketoconazole in tablet form, 200 mg once daily, is a systemic antifungal agent that can be used as an alternative. It is effective if absorbed. Fluconazole (Diflucan) is a systemic antifungal agent. The recommended dose is a 100-mg tablet, once daily for 9 to 14 days. Oral fluconazole[61,106] is the latest systemic antifungal agent and is an extremely effective treatment for oral candidiasis, although resistance has been reported.[31] Two 100-mg tablets are used on the first day, followed by one 100-mg tablet daily until the lesions disappear. Antifungal therapy should be maintained for 1 to 2 weeks, and some patients may need maintenance therapy because of frequent relapse. Angular cheilitis usually responds to topical antifungal creams, such as nystatin-triamcinolone (Mycolog II), clotrimazole (Mycelex), or ketoconazole (Nizoral).

Occasionally, other and unusual oral fungal lesions are seen. They include histoplasmosis,[51,61,75,122] geotrichosis,[52] aspergillosis[111] and cryptococcosis.[30,69,78,118]

GINGIVITIS AND PERIODONTITIS

Unusual forms of gingivitis and periodontal disease are seen in association with HIV infection. The gingiva may show a fiery red marginal line, known as linear gingival erythema (Fig. 12–4), even in mouths showing absence of significant accumulations of plaque.[70,125] The periodontal disease, necrotizing ulcerative periodontitis, occurs in approximately 30% to 50% of AIDS clinic patients[82] but is rarely seen in asymptomatic HIV-positive individuals.[126] It resembles, in some respects, acute necrotizing ulcerative gingivitis (ANUG) superimposed on rapidly progressive periodontitis (Fig. 12–5).

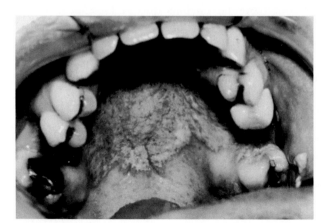

FIGURE 12–1. Pseudomembranous candidiasis.

TABLE 12–2. DIAGNOSIS AND MANAGEMENT OF ORAL HIV DISEASE

Condition	Diagnosis	Management
Fungal		
Candidiasis	Clinical appearance KOH preparation Culture	Antifungals
Histoplasmosis	Biopsy	Systemic therapy
Geotrichosis	KOH preparation Culture	Polyene antifungals
Cryptococcosis	Culture Biopsy	Systemic therapy
Aspergillosis	Culture Biopsy	Systemic therapy
Bacterial		
Linear gingival erythema	Clinical appearance	Plaque removal, chlorhexidine
Necrotizing ulcerative periodontis	Clinical appearance	Plaque removal, débridement, povidone-iodine, metronidazole, chlorhexidine
Necrotizing stomatitis	Clinical appearance Culture and biopsy (to exclude other causes) Culture Biopsy	Débridement, povidone-iodine, metronidazole, chlorhexidine
Mycobacterium avium complex	Culture Biopsy	Systemic therapy
Klebsiella stomatitis	Culture	Systemic therapy (based on antibiotic sensitivity testing)
Viral		
Herpes simplex	Clinical appearance Immunofluorescence on smears	Most cases are self-limiting Oral acyclovir for prolonged cases (>10 days)
Herpes zoster	Clinical appearance	Oral or intravenous acyclovir
Cytomegalovirus ulcers	Biopsy, immunohistochemistry for CMV	Ganciclovir
Hairy leukoplakia	Clinical appearance Biopsy; in situ hybridization for Epstein-Barr virus	Not routinely treated Oral acyclovir for severe cases
Warts	Clinical appearance Biopsy	Excision
Neoplastic		
Kaposi's sarcoma	Clinical appearance	Palliative surgical or laser excision for some bulky or unsightly lesions; intralesional chemotherapy or sclerosing agents; radiation therapy; chemotherapy
Non-Hodgkin's lymphoma	Biopsy	Chemotherapy
Squamous cell carcinoma	Biopsy	Excision or radiation therapy or both
Other		
Recurrent aphthous ulcers	History Clinical appearance Biopsy (to exclude other causes)	Topical steroids Thalidomide for most severe cases
Immune thrombocytopenic purpura	Clinical appearance Hematologic workup	
Salivary gland disease	History, clinical appearance, salivary flow measurements Biopsy (to exclude other causes—needle or labial salivary gland biopsy)	Salivary stimulants or change in systemic medication or both Topical fluorides

Thus, there may be halitosis in some cases and a history of rapid onset. There is necrosis of the tips of interdental papillae, with the formation of cratered ulcers. However, in contrast to patients with ANUG, these patients complain of spontaneous bleeding and severe, deep-seated pain that is not readily relieved by analgesics. There may be rapid progressive loss of gingival and periodontal soft tissues and extraordinarily rapid destruction of supporting bone. Teeth may, therefore, loosen and even exfoliate. The periodontal disease often demonstrates a severity and a rapid rate of progression that were not seen by the major-

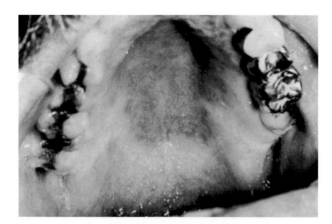

FIGURE 12–2. Erythematous candidiasis.

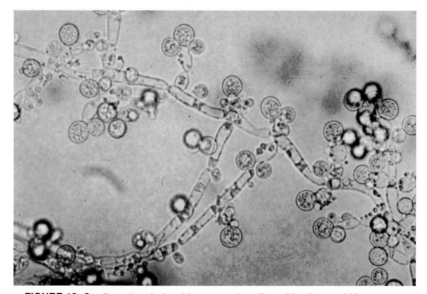

FIGURE 12–3. Potassium hydroxide preparation. Fungal hyphae and blastospores.

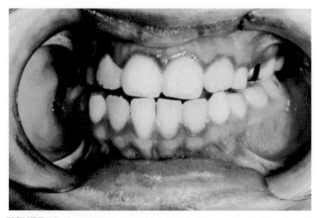

FIGURE 12–4. HIV-associated gingivitis (linear gingival erythema).

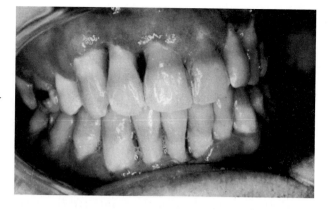

FIGURE 12–5. HIV-associated periodontitis (necrotizing ulcerative periodontitis).

ity of practicing dentists and periodontists prior to the AIDS epidemic. Exposure and even sequestration of bone may occur, producing necrotizing stomatitis lesions[124] similar to the noma seen in severely malnourished persons in World War II and more recently in developing countries in association with malnutrition and chronic infection, such as malaria. The pathologic and microbiologic features of these remarkable periodontal lesions are under investigation.[44,84,86,87,130,131] Standard therapy for gingivitis and periodontitis is ineffectual. Instead, the therapeutic regimen that is effective[32,91] involves thorough débridement and curettage, followed by application of a combination of topical antiseptics, notably povidone-iodine (Betadine) irrigation followed with chlorhexidine (Peridex) mouthwashes, sometimes supplemented with a 4- to 5-day course of antibiotics, such as metronidazole (Flagyl) 250 mg qid, Augmentin 250 mg (1 tab tid), or clindamycin 300 mg tid. Treatment will fail if thorough local removal of bacteria and diseased hard and soft tissue is not achieved during the initial treatment phase and maintained long term.

OTHER BACTERIAL LESIONS

A few cases have occurred of oral mucosal lesions associated with unusual bacteria, including *Klebsiella pneumoniae* and *Enterobacter cloacae*.[42,109] These have been diagnosed using aerobic and anaerobic cultures and have responded to antibiotic therapy based on in vitro sensitivity assays. Oral ulcers caused by *Mycobacterium avium* have also been described,[119] as have lesions of bacillary angiomatosis (Chapter 25).[114]

HERPES SIMPLEX (Chapter 26)

Oral lesions due to herpes simplex virus (HSV) are a common feature of HIV infection. The condition usually occurs as recurrent intraoral lesions with crops of small, painful vesicles that ulcerate. These lesions commonly appear on the palate or gingiva. Smears from the lesions may reveal giant cells, and HSV can be identified using monoclonal antibodies and immunofluorescence.[70] The lesions usually heal, although they may recur. In patients with a history of prolonged bouts (10 days) of such lesions, it may be considered appropriate to treat them with oral acyclovir as soon as symptoms are reported. Usually one 200-mg capsule taken five times a day is effective. Acyclovir-resistant herpes of the lips and perioral structures have been described.[20,22,81] The lesions responded to foscarnet.

HERPES ZOSTER (Chapter 26)

Both chickenpox and herpes zoster (shingles) have occurred in association with HIV infection.[83,108] In orofacial zoster, the vesicles and ulcers follow the distribution of one or more branches of the trigeminal nerve on one side. Facial nerve involvement with facial palsy (Ramsay Hunt syndrome) also may occur. Prodromal symptoms may include pain referred to one or more teeth, which often prove to be vital and noncarious. The ulcers usually heal in 2 to 3 weeks, but pain may persist. Oral acyclovir in doses up to 4 g/day may be used in severe cases, but occasionally patients must be hospitalized to receive intravenous acyclovir therapy.

CYTOMEGALOVIRUS ULCERS

(Chapter 26)

Oral ulcers caused by cytomegalovirus (CMV) occasionally occur.[50,60] These ulcers can occur on any oral mucosal surface, and diagnosis is made by biopsy and immunohistochemistry. Oral ulcers due to CMV are usually seen in the presence of disseminated disease, but cases have occurred in which the oral ulcer was the first presentation. Whether to treat with 3,4-dihydroxyphenylglycol (DHPG) depends on the severity of the viral infection, and full workup is indicated. Ulcers simultaneously infected by both HSV and CMV also occur.[53,61]

HAIRY LEUKOPLAKIA

First seen on the tongue in homosexual men,[37] hairy leukoplakia has since been described in several oral mucosal locations, including the buccal mucosa, soft palate, and floor of mouth and in all risk groups for AIDS.[9,23,24,36,40,48,49,62,68,99] Hairy leukoplakia produces white thickening of the oral mucosa, often with vertical folds or corrugations (Fig. 12–6 and Color Plate 1B). The lesions range in size from a few millimeters to involvement of the entire dorsal surface of the tongue. The differential diagnosis includes pseudomembranous candidiasis, smoker's leukoplakia, epithelial dysplasia or oral cancer, white sponge nevus, and the plaque form of lichen planus. Biopsy reveals epithelial hyperplasia with a thickened parakeratin layer showing surface irregularities, projections or "hairs," vacuolated prickle cells, and very little inflammation.[12,37,47,106] Epstein-Barr virus (EBV) can be identified in vacuolated and other prickle cells and in the superficial layers of the epithelium by using cytochemistry, electron microscopy, Southern blot test, and in situ hybridization[5,7,12,47,48,76] For cases in which biopsy is not considered appropriate (e.g., hemophiliacs, children, large-scale epidemiologic studies), we have developed cytospin and filter in situ hybridization techniques.[11] Langerhans' cells are sparse or absent from the lesion.[8] Hairy leukoplakia is not premalignant.[36,48] Indeed, the keratin profile of the lesions suggests reduced, rather than increased, cell turnover.[117,123]

Almost all patients with hairy leukoplakia are HIV seropositive, and many subsequently develop AIDS (median time 24 months) and die (median time 44 months).[39,41,64] Patients with tiny or extensive lesions show no difference in this tendency.[106] Rare cases have been described in HIV-negative individuals, usually in association with immunosuppression associated with organ transplantation.[21,38,59,115] Hairy leukoplakia has not been seen on other than oral mucosal surfaces.[54]

Hairy leukoplakia apparently is an EBV-induced benign epithelial thickening. High doses of oral acyclovir appear to reduce the lesion clinically,[1,6,27,98] and we have shown that the acyclovir prodrug desciclovir can eliminate both the lesion and the EBV infection present in the epithelial cells.[34] However, these effects are soon reversed after cessation of acyclovir or desciclovir therapy. Hairy leukoplakia occasionally may regress spontaneously, and zidovudine does not appear to increase regression.[63]

It is not clear whether hairy leukoplakia is caused by direct infection or reinfection of maturing epithelial cells by EBV from the saliva, by EBV-infected B cells infiltrating the epithelium, or by latent infection of the basal cell layer.[4,88,124] EBV variants, unusual EBV types,

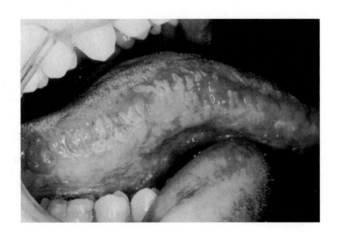

FIGURE 12–6. Hairy leukoplakia.

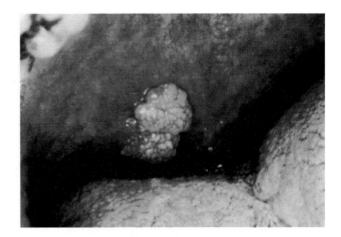

FIGURE 12–7. Wart on the palate.

and even multiple strains of EBV have been found in the lesion.[28,90,93,102,121]

WARTS

Oral lesions caused by human papillomavirus (HPV) can occur as single or multiple papilliferous warts with multiple white and spikelike projections, as pink cauliflower-like masses (Fig. 12–7), as single projections, or as flat lesions resembling focal epithelial hyperplasia.[42,43] In patients with HIV infection, we have seen numerous examples of each type. Southern blot hybridization has not revealed (as would be expected) HPV types 6, 11, 16, and 18, which usually are associated with anogenital warts, but HPV type 7, which usually is found in butcher's warts of the skin, or HPV types 13 and 32, previously associated with focal epithelial hyperplasia.[35,116] Venereal transmission thus seems not involved in these warts. Instead, they may be attributable to activation of latent HPV infection or perhaps autoinfection from skin and face lesions. Dysplastic warts due to novel HPV types also have been described.[96,120]

If large, extensive, or otherwise troublesome, these oral warts can be removed using surgical or laser excision. In some cases, we have seen recurrence after therapy and even extensive spread throughout the mouth.

NEOPLASTIC DISEASE

Kaposi's Sarcoma (Chapter 28)

Kaposi's sarcoma (KS) in patients with AIDS produces oral lesions in many cases.[13,25,97,] [110,112] The lesions occur as red or purple macules, papules, or nodules. Occasionally, the lesions are the same color as the adjoining normal mucosa. Although frequently they are asymptomatic, pain may occur because of traumatic ulceration with inflammation and infection. Bulky lesions may be visible or may interfere with speech and mastication. Diagnosis involves biopsy.

Lesions at the gingival margin frequently become inflamed and painful because of plaque accumulation. Excision, by surgical means or by laser, is readily performed and can be repeated if the lesion again produces problems. Local radiation therapy has been used to reduce the size of such lesions. Oral lesions usually regress when patients receive chemotherapy for aggressive KS, and individual lesions may respond to local injection of vinblastine[19] or even of sclerosing agents.[77]

Lymphoma (Chapter 28)

Although not seen as frequently as with oral KS, oral lesions are a common feature of HIV-associated lymphoma.[14,16,66,132] A biopsy may prove that poorly defined alveolar swellings or discrete oral masses in individuals who are HIV seropositive are non-Hodgkin's lymphoma. No treatment is provided for the oral lesions separate from the systemic chemotherapy regimen that usually is used in such cases.

Carcinoma

Several cases have been seen of oral squamous cell carcinoma, particularly of the tongue,

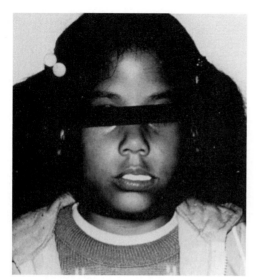

FIGURE 12–8. Parotid enlargement.

in young homosexual males.[112] It is not clear whether these lesions are related to HIV infection; population-based and cancer registry epidemiologic studies have not produced evidence to support such a link.

OTHER LESIONS [100,101]

Recurrent aphthous ulcers (RAU) are a common finding in the normal population. There is an impression,[75,79,80,94,112] not as yet substantiated by prospective studies of incidence, that RAU are more common among HIV-seropositive individuals. These lesions occur as recurrent crops of small (1- to 2-mm) to large (1-cm) ulcers on the nonkeratinized oral and oropharyngeal mucosa. They can interfere significantly with speech and swallowing and may present considerable problems in diagnosis. When they are large and persistent, biopsy may be indicated to exclude lymphoma. The histopathologic features of RAU are those of nonspecific inflammation. Treatment with topical steroids often is effective in reducing pain and accelerating healing. Valuable agents include fluocinonide (Lidex), 0.05% ointment, mixed with equal parts of Orabase applied to the lesion up to six times daily, or clobetasol (Temovate), 0.05% mixed with equal parts of Orabase applied three times daily. These are particularly effective treatments for early lesions. Dexamethasone (Decadron) elixir, 0.5 mg/ml used as a rinse and expectorated, is also helpful, particularly when the location of the lesion makes it difficult for the patient to apply fluocinonide. Recently, thalidomide has been found to be useful in the management of steroid-resistant ulcers.[89,92,101,127,128]

Immune thrombocytopenic purpura may produce oral mucosal ecchymoses or small blood-filled lesions.[43] Spontaneous gingival bleeding may occur. Diagnosis by hematologic evaluation is usually straightforward, but, as with any systemic condition presenting as oral lesions, full workup is indicated.

We have seen several cases of parotid enlargement in pediatric AIDS patients[65,71–73] (Fig. 12–8) and, more recently, among adults who are HIV seropositive.[26,55–58,103–105] HIV-infected children with parotid enlargement progress less rapidly than those without parotid enlargement.[65] No specific cause for HIV-associated salivary gland disease has been determined, although viral causes are suspected. Diagnosis to exclude lymphoma, leukemia, and other causes of salivary gland enlargement may involve labial salivary gland biopsy and major salivary gland needle biopsy. Some of these cases show xerostomia. Furthermore, the latter condition may be seen in association with HIV infection in the absence of salivary gland enlargement. The patient may complain of oral dryness, and there may be signs of xerostomia, such as lack of pooled saliva, failure to elicit salivary expression from Stensen's or Wharton's ducts, and obvious mucosal dryness. Tests of salivary function, notably stimulated parotid flow-rate determination, show reduced salivary flow. Some of these cases are attributable to side effects of medications that reduce salivation. In such cases, it may be possible to arrange to change the medications or their doses. In other cases, stimulation of salivary flow by use of sugarless candy may alleviate some of the discomfort. Topical fluorides and other preventive dentistry approaches are used to reduce the frequency of caries.

SUMMARY

The oral manifestations of HIV infection occur as a variety of opportunistic infections, neoplasms, and other lesions. Some of them are common, perhaps the most common, features of HIV disease and are highly predictive of the development of AIDS. Clinicians caring for HIV-infected persons should become familiar with the diagnosis and management of this group of conditions.

The oral lesions of HIV infection present

challenges of diagnosis and therapy. They also offer unrivaled opportunities to investigate the epidemiology, cause, pathogenesis, and treatment of mucosal diseases. As the epidemic progresses, it can be expected that further lesions will be observed and that additional rational and effective therapeutic approaches will be developed.

REFERENCES

1. Barr C: Treatment of HIV-associated oral diseases. In Greenspan JS, Greenspan D, eds. Oral manifestations of HIV infection. Carol Stream, IL, Quintessence Publishing Co, Inc, 1995, pp 362–365
2. Barrett AP: Clinical characteristics and mechanisms involved in chemotherapy-induced oral ulceration. J Oral Med 41:424, 1983
3. Barrett AP: Oral changes as initial diagnostic indicators in acute leukemia. J Oral Med 41:234, 1986
4. Becker J, Leser U, Marschall M, et al: Expression of proteins encoded by Epstein-Barr virus trans-activator genes depends on the differentiation of epithelial cells in oral hairy leukoplakia. Proc Natl Acad Sci U S A 88:8332–8336, 1991
5. Belton CM, Eversole LR: Oral hairy leukoplakia: Ultrastructural features. J Oral Pathol 15:493, 1986
6. Brockmeyer NH, Kreuzfelder E, Mertins L, et al: Zidovudine therapy of asymptomatic HIV-1-infected patients and combined zidovudine-acyclovir therapy of HIV-1-infected patients with oral hairy leukoplakia. J Invest Dermatol 92:647, 1989
7. Corso B, Eversole LR, Hutt-Fletcher L: Hairy leukoplakia: Epstein-Barr virus receptors on oral keratinocyte plasma membranes. Oral Surg Oral Med Oral Pathol 67:416–421, 1989
8. Daniels TE, Greenspan D, Greenspan JS, et al: Absence of Langerhans cells in oral hairy leukoplakia, an AIDS-associated lesion. J Invest Dermatol 89:178–182, 1987
9. De Maubeuge J, Ledoux M, Feremans W, et al: Oral "hairy" leukoplakia in an African AIDS patient. J Cutan Pathol 13:235, 1986
10. DePaola LG, Peterson EE, Overholser DJJ, et al: Dental care for patients receiving chemotherapy. J Am Dent Assoc 112:198, 1986
11. DeSouza YG, Freese UK, Greenspan D, Greenspan JS: Diagnosis of Epstein-Barr virus infection in hairy leukoplakia by using nucleic acid hybridization and noninvasive techniques. J Clin Microbiol 28:2775–2778, 1990
12. DeSouza YG, Greenspan D, Gelton JR, et al: Localization of Epstein-Barr virus DNA in the epithelial cells of oral hairy leukoplakia using in-situ hybridization on tissue sections (Letter). N Engl J Med 320:1559–1560, 1989
13. Dodd CL, Greenspan D, Greenspan JS: Oral Kaposi's sarcoma in a woman as a first indication of infection with the human immunodeficiency virus. J Am Dent Assoc 122:61–63, 1991
14. Dodd CL, Greenspan D, Heinic GS, et al: Multifocal oral non-Hodgkin's lymphoma in an AIDS patient. Br Dent J 175:373–377, 1993
15. Dodd CL, Greenspan D, Katz MH, et al: Oral candidiasis in HIV infection: Pseudomembraneous and erythematous candidiasis show similar rates of progression to AIDS. AIDS 5:1339–1343, 1991
16. Dodd CL, Greenspan D, Schiodt M, et al: Unusual oral presentation of non-Hodgkin's lymphoma in association with HIV infection. Oral Surg Oral Med Oral Pathol 73:603–608, 1992
17. Dreizen S, McCredie KB, Bodey GP, et al: Quantitative analysis of the oral complications of antileukemia chemotherapy. Oral Surg 62:650, 1986
18. EC-Clearinghouse on Oral Problems Related to HIV Infection and WHO Collaborating Centre on Oral Manifestations of the Human Immunodeficiency Virus: Classification and diagnostic criteria for oral lesions in HIV infection. J Oral Pathol Med 22:289–291, 1993
19. Epstein JB, Scully C: Intralesional vinblastine for oral Kaposi's sarcoma in HIV infection. Lancet 2:1100–1101, 1989
20. Epstein JB, Scully C: HIV infection: Clinical features and treatment of thirty-three homosexual men with Kaposi's sarcoma. Oral Surg Oral Med Oral Pathol 71:38–41, 1991
21. Epstein JB, Sherlock CH, Greenspan JS: Hairy leukoplakia-like lesions following bone marrow transplantation (Letter). AIDS 5:101–102, 1991
22. Erlich KS, Mills J, Chatis P, et al: Acyclovir-resistant herpes simplex virus infections in patients with the acquired immunodeficiency syndrome. N Engl J Med 320:293–296, 1989
23. Feigal DW, Katz MH, Greenspan D, et al: The prevalence of oral lesions in HIV-infected homosexual and bisexual men: Three San Francisco epidemiological cohorts. AIDS 5:519–525, 1991
24. Ficarra G, Barone R, Gaglioti D: Oral hairy leukoplakia among HIV-positive intravenous drug abusers: A clinico-pathologic and ultrastructural study. Oral Surg Oral Med Oral Pathol 65:421–426, 1988
25. Ficarra G, Person AM, Silverman S, et al: Kaposi's sarcoma of the oral cavity: A study of 134 patients with a review of the pathogenesis, epidemiology, clinical aspects, and treatment. Oral Surg Oral Med Oral Pathol 66:543–550, 1988
26. Finfer MD, Schinella RA, Rothstein SG, Persky MS: Cystic parotid lesions in patients at risk for the acquired immunodeficiency syndrome. Arch Otolaryngol Head Neck Surg 144:1290–1294, 1988
27. Friedman-Kein AE: Viral origin of hairy leukoplakia (Letter). Lancet 2:694, 1986
28. Gilligan K, Rajadurai P, Resnick L, Raab-Traub N: Epstein-Barr virus small nuclear RNAs are not expressed in permissively infected cells in AIDS-associated leukoplakia. Proc Natl Acad Sci U S A 87:8790–8794, 1990
29. Glavind L, Lund B, Loe H: The relationship between periodontal state and diabetes duration, insulin dosage and retinal changes. J Periodontol 39:341, 1968
30. Glick M, Cohen SG, Cheney RT, et al: Oral manifestations of disseminated *Cryptococcus neoformans* in a patient with acquired immunodeficiency syn-

drome. Oral Surg Oral Med Oral Pathol 64: 454–459, 1987

31. Gottlieb MS, Schroff R, Schantez HM: *Pneumocystis carinii* pneumonia and mucosal candidiasis in previously healthy homosexual men: Evidence of a new acquired cellular immunodeficiency. N Engl J Med 305:1425–1431, 1981

32. Grassi M, Williams CA, Winkler JR, Murray PA: Management of HIV-associated periodontal diseases. In Robertson PB, Greenspan JS, eds. Perspectives on oral manifestations of AIDS: Diagnosis and management of HIV-associated infections. Littleton, MA, PSG, 1988, pp 119–130

33. Greenspan D: Treatment of oral candidiasis in HIV infection. Oral Surg Oral Med Oral Pathol 78: 211–216, 1994

34. Greenspan D, DeSouza Y, Conant MA, et al: Efficacy of desciclovir in the treatment of Epstein-Barr virus infection in oral hairy leukoplakia. J Acquir Immune Defic Syndr 3:571–578, 1990

35. Greenspan D, de Villiers EM, Greenspan JS, et al: Unusual HPV types in the oral warts in association with HIV infection. J Oral Pathol 17:482–487, 1988

36. Greenspan D, Greenspan JS: The significance of oral hairy leukoplakia. Oral Surg Oral Med Oral Pathol 73:151–154, 1992

37. Greenspan D, Greenspan JS, Conant M, et al: Oral "hairy" leucoplakia in male homosexuals: Evidence of association with both papillomavirus and a herpes-group virus. Lancet 2:831–834, 1984

38. Greenspan D, Greenspan JS, DeSouza YG, et al: Oral hairy leukoplakia in an HIV-negative renal transplant recipient. J Oral Pathol Med 18:32–34, 1989

39. Greenspan D, Greenspan JS, Hearst NG, et al: Oral hairy leukoplakia; human immunodeficiency virus status and risk for development of AIDS. J Infect Dis 155:475–478, 1987

40. Greenspan D, Hollander H, Friedman-Kien A, et al: Oral hairy leukoplakia in two women, a hemophiliac and a transfusion recipient (Letter). Lancet 2: 978, 1986

41. Greenspan D, Greenspan JS, Overby G, et al: Risk factors for rapid progression from hairy leukoplakia to AIDS: A nested case control study. J Acquir Immune Defic Syndr 4:652–658, 1991

42. Greenspan D, Greenspan JS, Pindborg JJ, Schiodt M: AIDS and the dental team. Copenhagen, Munksgaard, 1986

43. Greenspan D, Greenspan JS, Pindborg JJ, Schiodt M: AIDS and the mouth. Copenhagen, Munksgaard, 1990

44. Greenspan JS: Periodontal complications of HIV infection. Compend Cont Educ Dent 18S: S694–S698, 1994

45. Greenspan JS, Barr CE, Sciubba JJ, Winkler JR, USA Oral AID Collaborative Group: Oral manifestations of HIV infection: Definitions, diagnostic criteria and principles of therapy. Oral Surg Oral Med Oral Pathol 73:142–144, 1992

46. Greenspan JS, Greenspan D, eds: Oral manifestations of HIV infection. Carol Stream, IL, Quintessence Publishing Co, Inc, 1995

47. Greenspan JS, Greenspan D, Lennette ET, et al: Replication of Epstein-Barr virus within the epithelial cells of "hairy" leukoplakia, an AIDS-associated lesion. N Engl J Med 313:1564–1571, 1985

48. Greenspan JS, Greenspan D, Palefsky JM: Oral hairy

leukoplakia after a decade. Epstein-Barr virus report 2:123–128, 1995

49. Greenspan JS, Mastrucci T, Leggott P, et al: Hairy leukoplakia in a child. AIDS 2:143, 1988

50. Heinic GS: Oral cytomegalovirus infection in association with HIV infection: A review. In Greenspan JS, Greenspan D, eds. Oral manifestations of HIV infection. Carol Stream, IL, Quintessence Publishing Co, Inc, 1995, pp 225–228

51. Heinic G, Greenspan D, MacPhail LA, et al: Oral *Histoplasma capsulatum* in association with HIV infection: A case report. J Oral Pathol Med 21:85–89, 1992

52. Heinic GS, Greenspan D, MacPhail LA, Greenspan JS: Oral *Geotrichum candidum* infection in association with HIV infection. Oral Surg Oral Med Oral Pathol 73:726–728, 1992

53. Heinic GS, Northfelt DW, Greenspan JS, et al: Concurrent oral cytomegalovirus and herpes simplex virus infection in association with HIV infection: A case report. Oral Surg Oral Med Oral Pathol 75: 488–494, 1993

54. Hollander H, Greenspan D, Stringari S, et al: Hairy leukoplakia and the acquired immunodeficiency syndrome. Ann Intern Med 104:892, 1986

55. Itescu S, Brancato LJ, Buxbaum J, et al: A diffuse infiltrative CD8 lymphocytosis syndrome in human immunodeficiency virus (HIV) infection: A host immune response associated with HLA-DR5. Ann Intern Med 112:3–10, 1990

56. Itescu S, Brancato LJ, Winchester R: A sicca syndrome in HIV infection: Association with HLA-DR5 and CD8 lymphocytosis (Letter). Lancet 466–468, 1989

57. Itescu S, Dalton J, Zhang HZ, Winchester R: Tissue infiltration in a CD8 lymphocytosis syndrome associated with human immunodeficiency virus-1 infection has the phenotypic appearance of an antigenically driven response. J Clin Invest 91(5): 2216–2225, 1993

58. Itescu S, Mathur-Wagh U, Skovron ML, et al: HLA-B35 is associated with accelerated progression to AIDS. J Acquir Immune Defic Syndr 5:37–45, 1991

59. Itin P, Rufli I, Rudlinser R, et al: Oral hairy leukoplakia in a HIV-negative renal transplant patient: A marker for immunosuppression. Dermatologica 17:126–128, 1988

60. Jones AC, Freedman PD, Phelan JA, et al: Cytomegalovirus infections of the oral cavity. Oral Surg Oral Med Oral Pathol 75:76–85, 1993

61. Jones AC, Migliorati CA, Baughman RA: The simultaneous occurrence of oral herpes simplex virus, cytomegalovirus, and histoplasmosis in an HIV-infected patient. Oral Surg Oral Med Oral Pathol 74:334–339, 1992

62. Kabani S, Greenspan D, de Souza Y, et al: Oral hairy leukoplakia with extensive oral mucosal involvement. Oral Surg Oral Med Oral Pathol 67: 411–415, 1989

63. Katz MH, Greenspan D, Heinic GS, et al: Resolution of hairy leukoplakia: An observational trial of zidovudine versus no treatment (Letter). J Infect Dis 164:1240–1241, 1991

64. Katz MH, Greenspan D, Westenhouse J, et al: Progression to AIDS in HIV-infected homosexual and bisexual men with hairy leukoplakia and oral candidiasis. AIDS 6:95–100, 1992

65. Katz MH, Mastrucci MT, Leggott PJ, et al: Prognostic

significance of oral lesions in children with perinatally acquired human immunodeficiency virus infection. Am J Dis Child 147(1):45–48, 1993

66. Kaugars GE, Burns JC: Non-Hodgkin's lymphoma of the oral cavity associated with AIDS. Oral Surg Oral Med Oral Pathol 67:433–436, 1989

67. Klein RS, Harris CA, Small CR, et al: Oral candidiasis in high-risk patients as the initial manifestation of the acquired immunodeficiency syndrome. N Engl J Med 311:354–358, 1984

68. Konrad K: Orale "haarige" Leukoplakie—Klinische Freuhmanifestation der HTLV-III-Infektion. Wien Klin Wochenschr 3 (Suppl):702, 1986

69. Kuruvilla A, Humphrey DM, Emko P: Coexistent oral cryptococcosis and Kaposi's sarcoma in acquired immunodeficiency syndrome. Cutis 49:260–264, 1992

70. Lamster I, Grbic J, Fine J, et al: A critical review of periodontal disease as a manifestation of HIV infection. In Greenspan JS, Greenspan D, eds. Oral Manifestations of HIV Infection: Proceedings of the Second International Workshop. Chicago, Quintessence Publishing Co, 1994

71. Leggott PJ: Oral manifestations of HIV infection in children. Oral Surg Oral Med Oral Pathol 73:187–192, 1992

72. Leggott PJ: Oral manifestations in pediatric HIV infection. In Greenspan JS, Greenspan D, eds. Oral manifestations of HIV infection. Carol Stream, IL, Quintessence Publishing Co, Inc, 1995, pp 234–239

73. Leggott PJ, Robertson PB, Culver KW: HIV infection in children. Calif Dent Assoc J 15:56–60, 1987

74. Leggott PJ, Robertson PB, Greenspan D, et al: Oral manifestations of primary and acquired immunodeficiency diseases in children. Pediatr Dent 9:89–104, 1987

75. Liang GS, Daikos GL, Serfling U, et al: An evaluation of oral ulcers in patients with AIDS and AIDS-related complex. J Am Acad Dermatol 29(4):563–568, 1993

76. Loning T, Henke R-P, Reichart P, Becker J: In situ hybridization to detect Epstein-Barr virus DNA in oral tissues of HIV-infected patients. Virchows Arch [A] 412:127–133, 1987

77. Lucatoto FM, Sapp JP: Treatment of oral Kaposi's sarcoma with a sclerosing agent in AIDS patients. Oral Surg Oral Med Oral Pathol 75:192–198, 1993

78. Lynch DP, Naftolin LZ: Oral *Cryptococcus neoformans* infection in AIDS. Oral Surg Oral Med Oral Pathol 64:449–453, 1987

79. MacPhail LA, Greenspan D, Feigal DW, et al: Recurrent aphthous ulcers in association with HIV infection: Description of ulcer types and analysis of T-cell subsets. Oral Surg Oral Med Oral Pathol 71:678–683, 1991

80. MacPhail LA, Greenspan D, Greenspan JS: Recurrent aphthous ulcers in association with HIV infection: Diagnosis and treatment. Oral Surg Oral Med Oral Pathol 73:283–288, 1992

81. MacPhail LA, Greenspan D, Schiodt M, et al: Acyclovir-resistant, foscarnet-sensitive oral herpes simplex type 2 lesion in a patient with AIDS. Oral Surg Oral Med Oral Pathol 67:427–432, 1989

82. Masouredis CM, Katz MH, Greenspan D, et al: Prevalence of HIV-associated periodontitis and gingivitis in HIV-infected patients attending an AIDS

clinic. J Acquir Immune Defic Syndr 5:479–483, 1992

83. Melbye M, Grossman RJ, Goedert JJ, et al: Risk of AIDS after herpes zoster. Lancet 1:728–731, 1987

84. Murray PA, Grassi M, Winkler JR: The microbiology of HIV-associated periodontal lesions. J Clin Periodontol 16:636–642, 1989

85. Murray HW, Hillman AD, Rubin BY, et al: Patients at risk for AIDS-related opportunistic infections. N Engl J Med 313:1504–1510, 1985

86. Murray PA, Winkler JR, Peros WJ, et al: DNA probe detection of periodontal pathogens in HIV-associated periodontal lesions. Oral Microbiol Immunol 6:34–40, 1991

87. Murray PA, Winkler JR, Sadkowski L, et al: Microbiology of HIV-associated gingivitis and periodontitis. In Robertson PB, Greenspan JS, eds. Perspectives on oral manifestations of AIDS: Diagnosis and management of HIV-associated infections. Littleton, MA, PSG, 1988, pp 105–118

88. Niedobitek G, Young LW, Lau R, et al: Epstein-Barr virus infection in oral hairy leukoplakia: Virus replication in the absence of a detectable latent phase. J Gen Virol 72:3035–3046, 1991

89. Oldfield ECR: Thalidomide for severe aphthous ulceration in patients with human immunodeficiency virus (HIV) infection. Am J Gastroenterol 89(12):2276–2277, 1994

90. Palefsky J, Berline J, Penaranda M-E, et al: Nucleotide sequence heterogeneity of Epstein-Barr virus latent membrane protein 1 gene in oral hairy leukoplakia. In Greenspan JS, Greenspan D, eds. Oral manifestations of HIV infection. Carol Stream, IL, Quintessence Publishing Co, Inc, 1995, pp 175–183

91. Palmer GD: Periodontal therapy for patients with HIV infection. In Greenspan JS, Greenspan D, eds. Oral Manifestations of HIV Infection: Proceedings of the Second International Workshop. Chicago, Quintessence Publishing Co, 1994

92. Paterson DL, Georghiou PR, Allworth AM, Kemp RJ: Thalidomide as treatment of refractory aphthous ulceration related to human immunodeficiency virus infection. Clin Infect Dis 20(2):250–254, 1995

93. Patton DF, Shirley P, Raab-Traub N, et al: Defective viral DNA in Epstein-Barr virus-associated oral hairy leukoplakia. J Virol 64:397–400, 1990

94. Phelan JA, Eisig S, Freedman PD, et al: Major aphthous-like ulcers in patients with AIDS. Oral Surg Oral Med Oral Pathol 71:68–72, 1991

95. Pindborg JJ: Classification of oral lesions associated with HIV infection. Oral Surg Oral Med Oral Pathol 67:292–295, 1989

96. Regezi JA, Greenspan D, Greenspan JS, et al: HPV-associated epithelial atypia in oral warts in HIV+ patients. J Cutan Pathol 21(3):217–223, 1994

97. Regezi JA, MacPhail LA, Daniels TE: Oral Kaposi's sarcoma: A 10-year retrospective histopathologic study. J Oral Pathol Med 22:292–297, 1993

98. Resnick L, Herbst JHS, Ablashi DV, et al: Regression of oral hairy leukoplakia after orally administered acyclovir therapy. JAMA 259:384–388, 1988

99. Rindum JL, Schiodt M, Pindborg JJ, Scheibel E: Oral hairy leukoplakia in three hemophiliacs with human immunodeficiency virus infection. Oral Surg Oral Med Oral Pathol 63:437–440, 1987

100. Royce RC, Luckmann RS, Fusaro RE, Winkelstein

WJ: The natural history of HIV-1 infection: Staging classifications of disease. AIDS 5:355–364, 1991

101. Ryan J, Colman J, Pedersen J, Benson E: Thalidomide to treat esophageal ulcer in AIDS (Letter). N Engl J Med 327:208–209, 1992

102. Sandvej KS, Krenacs L, Hamilton-Dutoit SJ, et al: Epstein-Barr virus latent and replicative gene expression in oral hairy leukoplakia. Histopathology 20: 387–395, 1992

103. Schiodt M: HIV-associated salivary gland disease—a new entity. Symposium in Oral Pathology. University of Rostock, 1990

104. Schiodt M, Dodd CL, Greenspan D, et al: Natural history of HIV-associated salivary gland disease. Oral Surg Oral Med Oral Pathol 74:326–331, 1992

105. Schiodt MS, Dodd CL, Greenspan D, Greenspan JS: HIV-associated salivary gland disease. In Greenspan JS, Greenspan D, eds. Oral manifestations of HIV infection. Carol Stream, IL, Quintessence Publishing Co, Inc, 1995, pp 145–151

106. Schiodt M, Greenspan D, Daniels TE, Greenspan JS: Clinical and histologic spectrum of oral hairy leukoplakia. Oral Surg Oral Med Oral Pathol 64: 716–720, 1987

107. Schiodt M, Pindborg JJ: AIDS and the oral cavity. Int J Oral Maxillofac Surg 16:1–14, 1987

108. Schiodt M, Rindum J, Bygbert I: Chickenpox with oral manifestations in an AIDS patient. Dan Dent J 91:316–319, 1987

109. Schmidt-Westhausen A, Fehrenbach FJ, Reichart PA: Oral Enterobacteriaceae in patients with HIV infection. J Oral Pathol 19:229–231, 1990

110. Scully C, Laskaris G, Pindborg J, et al: Oral manifestations of HIV infection and their management. I. More common lesions. Oral Surg Oral Med Oral Pathol 71:158–166, 1991

111. Shannon MT, Sclaroff A, Colm SJ: Invasive aspergillosis of the maxilla in an immunocompromised patient. Oral Surg Oral Med Oral Pathol 70:425–427, 1990

112. Silverman S, Migliorati CA, Lozada-Nur F, et al: Oral findings in people with or at risk for AIDS: A study of 375 homosexual males. J Am Dent Assoc 112: 187–192, 1986

113. Sokol-Anderson ML, Prelutsky DJ, Westblom TU: Giant esophageal aphthous ulcers in AIDS patients: Treatment with low-dose corticosteroids. AIDS 5:1537–1538, 1991

114. Speight PM: Epithelioid angiomatosis affecting the oral cavity as a first sign of HIV infection. Br Dent J 171:367–370, 1991

115. Syrjanen S, Laine P, Happoinen RP, Niemela M: Oral hairy leukoplakia is not a specific sign of HIV infection but related to suppression in general. J Oral Pathol Med 18:28–31, 1989

116. Syrjanen S, von Krogh G, Kellokoski J, Syrjanen K: Two different human papillomavirus (HPV) types associated with oral mucosal lesions in an HIV-seropositive man. J Oral Pathol Med 18:366–370, 1989

117. Thomas JA, Felix DH, Wray D, et al: Epstein-Barr

virus gene expression and epithelial cell differentiation in oral hairy leukoplakia. Am J Pathol 139: 1369–1380, 1991

118. Tzerbos F, Kabani S, Booth D: Cryptococcosis as an exclusive oral presentation. J Oral Maxillofac Surg 50:759–760, 1992

119. Volpe F, Schimmer A, Barr C: Oral manifestations of disseminated *Mycobacterium avium-intracellulare* in a patient with AIDS. Oral Surg 60:567, 1985

120. Volter C, He Y, Delius H, et al: Novel HPV types in oral papillomatous lesions from patients with HIV infection. Int J Cancer 66:453–456, 1996

121. Walling DM, Edmiston SN, Sixbey JW, et al: Coinfection with multiple strains of the Epstein-Barr virus in human immunodeficiency virus-associated hairy leukoplakia. Proc Natl Acad Sci U S A 89: 6560–6564, 1992

122. Werber JL: Histoplasmosis of the head and neck. Ear Nose Throat 67:841–845, 1988

123. Williams DM, Leigh IM, Greenspan D, Greenspan JS: Altered patterns of keratin expression in oral hairy leukoplakia: Prognostic implications. J Oral Pathol Med 20:167–171, 1991

124. Williams CA, Winkler JR, Grassi M, Murray PA: HIV-associated periodontitis complicated by necrotizing stomatitis. Oral Surg Oral Med Oral Pathol 69: 351–355, 1990

125. Winkler JR: Pathogenesis of HIV-associated periodontal diseases: What's known and what isn't. In Greenspan JS, Greenspan D, eds. Oral manifestations of HIV infection. Carol Stream, IL, Quintessence Publishing Co, Inc, 1995, pp 263–272

126. Winkler JR, Herrera C, Westenhouse J, et al: Periodontal disease in HIV-infected and uninfected homosexual and bisexual men (Letter). AIDS 6: 1041–1043, 1992

127. Youle M, Clarbour J, Farthing C, et al: Treatment of resistant aphthous ulceration with thalidomide in patients positive for HIV antibody. Br Med J 298: 432, 1989

128. Youle M, Hawkins D, Gazzard B: Thalidomide in hyperalgic pharyngeal ulceration of AIDS (Letter). Lancet 335:1591, 1990

129. Young LS, Lau R, Rowe M, et al: Differentiation-associated expression of the Epstein-Barr virus BZLF1 transactivator protein in oral hairy leukoplakia. J Virol 65:2868–2874, 1991

130. Zambon JJ, Reynolds HS, Genco RJ: Studies of the subgingival microflora in patients with acquired immunodeficiency syndrome. J Periodontol 61: 699–704, 1990

131. Zambon JJ, Reynolds H, Smutko J, et al: Are unique bacterial pathogens involved in HIV-associated periodontal diseases? In Greenspan JS, Greenspan D, eds. Oral Manifestations of HIV Infection: Proceedings of the Second International Workshop. Chicago, Quintessence Publishing Co, 1994

132. Ziegler JL, Beckstead JA, Volberding PA, et al: Non-Hodgkin's lymphoma in 90 homosexual men: Relation to generalized lymphadenopathy and the acquired immunodeficiency syndrome. N Engl J Med 311:565–570, 1984

Chapter *13*

Gastrointestinal Tract Manifestations of AIDS

JOHN P. CELLO

Over the past two decades millions of people throughout the world have become infected with the human immunodeficiency virus (HIV). More than 400,000 people have died already from the acquired immunodeficiency syndrome (AIDS). The full extent of the pandemic has not yet been elucidated. Hardly any organ system in the body is spared the ravages of AIDS. From the very outset of the AIDS epidemic, clinicians everywhere noted a high prevalence of gastrointestinal (GI) signs and symptoms. Some of these manifestations, such as weight loss, dysphagia, anorexia, and diarrhea, are almost universally found at some point in the course of the disease among patients with AIDS. Other GI signs and symptoms, such as odynophagia, hemorrhage, jaundice, or abdominal pain, are infrequent but important manifestations of AIDS-related conditions.

AIDS PATHOGEN AND MALIGNANCY DIAGNOSIS

In confirming individual AIDS-associated GI pathogens and malignancies (Table 13–1), considerable controversy remains about definitive diagnostic testing. Studies are needed detailing sensitivity, specificity, and diagnostic efficiency of the various tests. *Candida albicans* can be documented by using histopathology (and high-quality brush cytology) to demonstrate pseudomycelia. Serologic testing for *Candida* is not useful. Culture is rarely necessary except to differentiate *C. tropicalis* and *Torulopsis glabrata* from *C. albicans*, especially in patients for whom systemic antifungal drug fail.

Herpes simplex virus (HSV) is diagnosed definitively by using histopathology to demonstrate infected cells with classic Cowdry type A inclusions. Viral culture is confirmatory for HSV.

Cytomegalovirus (CMV) infection is pervasive among AIDS patients. Its true extent and nature remain undefined. Demonstration of CMV-infected endothelial cells is the hallmark of CMV disease in the immunocompromised patient. Tissue cultures positive for CMV alone are *not* definitive for CMV disease. The yield of CMV by histopathology is enhanced by special immunohistochemical stains, although these are rarely necessary.

Cryptosporidiosis and infection with *Isospora belli* are best confirmed by adequate stool analysis. Microsporidia no longer need electron microscopic analysis of enteric biopsies for diagnosis. Standard light microscopy and "fungifluor" stool stains are now sufficient. Finally, *Entamoeba histolytica* is best diagnosed on the basis of stool analysis. However, colonic biopsies can establish the diagnosis when stool analysis shows no abnormalities.

For the proper processing of specimens for microbiologic culture and histopathology, special attention should be paid to the last column in Table 13–1. It should be emphasized that this table represents current practice and may change with further clinical studies.

OVERVIEW OF SIGNS AND SYMPTOMS OF HIV INFECTIONS AND MALIGNANCIES

GI abnormalities are commonly encountered in the evaluation and treatment of patients with AIDS. Although some of these GI manifestations (e.g., weight loss, anorexia, and large-volume diarrhea) are often difficult to diagnose and treat specifically, many other manifestations of HIV infection, particularly those in the esophagus, liver, biliary tract, and rectosigmoid, can be expeditiously evaluated, definitively

TABLE 13–1. IDENTIFICATION OF AIDS-ASSOCIATED PATHOGENS

Disease Pathogen	Principal Diagnostic Test	Principal Feature	Supplementary Diagnostic Test
Candida albicans	Histopathology (H&E, silver stains), brush cytology	Tissue-invasive pseudomycelia (PAS or methenamine stains)	Fungal culture
Herpes simplex	Histopathology (H&E, immunofluorescent stains)	Cowdry type A inclusions	Viral tissue culture
Cytomegalovirus (CMV)	Histopathology (H&E stains)	CMV-infected endothelial cells	Viral tissue culture
Cryptosporidium/Isospora belli	Stool analysis	AFB stain–positive cysts	Small-bowel or colon biopsy
Entamoeba histolytica	Stool analysis	Erythrocytophagous ameba (use optical micrometer)	Colonic biopsy
Mycobacterium avium-intracellulare	Histopathology (H&E, Fite stains)	Poorly formed granulomata (massive AFB infection of macrophages)	AFB culture
Microsporidia	Light microscopy, ? fungifluor stain of stools	Microcysts-enterocytes or stool	Electron microscopy
Lymphoma	Histopathology (H&E stains)	Malignant lymphocytes	Immunohistochemical stains (B and T cell markers)
Kaposi's sarcoma	Histopathology (H&E stain)	Vascular "slits," malignant endothelial cells	Special stains (*Ulex europaeus* stain)

H&E, hematoxylin and eosin; AFB, acid-fast bacillus; PAS, periodic acid–Schiff.

diagnosed, and specifically treated. The most common GI manifestations of HIV infection are reviewed in the following organ-related scheme. Emphasis is placed on the diagnosis and management of treatable conditions.

Esophageal Diseases

Dysphagia, odynophagia, and retrosternal esophageal pain (esophagospasm) are common occurrences among patients with acute and chronic HIV infection. In addition, *acute AIDS esophagitis* was reported in eight patients during their initial illness from HIV infection.[41] These patients had dysphagia, odynophagia, and retrosternal pain lasting from 2 to 14 days, with spontaneous resolution thereafter.

The most common esophageal complaint among AIDS patients is dysphagia (difficulty swallowing, with a sensation of food sticking). The most common organism associated with dysphagia is *C. albicans*, with the majority of these patients having both thrush and esophageal candidiasis[26] (Table 13–2). For those patients with thrush and esophageal complaints, a course of antifungal therapy, including ketoconazole, 200 mg/day, or fluconazole, 100 mg/day, for 7 to 14 days is indicated (Chapter 12). Barium contrast radiography may support but not document the diagnosis of esophageal

candidiasis. Endoscopy should not be performed in AIDS patients with thrush and dysphagia simply to document esophageal involvement unless treatment with systemic antifungal drugs fails to produce significant improvement in symptoms. Large, yellow-white plaques throughout the esophagus are usually noted in patients with *Candida* esophagitis, and biopsies or direct cytology brushings should be performed to look for tissue-invasive pseudomycelia. Despite favorable symptomatic response to current antifungal therapy, esophageal lesions may not completely resolve despite months of therapy.[26,48]

Pain on swallowing (odynophagia) and retrosternal episodic pain without swallowing (esophagospasm), in addition to dysphagia, are more commonly encountered in patients with herpes esophagitis and CMV esophagitis than in those with *Candida* esophagitis.[50] Although discrete single ulcers have been reported in patients with CMV esophagitis, extremely large (2- to 10-cm-long) and/or multiple, shallow, superficial ulcerations extending throughout much of the esophagus also have been noted. Indeed, CMV ulcerations may be so extensive and circumferential that virtually no normal mucosa, only infected granulation tissue, is encountered. Although patients with CMV esophagitis may experience an initially favorable response to ganciclovir, relapses are common, and gan-

TABLE 13–2. CLINICAL FEATURES OF AIDS-ASSOCIATED ESOPHAGITIS

Parameter	*Candida*	Cytomegalovirus	Herpes Simplex Virus	Idiopathic Ulcers
Thrush	Usual	Occasional	Occasional	Occasional
Dysphagia	Severe	Moderate	Moderate	Moderate
Odynophagia	Rare	Moderate	Severe	Severe
Esophagospasm	Rare	Moderate	Severe	Severe
Localization	Poor	Good	Excellent	Good
Endoscopic feature	Diffuse plaques	Giant shallow ulcers	Deep ulcers	Shallow ulcers
Diagnostic tests	Histology, cytology	Histology	Histology, culture	Histology, culture
Therapy	Fluconazole	Ganciclovir, foscarnet	Acyclovir	Steroids, thalidomide
Response to therapy	Excellent	Fair	Excellent	Good

ciclovir maintenance therapy or foscarnet administration is usually needed (Chapter 26).[4,13,24,38] Oral agents effective against CMV are currently under study and urgently needed given the high relapse rate for enteric CMV infection after ganciclovir treatment.

Although sometimes indistinguishable from CMV ulcerations, HSV (type 1 and 2) ulcers are generally fewer and smaller in diameter, but deeper than those of CMV. Chronic AIDS-related herpetic esophageal ulcerations are usually deep, clean-based ulcerations, 1 to 2 cm in diameter. These large and deep chronic herpetic ulcerations usually are associated clinically with well-localized, intense esophagospasm, odynophagia, and dysphagia. Fortunately, the clinical response to acyclovir has been gratifying among patients with HSV esophagitis, although maintenance therapy is needed (Chapter 26).

Rarely, primary lymphoma, Kaposi's sarcoma (KS), histoplasmosis, or squamous cell carcinoma has been noted in the esophagus among patients with AIDS. On occasion, patients with AIDS have large geographic ulcers of the esophagus where no pathogens have been isolated by histopathology or viral cultures. These so-called *idiopathic aphthous esophageal ulcerations* look nearly identical to those associated with CMV, and their diagnosis requires careful specimen processing to exclude other disease entities. Repeat endoscopy is usually indicated for those patients with large idiopathic esophageal ulcers with negative initial biopsy results. Anecdotal reports suggest that these patients may respond to intralesional steroid injections (by endoscopy), oral steroid administration, or thalidomide. Before treating patients with steroids, however, multiple negative biopsy results from at least two endoscopies should be obtained.[50]

In addition to these AIDS-specific esophageal diseases, bedridden patients with advanced HIV infection may experience severe esophageal peptic acid reflux with esophagitis and esophageal ulcerations. Given the multiplicity of possible causes of esophagitis, the distinct possibility of specific therapy, and the relative ease of diagnosis, we strongly recommend performing endoscopy in AIDS patients with esophageal complaints except in those with classic thrush.

Gastric Diseases

Nausea, vomiting, hematemesis, melena, and early satiety are occasionally encountered in patients with AIDS or advanced HIV infection.[11,18] A thorough investigation is once again indicated, since many of these patients will be found to have non–AIDS-related GI diseases[11] (Table 13–3).

KS is noted frequently on endoscopy in patients with documented cutaneous or nodal KS (Chapter 28). In one prospective survey of 50

TABLE 13–3. CAUSE OF UPPER GASTROINTESTINAL BLEEDING IN 13 AIDS PATIENTS

Lesion	Number of Patients
Kaposi's sarcoma	
Gastric	3
Duodenal	1
Lymphoma, gastric	2
Cytomegalovirus	
Esophagitis	1
Gastritis	1
Gastric ulcer	1
Duodenal ulcer	1
Duodenitis	1
Mallory-Weiss tear	1
Variceal bleeding	1

patients with cutaneous or nodal KS, 20 (40%) had GI lesions noted on endoscopy or flexible sigmoidoscopy.[18] Only 7 of 30 (23%) visibly positive endoscopies or sigmoidoscopies could be confirmed histologically, however, probably because of the submucosal location of most KS lesions and the limited depth of endoscopic biopsy sampling.[18] AIDS-associated KS is rarely symptomatic. However, GI hemorrhage, perforation, and obstruction occasionally are encountered.

B-cell non-Hodgkin's lymphomas involving the antrum occasionally are associated with gastric outlet obstruction, hemorrhage, or both. Although non-AIDS gastric lymphomas commonly are confined initially to the stomach, AIDS-related gastric lymphomas are more commonly multifocal, with extensive disease throughout the abdomen in addition to gastric involvement. Although smaller lymphoma and KS lesions may go undetected by radiographic techniques and require endoscopy for detection, larger masses commonly are noted radiographically as target lesions with central umbilicated ulcerations. Specimens from these lesions should be obtained for biopsy directly by endoscopy.

Hepatobiliary Disease

Abnormal serum biochemical tests of liver function, right upper quadrant abdominal discomfort, and hepatomegaly increasingly are noted in patients with AIDS or advanced HIV infection.[6,9,12,14,21,27,32,36,43,44] Early and *complete* invasive and noninvasive evaluation of these patients should be undertaken, with particular attention to treatable non–HIV-associated biliary tract disease.

Acalculous cholecystitis, including gangrenous cholecystitis (an entity rarely encountered in young, ambulatory patients), has been reported in AIDS patients, the majority of whom have CMV, *Cryptosporidium*, or both noted on histologic sections.[6,21,31] The pathophysiology of this disease is uncertain. However, several patients have had CMV-infected endothelial cells together with mucosal necrosis and ulceration, suggesting, as with CMV enteritis, that necrotizing vasculitis is the mechanism of injury.

Hepatic parenchymal disease likewise is common in patients with HIV infection.[27,36,43] In a retrospective review of hepatic histology, clinical features, and laboratory data in 85 AIDS patients, only 1 of 26 (3.8%) percutaneous liver biopsy specimens and 9 of 58 (15%) postmortem liver specimens were normal[43] (Table 13–4). Steatosis, portal inflammation, and noncaseating, poorly formed granulomata were the most common histologic abnormalities (Table 13–5). AIDS-specific infections or malignancies were detected in 40% of both biopsy and autopsy groups.

In addition to a high frequency of KS (10 of 26 patients), CMV (10 of 26 patients), and *Mycobacterium avium-intracellulare* (5 of 26 patients), Nakanuma et al[36] also noted marked depletion of portal tract lymphocytes in livers of AIDS patients. In most instances, however, parenchymal liver disease in patients with AIDS is an anticipated feature of a previously diagnosed, widely disseminated disease process. Liver biopsy infrequently documents new AIDS-specific diagnoses.[1] Thus, performing percutaneous liver biopsy is not *usually* necessary in the

TABLE 13–4. HEPATIC HISTOLOGY IN 85 AIDS PATIENTS

Finding	Biopsy (% of total) (*N* = 26)	Autopsy (% of total) (*N* = 59)	Combined (% of total) (*N* = 85)
Normal	1 (3.8)	9 (15.3)	10 (11.8)
Steatosis	10 (38.5)	26 (44.1)	36 (42.4)
Portal inflammation	14 (53.8)	16 (27.1)	30 (35.3)
Congestion	1 (3.8)	18 (30.5)	19 (22.4)
Granulomata	10 (38.5)	2 (3.4)	12 (14.1)
Focal necrosis	5 (19.2)	5 (8.5)	10 (11.8)
Fibrosis or cirrhosis	4 (15.4)	4 (6.8)	8 (4.7)
Bile stasis	2 (7.7)	3 (5.1)	5 (5.9)
Kupffer cell hyperplasia	3 (11.5)	3 (5.1)	6 (7.1)
Piecemeal necrosis	2 (7.7)	1 (1.7)	3 (1.2)

From Schneiderman DJ, Arenson DM, Cello JP, et al: Hepatic disease in patients with acquired immune deficiency syndrome (AIDS). Hepatology 7:927, 1987, with permission.

TABLE 13–5. AIDS-SPECIFIC HEPATIC HISTOLOGIC FEATURES IN 85 PATIENTS

Finding	Biopsy (% of total) (N = 26)	Autopsy (% of total) (N = 59)	Combined (% of total) (N = 85)
No pathogens	15 (57.7)	34 (57.6)	49 (57.6)
Mycobacterium avium-intracellulare	8 (30.8)	6 (10.2)	14 (16.5)
Kaposi's sarcoma	0 (0.0)	11 (18.6)	11 (12.9)
Cytomegalovirus	2 (7.7)	6 (10.2)	8 (9.4)
Lymphoma	2 (7.7)	2 (3.4)	4 (4.7)
Cryptococcus	0 (0.0)	2 (3.4)	2 (2.4)
Histoplasma	0 (0.0)	1 (1.7)	1 (1.2)
Coccidioides	0 (0.0)	1 (1.7)	1 (1.2)

From Schneiderman DJ, Arenson DM, Cello JP, et al: Hepatic disease in patients with acquired immune deficiency syndrome (AIDS). Hepatology 7:927, 1987, with permission.

majority of patients with abnormal liver function tests.

Obstructive biliary tract disease should, however, be thoroughly and expeditiously evaluated in AIDS patients. We and others have noted profound abnormalities on ultrasound, computed tomography (CT), and endoscopic cholangiography in patients with HIV infection, and the full spectrum of HIV disease manifested in the biliary tree has yet to be elucidated.[6,9,12,14,21,32,44] Patients with AIDS-associated biliary tract disease often have fever, pain, and tenderness in the right upper quadrant and dramatic increases in serum alkaline phosphatase (2 to 20 times above the upper limits of normal).[12,14,44] Most patients with AIDS-associated biliary tract disease will be noted by ultrasound or CT abdominal scanning techniques to have prominent or dilated intrahepatic or extrahepatic bile ducts, or both, with dilation down to the periampullary area, together with marked thickening of the ductal walls.[14] Endoscopic retrograde cholangiopancreatography (ERCP) of 51 AIDS patients by our service at San Francisco General Hospital over the past 8 years demonstrated intrahepatic and extrahepatic sclerosing cholangitis changes (including irregular ductal mucosa) and papillary stenosis in 25 patients, intrahepatic ductal sclerotic changes alone in 6 patients, papillary stenosis alone in 5 patients, and high-grade extrahepatic bile duct obstruction in 4 patients (Figs. 13–1 to 13–3). Only 11 of 51 AIDS patients studied by ERCP because of pain and markedly elevated serum alkaline phosphatase levels had normal cholangiograms (Table 13–6). All 20 patients with papillary stenosis *and* abdominal pain underwent ERCP sphincterotomy, with multiple biopsies of the ampulla of Vater. Eighteen of 40 patients (45%) with abnormal cho-

langiograms had specific AIDS-related pathogens or malignancies in the regions of ductal disease as demonstrated by cholangiography (CMV, 7; *Cryptosporidium*, 5; CMV and *Cryptosporidium*, 1; KS, 1; *M. avium-intracellulare*, 3; lymphoma, 1) (Color Plate II*C*). The pathophysiology of AIDS-associated sclerosing cholangitis and papillary stenosis is uncertain, although CMV, microsporidial, or cryptosporidial ulceration and subsequent fibrotic stricturing of the bile duct have been suggested by our own studies and by some additional reports. Initial results of a prospective study being conducted at San Francisco General Hospital suggest that more than 40% of asymptomatic AIDS patients have abnormal bile duct morphology.

In a recently completed study evaluating the long-term outcome of ERCP sphincterotomy for 25 patients with AIDS-associated papillary stenosis, we noted sustained pain relief for up to 9 months.[12] Despite pain relief, serum alkaline phosphatase levels did not decrease, likely because of progressive *intrahepatic* sclerosing cholangitis[12] (Fig. 13–4).

AIDS-Related Diarrhea

Diarrhea is experienced by over 50% of patients with AIDS at some time during their illness and can be a major source of morbidity and mortality in nearly one quarter of patients. Specific pathogens may be isolated in up to 75% to 80% of patients with chronic diarrhea. A large number of pathogens may involve the small or large bowel or both, including bacteria, parasites, mycobacteria, and viruses.[1–3,5,10,13,15–17,19,20,22,25,28–30,33,34,37,39,40,45–47,49] The major etiologic infectious agents in patients with AIDS-associated diarrhea are listed in Ta-

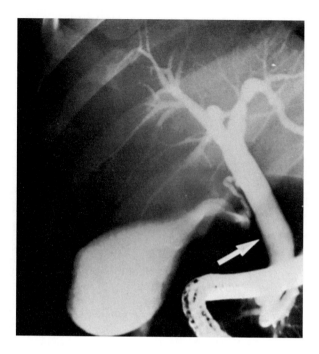

FIGURE 13–1. AIDS-associated papillary stenosis. Entire biliary tree is filled with contrast. Extrahepatic bile duct (*arrow*) is dilated, as evidenced by comparison to the endoscope (11.5 mm). A sphincterotomy was performed.

bles 13–7 and 13–8. The bacterial pathogens, including *Salmonella, Shigella,* and *Campylobacter,* usually cause an acute diarrheal illness. However, chronic diarrhea mimicking inflammatory bowel disease occasionally may be encountered. On rare occasions, patients may develop a bacterial toxin-associated diarrhea from *Clostridium difficile,* related to prior use of antibiotics. Diag-

nosis of *C. difficile*–associated colitis depends on identification of toxin in the stool as well as direct examination of the distal bowel demonstrating classic yellow-brown adherent pseudomembranes. Parasites, including *Cryptosporidium, Isospora, Entamoeba histolytica, Giardia, Microsporidia,* and *Strongyloides,* are collectively common causes of chronic diarrhea in pa-

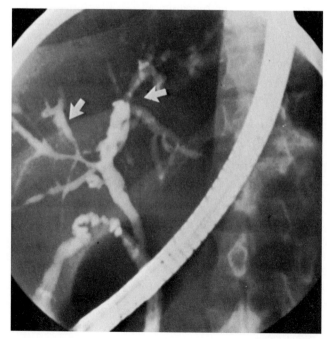

FIGURE 13–2. AIDS-sclerosing cholangitis. Intra- and extrahepatic ducts are markedly irregular. There are focal strictures and irregular dilations of the intrahepatic ducts (*arrows*).

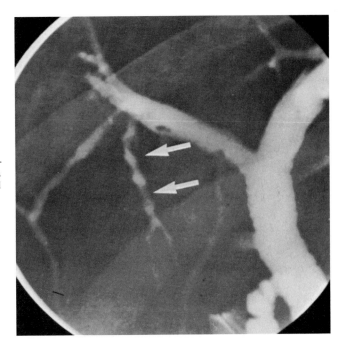

FIGURE 13–3. Intrahepatic sclerosing cholangitis. Intrahepatic ducts are irregular, with a beaded appearance (*arrows*). Extrahepatic ductal mucosa has a serrated appearance.

tients with HIV disease.[22,30,40,47] *Mycobacterium avium-intracellulare* and, less commonly, *Mycobacterium tuberculosis* may be associated with chronic diarrheal illnesses in patients with HIV disease. Cytomegalovirus, herpes, and adenovirus are also reportedly associated with chronic diarrheal illnesses. Grohmann et al[19] from the Centers for Disease Control and Prevention (CDC) reported identification of additional viral agents in the stools of HIV patients with chronic diarrhea. They noted that in addition to adenovirus, there were significant associations of the following agents with chronic diarrhea: astrovirus, caliciviridae, and picobirnaviruses. They noted one or more of these viral agents in over one third of stools submitted by patients with chronic diarrhea. The clinical

significance of these viruses remains to be clarified.

In patients with HIV-related diarrhea, the minimum evaluation should consist of a careful search for routine bacterial enteric pathogens by culture, examination of the stools for typical and atypical ova and parasites, and an examination of the stool for *C. difficile* toxin if the patient has received antibiotics within the past 2 to 3 months.[20,23] Furthermore, a Sudan stain for fecal fat, if positive, should direct the focus to small bowel rather than to colon, whereas the presence of fecal leukocytes more strongly suggests a colonic inflammatory disease.[19,22]

Several agents are so commonly encountered in the stools or bowel wall or both of patients with severe refractory AIDS-associated diarrhea

TABLE 13–6. AIDS CHOLANGIOPATHY: CLINICAL FEATURES OF 51 PATIENTS STUDIED AT SAN FRANCISCO GENERAL HOSPITAL

Features	Abnormal ERCP (N = 40)	Normal ERCP (N = 11)	p Value
Age (years)	36 ± 1.2	35.6 ± 3.0	NS
AIDS duration (months)	10.8 ± 2.2	11.2 ± 2.9	NS
Right upper quadrant pain	35/40 (88%)	8/11 (73%)	NS
Abnormal ultrasound	28/38 (74%)	1/10 (10%)	<0.001
Abnormal computed tomographic scan	12/17 (71%)	0/9 (0)	0.003
Alkaline phosphatase (IU/liter)	744 ± 120	700 ± 137	NS
Alanine aminotransferase (IU/liter)	95 ± 15	114 ± 30	NS
Bilirubin (mg/dl)	1.4 ± 0.5	2.5 ± 1.4	NS

ERCP, endoscopic retrograde cholangiopancreatography; NS, not significant.

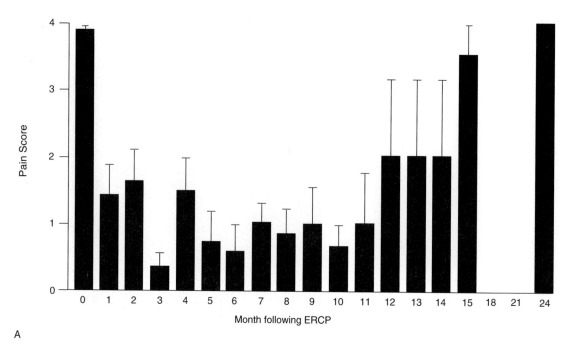

A

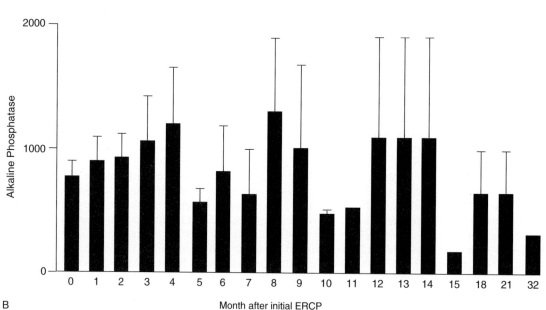

B

FIGURE 13–4. *A*, Pain scores in 25 patients undergoing ERCP sphincterotomy for AIDS-associated papillary stenosis. Scale: 0 = no pain, 4 = severe debilitating pain. There is a significant decrease in period pain scores for 9 months following sphincterotomy. *B*, Serum alkaline phosphates levels following ERCP sphinctero-tomy. No significant decrease was noted. (From Cello JP, Chan MF: Long-term followup of ERCP sphinctero-tomy for patients with AIDS papillary stenosis. Am J Med 99:600–603, 1995, with permission of the publisher. Copyright 1995 by Excerpta Medica Inc.)

that they deserve special mention. There is little question that the most common cause of chronic AIDS-associated diarrhea is infection with *Cryptosporidium*. This infestation produces profuse watery diarrhea, weight loss, paraumbil- ical abdominal pain, and nausea and vomiting without fever. The diagnosis usually depends on stool studies using concentration techniques and acid-fast stains. It is uncertain how many patients with *Cryptosporidium* are undiagnosed

TABLE 13–7. INFECTIOUS DIARRHEA IN 43 AIDS PATIENTS

Cause	No.*	Percent
Cytomegalovirus	15	20
Mycobacterium avium	10	14
Salmonella sp.	10	14
Cryptosporidium	8	11
Entamoeba histolytica	6	8
Giardia lamblia	4	5
Herpes simplex virus	4	5
Campylobacter jejuni	3	4
Isospora belli	2	3
Clostridium difficile	2	3
Candida sp.	2	3
Strongyloides	2	3
Kaposi's sarcoma	1	1
Other pathogens	5	7
TOTAL	74	

Data from Smith et al[47] and Antony et al.[1]
* Some with multiple pathogens.

by stool studies alone. However, in controlled clinical trials, we and others have clearly demonstrated cryptosporidia on intestinal biopsy in patients who have had multiple stools negative for the pathogen. Treatment of cryptosporidiosis is unsatisfactory at best, although the most promising agents include azithromycin, paromomycin and bovine immune concentrate from colostrum. Although spiramycin has been demonstrated to be beneficial in children with cryptosporidiosis, the results in adults have been less than satisfactory.[2,16,35,42,43]

Mycobacterium avium complex (MAC) produces a systemic illness not infrequently characterized by profound diarrhea, weight loss, and fever. Paraumbilical or right upper-quadrant pain with anorexia also is common. In most instances, MAC disease can be diagnosed by blood culture, but once again we and others have noted MAC on acid-fast stains of enteric biopsies in patients who have had blood cultures negative for mycobacteria. Endoscopic ex-

TABLE 13–8. AIDS DIARRHEA—ETIOLOGY

Infectious Agents	
Bacteria	*Salmonella, Shigella, Campylobacter* sp., *Clostridium difficile*
Parasites	*Cryptosporidium, Isospora, E. histolytica, Giardia, Microsporidia, Strongyloides*
Mycobacteria	*M. avium-intracellulare, M. tuberculosis*
Viruses	CMV, herpes, adenovirus, astrovirus, caliciviridae, HIV (AIDS enteropathy)

amination may demonstrate thickened valvulae conniventes or intramural mass effects in certain patients. As with cryptosporidiosis, MAC treatment is less than satisfactory, and even multiple-agent chemotherapeutic programs produce dismal responses.

Microsporidiosis is being identified increasingly in up to 15% to 20% of patients with previously documented refractory diarrhea.[5,15,34] At least two species, *Enterocytozoon bienusi* and *Encephalitozoon cuniculi,* have been noted principally. Patients with microsporidiosis have profuse watery diarrhea, profound weight loss, and paraumbilical abdominal pain but no fevers or profound anorexia. The definitive diagnosis of microsporidiosis remains problematic. Although stool analyses using formalin-fixed stools treated by the chromotrope-based technique or a "fungifluor" stain and examined by light microscopy appear promising, in most hands, enteric biopsies are required. Examination by electron microscopy is the most established technique, but it is cumbersome and expensive. Giemsa or hematoxylin and eosin (H& E)–stained specimens examined by light microscopy can be used to make the diagnosis.[39] Therapy of microsporidiosis is problematic, and the most promising drug appears to be albendazole.[5] Few studies, however, have documented treatment of microsporidiosis by albendazole or other agents.[5]

Cytomegalovirus may involve the gastrointestinal tract from mouth to anus and has been associated with intermittent or persistent diarrhea. Abdominal pain is a common phenomenon among patients with CMV enteritis, and on occasion patients experience substantial episodes of GI tract bleeding and even severe acute abdominal pain. The diagnosis of cytomegalovirus enteritis requires endoscopic examination and biopsy.[33] Hematoxylin and eosin stains are usually satisfactory for making the diagnosis, and little is gained by performing immunohistochemical stains or DNA in-situ hybridization techniques on specimens negative for CMV by H&E stains. Ideally, CMV enteritis should be evidenced by the demonstration of CMV-infected endothelial cells within the lamina propria or submucosa. Treatment for CMV enteritis is the subject of only a few prospective trials. However, in one double-blind placebo-controlled trial, ganciclovir 5 mg/kg bid for 14 days was associated with decreased tissue biopsy culture positivity, decreased positivity of urine cultures, decrease in new extraenteric sites, and an improvement in colonoscopy score.[13] Studies using foscarnet for CMV enteritis are limited and consist only of prospective open-label trials. Nonetheless, preliminary results suggest that nearly two thirds of patients respond at least temporarily to foscarnet therapy for CMV enteritis.[4,38]

HIV enteropathy has been described in 15% to 60% of patients with severe refractory diarrhea. By definition, these patients have histopathologic and functional abnormalities of the small bowel but no pathogens or malignancies identified by detailed evaluation.[25,37,49] Characteristically, these patients may have subtotal villous atrophy and abnormal tests of small bowel function, including 72-hour fecal fat, D-xylose, and PABA absorption. The mechanism of HIV-associated enteropathy is uncertain, although HIV clearly infects enterocytes as well as gut mononuclear, lymphocyte, and enterochromaffin cells.[3,25,37,49] Thus, HIV itself may be a direct gut pathogen, causing destruction of enterocytes or precipitating the release of hormonally active substances from lamina propria cells.[31] It should be recognized that with identification of newer agents from the feces and gut wall among patients with HIV disease-associated diarrhea, there has been a decrease in the number of patients given the designation HIV enteropathy.[19,22,29]

Initial studies with octreotide (Sandostatin), a somatostatin analog, suggest that some patients with dehydrating diarrhea had responses.[10,17,45,46] In our multicenter, open-label clinical trial of octreotide, 21 of 51 patients (41%) were partial or complete responders (decrease in daily stool weight to ≤50% baseline or <250 g/day)[10] (Fig. 13–5). Baseline laboratory studies (Tables 13–9 and 13–10) demonstrated defects in nutrient absorption, including altered D-xylose, bentiromide, and fat absorption. The latter nutrient absorption was profoundly abnormal (Table 13–11) as evidenced by nearly one quarter of dietary fat appearing as fecal fat in 72-hour collections (nl <7% malabsorption). Responders to subcutaneous octreotide (at dosages ranging from 50 to 500 μg every 8 hours) were significantly less likely to have enteric pathogens than were nonresponders (33% versus 70%, $p < 0.01$) (Table 13–11).

Recently, we completed a multicenter, double-blind, placebo-controlled trial of moderate-dose octreotide in patients with refractory AIDS-associated diarrhea.[45] Over this 3-week protocol, 129 patients with a stool weight of

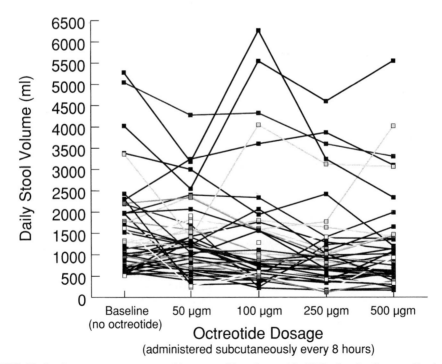

FIGURE 13–5. Dose response to octreotide among 51 patients with AIDS-related refractory diarrhea. By day 14 of subcutaneous octreotide therapy, mean stool volumes had decreased from 1604 ± 180 ml/day to 1084 ± 162 ml/day ($p < 0.01$).

TABLE 13–9. LABORATORY DATA

	Day 0	Day 14	Day 28
Hematocrit (%)	34.1 ± 0.9	32.3 ± 0.9	34.4 ± 1.3
		($n = 50$)	($n = 29$)
White blood count	3.5 ± 0.3	3.0 ± 0.2	3.3 ± 0.3
($\times 1000$)/mm^3		($n = 50$)*	($n = 29$)
Carotene (μmol/liter)	0.87 ± 0.1	0.79 ± 0.2	0.70 ± 0.09
	($n = 45$)	($n = 11$)	($n = 10$)
Albumin (g/liter)	35 ± 1	32 ± 2	35 ± 0.2
	($n = 19$)	($n = 19$)	($n = 14$)
Glucose (mmol/liter)	5.2 ± 0.2	5.9 ± 0.4†	5.1 ± 0.2
D-Xylose (mmol/liter)‡	0.63 ± 0.08	0.52 ± 0.11	($n = 31$)
	($n = 32$)	($n = 16$)	
Bentiromide (%)	45.2 ± 4.1	59.7 ± 8.2	
	($n = 20$)	($n = 9$)	
Patient weight (kg)	58.7 ± 1.3	59.1 ± 1.3	59.9 ± 1.4
			($n = 29$)
Karnofsky score	66 ± 2	69 ± 2	76 ± 2*
	($n = 50$)	($n = 50$)	($n = 32$)

NOTE: Day 14 (i.e., end of second week of drug) and day 28 (off drug) values not significantly different from day 0 unless indicated.

Normal values: carotene, 1.12–3.72 μmol/liter; glucose, 2.22–3.89 mmol/liter; D-xylose, >1.67 mmol/liter at 2 hours; bentiromide, >57% excretion in 6 hours.

$n = 51$ unless stated otherwise; all mean values ± SEM.

* $p < 0.01$.

† $p < 0.001$.

‡ After 25-g oral dose; 2-hour serum level.

greater than 500 g/day/despite routine antidiarrheal therapy were randomized to receive octreotide or placebo. The octreotide dose was increased to a maximum of 300 μg tid, during which 72-hour stool collections were obtained. After the placebo-controlled trial, all patients received open-label octreotide at doses of up to 500 μg tid. After 3 weeks of therapy, 48% of octreotide- and 39% of placebo-treated patients responded ($p = 0.43$). At 300 μg tid, 50% of octreotide and 30.1% of placebo-treated patients responded ($p = 0.12$) (Fig. 13–6). For those patients with baseline stool weights of between 1000 and 2000 g/day, however, 57% of octreotide and 25% of placebo-treated patients responded ($p = 0.06$). Response rates based upon diarrhea duration, body weight, CD4 counts, and presence or absence of pathogens showed no benefit of octreotide.[45] However,

during the open-label phase of the trial, employing a dose of octreotide of 500 μg tid, both stool weight and bowel movement frequency demonstrated progressive decreases. After 8 weeks of therapy, there was a 42.3% decrease in stool weight ($p < 0.001$) and a 38.9% decrease in stool frequency ($p < 0.001$) (Fig. 13–7). Future studies of high-dose octreotide with supplementary pancreatic enzymes are appropriate at this time, given the previously demonstrated increase in steatorrhea together with the improvement noted during open-label trials with higher dose octreotide.

Peritoneal Disease

On occasion, patients with AIDS or ARC develop ascites.[51] Since some HIV-infected pa-

TABLE 13–10. FAT ABSORPTION BALANCE STUDIES

Parameter	Day 0	Day 14	p Value
Fat ingested (72 hours; in grams)	282.5 ± 19.3	306.6 ± 23.3	NS
Fecal fat (72 hours; in grams)	53.2 ± 6.7	107.3 ± 18.0	<0.001
Fat malabsorption*	0.22 ± 0.03	0.30 ± 0.04	<0.001

NS, not significant; day 0, baseline; day 14, end of second week of drug administration.

* Calculated as 72-hour fecal fat (g) divided by 72-hour dietary fat intake.

TABLE 13–11. OCTREOTIDE RESPONDERS VERSUS NONRESPONDERS AT DAY 14

Parameter	Responders (N = 21)	Nonresponders (N = 30)	p Value
Stool volume (ml)	541 ± 105*	1471 ± 245	0.002
Stool frequency (per day)	2.54 ± 0.21	5.41 ± 0.58	<0.0001
Hematocrit (%)	35.6 ± 1.7	33.1 ± 0.9	NS
White blood count (× 1000)/mm³	3.5 ± 0.5	3.6 ± 0.3	NS
Carotene (μmol/liter)	1.03 ± 0.2 (n = 19)	0.71 ± 0.1 (n = 26)	NS
Glucose (mmol/liter)	5.1 ± 0.2	5.3 ± 0.3	NS
D-Xylose (mmol/liter)	0.65 ± 0.11 (n = 11)	0.62 ± 0.11 (n = 21)	NS
Fecal fat (72 hours; in grams at day 0)	56.1 ± 10.8	52.9 ± 8.4 (n = 29)	NS
Fecal fat (72 hours; grams at day 14)	96.7 ± 32.7	120 ± 17.5 (n = 27)	<0.05
Bentiromide (%)	48.1 ± 8.1 (n = 8)	43.3 ± 4.6 (n = 12)	NS
Patient weight (kg)	58.7 ± 1.6	58.7 ± 1.9	NS
Karnofsky score	70.7 ± 2.6	63.6 ± 2.6 (n = 29)	NS
Presence of cryptosporidia	5 (24%)	10 (33%)	NS
No pathogens identified	14 (67%)	9 (30%)	<0.01

NS, not significant.
* All values ± SEM.

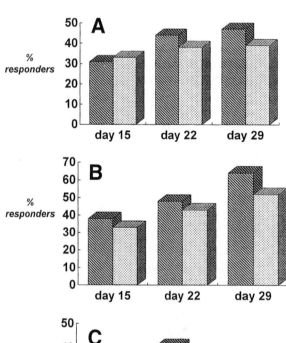

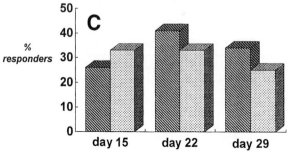

FIGURE 13–6. Percentage of patients responding to drug/placebo in each group based on study day. *A*, All patients. *B*, Patients with idiopathic diarrhea. *C*, patients with enteric pathogens. ▨, Octreotide; ⊡, placebo. (From Simon DM, Cello JP, Valenzuela J, et al: Multicenter trial of octreotide in patients with refractory acquired immunodeficiency syndrome-associated diarrhea. Gastroenterology 108:1753–1760, 1995, with permission.)

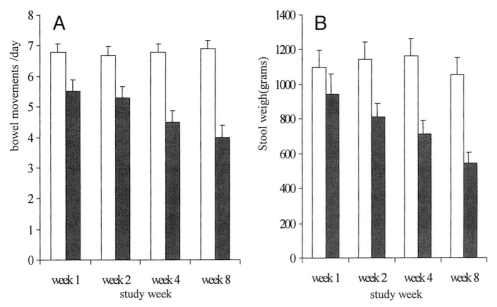

FIGURE 13–7. Changes in (*A*) bowel movement frequency and (*B*) stool weight in all patients studied during the open-label phase of study (mean ± SEM). All differences were statistically significant at $p < 0.001$ except for week 1 stool weight ($p = 0.1$). □, Baseline; ■, therapy.

tients may have underlying cirrhosis (caused by either alcohol consumption or viral hepatitis), a sizable percentage of them will have transudative ascites related to their chronic liver disease. Exudative ascites (ascites protein concentration >1.5 to 2.0 g/dl), however, should be thoroughly evaluated in patients with HIV infection. Careful evaluation of the ascites fluid, including cytological evaluations (sampling large volumes) and acid-fast stains, should be done early to exclude patients with malignancy and tuberculous peritonitis. In patients with new onset of exudative ascites and negative or equivocal evaluations by paracentesis or fine-needle aspiration biopsy or both, laparoscopic evaluations with directed biopsy of the peritoneum may be indicated particularly to include tuberculosis.

REFERENCES

1. Antony MA, Brandt LJ, Klein RS, Bernstein LH: Infectious diarrhea in patients with AIDS. Dig Dis Sci 33: 1141, 1988
2. Armitage K, Flanigan T, Carey J, et al: Treatment of cryptosporidiosis with paromycin. A new report of five cases. Arch Intern Med 152:2497, 1992
3. Bigornia E, Simon D, Weiss L, et al: Detection of HIV-1 protein and genomic sequences in enterochromaffin cells of HIV-1-seropositive patients. Am J Gastroenterol 87:1624, 1992
4. Blanshard C: Treatment of HIV-related cytomegalovirus disease of the gastrointestinal tract with foscarnet. J Acquir Immune Defic Syndr 5(Suppl 1):S25, 1992
5. Blanshard C, Ellis DS, Tovey DG, et al: Treatment of intestinal microsporidiosis with albendazole in patients with AIDS. AIDS 6:311, 1992
6. Blumberg RS, Kelsey P, Perrone T, et al: Cytomegalovirus- and *Cryptosporidium*-associated acalculous gangrenous cholecystitis. Am J Med 76:1118, 1984
7. Burke DS, Brundage JF, Herbold JR, et al: Human immunodeficiency virus infections among civilian applicants for United States Military Service, October 1985 to March 1986. N Engl J Med 317:131, 1987
8. Caccamo D, Perez NK, Marchevsky A: Primary lymphoma of the liver in the acquired immunodeficiency syndrome. Arch Pathol Lab Med 110:553, 1986
9. Cello JP: Acquired immunodeficiency syndrome cholangiopathy: Spectrum of disease. Am J Med 86: 539–546, 1989
10. Cello JP, Grendell JH, Basuk P, et al: Effect of octreotide on refractory AIDS-associated diarrhea. A prospective, multicenter clinical trial. Ann Intern Med 115:705–710, 1991
11. Cello JP, Wilcox CM: Evaluation and treatment of gastrointestinal tract hemorrhage in patients with AIDS. In Friedman SL, ed. Gastrointestinal Manifestations of AIDS. Gastroenterology Clinics of North America. Philadelphia, WB Saunders Co, 1988, pp 639–648

12. Cello JP, Chan MF: Long-term followup of endoscopic retrograde cholangiopancreatography (ERCP) sphincterotomy for patients with acquired immune deficiency syndrome papillary stenosis. Am J Med 1995 (In press)

13. Dieterich DT, Kotler DP, Busch DF, et al: Ganciclovir treatment of cytomegalovirus colitis in AIDS: A randomized, double-blind placebo-controlled multicenter study. J Infect Dis 167:278, 1993

14. Dolmatch BL, Laing FC, Federle MP, et al: AIDS-related cholangitis: Radiographic findings in nine patients. Radiology 163:313, 1987

15. Eeftinck-Schattenkerk JK, van Gool T, van Ketel RJ, et al: Clinical significance of small-intestinal microsporidiosis in HIV-II-infected individuals. Lancet 337:895, 1991

16. Fafard J, Lalonde R: Long-standing symptomatic cryptosporidiosis in a normal man: Clinical response to spiramycin. J Clin Gastroenterol 12:190, 1990

17. Fanning M, Monte M, Sutherland LR, et al: Pilot study of Sandostatin (octreotide) therapy of refractory HIV-associated diarrhea. Dig Dis Sci 36:476, 1991

18. Friedman SL, Wright TL, Altman DF: Gastrointestinal Kaposi's sarcoma in patients with acquired immunodeficiency syndrome—endoscopic and autopsy findings. Gastroenterology 89:102, 1985

19. Grohmann GS, Gloss RI, Pereira HG, et al: Enteric viruses and diarrhea in HIV-infected patients. N Engl J Med 329:14–20, 1993

20. Johanson JF, Sonnenberg A: Efficient management of diarrhea in the acquired immunodeficiency syndrome (AIDS). Ann Intern Med 112:942–948, 1990

21. Kavin H, Jonas RB, Chowdhury L, et al: Acalculous cholecystitis and cytomegalovirus infection in the acquired immunodeficiency syndrome. Ann Intern Med 104:53, 1986

22. Kearney DJ, Koch J, Cello JP: Prospective study of endoscopic evaluation of patients with AIDS-related diarrhea. Gastroenterology 108:A20, 1995

23. Koch J, Garcia-Shelton YL, Chan MF, et al: Steatorrhea—early manifestations of AIDS-related malnutrition. Gastroenterology 106:A614, 1994

24. Koretz SH, Collaborative DHPG Treatment Study Group: Treatment of serious cytomegalovirus infections with 9-(1,3 dihydroxy-2-propoxymethyl) guanine in patients with AIDS and other immunodeficiencies. N Engl J Med 314:801, 1986

25. Kotler DP, Gaetz HP, Lange M, et al: Enteropathy associated with the acquired immunodeficiency syndrome. Ann Intern Med 101:421, 1984

26. Laine L, Dretler RH, Conteas C, et al: Fluconazole compared with ketoconazole for the treatment of candida esophagitis in AIDS. Ann Intern Med 117:655, 1992

27. Lebovics E, Thung SN, Schaffner F, et al: The liver in the acquired immunodeficiency syndrome: A clinical and histologic study. Hepatology 5:293, 1985

28. Louie E, Borkowsky W, Klesius PH, et al: Treatment of cryptosporidiosis with oral bovine transfer factor. Clin Immunol Immunopathol 44:329, 1987

29. Lum DF, Hui SC, Cello JP: Flexible sigmoidoscopy (FS) in evaluating AIDS/HIV associated diarrhea: Are we wasting time and resources? Gastrointest Endosc 39:298, 1993 (Presented)

30. Lumb R, Hardiman R: *Isospora belli* infection. Med J Aust 155:194, 1991

31. Manfredi R, Vezzadini P, Costigliola P, et al: Elevated plasma levels of vasoactive intestinal peptide in AIDS patients with refractory diarrhea. Effects of treatment with octreotide. AIDS 7:223, 1993

32. Margulis SJ, Honig CL, Soave R, et al: Biliary tract obstruction in the acquired immunodeficiency syndrome. Ann Intern Med 105:207, 1986

33. Meiselman MS, Cello JP, Margaretten W: Cytomegalovirus colitis—report of the clinical, endoscopic and pathologic findings in two patients with the acquired immune deficiency syndrome. Gastroenterology 88:171, 1985

34. Molina JM, Sarfati C, Beauvais B, et al: Intestinal microsporidiosis in human immunodeficiency virus-infected patients with chronic unexplained diarrhea: Prevalence and clinical and biologic features. J Infect Dis 167:217, 1993

35. Moskovitz BL, Stanton TL, Kusmierek JJ: Spiramycin therapy for cryptosporidial diarrhea in immunocompromised patients. J Antimicrob Chemother 22(Suppl B):189, 1988

36. Nakanuma Y, Liew CT, Peters RL, et al: Pathologic features of the liver in acquired immune deficiency syndrome (AIDS). Liver 6:158, 1986

37. Nelson J, Wiley C, Reynolds-Kohler C, et al: Human immunodeficiency virus detected in the bowel epithelium from patients with gastrointestinal symptoms. Lancet 1:259, 1988

38. Nelson MR, Connolly GM, Hawkins DA, Gazzard BG: Foscarnet in the treatment of cytomegalovirus infection of the esophagus and colon in patients with the acquired immune deficiency syndrome. Am J Gastroenterol 86:876, 1991

39. Orenstein JM, Tenner M, Kotler DP: Localization of infection by the microsporidion *Enterocytozoon bieneusi* in the gastrointestinal tract of AIDS patients with diarrhea. AIDS 6:195, 1992

40. Pape JW, Johnson WD: *Isospora belli* infections. Prog Clin Parasitol 2:119, 1991

41. Rabeneck L, Boyko WJ, McLean DM, et al: Unusual esophageal ulcers containing enveloped virus-like particles in homosexual men. Gastroenterology 90:1882, 1986

42. Saez-Llorens X, Odio CM, Umana MA, Morales MV: Spiramycin vs placebo for treatment of acute diarrhea caused by cryptosporidium. Pediatr Infect Dis J 8:136, 1989

43. Schneiderman DJ, Arenson DM, Cello JP, et al: Hepatic disease in patients with acquired immune deficiency syndrome (AIDS). Hepatology 7:925, 1987

44. Schneiderman DJ, Cello JP, Laing FC: Papillary stenosis and sclerosing cholangitis in the acquired immunodeficiency syndrome. Ann Intern Med 106:546, 1987

45. Simon DM, Cello JP, Valenzuela J, et al: Multicenter trial of octreotide in patients with refractory acquired immunodeficiency syndrome-associated diarrhea. Gastroenterology 108:1753–1760, 1995

46. Simon D, Weiss L, Tanowitz H, Wittner J: Resolution of cryptosporidium infection in an AIDS patient after improvement of nutritional and immune status with octreotide. Am J Gastroenterol 86:615, 1991

47. Smith PD, Lane C, Vee J, et al: Intestinal infections in patients with the acquired immunodeficiency syndrome (AIDS). Ann Intern Med 108:328, 1988

48. Tavitian A, Raufman JP, Rosenthal LE, et al: Ketoconazole-resistant *Candida* esophagitis in patients with acquired immunodeficiency syndrome. Gastroenterology 90:443, 1986

49. Ullrich R, Zeitz M, Heise W, et al: Small intestinal

structure and function in patients infected with human immunodeficiency virus (HIV): Evidence for HIV-induced enteropathy. Ann Intern Med 111: 15, 1989

50. Wilcox CM: A pilot study of oral corticosteroid therapy for idiopathic esophageal ulcerations associated with human immunodeficiency virus infection. Am J Med 93(2):131, 1992

51. Wilcox CM, Forsmark CE, Darragh T, et al: High-protein ascites in patients with the acquired immunodeficiency syndrome. Gastroenterology 100:745, 1991

Chapter 14

Management of the Neurologic Complications of HIV-1 Infection and AIDS

RICHARD W. PRICE

Human immunodeficiency virus type 1 (HIV-1) infection, particularly its late phase, the acquired immunodeficiency syndrome (AIDS), is complicated by a variety of central nervous system (CNS) and peripheral nervous system (PNS) disorders (for general reviews, see references 28, 29, 107, and 193). Classification of these disorders according to their underlying pathophysiologic or pathogenetic process provides a rational framework for comprehending and managing the spectrum of conditions to which these patients are susceptible (Table 14–1) and also allows one to deal systematically with new or unusual conditions as they are encountered.

The most important pathogenetic determinant of susceptibility is the **stage of systemic HIV-1 infection** and particularly the resultant degree of immunosuppression. The underlying immune status exerts a predominating effect on disease vulnerability and therefore strongly influences the probabilities of differential diagnosis. For this reason, in the following discussion the neurologic aspects of HIV-1 infection are first segregated according to the phase of systemic infection in which they develop, and the conditions that occur in early HIV-1 infection are considered before the more common conditions that complicate the late, severely immunocompromised phase of infection.

Discussion of the complications of late HIV-1 infection uses the empirically derived approach of the neurologist and a classification based upon **neuroanatomic localization.** This is founded upon the predilection of different disease processes to afflict selected parts of the CNS and PNS, thereby providing a rational starting point for differential diagnosis.

NERVOUS SYSTEM INVOLVEMENT EARLY IN HIV-1 INFECTION

Based upon their frequency, major clinical attention has focused on the common neurologic sequelae of late HIV-1 infection, but the earlier phases of systemic HIV-1 infection can, although less commonly, also be accompanied by clinically important neurologic disorders. This includes both the phase of acute infection with seroconversion and the middle "asymptomatic" period of "clinical latency." Indeed, a number of observations suggest that the CNS is commonly exposed to HIV-1 early in systemic infection and perhaps throughout its course.

Early Neurologic Complications of Acute HIV-1 Infection

A variety of CNS disorders have been described in the period after initial HIV-1 infection (Chapter 6) with their frequency ranging from 8% for encephalopathies and neuropathies to as high as 45% for less specific manifestations such as headache.[26,36,37,40,56,72,87,91,150,169,203,217] They may occur from several days to weeks after the seroconversion-related illness that resembles mononucleosis or, less often, in the absence of overt systemic illness. These early neurologic complications usually evolve subacutely and may take the form of focal or diffuse encephalitis or leukoencephalopathy, meningitis, ataxia, or myelopathy, either alone or together with PNS abnormalities. The latter include cranial neuropathy, brachial plexopathy, or neuropathy. They are characteristically monophasic, and most patients appear to recover

TABLE 14–1. CLASSIFICATION OF THE NEUROLOGIC COMPLICATIONS OF HIV-1 INFECTION ACCORDING TO UNDERLYING PATHOPHYSIOLOGIC AND PATHOGENETIC CATEGORIES

Underlying Process	Examples
Opportunistic infections	Cerebral toxoplasmosis
	Cryptococcal meningitis
	Progressive multifocal leukoencephalopathy (PML)
	Cytomegalovirus (CMV) encephalitis, polyradiculopathy and mononeuritis multiplex
Opportunistic neoplasms	Primary central nervous system lymphoma
	Metastatic lymphoma
Metabolic, toxic, and other complications of systemic disease	Hypoxic encephalopathy
	Sepsis
	Stroke
Functional (psychiatric) disorders	Anxiety disorder
	Psychotic depression
Unique conditions (?) related to a primary effect of HIV-1 itself	AIDS dementia complex
	Distal sensory polyneuropathy (DSPN)
Autoimmune disorders	Guillain-Barré syndrome
	Chronic inflammatory demyelinating polyneuropathy (CIDP)

within a number of weeks, although cognitive deficits may persist in some patients with encephalitis. The cerebrospinal fluid (CSF) usually shows a minor lymphocyte-predominant pleocytosis with a modest rise in protein. Results of neuroimaging using computed tomography (CT) have been normal, but experience with magnetic resonance imaging (MRI) has not been reported. The electroencephalogram (EEG) may be focally or diffusely slow. Although these early syndromes apparently are uncommon, it is possible that their incidence is underappreciated.

Neurologic Complications During the "Asymptomatic" Phase of Systemic HIV-1 Infection

Most common among the neurologic complications manifesting during the "asymptomatic" or clinically latent phase of HIV-1 infection are demyelinating neuropathies. These resemble the subacute Guillain-Barré syndrome or chronic inflammatory demyelinating polyneuropathy (CIDP) seen in other contexts, with the exception that the CSF often exhibits uncharacteristic, albeit mild, pleocytosis.[42,44] The pathophysiology of HIV-1-related demyelinating neuropathies probably parallels that of demyelinating neuropathies in other settings and has an autoimmune basis. Indeed, these disorders provide evidence that HIV-1 infection is accompanied by disordered immune regulation and not simply declining host defenses;

during this middle phase of infection autoimmunity is more important than the opportunistic infections that dominate the late phase. Patients with these demyelinating neuropathies appear to respond favorably to corticosteroids, plasmapheresis, and intravenous immunoglobulin (IVIg), with the latter two treatments currently preferred. The prognosis of demyelinating neuropathies in this setting may not be as good as that in patients who are not infected with HIV-1.[43,196]

A rare but intriguing multiple sclerosis–like illness also has been reported in HIV-1–infected patients in the latent phase of infection.[18,82] The presentation is in the setting of preserved CD4+ T-lymphocyte counts and may include remissions and exacerbations, along with corticosteroid responsiveness. Although these cases may represent the concurrence of two diseases, more likely, as with the demyelinating neuropathies, they relate to an autoimmune process triggered by HIV-1 infection with clinical (and perhaps pathogenetic) features similar to those of multiple sclerosis.

Asymptomatic HIV-1 Infection of the CNS

Although clinically overt nervous system involvement may occur early in the course of HIV-1 infection, neurologically asymptomatic infection is more common. Studies of CSF in clinically well patients have shown: (1) abnormalities of routine studies, including cell count, total protein, and immunoglobulin; (2) local, intra–blood-brain barrier synthesis of anti–HIV-1 antibody; and (3) culture isolation of virus or detection of viral nucleic acid after polymerase chain reaction (PCR) amplification.[41,62,78,91,116,120,171,172] These abnormalities have been noted in fully functional, asymptomatic patients who have remained well during follow-up care for a year or more. Such incidental abnormal levels in cell count, protein, immunoglobulin, oligoclonal bands, and HIV-1 detection must be taken into account when interpreting CSF results obtained for other diagnostic purposes or in following therapy.

These CSF findings and the rare demonstration of HIV-1 in the brain following initial infection[54] imply that entry into the nervous system is an intrinsic part of the ecology of the virus in the human host. They also indicate that HIV-1 can be relatively nonpathogenic for the CNS, underscoring the critical question of what leads to the subsequent conversion of this asymptomatic state in some patients to either aseptic meningitis or parenchymal encephalitis.[163,166,167]

LATE NERVOUS SYSTEM INVOLVEMENT BY HIV-1

In the late stages of HIV-1 infection, when immune defenses have been severely compromised and systemic complications begin to accumulate, the nervous system becomes highly susceptible to a wide array of disorders. These may involve all levels of the neuraxis, including meninges, brain, spinal cord, peripheral nerve, and muscle.

Meningitis and Headache

Several disorders involving the leptomeninges may afflict patients with advanced HIV-1 disease (Table 14–2), with symptomatology rang-

TABLE 14–2. MENINGITIDES COMPLICATING HIV-1 INFECTION

Common
Asymptomatic meningeal reaction
Cryptococcal meningitis
Aseptic (? HIV-1) meningitis
Uncommon
Tuberculous meningitis (*Mycobacterium tuberculosis*)
Syphilitic meningitis
Histoplasmosis
Coccidioidomycosis
Lymphomatous meningitis (metastatic)
Listeria monocytogenes

ing from frontal mild headache to severe disability with hydrocephalus and cranial nerve palsies. Additionally, a number of conditions can mimic meningitis or cause headache.[76,109] For example, parenchymal brain diseases, such as toxoplasmosis (Chapter 24) and primary CNS lymphoma (Chapter 28), may initially manifest with headache as an important symptom without clear focal brain dysfunction.

Headache also may occur without accompanying meningeal reaction. In some patients, this occurs as a complication of systemic illness. For example, patients with *Pneumocystis carinii* pneumonia (PCP) may have headache as an earlier and more prominent symptom than shortness of breath or cough. The headache may then resolve with treatment of the PCP. In other patients, however, a precipitating opportunistic infection is not identified, and the term *HIV headache* has been used to describe this condition, which may be severe and protracted.[31] It is speculated that circulating vasoactive cytokines may be involved in the pathogenesis of this headache. Although some of these patients seem to be helped by tricyclic antidepressants, others are not and may even require narcotic analgesics.

Among the true meningitides, a syndrome of aseptic meningitis, presumably related to direct HIV-1 infection of the meninges, can occur acutely in the setting of seroconversion as described previously, but is more common in patients with advanced HIV-1 infection.[94,95] Clinically, this may segregate into two types: an acute form and a chronic form. Both occur in late HIV-1 infection, usually in the transitional phase (CD4+ T-lymphocyte count 200 to 500/mm^3) or, somewhat less frequently, in the phase of overt AIDS (CD4+ cell count <200/mm^3). Both are accompanied by meningeal symptoms (e.g., headache and photophobia), although meningeal signs (e.g., nuchal rigidity) are more characteristic of the acute group. Cranial nerve palsies can complicate the course, affecting cranial nerves V, VII, and VIII, with Bell's palsy sometimes recurring. The CSF shows mild mononuclear pleocytosis, usually with normal or mildly depressed glucose and slightly elevated protein levels. The presumption that this condition is due to direct HIV-1 infection of the meninges relates to two observations: the virus can be isolated from the CSF of some, and no other cause has been identified. However, whether HIV-1 infection is the sole or even major cause of the disorder can be questioned, since other causes of aseptic meningitis might be expected to provoke an influx of HIV-1–infected lymphocytes and monocytes into the CSF, thereby increasing the likelihood of viral isolation. Additionally, because of the high prevalence of mild abnormalities in the CSF of HIV-1–infected individuals described earlier, the definition of aseptic meningitis becomes ambiguous in some patients. Difficulties arise when one tries to distinguish HIV-1–related aspetic meningitis from the HIV headache discussed previously. Although the degree of pleocytosis might be used as a guide, presuming that the cellular reaction is involved in the genesis of symptoms, how is the cell count of 5 to 20/mm³ in the fluid of a patient with headache interpreted? Further study is needed to clarify this issue. The syndrome itself is benign but may imply a poor prognosis in relation to impending progression to AIDS in some patients. There have been no reports on the effects of antiretroviral therapy on this disorder.

The most important meningeal infection in AIDS patients is caused by *Cryptococcus neoformans*, also the most common CNS fungal infection in these patients[2,58,143,159,181,201] (Chapter 23). This infection may present as subacute meningitis or meningoencephalitis with headache, nausea, vomiting, and confusion, just as in non-AIDS patients. However, in many AIDS patients, symptoms are remarkably mild, and the CSF formula may, likewise, contain few or no cells and little or no perturbation in glucose or protein levels. Hence, it is imperative that in such patients cryptococcal antigen is assessed and fungal cultures obtained. An India ink study of the CSF may be helpful to visualize the organism's capsule, especially if the CSF cryptococcal antigen is not immediately available. Of note, the serum cryptococcal antigen is almost always positive, thereby serving as a screen in patients in whom the diagnostic suspicion is low or in whom a lumbar puncture is contraindicated. Therapeutic management of cryptococcal meningitis is considered in Chapter 23.

Meningitis appears to be an uncommon complication of tuberculosis in HIV-1–infected patients, and it is not yet certain whether in these patients there is a difference in clinical presentation and response to therapy compared to other settings in which subacute or chronic meningitis manifests with neck stiffness, cranial nerve palsies, hydrocephalus, and vascular occlusions.[14,59] Differentiation from cryptococcal meningitis is aided by the tendency of tuberculous meningitis: (1) to occur with higher CD4+

lymphocyte counts and in patients from lower socioeconomic circumstances; (2) to induce a partial polymorphonuclear cell response in the CSF; and (3) to be accompanied by evidence of systemic infection. Other diagnostic and treatment aspects of *Mycobacterium tuberculosis* are discussed in Chapter 22.

Meningeal involvement by syphilis in HIV-1–infected individuals may take the form of acute meningitis or meningovascular syphilis. However, there is some evidence suggesting that HIV-1 infection may alter the natural course of neurosyphilis and that meningovascular syphilis may occur both more commonly and earlier in those with HIV-1 infection.[15,21,53,102,104,114] The full extent to which underlying HIV-1 infection alters the presentation, clinical course, or response to therapy of CNS syphilis is unsettled.[77,192] The previously discussed CSF abnormalities common in asymptomatic seropositive patients, including elevated protein and cell counts, render interpretation of such findings in patients with positive syphilis serologies or those undergoing treatment more difficult. Most clinicians now favor more aggressive treatment of new or previously untreated syphilis seropositivity. These issues are discussed in more detail in Chapter 27.

Systemic lymphoma complicating HIV-1 infection may spread secondarily to the CNS, usually involving the meninges.[19,23,63,64,68] Clinical manifestations may be cryptic but often include cranial nerve palsies, headaches, or increased intracranial pressure (ICP).

Other causes of meningitis are uncommon in AIDS patients. Pyogenic meningitis is usually a complication of systemic sepsis, often related to iatrogenic manipulations including indwelling venous catheters, systemic antibiotics, and other predisposing factors. *Listeria monocytogenes* meningitis has been identified but seems to be rare. In these cases, as in the more common causes of meningitis discussed earlier, specific therapy should be combined with management of secondary sequelae such as elevated intracranial pressure due to CSF outflow obstruction. This often can be remedied with repeated lumbar punctures, but in some patients may also require ventricular shunt placement.

Diffuse Brain Disease and Dementia

Affliction of the brain parenchyma in AIDS can be usefully divided into conditions that

TABLE 14–3. DIFFUSE BRAIN DISEASE COMPLICATING HIV-1 INFECTION

With Concomitant Depression of Alertness
Metabolic/toxic encephalopathies (alone or as an exacerbating influence on AIDS dementia complex)
Toxoplasmosis—"encephalitic" form
Cytomegalovirus encephalitis
Secondary to fungal, bacterial, or mycobacterial meningitis (as in Table 14–2)
Herpes simplex encephalitis
With Preservation of Alertness
AIDS dementia complex

cause predominantly focal symptoms and those accompanied by more diffuse dysfunction (Table 14–3). Although there is some overlap in these disorders (e.g., cerebral toxoplasmosis may have both an "encephalitic" and a more common focal picture), this division is generally valuable as the first step in differential diagnosis. The nonfocal disorders can, in turn, be subdivided into: (1) those with parallel impairment of both alertness and cognition and (2) a disorder, the AIDS dementia complex, in which alertness is characteristically spared, but cognition, motor function, and behavior are impaired.

Diffuse Encephalopathies

The various meningitides discussed earlier may cause diffuse brain dysfunction. Additionally, the metabolic or toxic encephalopathies developing as sequelae to the systemic nonneurologic diseases suffered by AIDS patients, such as pneumonias with hypoxia and systemic sepsis, may cause generalized encephalopathy. Clinicians should be alert to the development of Wernicke's encephalopathy, which may complicate AIDS, usually in the setting of severe systemic disease.[22,35] CNS-active drugs, including sedatives and narcotic analgesics, may cloud mentation or alertness just as in non-AIDS patients; these effects can occur alone but also may manifest as an exacerbating or unmasking influence on the AIDS dementia complex, resulting in a mixture of the two conditions and exaggerating medication effects. HIV-1–infected patients may be more sensitive to neuroleptics and thereby manifest parkinsonism or other movement disorders at seemingly lower doses.[93]

Certain brain infections also can produce diffuse brain dysfunction. CNS toxoplasmosis, which usually causes focal neurologic symptoms and signs, may present as a generalized encephalopathy with clouding of consciousness and diffuse cerebral dysfunction.[83,137] This may be a particularly fulminating illness and relates to the presence of abundant toxoplasmic microabscesses, which may be poorly imaged by CT or MRI scan. Similarly, CNS lymphoma can infiltrate deep structures and impair cognition, alertness, and motor function without prominent focal symptoms or signs.

The overall clinical importance of cytomegalovirus (CMV) encephalitis remains imprecisely defined. Systemic CMV infection is very common in AIDS patients, and the brain is frequently infected. Thus, evidence of mild brain infection is a frequent finding at autopsy. In perhaps one quarter of patients dying of AIDS, CMV infection is marked by scattered microglial nodules with occasional characteristic intranuclear inclusion bodies noted by routine histologic examination or by CMV antigens and nucleic acid when immunocytochemical or in situ hybridization techniques are used. However, clinicopathologic correlation suggests that this type of CMV infection plays, at most, only a minor role in causing overt CNS symptoms.[133,135,145,209,216] However, it is also clear that a small number of patients can manifest more severe CMV encephalitis, with subacute clouding of consciousness, confusion, or seizures.[20,92,103] The clinical diagnosis in such patients is often difficult. The suspicion is raised by the subacute development of diffuse encephalopathy affecting both cognition and alertness; hyponatremia is common in these patients and should help to alert clinicians to CMV diagnosis as well. More directly, the presence of ventricular ependymitis, with local signal alteration or contrast enhancement detected by CT or MRI, can aid diagnosis.[92,158] While CSF culture results are usually negative in this setting, PCR may identify the presence of CMV nucleic acid. This will likely evolve to become the most practical approach to rapid diagnosis, although further experience is needed to clarify its specificity and sensitivity.[39,79,210,218] The efficacy of ganciclovir and foscarnet in treating CMV encephalitis remains to be defined, but until shown otherwise, such antiviral therapy probably should be instituted rapidly in this setting (see more detailed discussion of therapy in Chapter 26).

Encephalitis related to herpes simplex virus types 1 (HSV-1) and 2 (HSV-2) also occurs in AIDS patients and may present as a subacute nonfocal or focal encephalopathy, although neither the frequency nor the core of the clinical presentation is clearly defined.[107,173]

AIDS Dementia Complex

The AIDS dementia complex is characterized by a triad of cognitive, motor, and behavioral dysfunction.[135,136,139,164,165,167,168] It is perhaps the most common CNS complication of HIV-1 infection and, if its mild form is included, may eventually afflict the majority of AIDS patients. It is generally a late complication of HIV-1 infection and characteristically manifests during the same phase as the major opportunistic infections and neoplasms that define systemic AIDS, although patients can present with this syndrome before these major systemic complications.[138] However, results of larger cohort studies indicate that this syndrome is uncommon in patients who are systematically well.[6,121,126,139,186,187] It was the impression of our group that, prior to the widespread use of zidovudine, the majority of patients with very low CD4+ T-lymphocyte counts either exhibited frank mild to severe AIDS dementia complex or subclinical brain dysfunction. Early and widespread use of zidovudine and perhaps other antiretrovirals appears to have reduced the prevalence of the AIDS dementia complex.[153,154]

TERMINOLOGY AND CLASSIFICATION. The term *AIDS dementia complex* was introduced to describe a cohesive constellation of symptoms and signs rather than an established disease entity of uniform etiopathogenesis.[136,162,164–166,168] Each of the three component terms was included for a defined reason. *AIDS* was included because the morbidity and prognosis of the condition can be comparable to those of other clinical AIDS-defining complications of HIV-1 infection. *Dementia* was included because of the acquired and persistent cognitive decline, marked by prominent mental slowing and inattention. The dementia is characteristically unaccompanied by alterations in the level of alertness. The third component, *complex,* was added because the syndrome also, importantly, includes impaired motor performance and, at times, characteristic behavioral changes. Myelopathy and organic psychosis are encompassed within this term, but neither neuropathy nor functional psychiatric disturbance is included.

We have used a five-part staging system for describing the severity of the AIDS dementia complex based on functional and motor status for adult patients.[165,191] It provides a common descriptive vocabulary for both clinical and investigative purposes. Although the World Health Organization (WHO) and the American Academy of Neurology (AAN) have introduced additional terminologies with certain useful features, including segregation of predominating myelopathy and predominating dementia and requiring greater severity when using the term dementia,[3,220] we have continued to use the AIDS dementia complex staging scheme in our own studies and clinical practice because of its simplicity and parsimony.

The AIDS dementia complex staging and the WHO/AAN classification can be cross-translated as outlined in Table 14–4. The WHO/AAN classification introduced the term *HIV-1–associated cognitive/motor complex* to encompass the full constellation of the AIDS dementia complex and added subcategories to refer to patients with predominantly cognitive (HIV-associated dementia) or myelopathic (HIV-1–associated myelopathy) presentations of sufficient severity to interfere with work or activities of daily living (ADL) (hence severe enough to qualify as stage 2 or greater in AIDS dementia complex staging). The term *HIV-associated minor cognitive/motor disorder* was introduced to designate patients with mild symptoms and signs and only minimal functional impairment of work or ADL (stage 1 AIDS dementia complex).

CLINICAL PRESENTATION. The clinical features of the AIDS dementia complex are summarized briefly in Table 14–5. Patients' earliest symptoms usually consist of difficulties with concentration and memory. They begin to lose track of their train of thought or conversation. Many complain of "slowness" in thinking. Complex tasks become more difficult and take longer to complete, and memory impairment or difficulty in concentration lead to missed appointments and the need to keep lists of daily chores.

Despite these complaints, early in the evolution of the illness the relatively insensitive bedside mental status examination may be within normal limits; responses may be correct although they are characteristically slowed. As the condition progresses, however, patients begin to perform poorly on tasks requiring concentration and attention, such as word and digit reversals and subtracting serial 7s. With further worsening a larger array of mental status tests becomes abnormal. Nonetheless, the core difficulty of slowing, poor attention and concentration, remains most prominent. Afflicted individuals also may appear apathetic, with poor insight and indifference to their illness.

Symptoms of motor dysfunction usually lag behind those of intellectual impairment. When

TABLE 14–4. COMPARISON OF AIDS DEMENTIA COMPLEX AND WORLD HEALTH ORGANIZATION/AMERICAN ACADEMY OF NEUROLOGY (WHO)/(AAN) CLASSIFICATIONS

AIDS Dementia Complex Staging	WHO/AAN Classification: HIV-Associated Cognitive-Motor Complex
Stage 0: Normal	
Stage 0.5: Subclinical or Equivocal	No corresponding classification
Minimal or equivocal symptoms	
Mild (soft) neurologic signs	
No impairment of work or activities of daily living (ADL)	
Stage 1: Mild	HIV-1–Associated Minor Cognitive-Motor Disorder
Unequivocal intellectual or motor impairment	Symptoms: two of five types in cognitive, motor, behavioral spheres
	Examination: neurologic or neuropsychologic abnormalities
Able to do all but the more demanding work or ADL	
	Mild impairment of work or ADL
	HIV-Associated Dementia and HIV-Associated Myelopathy
Stage 2: Moderate	*Mild*
Cannot work or perform demanding ADL	Impaired work and ADL
Capable of self-care	Capable of basic self-care
Ambulatory but may need a single prop	Ambulatory but may need a single prop
Stage 3: Severe	*Moderate*
Major intellectual disability	Unable to work or function unassisted
or	*or*
Cannot walk unassisted	Cannot walk unassisted
Stage 4: End Stage	*Severe*
Nearly vegetative	Unable to perform ADL unassisted
Rudimentary cognition	Confined to bed or wheelchair
Para- or quadriplegic	

present, complaints most often include poor balance or incoordination. Gait incoordination can result in more frequent tripping and falling or a perceived need to exercise new care in walking. Similarly, patients may drop things more frequently or become slower and less precise with normal hand activities, such as eating or writing. However, even when such symptoms are lacking, motor abnormalities can almost al-

TABLE 14–5. MAJOR CLINICAL MANIFESTATIONS OF THE AIDS DEMENTIA COMPLEX, A SUBCORTICAL DEMENTIA AFFECTING COGNITION, MOTOR PERFORMANCE, AND BEHAVIOR

Early	Late
Cognition	
Inattention	Global dementia
Reduced concentration	
Forgetfulness	
Motor Performance	
Slowed movements	Paraplegia
Clumsiness	
Ataxia	
Behavior	
Apathy	Mutism
Altered personality	
(Agitation)	

ways be detected on examination early in the course of the disease. These include slowing of rapid successive and alternating movements of the extremities (e.g., attempts at rapid opposition of index finger and thumb or foot tapping) and impaired ocular smooth pursuits and saccadic eye movements. Abnormal reflexes also may be present, with generalized hyperreflexia and the development of release signs, such as snout, glabellar, and, less commonly, grasp responses. As the disease evolves, spastic ataxia and, subsequently, leg weakness may limit walking. Patients with an early or predominating spastic-ataxic gait usually have vacuolar myelopathy pathologically. Bladder and bowel incontinence may develop in the later stages of the condition but are uncommon early. At the end stage of the AIDS dementia complex patients are nearly vegetative, lying in bed with a vacant stare, seemingly unaware of their surroundings, unable to ambulate, and incontinent. However, unless intercurrent illness develops, the level of arousal is usually preserved so that they appear awake.

Psychologic depression is surprisingly infrequent in these patients, despite the prominence of psychomotor slowing. Patients appear uninterested and lack initiative but are without dys-

TABLE 14–6. SOME COMPARATIVE FEATURES

	Clinical Features		
	Temporal Profile	Level of Alertness	Fever
Cerebral toxoplasmosis	Days	Reduced	Common
Primary CNS lymphoma	Days to weeks	Variable	Absent
Progressive multifocal leukoencephalopathy (PML)	Weeks	Preserved	Absent
AIDS dementia complex	Weeks to months	Preserved	Absent
CMV encephalitis	Days to weeks	Reduced	Common
Cryptococcal meningitis	Days	Variable	Common

phoria. In a minority, a more agitated organic psychosis may be the presenting or predominant aspect of the illness.[88] Such patients are irritable and hyperactive and may be overtly manic; however, there is always an element of confusion and when their hyperactive state comes under control, the underlying cognitive impairment is evident.

In children, the disorder has the same general features, although the course may vary somewhat and occur in either a progressive or static form.[11,12,66,129] The progressive form is characterized by the gradual loss of previously acquired motor skills in conjunction with the evolution of motor abnormalities ranging from spastic paraparesis to quadriplegia with pseudobulbar palsy and rigidity. Acquired microcephaly is almost universal.

NEUROPSYCHOLOGICAL TEST PROFILE. Formal neuropsychologic studies quantitatively support the clinical findings of the AIDS dementia complex and are, at times, helpful in confirming both the presence and characteristic profile of its cognitive impairment. They are perhaps most useful in longitudinally following the course of disease or response to therapy. In general, the neuropsychologic tests most sensitive to AIDS dementia complex include some or all of the following characteristics: performance under time pressure, motor speed, and alternation between two performance rules or stimulus sets.[126,186,189,191,205]

NEUROIMAGING STUDIES. Neuroimaging procedures and CSF examination usually are essential to the evaluation of AIDS patients with CNS dysfunction, including those with the AIDS dementia complex. Imaging may be needed to exclude other neurologic conditions that can present with overlapping symptoms and signs, and also often shows characteristic, although perhaps unspecific, abnormalities (Table 14–6). These include the nearly universal finding of cerebral atrophy with widened cortical sulci and enlarged ventricles found on either CT scanning or MRI.[47,73,136,148,156,157] Basal ganglia are also reduced in volume.[5] Additionally, some patients have patchy or diffuse T2-weighted abnormalities on MRI in the hemispheric white matter and, less commonly, the basal ganglia or thalamus.[100,101,131,156,160] Children with AIDS-related dementia often have basal ganglion calcification and atrophy.[13]

CSF. Examination of the CSF in patients with AIDS dementia complex reveals abnormalities in both routine and more specialized tests. However, routine analysis is confounded by the CSF abnormalities described earlier in patients with asymptomatic HIV-1 infection, including HIV-1 isolation or detection of amplified nucleic acid. The likelihood of detecting HIV-1 p24 core antigen in the CSF increases with AIDS dementia complex severity, although free antigen is still a relatively infrequent finding and thus of lower sensitivity diagnostically.[32,155] Whether quantitative studies of the CSF viral burden using quantitative PCR amplification will prove useful in the diagnosis and longitudinal evaluation of patients awaits assessment of this newer technology on this fluid. More useful as surrogate markers in the CSF at this time are indicators of immune activation, including β_2-microglobulin and neopterin, whose concentrations correlate with the presence and severity of the AIDS dementia complex.[24,25,30,85] Although nonspecific in that they are elevated in other CNS opportunistic infections and primary CNS lymphoma, these markers may be useful in efforts to distinguish mild AIDS dementia complex from psychiatric disease as well as in following responses to therapy.

NEUROPATHOLOGY. Histologic abnormalities in demented AIDS patients are most prominent in the subcortical structures and the find-

OF MAJOR CNS PROCESSES IN AIDS

	Neuroimaging Features	
No. of Lesions	Type of Lesions	Location of Lesions
Multiple	Mass effect; spherical ring enhancing	Basal ganglia, cortex
One or few	Mass effect; irregular; weakly enhancing	Often periventricular with subependymal spread, white matter
Multiple	No mass effect; nonenhancing; white on T2, black on T1 MRI	White matter, usually subcortical involving U-fibers
None, diffuse, or multiple	Cerebral atrophy; fluffy or diffuse T2 signal, no mass effect or enhancement	Central white matter (sparing U-fibers), basal ganglia
Few	Small, T2 signal, enhancement	Ependymal, small cortical
Variable	Dilated perivascular spaces	Basal ganglia

ings on routine examination can be segregated into three seemingly discontinuous but frequently overlapping sets: (1) gliosis and diffuse white matter pallor, (2) multinucleated-cell encephalitis, and (3) vacuolar myelopathy. A less common additional finding is diffuse or focal spongiform change of the cerebral white matter.[34,84,135,145,175] The most common of these abnormalities is the central astrocytosis and accompanying diffuse white matter pallor that, in isolation, correlate with milder AIDS dementia complex. Inflammation is characteristically scant, consisting of a few perivascular lymphocytes and brown-pigmented macrophages accompanying the astrocytosis. This is accompanied by disruption of the blood-brain barrier.[160]

Multinucleated cells characteristically are found in patients with more severe clinical disease.[27,135] The multinucleated cells derive from macrophages and microglia and are accompanied by neighboring macrophage and microglial reaction, along with local edema and white matter rarefaction. They are concentrated most often in the white matter and deep gray structures. It is in these severe cases that neuronal changes have been detected, including both loss of selected cortical neurons and alterations in neuronal dendritic structures.[117,118]

Although inflammation with multinucleated cells also may occur in the spinal cord, vacuolar myelopathy is more common.[146] The latter pathologically resembles subacute combined degeneration resulting from vitamin B_{12} deficiency, but levels of this vitamin generally are normal in serum. Although there is a general correlation between the incidence of vacuolar myelopathy and the other pathologic abnormalities found in the brain, the myelopathy can occur in the absence of the multinucleated cells and, indeed, does not correlate with local productive HIV-1 infection.[46,147,177,202]

ETIOLOGY AND PATHOGENESIS. Evidence from a growing number of studies supports a primary role for HIV-1 in the AIDS dementia complex, at least in the subset of patients with more severe dysfunction.[27,162,163,166,167] There is also a growing consensus that macrophages and microglia, along with multinucleated cells derived from these two cell types, are the principal participants in *productive* infection. Recent observations using combined PCR amplification in concert with in situ localization and other techniques to detect expression of nonstructural viral gene products suggest that other cell types in the brain, including the native astrocytes and neurons as well as vascular endothelial cells, may be infected, although perhaps without the capacity to produce progeny virus.[141,183,204] This is consistent with some cell culture studies that have demonstrated low-level infection of astrocytic and other neuroectodermal cells and cell lines, involving a non-CD4 virus–cell interaction.

Having said that HIV-1 can be found in the brains of demented individuals, it should be emphasized that this is not an invariant finding, and there are various opinions regarding the correlation of this viral load with the stage of the AIDS dementia complex.[27,75,215] Characteristically, it is only in the more severely affected patients (stages 2 and greater) that multinucleated-cell encephalitis or severe productive HIV-1 infection is commonly found. Of note, the viral "strains" cultured or cloned from brains of these patients exhibit a macrophage-tropic phenotype and may even have genetic characteristics that favor replication in *brain* macrophages and microglia.[142,161,188,214] As a consequence of the discrepancy between clinical deficits, on the one hand, and these pathologic and virologic features, on the other, indirect pathogenetic processes relating infection and brain injury have been proposed (for reviews, see references 65, 111, 163, 166, 167 and 207). These processes may involve virus-coded toxins (e.g., gp120) or cell-coded toxins, particularly cytokines.

TREATMENT. Several studies have indicated that the AIDS dementia complex and its pediatric counterpart respond to zidovudine therapy.[33,151,185,190,222] However, optimum dosing has not been established, since the doses used in a placebo-controlled trial were higher than those currently recommended for systemic disease.[190] Moreover, there are currently no clear guidelines regarding the efficacy of other antiretroviral drugs (including the other nucleosides, nonnucleoside reverse transcriptase inhibitors, or protease inhibitors) in this condition, although one hopes that such information might soon be forthcoming. The possible role of toxins in the genesis of AIDS dementia complex has given rise to proposals to attempt to block the effects of these putative intermediaries (for review, see reference 164). For example, the calcium channel blocker nimodipine and the N-methyl-D-aspartate receptor inhibitor memantine, both of which appear to block the neurotoxicity of HIV-1 gp120 in cell culture, have been the focus of early-phase clinical trials.[110–112]

FOCAL BRAIN DISEASES

A number of focal brain disorders can afflict AIDS patients (Table 14–7). Evaluation of these conditions begins with the recognition of their focal nature along with associated background

TABLE 14–7. FOCAL BRAIN DISEASE COMPLICATION HIV-1 DISEASE

Acute
Vascular disorders
Seizures*
Subacute
Cerebral toxoplasmosis
Primary central nervous system lymphoma (PCNSL)
Progressive multifocal leukoencephalopathy (PML)
Tuberculous brain abscess (*Mycobacterium tuberculosis*)
Cryptococcoma
Varicella-zoster virus encephalitis
Herpes encephalitis

* Secondary to subacute focal (macroscopic) disorders or to nonfocal (microscopic or toxic-metabolic) processes.

systemic symptoms and signs (e.g., fever, headache). Initial evaluation often focuses on distinguishing the three most common causes of focal brain disease: cerebral toxoplasmosis, primary CNS lymphoma (PCNSL), and progressive multifocal leukoencephalopathy (PML). Investigations include neuroradiologic characterization and often a strategy involving therapeutic trial, followed in some by brain biopsy.

The temporal profile of the onset and evolution of these focal brain disorders is an important aspect of their clinical presentation. An abrupt onset suggests either a vascular cause or seizure. AIDS patients may suffer transient ischemia or even stroke, leaving residual brain injury.[63,134,149] Fortunately, most have a benign outcome. Seizures may be related to HIV-1 infection (AIDS dementia complex) or may result from focal opportunistic infections and neoplasms. Careful clinical and neuroimaging investigations are warranted to evaluate for focal diseases.[8,96,198,208,219]

The most common focal disorders all characteristically have a subacute onset and evolve over days or, at times, weeks. Of these, cerebral toxoplasmosis characteristically progresses most rapidly (days) and PML most slowly (weeks), whereas primary CNS lymphoma lies somewhere in between. A comparison of some of the major clinical and neuroradiologic features of the common CNS complications of AIDS is outlined in Table 14–6. There are group differences in the associated findings that distinguish the three major focal disorders, although each may cause similar neurologic deficits with individual cases being clinically overlapping. Thus, patients with toxoplasmosis commonly present with a combination of focal deficits and a generalized encephalopathy that includes confusion or clouding of consciousness[113,137] (Chapter 24). This contrasts with patients suffering from PML, at least at the onset, in which focal neurologic deficits are unaccompanied by either diffuse brain dysfunction or evidence of a systemic toxic state. The CNS lymphomas, when accompanied by significant mass effect or when located deep in the frontal or periventricular region, can cause more global mental dysfunction. Cryptococcoma is usually a complication of cryptococcal meningitis, but when it occurs alone, cryptococcal antigen testing may occasionally be negative in the CSF, making diagnosis difficult.[2,105]

In approaching patients with focal disease, neuroimaging, particularly MRI, is critical both to confirm the presence of macroscopic focal disease and to determine the morphology and character of the "lesion." Multiple lesions, involving the cortex or deep brain nuclei (thalamus, basal ganglia) with mass effect and surrounded by edema, strongly favor a diagnosis of cerebral toxoplasmosis. In most cases, toxoplasmic abscesses exhibit ringlike contrast enhancement on CT or MRI scans, but rarely, either homogeneously enhancing or nonenhancing, hypodense lesions may be noted. In general, MRI is the preferred modality for more clearly detecting and defining the multiple spherical lesions characteristic of the disease. Only very rarely are the CT or, more particularly, the MRI scans normal.[67,137]

Primary CNS lymphomas of B-cell origin are opportunistic neoplasms that complicate the course of AIDS in approximately 5% of patients[6,10,55,68,106,123,170,197] (see Chapter 28). When symptomatic, patients with primary brain lymphomas present with progressive focal or multifocal neurologic deficits similar to those with toxoplasmosis, although the tempo of disease evolution is often slower. Neuroradiologic studies are usually sensitive in detecting primary brain lymphomas, but do not establish a definitive diagnosis. Characteristically, these tumors are multicentric but often show only one or two lesions on CT or MRI. Their location is usually deep in the brain in proximity to the lateral ventricles, where they may spread under the ependymal lining; they occur most often in the white rather than gray matter. On CT they may enhance after contrast administration, but very often such enhancement is either weak or absent; again, MRI scanning is more sensitive. However, final diagnosis relies on brain biopsy. Recently, thallium single-photon-emission computed tomography (SPECT) imaging has been applied to help distinguish cerebral toxoplasmosis from primary CNS lymphoma, with the former characterized by decreased uptake of the radionuclide and the latter by increased uptake.[179]

Toxoplasma serology is of diagnostic help when attempting to distinguish among causes of focal brain lesions with mass effect. Because the disease typically is due to reactivation of the organism, patients with cerebral toxoplasmosis rarely have negative serum IgG antibody titers.[80,113,137] However, these titers may be low (occasionally, an apparently negative titer will be positive when a more concentrated specimen such as a 1:4 dilution is tested) and frequently do not rise during the course of the illness. Thus, a positive titer indicates suscepti-

bility, and a negative titer casts doubt on the diagnosis and pushes the clinician for an earlier biopsy. Because of its frequency (5% to 15% of AIDS patients) and gratifying response to therapy, initial diagnosis of patients with focal brain disease is targeted to cerebral toxoplasmosis. In treating patients with cerebral toxoplasmosis and indeed all AIDS patients, the use of **corticosteroids should be avoided when possible.** This is particularly important when considering a therapeutic trial to differentiate between toxoplasmosis and CNS lymphoma. Since the latter may respond symptomatically to corticosteroids alone, clinical or CT improvement on a combination antibiotic-steroid treatment is difficult to interpret. More generally, corticosteroids intensify the impairment of immune defenses in AIDS patients, potentially worsening not only toxoplasmosis but also other systemic opportunistic infections. However, if cerebral edema threatens brain herniation, judicious short-term corticosteroid therapy may be instituted along with appropriate specific therapy and subsequently tapered rapidly once the patient improves.

PML is an opportunistic infection caused by a human papovavirus, JC virus.[16,98,174,184] It develops in approximately 4% of AIDS patients, and in some, it will be their presenting illness. The disease is characterized by selective white matter destruction. Clinical evolution usually is more protracted than that of either toxoplasmosis or CNS lymphoma, and altered consciousness related to brain swelling is not a feature. Definitive diagnosis is made by brain biopsy or autopsy, although suspicion is aroused by the clinical history and an examination suggesting more than one cerebral focus, along with a CT scan or MRI demonstrating white matter lesions without mass effect and usually without contrast enhancement (Table 14–6). Application of PCR to CSF may be helpful, but studies thus far have shown some limitations with respect to both sensitivity and specificity.[122,211,212] There is no proven effective therapy for the disease, although anecdotal experience has raised the question of whether cytosine arabinoside might be helpful in some patients.[152] It is notable that spontaneous remission of PML in AIDS patients has been clearly documented.[17]

Although unusual, varicella-zoster virus (VZV) and, to a lesser extent, HSV-1 and HSV-2 have been reported as causes of CNS disease in AIDS patients. VZV infections are of at least three types, and sometimes admixed[81]: (1) multifocal direct brain infection affecting principally the white matter and partially mimicking PML[97,132,180]; (2) cerebral vasculitis, which characteristically follows ophthalmic herpes zoster and causes contralateral hemiplegia, but may occur after zoster in other locations and be more widespread in the brain[60,90]; and (3) myelopathy complicating herpes zoster with both vasculitic and parenchymal elements.[57] These may occur temporally remote from or in the absence of herpes zoster. As noted earlier, both HSV-1 and HSV-2 have been identified in brains of some AIDS patients,[107,173] but the clinical correlates of these infections in AIDS patients have not been wholly delineated.

MYELOPATHIES

Myelopathies complicating HIV-1–infected individuals can be classified into segmental and diffuse forms (Table 14–8). The segmental forms tend to follow an acute or subacute time course and are relatively rare. VZV, toxoplasmosis, and spinal epidural or intradural lymphoma may all give a clinical picture of partial or complete transverse myelitis.[57,89,124] In addition, CMV polyradiculopathy may also involve the spinal cord in a segmental manner, typically evolving over a number of weeks.[127,200] Combined CMV and HSV infection of the spinal cord has been described, although antemortem recognition may be exceptionally difficult.[206]

The more slowly progressive **vacuolar myelopathy** is far more common.[46,146,202] Usually, it is accompanied by varying degrees of cognitive and upper extremity affliction. Therefore, it has been included under the umbrella of the clinical term, AIDS dementia complex, discussed previously. In some patients, however, it occurs in relative isolation or with a marked preponderance. These patients exhibit progressive, painless gait disturbance with ataxia and

TABLE 14–8. MYELOPATHIES COMPLICATING HIV-1 INFECTION

Segmental (Focal), Acute or Subacute
Transverse Myelitis
  Varicella-zoster virus (herpes zoster) myelopathy
  Spinal epidural or intradural lymphoma
  Toxoplasmosis
With Polyradiculopathy
  CMV
Subacute or Chronic, Progressive, and Diffuse Form
Vacuolar myelopathy
HTLV-I–associated myelopathies

spasticity. Bladder and bowel difficulty usually becomes significant only after considerable gait symptoms appear, and sensory disturbance is less conspicuous unless there is concomitant neuropathy. Patients do not usually manifest a distinct sensory or motor level as in patients with transverse myelopathy. Even in those patients with seemingly isolated lower extremity symptoms, examination usually reveals some evidence of disturbance higher in the neuraxis, including, most often, slowed rapid alternating finger movements and hyperactive deep tendon reflexes, including the jaw jerk. In typical cases, we do not recommend performance of either spinal MRI or myelography, since both are usually negative in vacuolar myelopathy. These studies are needed only if there is question of another type of myelopathy, usually one with segmental features.

An additional cause of myelopathy in HIV-1–infected patients relates to coinfection with a second type of retrovirus, human T-cell lymphotropic virus type I (HTLV-I).[1,176] This relates principally to the convergent epidemiologies of these infections related to intravenous injection and heterosexual transmission rather than to increased disease susceptibility resulting from immunosuppression and, as a result, is likely to occur principally in intravenous drug users and their sexual contacts. Clinically, the disorder is very similar to vacuolar myelopathy but can be distinguished pathologically. Clinical diagnosis is suspected when positive HTLV-I serology is present. Specific diagnosis may be important, since HTLV-I–associated myelopathy (HAM), at least in the non-AIDS patient, may respond to immunosuppressive therapies, including plasmapheresis.[119]

PERIPHERAL NEUROPATHIES

Peripheral neuropathies of several types can complicate the various stages of HIV-1 infection (Table 14–9) (for reviews, see references 42, 71, 86, and 196). Those occurring in the acute and latent phases of infection have been discussed previously. Neuropathies during the transitional phase include herpes zoster and one of two types of mononeuritis multiplex that can develop as complications of HIV-1. Both of the latter are unusual, but are important to recognize.[182,199] The type that occurs in the transitional setting (usually with CD4+ counts of 200 to 500 cells/mm^3) appears to have a more benign outcome and may have an autoimmune,

TABLE 14–9. PERIPHERAL NEUROPATHIES COMPLICATING HIV-1 INFECTION

Acute or Seroconversion Phase of Systemic HIV-1 Infection
Mononeuritides, brachial plexopathy
Acute demyelinating polyneuropathy
Clinical Latent ("Asymptomatic") Phase (CD4+ T Lymphocytes >500/mm³)
Acute demyelinating polyneuropathy (Guillain-Barré syndrome)
Chronic inflammatory demyelinating polyneuropathy (CIDP)
Transition Phase (200 to 500 CD4+ Cells)
Herpes zoster neuropathy
Mononeuritis multiplex, "benign" type
Late Phase (<200 CD4+ Cells)
Predominantly sensory polyneuropathy
Autonomic neuropathy
CMV polyradiculopathy
CMV mononeuritis multiplex, severe type
Cranial mononeuropathies associated with aseptic meningitis
Mononeuropathies-radiculopathies secondary to lymphomatous meningitis
Nucleoside (ddI, ddC) toxicity

vasculitic pathogenesis. It involves fewer nerves and appears to remit; whether or not plasma exchange or other measures are helpful is uncertain.

The second form of mononeuritis multiplex occurs later in the course of systemic HIV-1 infection when CD4+ counts are lower and is more aggressive, leading to progressive paralysis and death in some patients. Accumulating evidence suggests that this more malignant mononeuritis multiplex is caused by multifocal CMV infection of nerve.[70,178,182,196,199] For this reason, clinical diagnosis of this neuropathy should be followed by aggressive anti-CMV therapy unless another etiology is proven (Chapter 26). CMV also causes another important neuropathic syndrome, a severe ascending polyradiculopathy that usually begins with painful lumbosacral root involvement and progresses rostrally to involve sensory, motor, and autonomic components.[61,69,127] Diagnosis of the latter is aided by finding polymorphonuclear pleocytosis in the CSF. Thickened spinal roots revealed by myelography or MRI scanning also have been reported. Although CMV can be cultured from the spinal fluid of these patients, viral replication and the appearance of cytopathology in culture are too slow to rely on as guides for therapy; PCR accelerates identification of this herpesvirus, but processing laboratory specimens for this assay may also take unduly long. Therefore, clinical diagnosis should

lead to rapid institution of specific antiviral therapy with ganciclovir, foscarnet, or a combination of these therapies.

The most common neuropathy in AIDS patients is a distal, predominantly sensory and axonal neuropathy.[6,44,86,108,128,207] Characteristically, in this neuropathy the sensory symptoms far exceed either sensory or motor dysfunction. The prevalence of this disorder is uncertain, but in mild form it is very common in late infection. Patients complain of numb or painful, burning feet, and inability to walk is more often due to discomfort than to either sensory ataxia or weakness. The pathogenesis of this neuropathy is uncertain. The suspicion that it may relate to direct HIV-1 infection of either nerve or dorsal root ganglion has not been substantiated, and anecdotal experience suggests that it does not generally respond to zidovudine or other antiretroviral therapy. Cytokine dysregulation and axonal toxicity may be implicated in its causation.[86,207] Treatment now relies on symptom management with tricyclics and various analgesics, including narcotics in severe cases.

Autonomic neuropathy of varying severity has also been reported in AIDS patients.[45,196,213] This may accompany sensory neuropathy, suggesting a common pathogenesis, but in some cases the severity of autonomic and sensory dysfunction diverges. The clinical features of the former range from mild positional hypotension to cardiovascular collapse during invasive procedures. In addition, autonomic neuropathy may contribute to chronic diarrhea in some HIV-1–infected individuals.[9]

Of increasing importance are the toxic peripheral neuropathies caused by certain antiretroviral nucleosides, particularly dideoxyinosine (ddI) and dideoxycytidine (ddC) (Chapter 8). Both of these drugs can cause axonal neuropathy in a dose-related fashion. Their clinical features are similar to the AIDS-related distal sensory polyneuropathy (DSPN) that usually begins with foot pain that is described as "aching," "burning," or "bruise-like." Although symptoms in many patients worsen for a few weeks after discontinuation of the drug, a phenomenon known as "coasting," these neuropathies are reversible if recognized early. Since they may be difficult to distinguish from the spontaneous AIDS-related DSPN and electrodiagnostic studies may be of little help in this differentiation, cessation or switch to alternative therapy may be necessary to confirm this diagnosis. Patients with underlying neuropathies of other types may be more vulnerable to this com-

TABLE 14–10. MYOPATHIES COMPLICATING HIV-1 INFECTION

Inflammatory myopathy (polymyositis)
Noninflammatory myopathies
Toxic myopathy: zidovudine therapy

---

plication, although this issue has not been well studied.

MYOPATHIES

Myopathies can occur at several stages of HIV-1 infection (Table 14–10) but are less common and less well-characterized than the neuropathies.[7,50,51,74,99,115,140,194,195,221] A wide range of presentations, from asymptomatic creatine kinase elevation to progressive severe proximal weakness, has been recognized. A polymyositis or dermatomyositis-like illness has been described in AIDS patients, although the pathogenesis is not clear but is suspected to involve autoimmunity. Viral antigens have been found in the inflammatory cells but not in myocytes,[99] and one report has identified multinucleated giant cells in the inflammatory infiltrate.[7]

Zidovudine therapy can also cause myopathy.[4,38,48,49,52,125,130,144,195] The clinical and laboratory features of this disorder have not been delineated fully, but proximal muscles, especially those of the legs, apparently are affected more often. In many of these patients, abnormalities of mitochondria are detected in muscle biopsy specimens. Clinical and laboratory improvement may occur after stopping zidovudine therapy.

CONCLUSION

As with other aspects of AIDS, precise diagnosis is important in patients with neurologic symptoms or signs, since an increasing number of these disorders can be treated, relieving morbidity or preventing death. Too often, physicians give up prematurely on patients because of their despair of reversing neurologic impairment before this is objectively justified by an established diagnosis and prognosis. The approach to diagnosis and management of the neurologic complications of HIV-1 infection and AIDS follows that used in general neurologic practice, but with an important difference that relates to the altered probabilities of differential diagnosis in this group of patients whose vulnerabilities to opportunistic and HIV-1–related neurologic diseases far overshadow the background incidence of ordinary neurologic diseases. When there is a diagnosis of underlying HIV-1 infection and an understanding of its systemic state, the neurologic history establishes the temporal profile of the neurologic disease and usually provides an initial impression of its anatomic localization. The neurologic examination refines this localization and uncovers additional, including asymptomatic, abnormalities. Neuroimaging studies using CT or MRI and, less commonly, angiography add further precision to anatomic localization and narrow the range of possible underlying pathologic processes. Electrodiagnosis using EEG or evoked potentials also can be helpful in delineating and localizing physiologic dysfunction, and nerve conduction studies and electromyography can similarly refine diagnosis of neuromuscular disease. Examination of CSF provides a direct view of inflammatory reactions in the meninges and can diagnose certain invading organisms or neoplasms. Therapeutic trial and tissue biopsy may be needed for exact diagnosis in some instances. These evaluations, pursued with a background understanding of the spectrum of neurologic disorders affecting these patients, allow accurate neurologic diagnosis in the great majority of patients.

REFERENCES

1. Aboulafia DM, Saxton EH, Koga H, et al: A patient with progressive myelopathy and antibodies to human T-cell leukemia virus type I and human immunodeficiency virus type I in serum and cerebrospinal fluid. Arch Neurol 47:477–479, 1990
2. Andreula CF, Burdi N, Carella A: CNS cryptococcosis in AIDS: Spectrum of MR findings. J Comput Assist Tomogr 17(3):438–441, 1993
3. Anonymous: Nomenclature and research case definitions for neurologic manifestations of human immunodeficiency virus-type 1 (HIV-1) infection. Report of a Working Group of the American Academy of Neurology AIDS Task Force [see comments] (Review). Neurology 41(6):778–785, 1991
4. Arnaudo E, Dalakas M, Shanske S, et al: Depletion of muscle mitochondrial DNA in AIDS patients with zidovudine-induced myopathy. Lancet 337(8740):508–510, 1991

5. Aylward EH, Henderer JD, McArthur JC, et al: Reduced basal ganglia volume in HIV-1-associated dementia: Results from quantitative neuroimaging. Neurology 43(10):2099–2104, 1993
6. Bacellar H, Munoz A, Miller EN, et al: Temporal trends in the incidence of HIV-1-related neurologic diseases: Multicenter AIDS Cohort Study, 1985–1992. Neurology 44(10):1892–1900, 1994
7. Bailey RO, Turok DI, Jaufmann BP, Singh JK: Myositis and acquired immunodeficiency syndrome. Hum Pathol 18(7):749–751, 1987
8. Bartolomei F, Pellegrino P, Dhiver C, et al: Epilepsy seizures in HIV infection. 52 cases (Review) [French]. Presse Med 20(42):2135–2138, 1991
9. Batman P, Miller A, Sedgewick P, Griffin G: Autonomic denervation in jejunal mucosa of homosexual men infected with HIV. AIDS 5:1247–1252, 1991
10. Baumgartner JE, Rachlin JR, Beckstead JH, et al: Primary central nervous system lymphomas: Natural history and response to radiation therapy in 55 patients with acquired immunodeficiency syndrome. J Neurosurg 73(2):206–211, 1990
11. Belman A, Ultmann M, Horoupian D, et al: Neurological complications in infants and children with acquired immune deficiency syndrome. Ann Neurol 18:560, 1985
12. Belman AL: HIV-1-associated CNS disease in infants and children (Review). Res Pub Assoc Res Nerv Ment Dis 72:289–310, 1994
13. Belman AL, Lantos G, Horoupian D, et al: AIDS: Calcification of the basal ganglia in infants and children. Neurology 36(9):1192–1199, 1986
14. Berenguer J, Moreno S, Laguna F, et al: Tuberculous meningitis in patients infected with the human immunodeficiency virus [see comments]. N Engl J Med 326(10):668–672, 1992
15. Berger J: Neurosyphilis in human immunodeficiency virus type 1-seropositive individuals. Arch Neurol 48:700, 1991
16. Berger J, Kaszovitz B, Donovan Post M, Dickinson G: Progressive multifocal leukoencephalopathy in association with human immunodeficiency virus infection: A review of the literature with a report of sixteen cases. Ann Intern Med 107:78, 1987
17. Berger J, Mucke L: Prolonged survival and partial recovery in AIDS-associated progressive multifocal leukoencephalopathy. Neurology 38:1060, 1988
18. Berger J, Sheremata W, Resnick L, et al: Multiple sclerosis-like leukoencephalopathy revealing human immunodeficiency virus infection. Neurology 39:324, 1989
19. Berger JR, Flaster M, Schatz N, et al: Cranial neuropathy heralding otherwise occult AIDS-related large cell lymphoma. J Clin Neuroophthalmol 13(2):113–118, 1993
20. Berman SM, Kim RC: The development of cytomegalovirus encephalitis in AIDS patients receiving ganciclovir. Am J Med 96(5):415–419, 1994
21. Berry C, Hooton T, Collier A, Lukehart S: Neurologic relapse after benzathine penicillin therapy for secondary syphilis in a patient with HIV infection. N Engl J Med 316:1587, 1987
22. Boldorini R, Vago L, Lechi A, et al: Wernicke's encephalopathy: Occurrence and pathological aspects in a series of 400 AIDS patients. Acta Biomed l Ateneo Parmense 63(1–2):43–49, 1992
23. Bomfim da Paz R, Kolmel HW: Meningitis with Burkitt like B-cell lymphoma in HIV infection. J Neurooncol 13(1):73–79, 1992
24. Brew B, Bhalla R, Fleisher M, et al: Cerebrospinal fluid B2 microglobulin in patients infected with human immunodeficiency virus. Neurology 39:830–834, 1989
25. Brew B, Bhalla R, Paul M, et al: Cerebrospinal fluid neopterin in human immunodeficiency virus type 1 infection. Ann Neurol 28:556–560, 1990
26. Brew B, Perdices M, Darveniza P, et al: The neurological features of early and 'latent' human immunodeficiency virus infection. Aust N Z J Med 19:700, 1989
27. Brew B, Rosenblum M, Cronin K, Price R: The AIDS dementia complex and HIV-1 brain infection: Clinical-virological correlations. Ann Neurol 38:563–570, 1995
28. Brew B, Sidtis J, Petito C, Price R: The neurological complications of AIDS and human immunodeficiency virus infection. In Plum F, ed. Advances in Contemporary Neurology. Philadelphia, FA Davis Co, 1988, pp 1–49
29. Brew BJ. Medical management of AIDS patients. Central and peripheral nervous system abnormalities (Review). Med Clin North Am 76(1):63–81, 1992
30. Brew BJ, Bhalla RB, Paul M, et al: Cerebrospinal fluid beta 2-microglobulin in patients with AIDS dementia complex: An expanded series including response to zidovudine treatment. AIDS 6(5):461–465, 1992
31. Brew BJ, Miller J: Human immunodeficiency virus-related headache. Neurology 43(6):1098–1100, 1993
32. Brew BJ, Paul MO, Nakajima G, et al: Cerebrospinal fluid HIV-1 p24 antigen and culture: Sensitivity and specificity for AIDS-dementia complex. J Neurol Neurosurg Psychiatry 57(7):784–789, 1994
33. Brouwers P, Moss H, Wolters P, et al: Effect of continuous-infusion zidovudine therapy on neuropsychologic functioning in children with symptomatic human immunodeficiency virus infection. J Pediatr 116:980–985, 1990
34. Budka H: Neuropathology of human immunodeficiency virus infection (Review). Brain Pathol 1(3):163–175, 1991
35. Butterworth RF, Gaudreau C, Vincelette J, et al: Thiamine deficiency and Wernicke's encephalopathy in AIDS. Metab Brain Dis 6(4):207–212, 1991
36. Calabrese L, Proffitt M, Levin K, et al: Acute infection with the human immunodeficiency virus (HIV) associated with acute brachial neuritis and exanthematous rash. Ann Intern Med 107:849, 1987
37. Carne C, Smith A, Elkington S, et al: Acute encephalopathy coincident with serocoversion for anti HTLV-III. Lancet 2:1206, 1985
38. Chalmers A, Greco C, Miller R: Prognosis in AZT myopathy. Neurology 41:1181, 1991
39. Cinque P, Vago L, Brytting M, et al: Cytomegalovirus infection of the central nervous system in patients with AIDS: Diagnosis by DNA amplification from cerebrospinal fluid. J Infect Dis 166(6):1408–1411, 1992
40. Clark SJ, Saag MS, Decker WD, et al: High titers of cytopathic virus in plasma of patients with symptomatic primary HIV-1 infection. N Engl J Med 324:954–960, 1991
41. Conrad DI, Schmid P, Syndulko K, et al: Quantifying

HIV-1 RNA using the polymerase chain reaction on cerebrospinal fluid and serum of seropositive individuals with and without neurologic abnormalities. J Acquir Immune Defic Syndr 10: 425–435, 1995

42. Cornblath D: Treatment of the neuromuscular complications of human immunodeficiency virus infection. Ann Neurol 23(Suppl):S88, 1988

43. Cornblath D, Chaudhry V, Griffin J: Treatment of chronic inflammatory demyelinating polyneuropathy with intravenous immunoglobin. Ann Neurol 30:104, 1991

44. Cornblath D, McArthur J: Predominantly sensory neuropathy in patients with AIDS and AIDS-related complex. Neurology 38:794, 1988

45. Craddock C, Pasvol G, Bull R, et al: Cardiorespiratory arrest and automatic neuropathy in AIDS. Lancet 2:16, 1987

46. Dal Pan GJ, Glass JD, McArthur JC: Clinicopathologic correlations of HIV-1-associated vacuolar myelopathy: An autopsy-based case-control study. Neurology 44(11):2159–2164, 1994

47. Dal Pan GJ, McArthur JH, Aylward E, et al: Patterns of cerebral atrophy in HIV-1-infected individuals: Results of a quantitative MRI analysis. Neurology 42(11):2125–2130, 1992

48. Dalakas M, Illa I, Pezeshkpour G, et al: Mitochondrial myopathy caused by long term zidovudine therapy. N Engl J Med 322:1098, 1990

49. Dalakas MC, Leon-Monzon ME, Bernardini I, et al: Zidovudine-induced mitochondrial myopathy is associated with muscle carnitine deficiency and lipid storage. Ann Neurol 35(4):482–487, 1994

50. Dalakas MC, Pezeshkpour GH: Neuromuscular diseases associated with human immunodeficiency virus infection (Review). Ann Neurol 23(48): S38–S48, 1988

51. Dalakas MC, Pezeshkpour GH, Gravell M, Sever JL: Polymyositis associated with AIDS retrovirus. JAMA 256(17):2381–2383, 1986

52. Damati G, Lewis W: Zidovudine causes early increases in mitochondrial ribonucleic acid abundance and induces ultrastructural changes in cultured mouse muscle cells. Lab Invest 71(6):879–884, 1994

53. Davis L: Neurosyphilis in the patient infected with human immunodeficiency virus. Ann Neurol 27: 211, 1990

54. Davis LE, Hjelle BL, Miller VE, et al: Early viral brain invasion in iatrogenic human immunodeficiency virus infection. Neurology 42(9):1736–1739, 1992

55. DeAngelis L: Primary CNS lymphoma: A new clinical challenge. Neurology 41:619, 1991

56. Denning D, Anderson J, Rudge P, et al: Acute myelopathy associated with primary infection with human immunodeficiency virus. Br Med J 294: 143, 1987

57. Devinsky O, Cho E, Petito C, Price R: Herpes zoster myelitis. Brain 114:1181, 1991

58. Dismukes WE: Management of cryptococcosis (Review). Clin Infect Dis 17(2):S507–S512, 1993

59. Dube MP, Holtom PD, Larsen RA: Tuberculous meningitis in patients with and without human immunodeficiency virus infection. Am J Med 93(5): 520–524, 1992

60. Eidelberg D, Sotrel A, Horopian D, et al: Thrombotic cerebral vasculopathy associated with herpes zoster. Ann Neurol 19:7, 1986

61. Eidelberg D, Sotrel A, Vogel H, et al: Progressive po-

lyradioculopathy in acquired immune deficiency syndrome. Neurology 36:912, 1986

62. Elovaara I, Nykyri E, Poutiainen E, et al: CSF followup in HIV-1 infection: Intrathecal production of HIV-specific and unspecific IGG, and beta-2-microglobulin increase with duration of HIV-1 infection. Acta Neurol Scand 87(5):388–396, 1993

63. Engstrom JW, Lowenstein DH, Bredesen DE: Cerebral infarctions and transient neurologic deficits associated with acquired immunodeficiency syndrome. Am J Med 86:528–532, 1989

64. Enting RH, Esselink RA, Portegies P: Lymphomatous meningitis in AIDS-related systemic non-Hodgkin's lymphoma: A report of eight cases. J Neurol Neurosurg Psychiatry 57(2):150–153, 1994

65. Epstein LG, Gendelman HE: Human immunodeficiency virus type 1 infection of the nervous system: Pathogenetic mechanisms [see comments] (Review). Ann Neurol 33(5):429–436, 1993

66. Epstein LG, Sharer LR, Oleske JM, et al: Neurologic manifestations of human immunodeficiency virus infection in children. Pediatrics 78(4):678–687, 1986

67. Falangola MF, Reichler BS, Petito CK: Histopathology of cerebral toxoplasmosis in human immunodeficiency virus infection: A comparison between patients with early-onset and late-onset acquired immunodeficiency syndrome. Hum Pathol 25(10):1091–1097, 1994

68. Formenti SC, Gill PS, Lean E, et al: Primary central nervous system lymphoma in AIDS. Results of radiation therapy. Cancer 63(6):1101–1107, 1989

69. Fuller G, Gill S, Guilloff R, et al: Ganciclovir treatment of lumbosacral polyradiculopathy in AIDS. Lancet 335:48, 1990

70. Fuller GN: Cytomegalovirus and the peripheral nervous system in AIDS (Review) J Acquir Immune Defic Syndr 5(1):S33–S36, 1992

71. Fuller GN, Jacobs JM, Guiloff RJ: Nature and incidence of peripheral nerve syndromes in HIV infection. J Neurol Neurosurg Psychiatry 56(4): 372–381, 1993

72. Gaines H, von Sydow M, Pehrson PO, Lundbergh P: Clinical pricure of primary HIV-1 infection presenting as a glandular-fever-like illness. Lancet 297:1363–1368, 1988

73. Gelman B, Guinto FJ: Morphometry, histopathology, and tomography of cerebral atrophy in the acquired immunodeficiency syndrome. Ann Neurol 31:32–40, 1992

74. Gherardi RK: Skeletal muscle involvement in HIV-infected patients (Review) Neuropathol Appl Neurobiol 20(3):232–237, 1994

75. Glass JD, Fedor H, Wesselingh SL, McArthur JC: Immunocytochemical quantitation of human immunodeficiency virus in the brain: Correlations with dementia. Ann Neurol 38:755–762, 1995

76. Goldstein J: Headache and acquired immunodeficiency syndrome. Neurol Clin 8:947, 1990

77. Gordon SE, Eaton ME, George R, et al: The response of symptomatic neurosyphilis to high-dose intravenous penicillin G in patients with human immunodeficiency virus infection. N Engl J Med 331: 1469–1473, 1994

78. Goudsmit J, Wolters E, Bakker M, et al: Intrathecal synthesis of antibodies to HTLV-III in patients without AIDS or AIDS related complex. Br Med J 292:1231, 1986

79. Gozlan J, Salord JM, Roullet E, et al: Rapid detection of cytomegalovirus DNA in cerebrospinal fluid of AIDS patients with neurologic disorders [published erratum appears in J Infect Dis 167(4):995, 1993]. J Infect Dis 166(6):1416–1421, 1992

80. Grant I, Gold J, Rosemblum M, et al: Toxoplasma gondii serology in HIV-infected patients: The development of central nervous system toxoplasmosis in AIDS. AIDS 4:519, 1990

81. Gray F, Belec L, Lescs MC, et al: Varicella-zoster virus infection of the central nervous system in the acquired immune deficiency syndrome (Review) Brain 117(Pt 5):987–999, 1994

82. Gray F, Chimelli L, Mohr M, et al: Fulminating multiple sclerosis-like leukoencephalopathy revealing human immunodeficiency virus infection. Neurology 41:105, 1991

83. Gray F, Gherardi R, Wingate E, et al: Diffuse "encephalitic" cerebral toxoplasmosis in AIDS: Report of four cases. J Neurol 236:273, 1989

84. Gray F, Haug H, Chimelli L, et al: Prominent cortical atrophy with neuronal loss as correlate of human immunodeficiency virus encephalopathy. Acta Neuropathol 82(3):229–233, 1991

85. Griffin DE, McArthur JC, Cornblath DR: Neopterin and interferon-gamma in serum and cerebrospinal fluid of patients with HIV-associated neurologic disease. Neurology 41(1):69–74, 1991

86. Griffin JW, Wesselingh SL, Griffin DE, et al: Peripheral nerve disorders in HIV infection. Similarities and contrasts with CNS disorders (Review). Res Pub Assoc Res Nerv Ment Dis 72:159–182, 1994

87. Hagberg L, Malmval B, Svennerholm L, et al: Guillain-Barre syndrome as an early manifestation of HIV central nervous system infection. Scand J Infect Dis 18:591, 1987

88. Harris MJ, Jeste DV, Gleghorn A, Sewell DD: New-onset psychosis in HIV-infected patients [see comments] (Review). J Clin Psychiatry 52(9):369–376, 1991

89. Harris TM, Smith RR, Bognanno JR, Edwards MK: Toxoplasmic myelitis in AIDS: Gadolinium-enhanced MR. J Comput Assist Tomogr 15(5): 809–811, 1990

90. Hilt D, Bucholz D, Krumholz A, et al: Herpes zoster ophthalmicus and delayed contralateral hemiparesis caused by cerebral angitiis: Diagnosis and management approaches. Ann Neurol 14:543, 1983

91. Ho D, Sarngadhara M, Resnick L, et al: Primary human T lymphotropic virus type III infection. Ann Intern Med 103:880, 1985

92. Holland NR, Power C, Mathews VP, et al: Cytomegalovirus encephalitis in acquired immunodeficiency syndrome (AIDS). Neurology 44(3 Pt 1): 507–514, 1994

93. Hollander H, Golden J, Mendelson T, Cortland D: Extrapyramidal symptoms in AIDS patients given low dose metoclopramide or chlorpromazine. Lancet 2:1186, 1985

94. Hollander H, McGuire D, Burack JH: Diagnostic lumbar puncture in HIV-infected patients: Analysis of 138 cases. Am J Med 96(3):223–228, 1994

95. Hollander H, Stringari S: Human immunodeficiency virus-associated meningitis: Clinical course and correlations. Am J Med 83:813, 1987

96. Holtzman D, Kaku D, So Y: New onset seizures associated with human immunodeficiency virus infection: Causation and clinical features in 100 cases. Am J Med 87:173, 1989

97. Horten B, Price R, Jimenez D: Multifocal varicella-zoster virus leukoencephalitis temporally remote from herpes zoster. Ann Neurol 9:251, 1981

98. Houff S, Major E, Katz D, et al: Involvement of JC virus-infected mononuclear cells from the bone marrow and spleen in the pathogenesis of progressive multifocal leukoencephalopathy. N Engl J Med 318:301, 1988

99. Illa I, Nath A, Dalakas M: Immunocytochemical and virological characteristics of HIV-associated inflammatory myopathies: Similarities with seronegative polymyositis. Ann Neurol 29:474, 1991

100. Jakobsen J, Gyldensted C, Brun B, et al: Cerebral ventricular enlargement relates to neuropsychological measures in unselected AIDS patients. Acta Neurol Scand 79:59, 1989

101. Jarvik J, Hesselink J, Kennedy C, et al: Acquired immunodeficiency syndrome: Magnetic resonance patterns of brain involvement with pathologic correlation. Neurology 45:731, 1988

102. Johns D, Tierney M, Felsenstein D: Alteration in the natural history of neurosyphilis by concurrent infection with the human immunodeficiency virus. N Engl J Med 316:1569, 1987

103. Kalayjian RC, Cohen ML, Bonomo RA, Flanigan TP: Cytomegalovirus ventriculoencephalitis in AIDS. A syndrome with distinct clinical and pathologic features (Review) Medicine 72(2):67–77, 1993

104. Katz D, Berger J: Neurosyphilis in acquired immunodeficiency syndrome. Arch Neurol 46:895, 1989

105. Kovacs J, Kovacs A, Polis M, et al: Cryptococcosis in the acquired immunodeficiency syndrome. Ann Intern Med 103:533, 1985

106. Levine AM: Non-Hodgkin's lymphomas and other malignancies in the acquired immune deficiency syndrome (Review). Semin Oncol 14(2 Suppl 3): 34–39, 1987

107. Levy RM, Bredesen DE, Rosenblum ML: Neurological manifestations of the acquired immunodeficiency syndrome (AIDS): Experience at UCSF and review of the literature (Review). J Neurosurg 62(4):475–495, 1985

108. Lipkin W, Parry G, Kiprov D, Abrams D: Inflammatory neuropathy in homosexual men with lymphadenopathy. Neurology 35:1479–1483, 1985

109. Lipton RB, Feraru ER, Weiss G, et al: Headache in HIV-1-related disorders. Headache 31(8): 518–522, 1991

110. Lipton SA: Neuronal injury associated with HIV-1 and potential treatment with calcium-channel and NMDA antagonists. Dev Neurosci 16(3–4): 145–151, 1994

111. Lipton SA, Gendelman HE: Seminars in medicine of the Beth Israel Hospital, Boston. Dementia associated with the acquired immunodeficiency syndrome (Review). N Engl J Med 332(14):934–940, 1995

112. Lipton SA, Stamler JS: Actions of redox-related congeners of nitric oxide at the NMDA receptor. Neuropharmacology 33(11):1229–1233, 1994

113. Luft BJ, Hafner R, Korzun AH, et al: Toxoplasmic encephalitis in patients with the acquired immunodeficiency syndrome. Members of the ACTG 077p/ANRS 009 Study Team. N Engl J Med 329(14):995–1000, 1993

114. Lukehart S, Hook E, Baker-Zander S: Invasion of the

central nervous system by *Treponema pallidum:* Implications for the diagnosis and treatment. Ann Intern Med 109:855, 1988

115. Manji H, Harrison MJ, Round JM, et al: Muscle disease, HIV and zidovudine: The spectrum of muscle disease in HIV-infected individuals treated with zidovudine. J Neurol 240(8):479–488, 1993

116. Marshall D, Brey R, Cahill W, et al: Spectrum of cerebrospinal fluid findings in various stages of human immunodeficiency virus infection. Arch Neurol 45:954–958, 1988

117. Masliah E, Achim CL, Ge N, et al: Cellular neuropathology in HIV encephalitis (Review) Res Pub Assoc Res Nerv Ment Dis 72:119–131, 1994

118. Masliah E, Ge N, Achim C, et al: Patterns of neurodegeneration in HIV encephalitis. J Neuro-AIDS 1: 161–173, 1996

119. Matsuo H, Nakamura T, Tsujihata M, et al: Plasmapheresis in treatment of human T-lymphotropic virus type-I associated myelopathy. Lancet 2(8620):1109–1113, 1988

120. McArthur J, Cohen B, Farzadegan H, et al: Cerebrospinal fluid abnormalities in homosexual men with and without neuropsychiatric findings. Ann Neurol 23(Suppl):S34–S37, 1988

121. McArthur JC, Hoover DR, Bacellar H, et al: Dementia in AIDS patients: Incidence and risk factors. Multicenter AIDS Cohort Study. Neurology 43(11): 2245–2252, 1993

122. McGuire D, Barhite S, Hollander H, Miles M: JC virus DNA in cerebrospinal fluid of human immunodeficiency virus-infected patients: Predictive value for progressive multifocal leukoencephalopathy. Ann Neurol 37(3):395–399, 1995

123. Meeker TC, Shiramizu B, Kaplan L, et al: Evidence for molecular subtypes of HIV-associated lymphoma: Division into peripheral monoclonal, polyclonal and central nervous system lymphoma. AIDS 5(6):669–674, 1991

124. Mehren M, Burns PJ, Mamani F, et al: Toxoplasmic myelitis mimicking intramedullary spinal cord tumor. Neurology 38:1648–1650, 1988

125. Mhiri C, Baudrimont M, Bonne G, et al: Zidovudine myopathy: A distinctive disorder associated with mitochondrial dysfunction. Ann Neurol 29:606, 1991

126. Miller E, Selnes O, McArthur J, et al: Neuropsychological performance in HIV-1-infected homosexual men: The Multi-center AIDS Cohort Study (MACS). Neurology 40:197–203, 1990

127. Miller R, Parry G, Lang W, et al: AIDS-related inflammatory polyradiculoneuropathy: Successful treatment with plasma exchange (Abstract). Neurology 36:206, 1986

128. Miller R, Parry G, Pfaeffl W, et al: The spectrum of peripheral neuropathy associated with ARC and AIDS. Muscle Nerve 11:857, 1988

129. Mintz M: Clinical comparison of adult and pediatric NeuroAIDS (Review). Adv Neuroimmunol 4(3): 207–221, 1994

130. Modica-Napolitano JS: AZT causes tissue-specific inhibition of mitochondrial bioenergetic function. Biochem Biophys Res Commun 194(1):170–177, 1993

131. Moeller AA, Backmund HC: Ventricle brain ratio in the clinical course of HIV infection. Acta Neurol Scand 81(6):512–515, 1990

132. Morgello S, Block G, Price R, et al: Varicella-zoster virus leukoencephalitis and cerebral vasculopathy. Arch Pathol Lab Med 112:173, 1988

133. Morgello S, Cho E, Neilsen S, et al: Cytomegalovirus encephalitis in patients with acquired immunodeficiency syndrome. Hum Pathol 18:289–297, 1987

134. Moriarty DM, Haller JO, Loh JP, Fikrig S: Cerebral infarction in pediatric acquired immunodeficiency syndrome. Pediatr Radiol 24(8):611–612, 1994

135. Navia B, Cho E-W, Petito C, Price R: The AIDS dementia complex: II. Neuropathology. Ann Neurol 19:525–535, 1986

136. Navia B, Jordan B, Price R: The AIDS dementia complex: I. Clinical features. Ann Neurol 19:517–524, 1986

137. Navia B, Petito C, Gold J, et al: Cerebral toxoplasmosis complicating the acquired immune deficiency syndrome: Clinical and neuropathological findings in 27 patients. Ann Neurol 19:224, 1986

138. Navia B, Price R: The acquired immunodeficiency syndrome dementia complex as the presenting or sole manifestation of human immunodeficiency virus infection. Arch Neurol 44:65–69, 1987

139. Neaton J, Wentworth D, Rhane F, et al: Methods of studying interventions. Considerations in choice of a clinical endpoint for AIDS clinical trials. Stat Med 13:2107–2125, 1994

140. Nordstrom DM, Petropolis AA, Giorno R, et al: Inflammatory myopathy and acquired immunodeficiency syndrome. Arthritis Rheum 32(4):475–479, 1989

141. Nuovo G, Gallery F, MacConnel P, Braun A: In situ detection of polymerase chain reaction-amplified HIV-1 nucleic acids and tumor necrosis factor-a RNA in the central nervous system. Am J Pathol 144:659–666, 1994

142. O'Brien W: Genetic and biologic basis of HIV-1 neurotropism. In Price R, Perry S, eds. HIV, AIDS and the Brain. New York, Raven Press, Ltd, 1994, pp 47–70

143. Panther L, Sande M: Cryptococcal meningitis in AIDS. In Sande M, Volverding P, eds. The Medical Management of AIDS. Philadelphia, WB Saunders Co, 1990

144. Peters BS, Winer J, Landon DN, et al: Mitochondrial myopathy associated with chronic zidovudine therapy in AIDS. Q J Med 86(1):5–15, 1993

145. Petito C, Cho E-S, Lemann W, et al: Neuropathology of acquired immunodeficiency syndrome (AIDS): An autopsy review. J Neuropathol Exp Neurol 45: 635–646, 1986

146. Petito C, Navia B, Cho E, et al: Vacuolar myelopathy pathologically resembling subacute combined degeneration in patients with acquired immunodeficiency syndrome (AIDS). N Engl J Med 312:874, 1985

147. Petito CK, Vecchio D, Chen YT: HIV antigen and DNA in AIDS spinal cords correlate with macrophage infiltration but not with vacuolar myelopathy. J Neuropathol Exp Neurol 53(1):86–94, 1994

148. Petty RK: Recent advances in the neurology of HIV infection (Review). Postgrad Med J 70(824): 393–403, 1994

149. Philippet P, Blanche S, Sebag G, et al: Stroke and cerebral infarcts in children infected with human immunodeficiency virus. Arch Pediatr Adolesc Med 148(9):965–970, 1994

150. Piette A, Tusseau F, Vignon D, et al: Letter to the editor. Lancet 1:852, 1986
151. Pizzo P, Eddy J, Fallon J, et al: Effect of continuous intravenous infusion of zidovudine (AZT) in children with symptomatic HIV infection. N Engl J Med 319:889–896, 1988
152. Portegies P, Algra P, Hollak C, et al: Response to cytarabine in progressive multifocal leukoencephalopathy in AIDS. Lancet 1:680, 1991
153. Portegies P, de Gans J, Derix M, et al: Declining incidence of AIDS dementia complex after introduction of zidovudine treatment. Br Med J 299:819–821, 1989
154. Portegies P, Enting RH, de Gans J, et al: Presentation and course of AIDS dementia complex: 10 years of follow-up in Amsterdam, The Netherlands. AIDS 7(5):669–675, 1993
155. Portegies P, Epstein L, Hung S, et al: Human immunodeficiency virus type 1 antigen in cerebrospinal fluid: Correlation with clinical neurological status. Arch Neurol 46:261–264, 1989
156. Post M, Tate L, Quencer R, et al: CT, MR, and pathology in HIV encephalitis and meningitis. AJR Am J Roentgenol 151:373, 1988
157. Post MJ, Berger JR, Quencer RM: Asymptomatic and neurologically symptomatic HIV-seropositive individuals: Prospective evaluation with cranial MR imaging [see comments]. Radiology 178(1):131–139, 1991
158. Post MJ, Hensley GT, Moskowitz LB, Fischl M: Cytomegalic inclusion virus encephalitis in patients with AIDS: CT, clinical, and pathologic correlation. AIR Am J Roentgenol 146(6):1229–1234, 1986
159. Powderly WG: Cryptococcal meningitis and AIDS (Review). Clin Infect Dis 17(5):837–842, 1993
160. Power C, Kong PA, Crawford TO, et al: Cerebral white matter changes in acquired immunodeficiency syndrome dementia: Alterations of the blood-brain barrier. Ann Neurol 34(3):339–350, 1993
161. Power C, McArthur JC, Johnson RT, et al: Demented and nondemented patients with AIDS differ in brain-derived human immunodeficiency virus type 1 envelope sequences. J Virol 68(7):4643–4649, 1994
162. Price R: AIDS dementia complex and HIV-1 brain infection: A pathogenetic framework for treatment and evaluation. Curr Top Microbiol Immunol 202:33–54, 1995
163. Price R: The cellular basis of central nervous system HIV infection and the AIDS dementia complex: Introduction. J Neuro-AIDS 1(1):1–28, 1995
164. Price R: Management of AIDS dementia complex and HIV-1 infection of the nervous system. AIDS 9(Suppl A):S221–S236, 1995
165. Price R, Brew B: The AIDS dementia complex. J Infect Dis 158:1079–1083, 1988
166. Price R, Brew B, Sidtis J, et al: The brain in AIDS: Central nervous system HIV-1 infection and AIDS dementia complex. Science 239:586–592, 1988
167. Price RW: Understanding the AIDS dementia complex (ADC). The challenge of HIV and its effects on the central nervous system (Review). Res Pub Assoc Res Nerv Ment Dis 72:1–45, 1994
168. Price RW, Sidtis JJ, Brew BJ: AIDS dementia complex and HIV-1 infection: A view from the clinic (Review). Brain Pathol 1(3):155–162, 1991
169. Rabeneck L, Popovic M, Gartner S, et al: Acute HIV-1 infection presenting with painful swallowing and esophageal ulcers. JAMA 263:2318–2322, 1990
170. Remick S, Diamond C, Migliozzi J, et al: Primary central nervous system lymphoma in patients with and without the acquired immune deficiency syndrome: A retrospective analysis and review of the literature. Medicine 69:345, 1990
171. Resnick L, Berger J, Shapshak P, Tourtellotte W: Early penetration of the blood-brain-barrier by HIV. Neurology 38:9–14, 1988
172. Resnick L, diMarzo-Veronese F, Schupbach J, et al: Intra-blood-brain-barrier synthesis of HTLV-III-specific IgG in patients with neurologic symptoms associated with AIDS or AIDS-related complex. N Engl J Med 313(24):1498–1504, 1985
173. Rhodes R: Histopathology of the central nervous system in the acquired immunodeficiency syndrome. Hum Pathol 18:636, 1987
174. Richardson E: Progressive multifocal leukoencephalopathy. In Vinken P, Bruyn G, eds. Handbook of Clinical Neurology, vol 34. Amsterdam, Elsevier, 1978, p 307
175. Rosenblum M: Infection of the central nervous system by the human immunodeficiency virus type 1: Morphology and relation to syndromes of progressive encephalopathy and myelopathy in patients with AIDS. Pathol Ann 25:117–169, 1990
176. Rosenblum M, Brew B, Hahn B, et al: Human T-lymphotropic virus type I associated myelopathy in patients with the acquired immune deficiency syndrome. Hum Pathol 23:513–519, 1992
177. Rosenblum M, Scheck A, Cronin K, et al: Dissociation of AIDS-related vacuolar myelopathy and productive human immunodeficiency virus type 1 (HIV-1) infection of the spinal cord. Neurology 39:892–896, 1989
178. Roullet E, Assuerus V, Gozlan J, et al: Cytomegalovirus multifocal neuropathy in AIDS: Analysis of 15 consecutive cases. Neurology 44(11):2174–2182, 1994
179. Ruiz A, Ganz WI, Post MJ, et al: Use of thallium-201 brain SPECT to differentiate cerebral lymphoma from toxoplasma encephalitis in AIDS patients. AJNR Am J Neuroradiol 15(10):1885–1894, 1994
180. Ryder JW, Croen K, Kleinschmidt-DeMasters BK, et al: Progressive encephalitis three months after resolution of cutaneous zoster in a patient with AIDS. Ann Neurol 19(2):182–188, 1986
181. Saag MS, Powderly WG, Cloud GA, et al: Comparison of amphotericin B with fluconazole in the treatment of acute AIDS-associated cryptococcal meningitis. The NIAID Mycoses Study Group and the AIDS Clinical Trials Group [see comments]. N Engl J Med 326(2):83–89, 1992
182. Said G, Lacroix C, Chemouilli P, et al: CMV neuropathy in AIDS: A clinical and pathological study. Ann Neurol 29:139, 1991
183. Saito Y, Sharer L, Epstein L, et al: Overexpression of nef as a marker for restricted HIV-1 infection of astrocytes in postmortem pediatric central nervous system tissues. Neurology 44:474–481, 1994
184. Schmidbauer M, Budka H, Shah K: Progressive multifocal leukoencephalopathy (PML) in AIDS and in the pre-AIDS era. Acta Neuropathol 80:375, 1990
185. Schmitt F, Bigleg J, McKinnis R, et al: Neuropsychological outcome of azidothymidine (AZT) in the treatment of AIDS and AIDS-related complex: A double blind, placebo-controlled trial. N Engl J Med 319:1573–1578, 1988

186. Selnes O, Miller E, McArthur J, et al: No evidence of cognitive decline during the asymptomatic stages. Neurology 40:204, 1990

187. Selnes OA, Galai N, Bacellar H, et al: Cognitive performance after progression to AIDS: A longitudinal study from the Multicenter AIDS Cohort Study. Neurology 45(2):267–275, 1995

188. Sharpless N, O'Brien W, Verdin E, et al: Human immunodeficiency virus type 1 tropism for brain microglial cells is determined by a region of the env glycoprotein that also controls macrophage tropism. J Virol 66:2588–2593, 1992

189. Sidtis JJ: Evaluation of the AIDS dementia complex in adults (Review). Res Pub Assoc Res Nerv Ment Dis 72:273–287, 1994

190. Sidtis JJ, Gatsonis C, Price RW, et al: Zidovudine treatment of the AIDS dementia complex: Results of a placebo-controlled trial. AIDS Clinical Trials Group. Ann Neurol 83(4):343–349, 1993

191. Sidtis JJ, Price RW: Early HIV-1 infection and the AIDS dementia complex (Comment). Neurology 40(2):323–326, 1990

192. Simon R: Neurosyphilis. Neurology 44:2228–2230, 1994

193. Simpson D, Tagliati M: Neurologic manifestations of HIV infection. Ann Intern Med 121:7769–7785, 1994

194. Simpson DM, Bender AN: Human immunodeficiency virus-associated myopathy: Analysis of 11 patients. Ann Neurol 24(1):79–84, 1988

195. Simpson DM, Citak KA, Godfrey E, et al: Myopathies associated with human immunodeficiency virus and zidovudine: Can their effects be distinguished? Neurology 43:971–976, 1993

196. Simpson DM, Olney RK: Peripheral neuropathies associated with human immunodeficiency virus infection (Review). Neurol Clin 10(3):685–711, 1992

197. So Y, Beckstead J, Davis R: Primary central nervous system lymphoma in acquired immune deficiency syndrome: A clinical and pathological study. Ann Neurol 20:566, 1986

198. So Y, Holtzman D, Abrams D, Olnery R: Peripheral neuropathy associated with acquired immunodeficiency syndrome: Prevalence and clinical features from a population based survey. Arch Neurol 45: 945, 1988

199. So Y, Olney R: The natural history of mononeuropathy multiplex and simplex in patients with HIV infection (Abstract). Neurology 41(Suppl):374, 1991

200. So YT, Olney RK: Acute lumbosacral polyradiculopathy in acquired immunodeficiency syndrome: Experience with 23 patients. Ann Neurol 35:53–58, 1994

201. Sugar AM: Overview: Cryptococcosis in the patient with AIDS (Review). Mycopathologia 114(3): 153–157, 1991

202. Tan SV, Guiloff RJ, Scaravilli F: AIDS-associated vacuolar myelopathy. A morphometric study. Brain 118:1247–1261, 1995

203. Tindall B, Cooper D: Primary HIV infection: Host responses and intervention strategies. AIDS 5:1, 1991

204. Tornatore C, Chandra R, Berger JR, Major EO: HIV-1 infection of subcortical astrocytes in the pediatric central nervous system. Neurology 44(3 Pt 1): 481–487, 1994

205. Tross S, Price R, Navia B, et al: Neuropsychological characterization of the AIDS dementia complex: A preliminary report. AIDS 2:81–88, 1988

206. Tucker T, Dix RD, Katzen C, et al: Cytomegalovirus and herpes simplex virus ascending myelitis in a patient with acquired immune deficiency syndrome. Ann Neurol 18:74–79, 1985

207. Tyor W, Wesselingh S, Griffin J, et al: Unifying hypothesis for the pathogenesis of HIV-associated dementia complex, vacuolar myelopathy, and sensory neuropathy. J Acquir Immune Defic Syndr Hum Retrovirol 9:379–388, 1995

208. Van Paesschen W, Bodian C, Maker H: Metabolic abnormalities and new-onset seizures in human immunodeficiency virus-seropositive patients. Epilepsia 36(2):146–150, 1995

209. Vinters H, Kwok M, Ho H, et al: Cytomegalovirus in the nervous system of patients with the acquired immunodeficiency syndrome. Brain 112:245, 1989

210. Weber T, Beck R, Stark E, et al: Comparative analysis of intrathecal antibody synthesis and DNA amplification for the diagnosis of cytomegalovirus infection of the central nervous system in AIDS patients. J Neurol 241(7):407–414, 1994

211. Weber T, Turner RW, Frye S, et al: Progressive multifocal leukoencephalopathy diagnosed by amplification of JC virus-specific DNA from cerebrospinal fluid. AIDS 8(1):49–57, 1994

212. Weber T, Turner RW, Frye S, et al: Specific diagnosis of progressive multifocal leukoencephalopathy by polymerase chain reaction. J Infect Dis 169(5): 1138–1141, 1994

213. Welby SB, Rogerson SJ, Beeching NJ: Autonomic neuropathy is common in human immunodeficiency virus infection. J Infect 23(2):123–128, 1991

214. Westervelt P, Trowbridge D, Epstein L, et al: Macrophage tropism determinants of HIV-1 in vivo. J Virol 66:2577–2582, 1992

215. Wiley CA, Achim CL: Human immunodeficiency virus encephalitis and dementia. Ann Neurol 38: 559–560, 1995

216. Wiley CA, Nelson JA: Role of human immunodeficiency virus and cytomegalovirus in AIDS encephalitis. Am J Pathol 133(1):73–81, 1988

217. Wiselka M, Nicholson K, Ward S, Flower A: Acute infection with human immunodeficiency virus associated with facial nerve palsy and neuralgia. J Infect 15:189, 1987

218. Wolf DG, Spector SA: Diagnosis of human cytomegalovirus central nervous system disease in AIDS patients by DNA amplification from cerebrospinal fluid. J Infect Dis 166:1412–1415, 1992

219. Wong M, Suite N, Labar D: Seizures in human immunodeficiency virus infection. Arch Neurol 47:640, 1990

220. World Health Organization: 1990 World Health Organization consultation on the neuropsychiatric aspects of HIV-1 infection. AIDS 4 9:935–936, 1990

221. Wrzolek MA, Sher JH, Kozlowski PB, Rao C: Skeletal muscle pathology in AIDS: An autoposy study. Muscle Nerve 13(6):508–515, 1990

222. Yarchoan R, Berg G, Brouwers P, et al: Response of human immunodeficiency virus associated neurological disease to 3'-azido-3'-deoxythymidine. Lancet 1:132, 1987

Chapter 15

HIV Disease: Psychosocial Issues and Psychiatric Complications

LISA CAPALDINI

People with human immunodeficiency virus (HIV) disease are confronted with multiple psychosocial stressors at all stages of their illness. Sometimes, these stressors are life changes that are brought on by disease and require accommodations, such as dealing with finances, preparing a will, or transferring to a residential housing unit. Sometimes, they manifest themselves as psychiatric complications, such as depression, anxiety, and substance abuse. Patients' ability to cope with or prevent these complications depends on their pre-HIV psychologic status, their social and psychologic support network, and their stage of HIV disease.

Many of the psychosocial complications of HIV disease—including social isolation, personal distress, and specific psychiatric syndromes such as depression and panic disorder—are treatable. For this reason, all HIV caregivers should learn to recognize patients with these conditions and either treat such patients or refer them for treatment. For example, depression is one of the most common and treatable complications of advanced HIV disease. Even in patients with advanced acquired immunodeficiency syndrome (AIDS), effective treatment of depression may result in fewer physical symptoms, better sleep, and overall improvement in quality of life.

The optimal treatment of the psychosocial sequelae of HIV disease requires communication between the primary medical provider and mental health and social work consultants. The role of primary care providers includes:

- Familiarizing themselves with drug side effects that may cause complications, such as anxiety, depression, delirium, and mania.
- Identifying patients' coping styles and social resources.

- Referring patients when distress results in decreased compliance with medical treatment, significant psychologic problems, or decreased quality of life.

Because primary care providers are usually the first practitioners to witness these complications, they need to be familiar with the full range of medical and psychotherapeutic resources available to their patients. Finally, medical practitioners need to develop a referral network for mental health consultation or management if and when their patients develop a psychiatric syndrome that requires special management by mental health professionals.

By the same token, mental health professionals need to recognize that many HIV psychiatric syndromes mimicking pure functional disorders are likely to be of organic etiology. They need to be aware not only of medication side effects that result in psychiatric symptoms but also of the spectrum and natural history of HIV disease. In this way, primary caregivers and mental health professionals play complementary roles in counseling patients and their loved ones.

This chapter has three major sections. The first is a review of the major psychiatric syndromes seen with HIV disease: depression, anxiety/panic disorder, delirium, mania, and psychosis. The second is a summary of the issues that patients coping with HIV disease must face, with emphasis on caregivers' ability to help patients address multiple losses, helplessness, and role and lifestyle adjustments. The third section is a review of ethical/legal issues, pain control, sleep disorders, and caregiver coping issues.

MAJOR PSYCHIATRIC SYNDROMES

Like other life-threatening and chronic diseases, AIDS may be complicated by psychiatric symptoms. In some cases, these may be precipitated by discrete biologic or psychosocial stressors.[62] In other cases, substance abuse or mood disorder may predate actual HIV infection.[2,104] Diagnosis of psychiatric syndromes may be complicated by the significant overlap between symptoms of HIV disease per se (fatigue, weight loss, sleep disorder, decreased libido, concentration impairment) and symptoms of depression. Finally, organic HIV disease may mimic a purely functional syndrome. For instance, HIV organic brain disease may cause symptoms indistinguishable from functional psychosis.[17,120] Study of psychiatric syndromes seen in HIV disease is complicated by methodologic ambiguities both in psychiatric nomenclature and in the changing nomenclature used to describe stages of HIV disease itself. For example, certain studies do not make clear distinctions between major depression as defined by Diagnostic and Statistical Manual of Mental Disorders (DSM-III-R) criteria, dysthymia with acute depressed mood, adjustment disorder with depressed mood, and organic affective disorder due to either underlying HIV organic brain disease (OBD) or medication side effects.[123]

Classification of HIV disease has been modified several times over the last half decade. Older studies using terms such as ARC and AIDS are difficult to compare to more recent studies that use such characteristics as T-cell count, CDC stages, or Walter Reed classifications. With the recognition that there is wide variability in the functional status of HIV-infected people within given T-cell subsets and with specific complications of HIV disease (e.g., Kaposi's sarcoma), it has been increasingly difficult to compare patient cohorts between studies with any assurance of equivalent patient subgroups.

An examination of the nomenclature of HIV psychiatry shows inconsistencies in the differentiation of primary from second diagnoses. For example, many patients with HIV dementia (i.e., organic brain disease) may have disorders of mood and behavior rather than obvious disorders of cognition. In fact, the standard mental status examination is insensitive to the neuropsychiatric impairment present in many patients with HIV-related neurocognitive symptoms.[101] Some researchers may label the patients in one study cohort as "demented," whereas others may label them as "depressed with cognitive impairment." Despite these methodologic problems, it is clear that at least six significant neuropsychiatric syndromes complicate HIV disease. In a majority of cases, these occur as a complication of HIV OBD rather than as sequelae of non-HIV factors, such as substance abuse or pre-HIV psychiatric or morbid status.

HIV-related neuropsychologic impairment can precede a diagnosis of otherwise symptomatic HIV disease.[94] In a review of organic mental disorders caused by HIV, Perry[101] identifies six observations suggesting that organic mental changes due to HIV could precede other symptoms of HIV infection. First, the symptoms of mental slowing, social withdrawal, impaired concentration, and lethargy, which could be interpreted purely psychologically as an adjustment disorder, were found after more extensive testing to be a complication of subcortical dementia. Less frequently, acute psychosis, delirium, and depressive or manic episodes have been seen as the initial presentation of HIV disease. Second, multiple studies have demonstrated that HIV is present in the nervous system shortly after infection and recoverable in the cerebrospinal fluid of patients with no neurocognitive symptoms within months of infection. These data suggest that HIV may affect the central nervous system (CNS) long before other symptoms of HIV infection appear. Third, Perry notes that certain developmental abnormalities found in children do not necessarily parallel their physical illness pattern. Fourth, brain abnormalities on imaging studies have been identified in many patients with symptomatic HIV disease but without CNS symptoms. Fifth, subcortical abnormalities have been identified on neuropathologic studies. Investigators believe that these subcortical abnormalities might explain some of the ill-defined psychiatric abnormalities that are not consonant with a purely cortical (cognitive) disorder. Last, Perry notes that increased neuropsychologic impairment has been identified in HIV-infected people relative to seronegative control subjects, even in patients who were free of clinically identifiable illness.

The actual prevalence of neuropsychiatric disorders among HIV-infected people is not known with precision. Conversely, the incidence of HIV infection in psychiatric outpatients and inpatients has not been well defined either. One study[117] demonstrated that 7% of inpatients admitted to a voluntary psychiatric facility were HIV-positive. HIV dementia, which may be the sole manifestation of HIV disease in some patients, may in turn be complicated by personality changes or organic psychosis. Navia and Price[94] note in their study of 29 patients with AIDS dementia that 11 had concomitant personality changes, and 2 had a concomitant organic psychosis.

Two investigators have suggested that psychiatric disorders may be seen with increased prevalence in people at risk for HIV but who are not necessarily HIV-positive. In a study of 56 ambulatory gay men, some of whom were HIV-positive, Atkinson et al[2] found that gay men had an increased lifetime rate of alcohol or nonopiate drug abuse, generalized anxiety disorder, and major depression, which often preceded symptomatic HIV disease or knowledge of HIV status, compared to 22 healthy heterosexual controls. Perry et al[104] studied 207 physically asymptomatic adults who were attending a center for serologic testing for the HIV virus. They found that these subjects had a high lifetime rate of mood disorder and nonalcohol substance abuse. Significantly, however, Perry et al note that although these subjects had relatively higher lifetime rates of mood and substance abuse disorders, they did not show evidence of current DSM-III-R Axis I psychopathology. They emphasize that their data do not support the conclusion that individuals at risk for AIDS are a psychiatrically morbid population.

Psychiatric syndromes may complicate any of the stages of HIV disease. Even individuals who have not been tested and individuals who are known to be HIV-negative may experience HIV-related psychologic distress. Some experience anxiety about being tested, and even those who receive negative test results may still develop anxiety, depression, or even delusional disorders related to AIDS fears.[138]

Patients who recently have tested seropositive may experience transient anxiety and depression, adjustment disorder (i.e., a maladaptive reaction that interferes with functioning occurring within 3 months of testing and resolving within 6 months), anxiety disorder, major depression, or even brief reactive psychosis.[124] Shortly after testing, HIV-positive people are at increased risk of suicide. A study of active-duty Air Force members who were HIV-positive and attempted suicide showed that 46.7% attempted suicide within 3 months of learning they were seropositive, and four of the seven attempted suicide within the first week of notification.[115]

Focused psychoeducational interventions may help reduce the distress of patients who learn they are HIV seropositive.[103] At this time, counselors can also assist patients with medical referrals and address patients' questions about safe sex, confidentiality, and partner notification.

Many patients with HIV disease develop an emotional crisis at the time they first recognize HIV-related symptoms. Although the symptoms may be relatively insignificant (e.g., hairy leukoplakia), the psychologic meaning of these ostensibly mild symptoms may be overwhelming to the patient. For many patients with HIV disease, their first physical symptom is a concrete reminder that they are infected with a previously dormant virus that usually is lethal and that their life expectancy is, therefore, limited. It is at this time that many HIV-infected people may first seek medical care.

It is essential for the initial care provider to assess the patient's physical status and equally important to assess the impact and meaning of the patient's physical symptoms on his or her emotional well-being. Patients at this time may need guidance about coping with disease progression. This may include developing a personal and social support system, voicing fears about disability, learning about financial support in the event of progressive disability, and even discussing options about life-sustaining treatment in the event of rapid disease progression (J. Clarke, personal communication, 1993). Non–mental health specialists can provide patients with brief psychotherapeutic interventions during regular office appointments.[38] These interventions include clarifying the meaning of illness by helping to elucidate the meaning of specific symptoms for the patient. Sharing their concerns about and reactions to their symptoms often helps patients cope with their fears and limitations.[38] Reframing involves allowing a patient to interpret a situation in a manner that is more psychologically empowering. For example, when patients are diagnosed with cytomegalovirus (CMV) retinitis, they tend to focus on the fear of losing their vision and on the inconvenience of receiving chronic parenteral medication. Pointing out that treatment of their CMV eye disease may well result in overall physical improvement, such as weight gain, increased energy, and decreased fevers, may help patients see the treatment not just as a burden but as an opportunity to improve their overall health.

The aim of role reversal or projection of the problem is to have patients view their own problems with compassion or objectivity. Many patients worry about burdening their loved ones and may thus be reluctant to ask for help or disclose the complications of their illness. Sometimes, placing the patient in the loved one's position (e.g., "If your mother had a serious disease, would you want her to tell you so that you would have the opportunity to help her?") gives patients the insight to help them interact with their support network and caregivers more constructively. Eisendrath[38] notes that problem- and solution-oriented approaches like these may not always be successful but can be useful for many patients and readily applied by a variety of practitioners. Many times, other members of the health care team, such as a physical therapist, home care nurse, or social worker, may be able to profoundly palliate the patient's feeling of loss of control and meaninglessness by addressing these concerns in such a pragmatic, solution-oriented way.

The importance of all caregivers helping their clients develop coping strategies cannot be overestimated.[23,60,75] Isolation, fear, anxiety, and marginalization are common psychosocial complications of chronic or disabling diseases. In a groundbreaking study of the effect of psychosocial treatment on the survival of patients of metastatic breast cancer, Spiegel et al[125] demonstrate that a psychosocial intervention could significantly improve the life expectancy of women with a systemic advanced disease. Other researchers[21,40,65] have elucidated a connection between immunologic function and stressors and have suggested that immunocompetence in HIV-infected people may be related to primary neuropsychiatric parameters, such as depression and distress.[65,112] One study of upwardly mobile gay men notes that psychologic resilience correlated with long-term survival.[111] Taylor et al[129] note that psychologic optimism correlated with a psychologically adaptive response to being HIV infected. Folkman et al[48] note that coping styles correlated well with the presence or absence of high-risk sexual behavior. Coping style may of itself affect the social support the patient may seek in an effort to adapt to HIV disease.[23,139] To date, no controlled, randomized studies definitively prove that psychosocial intervention can favorably alter the history of HIV disease[18,80,102] or prevent morbid psychiatric outcomes, such as substance abuse or suicide. Given the established prevalence and profound psychosocial and physical impact of these psychiatric complications, however, an active effort toward recognition, prevention, and treatment of psychiatric disease is warranted.

Six major neuropsychiatric syndromes have been identified as complications of HIV disease. They are depression, dementia/organic brain disease, anxiety/panic disorder, delirium, mania, and psychosis. Each complication is addressed separately, although many of these conditions may overlap in any given patient (e.g., patients with organic brain disease with prominent cognitive defects may also have features of depression or psychosis).

Wolcott et al[138] outline five general principles of assessment of suspected neuropsychiatric disorders in patients with HIV disease:

- All new psychiatric disorders should be considered secondary to a neuropsychiatric complication of HIV disease until thorough evaluation indicates otherwise.
- Organic mental disorder may appear weeks to months before an underlying primary CNS disease becomes apparent.
- Neurodiagnostic tests may be normal or nondiagnostic in patients with HIV-related organic mental disease or underlying primary CNS disease or both.
- Careful preventive screening is crucial to the early diagnosis of organic mental disease because mental status changes are often the first clinical sign of primary CNS changes, many of which are treatable.
- Primary care physicians and practitioners should consider early patient referral when HIV-related neuropsychiatric disorder is suspected.

Depression

Depression may be especially prevalent and difficult to diagnose in medically ill patients.[25,105] This is particularly true of HIV disease, where life stressors, premorbid psychiatric predispositions, specific organic complications, and centrally acting medications may all predispose to depression. Several studies have established that depression is more common in medical outpatients, patients with cancer, and especially patients with diseases affecting the CNS.[24,71] Other studies have established that in the primary care setting, practitioners tend to underrecognize and misdiagnose depression.[52,100] Finally, studies of patients with depression and comorbid medical illnesses have demonstrated that depression and chronic medical conditions have additive, even synergistic effects on physical and social functioning[11,16,41,136] and that failure to identify and treat even milder forms of depression may result in increased social morbidity.[14,15]

Early reports of depression and HIV disease suggested that depression was a widespread syndrome in HIV disease. These studies, however, were not well controlled and essentially relied on self-reporting. More recent studies using standardized depression rating scales suggest that the current prevalence of depression is between 4% and 14% in non–drug-using HIV-positive of 5% people, compared to a general prevalence rate in the population.[109]

The psychiatric diagnosis of major depression as currently defined cannot be made unless the patient exhibits five of the nine following symptoms during a 2-week period. In addition, either one of the first two symptoms must be present. The symptoms are (1) depressed mood, (2) markedly diminished pleasure in all activities, (3) significant and unintentional weight loss or gain, (4) insomnia or oversleeping, (5) fidgetiness or slowed movement or speech (psychomotor agitation or slowing), (6) fatigue or loss of energy, (7) feelings of worthlessness or excessive inappropriate guilt, (8) diminished ability to think or concentrate, and (9) recurrent suicidal thoughts. Clearly, many of these symptoms are also symptoms of primary HIV disease, specifically weight loss, increased sleeping or difficulty sleeping, psychomotor slowing (which may be a symptom of primary HIV dementia), fatigue, and diminished ability to think or concentrate. Thus, there is a significant overlap between common organic complications of HIV disease and the screening symptoms for depression.[98] Noting this diagnostic and methodologic difficulty, Fernandez and Levy recommend screening for depression in a diagnostically inclusive way.[46] With this method, all symptoms consistent with either depression or primary physical disease are included as possible symptoms of depression until proven otherwise. In patients with psychologic symptoms that improve after treatment of a primary disease, it can be safely concluded that the neuropsychiatric syndrome was indeed secondary to primary organic physical disease. Without such an inclusive approach to diagnosis, depression will go unrecognized in most patients with HIV disease because all their symptoms can be "accounted for" by the progression of their disease.

Another methodologic problem in diagnosing depression in patients with HIV disease is the significant overlap between symptoms of depression and symptoms of encephalopathy/OBD.[55] Like the geriatric population,[141] HIV-positive patients are at risk for both depression and dementia. Many of the symptoms of these two diseases overlap, such as forgetfulness, decreased concentration, sleep disturbance, behavioral abnormalities, and depressed mood. Early signs of HIV organic brain disease, such as forgetfulness, loss of interest in work, decreased libido, blunted affect, withdrawal, and poor concentration, can be easily misdiagnosed as a primary depressive problem.[62] Although surrogate markers for HIV disease, such as T-cell testing and viral load measurement, are clearly not adequately sensitive to rule out OBD in HIV-positive patients with high T-cell counts and low or undetectable viral load, the presence of cognitive symptoms in patients with relatively good physical health and good surrogate marker parameters is more consistent with a depressive reaction than a demential disorder. Researchers in the geriatric population have developed special geriatric depression scales to help differentiate the expected physical symptoms of aging, such as sleep disorder and concern about health status, from specific symptoms of depression, determinable by responses to such questions as "Do you often get bored?" and "Are you in good spirits most of the time?"[141] At this time, no specific depression screening scales like these have been used in the HIV-positive population. Clearly, they would be a useful diagnostic instrument to help clinicians differentiate core physical symptoms of HIV disease from affective complications of OBD and both of these from cognitive complications of OBD.

Finally, depression is often overlooked as a comorbid complication of medical disease because it may seem situationally appropriate: "I'd be depressed, too, if I had AIDS." Although clinical depression is more frequent in the medically ill, clinical depression is never a normal finding in people with HIV disease, any more than mechanical falls are normal in the elderly. Even when depression is a sequela of life-threatening, multisystem diseases like AIDS or cancer, it can be effectively diagnosed and treated.[41,105]

The causes of depression in HIV-positive patients are multiple. All patients with HIV disease, regardless of physical health status, face fundamental questions regarding the quality and length of their lives. Specific stressors experienced by HIV-positive people may include prolonged periods of physical discomfort, disability, and dependence; lifestyle disruption; loss of work and reduced socioeconomic status; disruption of support networks including family supports; decreased self-esteem; and sustained periods of loss of personal autonomy.[26,138] Also, some medications used to treat HIV disease may themselves cause depression, including zidovudine (Retrovir or AZT),[132,136] acyclovir,[134] anticonvulsants,[134] corticosteroids,[134] dapsone,[134] H_2-receptor antagonists,[134] interferon-α,[134] isoniazid,[134] metoclopramide,[134] nonsteroidal antiinflammatory drugs,[134] and sulfonamides.[134] In evaluation of HIV-positive patients with symptoms of depression, it is critical to rule out intercurrent primary CNS complications, such as meningitis, encephalitis, or space-occupying CNS lesions. All of these aforementioned complications are extremely rare in patients with CD4 (helper) counts greater than $200/mm^3$. HIV-positive patients with depressive symptoms also need to be carefully screened for substance abuse because chronic substance abuse also can cause depressive symptoms.

Although medical and social advances may help people with HIV disease live longer, these long-term survivors often must cope with more physical limitations (fatigue, pain, medication side effects), emotional stressors (loss of many friends to AIDS, isolation, fear of overtaxing caregivers), and spiritual struggles (struggling with the meaning of suffering, when/if ''to give up'') (R. Arpin, personal communication, 1993). Long-term survivors of HIV disease, although often temperamentally very psychologically hardy, are at high risk for depression as they cope with survivor's guilt, uncertainty about their ultimate prognosis, or multiple medical problems.

Depression can be safely and effectively treated by non–mental health professionals if the primary care practitioner is able to direct the time and attention to the recognition and management of this disorder.[37] In the Western industrialized world, the majority of patients with depression are treated in the primary care setting by general practitioners, family practitioners, and general internists. The principles of treating depression in HIV-positive patients are quite similar to those of treating depression in the general population and in medically ill patients. Some specific caveats in this setting are that HIV-positive patients may be especially

prone to disorientation with anticholinergic agents, such as sedating tricyclic antidepressants, especially if the patient has a preexisting cognitive impairment.[45] Second, patients with AIDS seem to be more prone to drug side effects and incomplete therapeutic responses than are seronegative patients.[46] Third, as noted below, stimulants may be a particularly effective treatment for depression in physically fatigued or cognitively impaired HIV-positive patients with depressive symptoms.[45]

Non–mental health professionals may be understandably reluctant to treat depression because it is a complication outside of their usual range of practice. Nonetheless, it is important to recognize that many physicians who treat HIV-positive patients have learned in effect to practice subspecialty care (i.e., in diagnosing and treating complex infections, dermatologic, neurologic, and hematologic complications of HIV disease). It is important for primary practitioners treating HIV-positive patients to familiarize themselves with the recognition and, ideally, the treatment of depression because many HIV-positive patients may not have the personal resources to obtain specific mental health care or may be unwilling to be treated in a mental health setting. More importantly, the primary care practitioner, being aware of the full spectrum of the patient's medical diagnoses, is in the ideal situation to help select medical therapy when pharmacologic intervention is appropriate for the treatment of depression.

As with seronegative patients who manifest depression, the consideration governing the choice of an antidepressant is not so much to optimize efficacy as to avoid or exploit medication side effects.[27,46] Parallels can be drawn between the treatment of depression in HIV-positive patients with symptomatic complications of HIV disease and, for example, common management of hypertension in patients with other medical disorders. For example, in treating hypertension in the elderly patient with postural hypertension, a physician would avoid drugs likely to aggravate orthostatic hypotension, such as centrally acting agents or α-adrenergic blockers. Similarly, a physician treating a patient with hypertension and angina would tend to use a β-blocker or calcium channel blocker because it would ameliorate both medical conditions. Similarly, in the case of depression, physicians should pick a medication that does not exacerbate prior symptoms and has the potential of ameliorating other symptoms of HIV disease (Table 15–1). For example, some patients

TABLE 15–1. ANTIDEPRESSANTS

Name (Trade Name)	Starting Dose	Therapeutic Dose (Oral)	Comments
Tricyclic Antidepressants (TCA)			
Amitriptylene (Elavil)	10–25 mg qhs	125–250 mg	Very sedating, very anticholinergic
Doxepin (Sinequan)	10–25 mg qhs	150–300 mg	Very sedating, an excellent antihistamine (can treat bid)
Nortriptylene (Aventyl, Pamelor)	25–50 mg qhs	75–200 mg	Has the least anticholinergic effects of tricyclics; established efficacy in neuropathy pain palliation
Desipramine (Norpramin)	25–50 mg	150–300 mg	The least sedating of tricyclics; good choice for treating peripheral neuropathy pain
Selective Serotonin Reuptake Inhibitors (SSRIs)			
Fluoxetine (Prozac)	10–20 mg qAM	20–80 mg	Has longest half-life of SSRIs and most prone to cause stimulant symptoms initially
Sertraline (Zoloft)	25–50 mg qAM	50–200 mg	Most likely to cause GI side effects
Paroxitene (Paxil)	10–20 mg qAM	25–50 mg	If daytime drowsiness occurs, initially can take qhs
Fluvoxamine (Luvox)	25 mg qhs	50–200 mg	*Note:* SSRIs as a class may be more prone to cause sexual dysfunction than other non-TCA antidepressants
Chloropropiophenones			
Bupropion (Wellbutrin)	75 mg bid	75–100 mg tid	Usually well-tolerated; tid dosing may compromise compliance; contraindicated in patients with unstable seizure disorders
Unclassified			
Venlafaxine (Effexor)	(1/2) 37.5 mg bid	50–100 mg bid	Start at very low doses to minimize agitation
Stimulants			
Methylphenidate (Ritalin)	5 mg qAM, early afternoon (bid)	10–60 mg daily	
Dextroamphetamine (Dexadrine)	5 mg qAM	5–40 mg daily	
MAO Inhibitors	Contraindicated		See text

with HIV disease have a syndrome of dry mouth similar to Sjögren's disease. In these patients, it is best to avoid tricyclic antidepressants with significant anticholinergic side effects because these are likely to aggravate the dry mouth condition. In patients with cognitive disorder along with depression, drugs with significant anticholinergic side effects should be avoided because they can aggravate cognitive impairment. Conversely, patients with HIV-related dermatitis and pruritus, whether due to underlying dry skin or idiopathic, may benefit from taking an antidepressant with significant antihistamine effects, such as doxepin, at bedtime. In this case, the clinician would have to weigh the benefits of reducing nighttime itching against the benefits and risks of inducing sedation and anticholinergic side effects.

With the advent of the newer antidepres-

sants, such as selective serotonin reuptake inhibitors (SSRIs) and bupropion (Wellbutrin), the clinician has a good range of well-tolerated antidepressants from which to choose.

In the case of tricyclic antidepressants, medications fall along a spectrum in which the most sedating medications tend also to have the most anticholinergic side effects. The prototype of this type of tricyclic antidepressant is amitriptyline (Elavil). Low doses of amitriptyline may help to induce sleep but may leave patients with morning somnolence or confusion. Low doses of amitriptyline occasionally are very helpful for chronic pain syndromes, but the same caveats regarding somnolence apply. In general, most consultants treating HIV-positive patients for depression recommend using less sedating medicines with fewer anticholinergic effects.[98] Dosing guidelines need to be based on the patient's overall physical and psychologic health. For example, in patients with advanced AIDS, who often have compromised hepatic and renal function and whose physiology may approximate that of geriatric patients, antidepressants should be begun in lower than standard dosages and be titrated upward very slowly until the desired clinical result is achieved. In HIV-positive patients in good physical health, standard doses of antidepressants may be safely initiated. In general, the optimal tricyclic antidepressant for people with HIV-related depression is either nortriptyline, which has the fewest anticholinergic side effects of all tricyclic antidepressants, beginning at a dosage of 25 mg/day, or desipramine, which has the least sedating effect of the tricyclic antidepressants, beginning at 50 mg/day.

The advent of SSRIs has provided physicians with three new and very helpful alternatives to tricyclic antidepressants. These new medications are paroxitene (Paxil), sertraline (Zoloft), fluoxetine (Prozac), and fluvoxamine (Luvox). In general, SSRIs have minimal anticholinergic side effects and rarely cause sustained sedation, although sedation occasionally may be a side effect in the induction phase of medication, particularly with paroxitene. These medications also tend not to exacerbate functional gastrointestinal and genitourinary symptoms, such as decreased gastric emptying and incomplete bladder emptying, which are commonly seen to complicate HIV disease.

The two main disadvantages of SSRIs are that they initially can have a stimulant effect, which patients with preexisting anxiety may find intolerable, and that they tend to cause sexual dysfunction, which may not recede with continued use of the medication. It is important to advise a patient of both of these potential side effects of SSRIs. In general, the initial stimulant effect tends to diminish with continued use of the medication, whereas symptoms of sexual dysfunction tend to be chronic. If the latter symptoms persist, an alternative medication may be indicated.

Unlike initial doses of tricyclic antidepressants, which are generally one third to one quarter of the final therapeutic dose, the initial starting dose of SSRIs as generally recommended may be also the final therapeutic dose. In patients who need to avoid the initial stimulant effect, it *can* be helpful to start at half-dose therapy. In the case of fluoxetine in capsule form, this can be accomplished by dissolving the 20-mg capsule in apple juice and drinking half the apple juice every other day to equal a 10-mg dose.

A significant benefit of the SSRIs is that they pose less risk of suicide in the overdose setting. The potential disadvantages are that, to date, SSRIs have not been shown in randomized controlled studies to ameliorate peripheral neuropathy as have some of the tricyclic antidepressants, such as nortriptyline (Pamelor), amitriptyline (Elavil), and desipramine. Additionally, these tricyclics have been shown to ameliorate chronic pain, which is a common symptom of depression in advanced HIV disease. An important area of future research addressing the treatment of depression in the setting of HIV disease is these other potential benefits of antidepressant therapy.

Bupropion (Wellbutrin) is another newer antidepressant that tends to have fewer sedating effects than the tricyclic antidepressants and milder stimulant effects than the SSRIs. A disadvantage is that it must be administered two to three times a day. This dosing schedule may pose problems for patients with dementia and for unsupervised patients. Bupropion is contraindicated in patients with unstable seizure disorders. Seizures have been noted in patients receiving over 300 mg/day of medication. It is known that advanced HIV disease may be complicated by seizures in the absence of known primary CNS disease. In patients with advanced HIV disease, higher doses of bupropion should be used cautiously because of the possibility of inducing seizures. To date, this specific complication has not been reported in HIV-positive patients.

Venlafaxine (Effexor) is a novel antidepressant that inhibits reuptake of both serotonin and norepinephrine. While most widely used to treat patients who have been refractory to other antidepressants,[96] it is also a well-tolerated first-line agent. Venlafaxine should be started at low doses to avoid severe agitation or anxiety that can occur with too rapid drug initiation.

Monoamine oxidase (MAO) inhibitors have been used for decades in the treatment of depression. Although highly effective, they are extremely risky to use in patients with cognitive deficits because patients using MAO inhibitors must be very careful about their diet and concomitant medication intake. Because patients with HIV disease generally take multiple medications and may be prone to dementia, MAO inhibitors should not be used in the treatment of affective disorders associated with HIV disease. If it is considered, MAO therapy should be initiated and monitored by a psychiatric consultant.

Stimulants such as methylphenidate (Ritalin) and dextroamphetamine have been used in the treatment of depression in the medically ill with good success. Stimulants tend to be more rapidly effective than standard antidepressants and are well tolerated in the medically ill.[4,45,49,73,97,119,140] Fernandez et al[43,63] have used stimulants in treating cognitive impairment due to AIDS-related OBD as well as cognitive impairment with attendant affective dysfunction. In their series, 90% of patients showed at least moderate response to stimulants, and no adverse effects were encountered. The maximum dose of methylphenidate used was 90 mg/day in divided doses. In the case of dextroamphetamine, 60 mg/day in divided doses was used.

Stimulants can be especially effective for patients with acute despondency related to acute medical disease. In this situation, stimulants may allow patients to mobilize their emotional resources to cope with the losses attendant with their disease and may enhance compliance with the therapeutic regimen. The standard initial dose of dextroamphetamine is 5 to 10 mg every morning with an optional supplemental dose at noon. Some patients experience a dysphoric stimulatory effect that they describe as being "wired." In these patients, stimulants are ineffective and should be discontinued. Although stimulants in general are not appropriate treatment for depression unrelated to medical illness, partly because tachyphylaxis is commonly seen, stimulants may be effective short- to moderate-term therapy for patients with advanced medical illness secondary to HIV disease. Stimulants are contraindicated in patients with a prior history of psychostimulant abuse.

Once an antidepressant is chosen, antidepressant therapy should be continued for 6 to 8 weeks to assess the patient's response to a specific dose. In cases where rapid amelioration of depression is necessary, dosages may be escalated more quickly with the understanding that dosages may need to be adjusted downward if and when medication side effects ensue.

Once an effective dosage is found, it should be continued for at least 6 months unless the patient develops a medication side effect or requires a dosage increase because of intercurrent stressors or drug malabsorption.

Depression, like hypertension, is a physiologically and biochemically heterogeneous disorder. The only medical information that can help predict medication efficacy in a given patient is a family history of favorable medication response to a particular medication. One advantage of tricyclic therapy is that serum levels may be obtained for some tricyclics to confirm that the patient is taking the medication and that the serum levels are in the therapeutic range. Mental health experts disagree as to the necessity and appropriateness of monitoring serum levels, with many arguing that in the absence of side effects and in the presence of a good clinical response, serum level determinations are not necessary. Serum levels are not obtainable in clinical practice for the SSRIs, bupropion, or stimulants. Medication titration in that setting is based on presence or absence of side effects and clinical response to the medication.

Anecdotal reports suggest that insomnia with early morning awakening may be a specific neuropsychiatric complication of HIV disease apart from any associated primary psychiatric disease, such as depression.[137] In this case, a low dose of a relatively sedating antidepressant such as doxepin or amitriptyline may be appropriate. In low doses (e.g., 50 mg) trazodone is also a useful sedating antidepressant but must be used with caution in men because it can cause priapism.

Psychotherapy and psychopharmocology play complementary roles in the treatment of HIV-associated depression.[86,88] While medication often relieves many of the physical and mood symptoms of depression, most patients can benefit from an opportunity to share their fears and suffering with a skilled therapist and/or within a support group. Traditional "open-ended" psychotherapeutic approaches are often inappropriate for people with HIV disease, especially those with advanced disease—therapeutic flexibility is especially important for these patients whose needs may rapidly change from session to session.[85,142]

Patients who do not respond to one or two antidepressants should be referred for psychiatric consultation. Causes of treatment resistance include comorbid psychiatric conditions, comorbid medical illness, and family issues.[36]

In summary, depression is extremely common in patients with chronic medical disorders, life-threatening diseases, and diseases affecting the central nervous system, all characteristic of HIV disease. Depression is common, is associated with significant morbidity, and is often partly if not fully reversible with appropriate intervention. Clinicians can best treat depression by screening all their patients with HIV disease for depression and by regularly assessing their patients for depression just as they might regularly assess a patient's PPD status or safe-sex practices.

Dementia

Several studies have established that AIDS dementia complex (ADC) or OBD is a common complication of AIDS and one that is quite variable in its presentation and severity.[9,35,62,93,101,138] The precise prevalence of ADC depends both on the overall stage of HIV disease of any given patient population and on the neuropsychiatric testing and criteria used to make the diagnosis. Researchers have reached conflicting conclusions about the prevalence of subtle neuropsychiatric impairment in functionally and clinically asymptomatic seropositive patients.[95,101] Overall, possibly 10% of people with AIDS have a comorbid neurologic disorder at the time of their index diagnosis, with 70% experiencing organic brain disease during the course of their illness, 66% experiencing moderate to severe impairment, and 33% having mild or subclinical symptoms. Autopsy studies show evidence of HIV-related CNS abnormalities in approximately 90% of patients with AIDS.[35,138]

Although on some level the subcortical dementia of HIV disease is technically a neurologic complication of AIDS, its clinical manifestations are often behavioral, cognitive, or psychiatric.[35,62] For example, in some patients with organic brain impairment, the primary presenting symptom may be psychomotor agitation, impaired social or occupational functioning, impairment of judgment, personality changes, mood and cognitive symptoms suggestive of depression, and even psychosis.[35,93,94] The overlap between these cognitive, affective, and functional symptoms may make accurate diagnosis difficult. Although neurocognitive examination may be helpful in identifying clinically occult cognitive impairment, standard neuropsychiatric examinations, including the standard mental status examinations, may not identify abnormalities in substantial numbers of patients with mild organic brain disease.[101] Moreover, the type and severity of symptoms a patient manifests may vary greatly with the clinical situation (e.g., a scheduled routine office visit versus hospitalization for an acute febrile illness), and with other confounding intercurrent factors, such as medication use, substance abuse, and intercurrent psychosocial stressors. Studies of patients with HIV-associated depression, mania, and delirium have established that many of these patients have comorbid OBD and that in many instances the actual etiology of these neuropsychiatric symptoms may indeed be OBD.[101,138] Thus, clinicians caring for patients manifesting any neuropsychiatric symptoms should screen the patient carefully for associated OBD. This screening should consist of administering standard basic mental status examinations as well as taking a careful history from family, friends, or co-workers who can provide useful information about the patient's functional status. Often, the first clue to function-threatening OBD may be inability to complete ordinary work tasks in a prompt manner or problems managing routine household responsibilities. In the case of children, OBD may be manifested by developmental abnormalities even in the absence of other symptoms of HIV disease.[101]

Clinicians treating HIV-associated dementia need to consider zidovudine therapy for potential reversal or slowing of the dementia process,[9,20] providing optimal milieu management for the patient, and providing appropriate practical and psychosocial support for the patient's loved ones. One published study[9] and several anecdotal reports (J. Clarke, personal communication, 1993) suggest that treatment with zidovudine may ameliorate the symptoms and natural history of HIV dementia. Some patients with even relatively severe cognitive impairments have been known to exhibit remarkable behavioral and cognitive improvement after receiving zidovudine therapy in supervised settings. Of note, the patients described in these anecdotal reports have taken doses of zidovudine larger than those now generally used, usually in the 800-mg/day range.[107] When HIV-associated OBD is complicated by symptoms of depression, the optimal treatment may not be standard antidepressant therapy but stimulant therapy.[43,63] Studies of stimulant therapy for patients with AIDS-related cognitive impairment and associated organic affective disorders have demonstrated that stimulants may improve both the cognitive status and mood of the patient and are safe even in patients with advanced AIDS. Symptoms of depression in patients with dementia may not take the form of standard mood changes but instead may be reflected in the patient's neglect of personal needs, such as hygiene and nutrition, or the patient's indifference to the environment, the disease, and medical treatments.[35] In patients with dementia, tricyclic antidepressants should be used with caution because those antidepressants with high anticholinergic receptor affinities are apt to increase confusion.[138]

Milieu management involves carefully assessing a patient's neurocognitive status (motor function, orientation, and memory) and adjusting the environment accordingly to maximize the patient's autonomy and to minimize the patient's risk.[10,22] The patient's need for supervision must be assessed carefully as well, be it by a health professional or by family members.[35] A home safety assessment should be conducted by a home nurse or social worker. The person making this assessment should check for the presence of reality-orientation cues, such as calendars and clocks, and ensure that hallways and living areas are brightly lit, that walkways are clear and free of electrical wires or unstable furniture, and that potentially dangerous items, such as sharp objects, chemicals and poisons, and power tools, are safely stored away. In addition, knobs should be removed from stoves to ensure that a confused patient will not inadvertently burn himself or herself or set fire to the home.

Milieu management also involves managing the patient's milieu on a communication level. Patients and their caregivers often find that communication difficulties are the most frustrating and heartwrenching complications of OBD. Many caregivers may feel inadequate in the face of an unpredictably angry, agitated, or incommunicative loved one despite their best efforts at compassionate and "36-hours-per-day" care. Helpful communication techniques include:

- Asking the patient simple yes-or-no questions. Avoiding lengthy explanations and instead giving short, pragmatic answers.
- Remembering that long-term memory is often intact and, thus, sharing remote reminiscences might be soothing—by contrast, immediate memory is likely to be quite impaired and, thus, immediate recall efforts may be frustrating for the patient.
- Speaking in a low-pitched, even tone of voice.

Caregivers need to be instructed in this technique as well as in specific techniques to help confused, agitated patients.

It is also critical for medical caregivers to assess the well-being of the patient's family and other caregivers. As brain disease advances, the patient may become less communicative. The caregiver may in effect lose his or her loved one before the patient's actual physical death. Some caregivers may respond to this loss by inappropriately increasing the time and intensity of their practical home efforts. Families and caregivers of patients with OBD need to be encouraged to take regular respites and to voice their needs. They, too, need to be monitored for signs of burnout or depression.[35]

The patient's home-based caregivers are much more likely to cope well and respond appropriately to the patient's increasing disability if they have some sense of understanding of the course of the disease and the types of measures they can take when problems arise. Simple instruction in basic techniques, such as managing patient transfers, dealing with incontinence, responding to agitation, and dealing with unpredictable behavior, can enhance caregivers' coping abilities and help them play a more practical and meaningful role in their loved one's care (C. Adams, personal communication, 1993).[4,50]

Wolcott et al[138] summarize the principles of management of patients with OBD as follows. First, clinicians should minimize drugs with CNS toxicity and recognize that some drugs used to treat HIV disease may in themselves cause or aggravate symptoms of ADC. Second, psychosocial treatment should begin early in the treatment of OBD. With appropriate intervention, a patient may develop "compensatory prostheses" to compensate for impaired cognitive function. In addition, at the time of recognition of OBD, early arrangements should be made for assessment of terminal care wishes and to arrange legal matters, such as wills and power of attorney. Social treatment also involves initiating appropriate home care services and, as importantly, appropriate respite services for home-based caregivers.

Wolcott et al also outline several principles of pharmacologic treatment of patients with OBD. First, medically ill patients with OBD should be begun on low doses of antidepressants or stimulants or medium to low doses of neuroleptics, with doses gradually adjusted to minimize CNS complications. Second, cognitively impaired patients manifesting depression may respond better to stimulants than to antidepressants, and psychotic syndromes, be they organic or functional, should be treated with the lowest effective dose of neuroleptics[45,138] (Table 15–2).

TABLE 15–2. NEUROLEPTIC/ANTIPSYCHOTIC MEDICATIONS

Relative Potency (Trade Name)	Starting (Oral) Adult Dose	Therapeutic Adult Daily Dose	Comments
Low potency (Thorazine, Mellaril)	25–50 mg q8–12h	50–800 mg	Very sedating/anticholinergic, low-risk EPS
Midpotency (Trilafon)	4 mg q8–12h	12–64 mg	Medium range risk for sedation/anticholinergic/EPS side effects
High potency (Haldol)	1–2 mg q6–8h	2–10 mg	Low risk for sedation, anticholinergic side effects, high EPS; case reports in AIDS patients of neuroleptic malignant syndrome

Clearly, dementia is one of the most heartbreaking and medically challenging complications of HIV disease. Effective disease recognition by the clinician requires a high index of suspicion of dementia whenever the patient manifests neurocognitive symptoms. Effective treatment of dementia in the AIDS setting requires a thorough understanding of the patient's medical status as well as his or her home situation and support network. Finally, patients with HIV-related dementia who remain at home need a well-coordinated interdisciplinary approach to make their home-based care safe, comprehensive, and humane.

Anxiety/Panic Disorder

Anxiety is commonly experienced by HIV-positive patients. When it is chronic and global, it is described as a generalized anxiety disorder. Manifestations of this may include trouble falling asleep, impaired concentration, psychomotor agitation, and fatigue. Anxiety also may be a complication of medications, including anticonvulsants, corticosteroids, ganciclovir, nonsteroidal antiinflammatory drugs, and sulfonamides.[134] Anxiety also may be due to drug withdrawal, and all patients with new symptoms of anxiety should be carefully screened for drug withdrawal or substance use. Discrete episodes of anxiety characterized by physiologic flight-or-fight symptoms, such as palpitations, shortness of breath, dizziness, headache, paresthesias, derealization, and depersonalization, are called panic attacks. Panic attacks are seen in increased frequency in the primary care setting relative to the population in general.[72] Panic disorder is also commonly seen with major depression, alcohol abuse, and posttraumatic stress disorders.[72]

In choosing therapy for anxiety or panic disorder, the clinician and patient must decide whether to use quick and short-acting medicines (e.g., alprazolam [Xanax] or lorazepam [Ativan]) to ameliorate intermittent symptoms or whether to use long-acting round-the-clock antianxiety medications (e.g., clonazepam [Klonopin]) to prevent chronic anxiety (Table 15–3). In general, patients with relatively infrequent and predictable anxiety, such as before an office visit, can be managed well with small doses of quick and short-acting antianxiety medicines. Conversely, patients with chronic anxiety are best managed with scheduled doses of long-acting antianxiety medicines to prevent breakthrough anxiety or anxiety secondary to withdrawal from anxiolytic agents. In these cases of chronic anxiety, buspirone (BuSpar)

TABLE 15–3. ANXIOLYTICS

Name (Trade Name)	Starting Dose	Therapeutic Dose	Comments
Clonazepam (Klonopin)	0.5 mg bid	0.5–2 mg bid	Excellent long-acting, round-the-clock anxiolytic; onset of action slow
Lorazepam (Ativan)	0.5–1 mg q8h prn	0.5–2 mg q8h prn	Rapid onset of action, no active metabolites
Alprazolam (Xanax)	0.5–1 mg q8h prn	0.5–2 mg q8h prn	Rapid onset of action
Buspirone (Buspar)	10 mg tid	10–15 mg tid	Nonsedating, nonaddictive; not useful for acute anxiety; suitable for patients with chronic anxiety

may be quite useful. Although it may take up to 2 to 3 weeks for buspirone to be fully effective as an anxiolytic, it has the great advantage of being nonaddictive and of not causing respiratory depression.[133] Buspirone has been shown in one study to help reduce anxiety and drug use in drug users with AIDS or AIDS-related complex.[5] Buspirone is not effective for treatment of acute anxiety. In cases where a long-acting anxiolytic is indicated, clonazepam can be titrated between 0.5 and 2 mg orally twice a day. Because many comorbid psychiatric conditions, such as substance abuse, can be seen with anxiety, patients need to be carefully screened for concomitant psychiatric conditions before anxiolytic therapy is undertaken.

Panic attacks, in particular, may mimic physiologic symptoms of HIV complications, such as shortness of breath or dizziness. Certain clues suggest that the symptoms stem from a panic attack rather than a primary organic complication of HIV disease. A panic attack is suspected if the physical symptoms are situational (e.g., occurring before an important laboratory study or on the anniversary of the death of a loved one) or if the symptoms produce significant apprehension out of proportion to the fear the patient experiences with analogous physical symptoms. Patients with panic disorder typically have multiple symptoms involving multiple organ systems during panic attacks. Panic attacks may last from minutes to hours and are often self-limited. Panic disorder is commonly complicated by agoraphobia. Clues to the presence of panic disorder include a previous patient history of depression or a family history of either panic disorder or depression.

Long-term therapy of panic disorder generally is best achieved with antidepressant medications. Tricyclic antidepressants have historically been the mainstay in treatment of panic disorder. However, the new agents, such as SSRIs and bupropion, theoretically also may be effective against panic disorders and should be considered in cases where tricyclic antidepressant therapy is contraindicated. It is important to recognize that although patients with panic disorder may not be overtly depressed, they are at high risk for suicide. Although there are no published reports of HIV-positive people with panic disorder committing suicide, it is clear that in the general population, patients with panic disorder are at significant risk for suicide and need to be monitored accordingly.

Patients receiving short-acting benzodiazepines need to be counseled about the possibility of drug withdrawal when these medicines are discontinued. In general, these medicines should be tapered rather than abruptly stopped. In the case of longer-acting benzodiazepines, tapering is partly achieved by the long-acting nature of the medicine, but a short taper should be considered when patients have been on long-acting benzodiazepines for a considerable period of time.

Delirium

Delirium is a serious complication of any illness, and HIV disease is no exception. The causes of delirium can include primary CNS opportunistic infections, drug side effects, systemic illness, and primary functional disease related to disorientation and confusion. Patients with delirium have a very guarded medical prognosis and should be managed accordingly, with an inclusive diagnostic approach that incorporates frequent reevaluation by the caregiver.

Important specific causes of delirium in the medically ill HIV-positive patient include hypoglycemia or hypotension due to intravenous pentamidine therapy, hyperkalemia secondary to high-dose trimethoprim-sulfamethoxazole (Septra) therapy, severe agitation due to high-dose corticosteroid therapy, electrolyte disorders due to renal tubular dysfunction secondary to foscarnet or amphotericin therapy, hypoxemia secondary to respiratory illness, hyponatremia secondary to syndrome of inappropriate antidiuretic hormone (SIADH) or hypotonic fluid administration, acute disinhibitory states due to use of benzodiazepines or other sedatives, and use of or withdrawal from recreational drugs.[46]

The general principles of treating delirium in HIV-positive patients are the same as those of patients in general.[1,45,47,51,128,138] General treatment measures include providing orienting information, minimizing disruption of the sleep/wake cycle, avoiding medications with CNS side effects, and treating agitation with appropriate pharmacologic intervention.[138]

Experts disagree as to the optimal pharmacologic treatment of HIV-related delirium. Current consensus follows the recomendations of Fernandez and Levy[46] for combining intravenous haloperidol (Haldol) with intravenous lorazepam, titrating the dosages and frequencies to achieve symptom control. However, Wolcott et al[138] advise treating delirium with minimal dosages of neuroleptics because HIV-positive patients appear to be more susceptible to both neuroleptic malignant syndrome and extrapyramidal side effects than otherwise medically comparable patients.[3,13,64,128,138] Patients with delirium need to be managed in a setting where regular, thorough neuropsychiatric assessments are undertaken by appropriate personnel. Drugs that can cause delirium include amphotericin, anticonvulsants, ciprofloxacin, corticosteroids, ganciclovir, interferon-α, and metoclopramide.[134]

Mania

Mania is characterized by persistently elevated expansive or irritable mood associated with less need for sleep, pressured speech, distractibility, flight of ideas, psychomotor agitation or increase in goal-directed activity, inflated self-esteem or grandiosity, and excessive involvement in pleasurable activities that have a high potential for painful consequences. Mania may occur as an initial manifestation of HIV disease, as a mood disorder superimposed on previously known advanced HIV disease, as hypomania, as a complication of Retrovir or other medications, or as a first manifestation of an opportunistic or systemic illness. In most cases, mania seems to be a complication of HIV-related OBD because it tends to occur late in the course of disease and to be commonly correlated with cognitive defects that often may not resolve when the manic episode recedes.[39,74] From the evidence of current case report studies, mania in AIDS carries a poor prognosis. In one study, over one quarter of the patients died within 6 months of their psychiatric presentation.[39]

Although patients with HIV disease are generally responsive to standard antimania medicines (Table 15–4),[53,70] their response may be incomplete, and they may be prone to more significant side effects.[39] Medications known to precipitate mania include anticonvulsants, bupropion, buspirone, corticosteroids, dapsone, H_2-receptor antagonists, metoclopramide, and zidovudine.[134] Lithium has generally been the mainstay of treatment of mania. However, lithium therapy poses many potential problems in patients with advanced HIV disease. Because these patients often take medicines that may alter renal function or affect tubular salt clearance, lithium dosing may be very difficult. Additionally, patients with HIV disease are prone to dehydration. They commonly experience protracted episodes of vomiting or diarrhea or both, placing them at increased risk for dehydration and thus lithium toxicity. Because of these potential problems, other agents, such as neuroleptics and anticonvulsants, should be considered for management of patients with both acute and chronic HIV-associated mania.

HIV-related mania should be treated as follows. First, potential offending medicines as noted should be decreased or stopped as soon as is medically feasible. Initial therapy may consist of a medium- or high-potency neuroleptic. Although low-potency neuroleptics are theoretically appealing because of their sedative effects, their usefulness is limited by their tendency to cause confusion even at low dosages (this probably reflects the underlying organic brain disease that predisposes patients with HIV disease to mania).[45] Anticonvulsants, such as carbamazepine and valproic acid, also have been used to stabilize mood in patients with HIV-associated mania. In the setting of HIV disease, mania is commonly associated with depressive disease and cognitive impairment, and all patients with HIV-associated mania should be carefully screened for both of these comorbid conditions. Hypomanic patients, although not at immediate risk regarding their medical

TABLE 15–4. ANTIMANIA DRUGS

Name (Trade Name)	Starting (Oral) Adult Dose	Therapeutic Adult Daily Dose	Comments
Lithium	(Onset 7–10 days) 300 mg tid (to start maintenance)	Acute 1200–2400 mg/day Maintenance 900–1500 mg/day	Avoid in patients with unstable volume status, fluctuating renal status, those receiving nephrotoxic drugs
Carbamazepine (Tegretol)	200 mg bid	400 mg bid	An increased risk of bone marrow effects has *not* been reported in AIDS patients; monitor LFTs, drug levels
Valproic acid (Depekoate)	250 mg bid	250 mg tid	Nausea is the main side effect limiting therapy

health, may have poor overall prognosis due to inability to comply with medical plans or treatment protocols because of unrealistic assessments about their health. These patients should receive aggressive treatment to enhance cooperation with the treatment program. When subject to intercurrent stressors, these hypomanic patients may develop symptoms consistent with full-blown mania and thus need to be carefully monitored.

Psychosis

Patients with HIV disease may present with organically based psychoses that are phenomenologically indistinguishable from functional psychoses.[120] All patients with a new psychosis disorder should, therefore, be carefully screened for risk factors for HIV disease, and appropriate workup should be undertaken for HIV-related problems when indicated. Medications that may cause psychosis and hallucinations include anabolic steroids, amphotericin, anticonvulsants, ciprofloxacin, buspirone, corticosteroids, dapsone, ganciclovir, H_2-receptor antagonists, interferon-α, isoniazid, chitaconizal, nonsteroidal antiinflammatory agents, metronidazole (Flagyl), salicylates, sulfonamides, and zidovudine.[134] Because of the increased risk of both neuroleptic malignant syndrome and extrapyramidal syndromes with high-dose and high-potency neuroleptics, both dosage and duration of neuroleptic therapy should be minimized. Midpotency neuroleptics, such as perphenazine (Trilafon), represent a good compromise between avoiding the anticholinergic side effects of low-potency neuroleptics and avoiding the higher risk of extrapyramidal symptoms with high-potency agents, such as haloperidol. However, most experts currently recommend haloperidol (Haldol), as midpotency agents tend to cause confusion in patients with advanced HIV disease. The same primary medical conditions noted previously as causes of mania and depression can precipitate psychosis. For this reason, the clinician should conduct a thorough medical evaluation and medication review to rule out a primary medical basis for any psychotic episode. Substance abuse should be carefully ruled out.

ETHICAL/LEGAL ISSUES

All patients with life-threatening illnesses, particularly those likely to affect CNS function and, therefore, legal competence,[83] need to make difficult decisions regarding their medical treatment in the last stages of their disease. These issues are best discussed when the patient is relaxed and cognitively intact, and the discussion is best initiated by the primary care provider with the broadest understanding of the patient's psychosocial circumstances and the tempo of his or her HIV disease.[34] Proactively broaching issues, such as designating a power of attorney and making a will, is especially important in patients who have nontraditional families (e.g., gay male couples) or in situations where the stress of the patient's illness has resulted in significant intrafamily conflict.[34,144] Studies of persons with AIDS show that most of them wish to discuss their preferences for life-sustaining measures with their physicians, and few actually have been given the opportunity.[59] Some patients on initially learning of their HIV positivity immediately have concerns about their ability to remain independent and autonomous if and when their disease progresses. These patients may wish to discuss this issue on the initial visit with their caregiver. Primary care practitioners need to be prepared for these discussions. It is important to reassure patients that they will not be abandoned as their condition progresses and that their wishes regarding life-sustaining treatment and palliative treatment will be respected should that time come.

Some patients with HIV disease want to discuss the option of rational suicide with their primary caregiver.[50,69,103] In one uncontrolled survey of HIV-infected patients, 67% of the respondents indicated that they had considered rational suicide as an option for themselves. In these respondents, suicidal feelings and depression were not necessarily related. Some reported that the ability to discuss this in an open setting, such as a support group, helped them normalize their feelings and to manage their suicidal thoughts.[69]

Rational suicide and euthanasia are extremely controversial issues within the medical profession. Nonetheless, practitioners must realize that many HIV-positive patients have at least considered suicide as an option for themselves. Thus, it is important for practitioners to examine their feelings about this issue because they are likely to be approached about it by their patients. In some cases, a candid and empathic discussion about terminal and palliative care issues may help relieve the patient's concerns about intractable physical or emotional suffering. In these discussions, it is appropriate for the clinician to carefully screen the patient for a reactive depression, especially one that is inappropriate to disease stage (e.g., a patient with no symptoms of HIV disease who is considering rational suicide).[8,69]

Estate planning and designation of power of attorney are important issues best mediated through professional legal counsel. These discussions are ideally undertaken during periods of relative good health between acute illnesses but occasionally may need to be undertaken in a hospital setting. Social workers may be an appropriate source of referral for legal assistance in cases where legal planning is deferred until relatively late. The attorney preparing legal documents in the acute medical setting needs to verify that the patient is legally competent to make or amend a will. Essentially, legal competence means the patient is aware of his or her setting and is aware of the changes or designations he or she is making in the will. Clinicians can help evaluate the patient's competency to assist legal counsel in the timing of legal planning. In the setting of even the intensive care unit where patients typically have multiorgan complications, clinical and formal assessments of cognition can be made to document a patient's cognitive status.[29] Since hospitalized and terminally ill patients with HIV disease are especially prone to delirium, it is critical that clinicians document a patient's mental status when legal documents are prepared or modified. Jones et al[68] have developed a straightforward bedside test of cognition for patients with HIV disease. In their study of 62 nondelirious patients with HIV infection, their Mental Alteration instrument took only 2 to 3 minutes to perform, and the results of this simple-to-perform and easily scored test correlated well with more complex instruments, such as the formal Mini-Mental State Examination and the Trail-Making Tests.

PAIN CONTROL

Chronic and acute pain are a common complications of HIV disease. These pain syndromes may include acute pain, such as that from a surgical incision or central line placement in the thorax, or chronic pain, such as peripheral neuropathy, chronic sinusitis, or chronic myalgias. The principles of pain management in HIV-positive patients are similar to those in other medically ill patients.[12] Pain may be easily overlooked in patients with multiple medical complications.[16,76,126] It can be helpful in both the inpatient and outpatient setting to take "pain vital signs" to assess the patient's degree of pain and his or her response to the current analgesic program.[77] In general, short-acting narcotics are best used for unpredictable or breakthrough pain, and longer-acting narcotics are best used for chronic pain. Newer narcotic medicine delivery systems include Roxanol, a liquid morphine solution that can be absorbed sublingually; fentanyl patches, a cutaneous delivery system that provides round-the-clock analgesia for 2 to 3 days; and portable patient-controlled analgesia units that deliver both constant and bolus infusions of parenteral narcotic medication. In addition, antidepressant therapy may be a very useful analgesia adjunct in patients with chronic pain, particularly neuropathic pain.

Peripheral neuropathy may respond to tricyclic antidepressant therapy alone. Lancinating or shooting neuropathic pain seems to respond best to carbamazepine therapy. Nontraditional pain-control interventions, such as body work, acupuncture, herbal therapy, and massage, may have very effective analgesic and psychosocial effects for some patients. Patients with advanced HIV disease receiving centrally acting medications, including narcotic therapy, should be closely monitored because these patients are particularly susceptible to confusion or delirium after receiving these agents. Postherpetic neuralgia may be palliated with tricyclic antidepressants. Postherpetic neuralgia has not been shown to be prevented by treating acute herpes zoster with high-dose acyclovir therapy.

GUILT SYNDROMES IN CAREGIVER ISSUES

Practitioners caring for HIV-positive patients need to recognize the psychiatric morbidity seen in HIV-negative caregivers of people with HIV disease. This morbidity may take the form of caregiver stress. Often, a fully employed spouse or partner may attempt to act as a primary practical caregiver to a loved one. Caregivers in this situation are extremely prone to burnout and depression and need active support from the primary practitioner. The primary medical practitioner should arrange for respite care and practical support at home to allow the home caregiver to focus on emotional and psychologic support rather than practical caregiving. The primary care practitioner can also provide invaluable support to HIV-negative caregivers by validating their difficult role and helping them manage priorities.[58] HIV-negative caregivers may experience survivor guilt and in some cases may develop frank adjustment disorders or major depression. In addition, primary care practitioners can help families share the burden of a family member's illness by encouraging them to seek help when they are feeling overwhelmed.

Ironically, within many families and communities, the primary home-based caregiver of an HIV-positive patient is also HIV-positive. In these situations, the practical difficulties involved in caregiving for an HIV-positive person may be compounded by the caregiver's understandable fears of future illness. It is natural for the caregiver to anticipate his or her illness, projecting his or her future course from the patient's present medical course. Additionally, in some communities, particularly the gay male community, many people with HIV disease and their caregivers have suffered multiple losses of friends, family, and even other caregivers. Standard models of coping with grief have emphasized a somewhat closed model of bereavement followed by resolution of grief. However, many HIV-positive people and their caregivers are in chronic mourning and never have the opportunity to fully resolve their grief from one loss before they must face yet another ill companion or friend.[58,87] No simple psychotherapeutic model has been developed to address these seemingly impossible psychologic burdens. Intuitively, however, it appears that simply giving patients and their loved ones an opportunity to air their difficulties and to receive emotional support may not only provide solace but also bond the relationship among the physician, the patient, and loved ones.

As importantly, caregivers and people with HIV disease need to find support in the community. These meaningful connections can include participating in public rituals, such as the AIDS Quilt and memorial services, belonging to a support group, receiving pastoral counseling, and participating in a religious congregation or other spiritual practices.[58] Because of the stigma associated with AIDS, especially the stigmas of intravenous drug use and nontraditional lifestyles, many people with AIDS-related grief may be reluctant to seek solace from their pastors. Social workers should identify sensitive and knowledgeable pastoral counselors in the community who can provide solace and guidance to these individuals and families.

Medical caregivers, too, need to recognize their high risk for burnout.[33,44] Caregivers may be confronted with fears of contagion or negative attitudes toward various populations at risk for HIV disease. Caregivers also may be in chronic mourning and may have suffered the cumulative loss of many patients and even colleagues.[58] Medical caregivers generally are not well prepared by their training programs to treat patients with progressive terminal illnesses. Instead, training programs tend to emphasize curative therapies rather than palliative therapies, which does not prepare trainees for the psychologic dilemmas and spiritual stress involved in caring for people with life-threatening or terminal illnesses.[50,81,92,113,114] Program administrators and clinic leaders can help their staffs cope with the psychologic and spiritual stress of working with people with HIV disease by setting up regular inservices for didactic training addressing the management of end-stage symptoms; by setting up informal group sessions to share feelings about difficult or beloved patients; and by ensuring regular respite from stressful care in the form of short work weeks, regular vacations, and regular mental health days.

Practitioners in solo practice settings need to ensure that they are well trained in all aspects of palliative care and have at least rudimentary training in assessment of the major psychiatric syndromes. Regular exercise, regular respites, and strict time off from work can physically and spiritually replenish medical caregivers, preparing them to provide optimal care for their patients.

CONCLUSION

A psychosocial approach to the care of HIV-positive patients involves a global, inclusive approach to the patient's life and to the patient's illness. Stoeckle et al[127] have characterized this type of global perspective as "the work of care." This work includes the standard information-gathering work and physical examination work involved in the standard history and physical examination but also involves emotional work (eliciting psychologic information), biographic work (understanding and knowing the patient), comfort work (personal support of patients in all stages of disease), negotiation and interpretive work (helping the patient understand the course of the disease), educational work (helping the patient prevent disease complications), brokering work (helping the patient negotiate the health care system), moral and ethical work (including eliciting preferences), collaborative colleague work (helping provide personal care in multispecialty settings), and self-reflective work (optimizing interpersonal relations among the patient, the family, and the practitioner).[127]

This inclusive model of the work of care is an excellent approximation to the ideal primary care model. Although mental health complications as discussed may have been managed traditionally by consultants, primary care practi-

tioners, given their comprehensive approach to the patient and the emphasis on continuity and coordination of care, are in an optimal position to assess and treat the neuropsychiatric complications of AIDS.[122] The actual impact of psychologic intervention in the care of HIV-positive patients has not been established.[66] However, actively investigating and compassionately treating the psychosocial complications of HIV disease will likely result in improved medical outcomes for the patient, better allocation of medical resources, increased comfort for patients and their loved ones, and increased satisfaction for the providers who can give comprehensive and compassionate care.

REFERENCES

1. Adams F: Emergency intravenous sedation of the delirious, medically ill patient. J Clin Psychiatry 49(Suppl):22–27, 1988
2. Atkinson J, Grant I, Kennedy C, et al: Prevalence of psychiatric disorders among men infected with human immunodeficiency virus. Arch Gen Psychiatry 45:859–864, 1988
3. Baer J: Study of 60 patients with AIDS or AID-related complex requiring psychiatric hospitalization. Am J Psychiatry 146:1285–1288, 1989
4. Bascom P, Tolle S: Care of the family when the patient is dying. West J Med 163(3):292–296, 1995
5. Batki S: Buspirone in drug users with AIDS or AIDS-related complex. J Clin Psychopharmacol 10(Suppl):111S–115S, 1993
6. Bennett J: Helping people with AIDS live well at home. Nurs Clin North Am 23:731–747, 1988
7. Bermon N: Family reproductive issues: Reproductive counseling. AIDS Clin Care 5:45–47, 1993
8. Block S, Billings JA: Patient requests for euthanasia and assisted suicide in terminal illness. Psychosomatics 36:445–457, 1995
9. Boccellari A, Dilley J, Shore M: Neuropsychiatric aspects of AIDS dementia complex: A report on a clinical series. Neurotoxology 9:381–390, 1988
10. Boccellari A, Zeifert P: Management of neurobehavioral impairment in HIV-1 infection. Psychiatr Clin North Am 17:183, 1994
11. Borson S, McDonald G, Gayle T, et al: Improvement in mood, physical symptoms, and function with nortriptyline for depression in patients with chronic obstructive pulmonary disease. Psychosomatics 33:190–201, 1992
12. Breitbart W: Psychiatric management of cancer pain. Cancer 63(Suppl):2336–2342, 1989
13. Breitbart W, Marotta R, Call P: AIDS and neuroleptic malignant syndrome. Lancet 2:1488–1489, 1988
14. Broadhead WE, Blazer DG, George LK, Tse CK: Depression, disability days, and days lost from work in a prospective epidemiologic survey: JAMA 264:2524–2528, 1990
15. Brody D, Larson D: The role of primary care physicians in managing depression. J Gen Intern Med 7:243–247, 1992
16. Bruera E, Miller J, Macmillan K, Kuehn N: Neuropsychological effects of methylphenidate in patients receiving a continuous infusion of narcotics for cancer pain. Pain 48:163–166, 1992
17. Buhrich N, Cooper D, Freed E: HIV infection associated with symptoms indistinguishable from functional psychosis. Br J Psychiatry 152:649–653, 1988
18. Burack J, Barrett D, Stall R, et al: Depressive symptoms and CD4 lymphocytes decline among HIV-infected men. JAMA 270:2568–2573, 1993
19. Burckhardt C: Coping strategies of the chronically ill. Nurs Clin North Am 22:543–550, 1987
20. Burger D, Kraaijeveld CL, Meenhorst PL, et al: Penetration of zidovudine into the cerebrospinal fluid of patients infected with HIV. AIDS 7:1581–1587, 1993
21. Calabrese J, Kling M, Gold P: Alterations in immunocompetence during stress, bereavement and depression: Focus on neuroendocrine regulation. Am J Psychiatry 144:1123–1134, 1987
22. Carlson D, Fleming K, Smith G, Evans J: Management of dementia-related behavioral disturbances: A nonpharmacologic approach. Mayo Clin Proc 70: 1108–1115, 1995
23. Carson V, Soekn K, Shanty J, et al: Hope and spiritual well-being: Essentials for living with AIDS. Perspect Psychiatr Care 26:28–34, 1990
24. Cassem E: Anxiety and depression as secondary phenomena. Psychiatr Clin North Am 13:597–612, 1990
25. Cassem E: Depressive disorders in the medically ill. Psychosomatics 36:S2–S10, 1995
26. Chesney M, Folkman S: Psychological impact of HIV disease and implications for intervention. Psychiatr Clin North Am 17:163, 1994
27. Choice of an antidepressant. Med Lett Drugs Ther 35:25–26, 1993
28. Chuang H, Jason G, Pajurkova E, et al: Psychiatric morbidity in patients with HIV infection. Can J Psychiatry 37:109–115, 1992
29. Coates T: Counseling patients seropositive for human immunodeficiency virus: An approach for medical practice. West J Med 153:629–634, 1990
30. Cohen L, McCue J, Green G: Do clinical and formal

assessments of the capacity of patients in the intensive care unit to make decisions agree? Arch Intern Med 153:2481–2485, 1993

31. Collier A, Marra C, Coombs R, et al: Central nervous system manifestations in human immunodeficiency virus infection without AIDS. J Acquir Immune Defic Syndr 5:229–241, 1992

32. Cote T, Biggar R, Dannenberg A: Risk of suicide among persons with AIDS. JAMA 268:2066–2068, 1992

33. Creagan E: Stress among medical oncologists: The phenomenon of burnout and a call to action. Mayo Clin Proc 68:614–615, 1993

34. Davis D: Rich cases: The ethics of thick description. Hastings Center Rep July–August:12–16, 1991

35. Donnell M: Nursing care of the patient with dementia. In Martin J, Hughes A, Franks P, eds. AIDS Home Care and Hospice Manual, ed 2. San Francisco, Visiting Nurses and Hospice of San Francisco, 1990, pp 103–111

36. Dubovsky S, Thomas M: Approaches to the treatment of refractory depression. J Pract Psychiatr Behav Health 2:14–22, 1996

37. Eisenberg L: Treating depression and anxiety in primary care: Closing the gap between knowledge and practice. N Engl J Med 326:1080–1083, 1992

38. Eisendrath S: Brief psychotherapy in medical practice: Keys to success. West J Med 158:376–378, 1993

39. El-Mallakh R: Mania in AIDS: Clinical significance and theoretical considerations. Int J Psychiatry Med 21:383–391, 1991

40. Evans D, Folds J, Petitto J, et al: Circulating natural killer cell phenotypes in men and women with major depression: Relation to cytotoxic activity and severity of depression. Arch Gen Psychiatry 49:388–395, 1992

41. Evans D, McCartney C, Haggerty J, et al: Treatment of depression in cancer patients is associated with better life adaptation: A pilot study. Psychosom Med 50:72–76, 1988

42. Evans D, McCartney C, Nemeroff C, et al: Depression in women treated for gynecological cancer: Clinical and neuroendocrine assessment. Am J Psychiatry 143:447–451, 1986

43. Fernandez F, Adams F, Levy J, et al: Cognitive impairment due to AIDS-related complex and its response to psychostimulants. Psychosomatics 29:38–46, 1988

44. Fernandez F, Holmes V, Levy J, et al: Consultation-liaison psychiatry and HIV-related disorders. Hosp Community Psychiatry 40:146–153, 1989

45. Fernandez F, Levy J: Psychopharmacology in HIV spectrum disorders. Psychiatr Clin North Am 17:135, 1994

46. Fernandez F, Levy J: Psychopharmacotherapy of psychiatric syndromes in asymptomatic and symptomatic HIV infection. Psychiatr Med 9:377–390, 1991

47. Fish N: Treatment of delirium in the critically ill patient. Clin Pharm 110:456–466, 1991

48. Folkman S, Chesney M, Pollack L, et al: Stress, coping, and high-risk sexual behavior. Health Psychol 11:218–222, 1992

49. Frierson RL, Wey JJ, Tabler JB: Psychostimulants for depression in the medically ill. Am Fam Physician 43:163–170, 1991

50. Garfield C: Sometimes My Heart Goes Numb: Love and Caring in a Time of AIDS. San Francisco, Jossey-Bass Publishers, 1995, pp 261–284

51. Gelfand S, Indelicato J, Benjamin J: Using intravenous haloperidol to control delirium. Hosp Community Psychiatry 43:215, 1992

52. Gerber P, Barrett J, Barrett J, et al: Recognition of depression by internists in primary care: A comparison of internist and "gold standard" psychiatric assessments. J Gen Intern Med 4:7–13, 1989

53. Gerner R: Treatment of acute mania. Psychiatr Clin North Am 16:443–456, 1993

54. Goldberg R: Diagnostic dilemmas presented by patients with anxiety and depression. Am J Med 98:278–284, 1995

55. Grant I, Olshen R, Atkinson JH, et al: Depressed mood does not explain neuropsychological deficits in HIV-infected persons. Neuropsychology 7:53–61, 1993

56. Gray J, Grant I, Atkinson H, et al: Incidence of AIDS dementia in a two-year follow-up of AIDS and ARC patients on an initial phase II AZT placebo-controlled study: San Diego cohort. J Neuropsychiatry Clin Neurosci 4:15–20, 1992

57. Grothe T, McKusick L: Coping with multiple loss. Focus, June 1992, 5–6

58. Gunnoe R: Coping with multiple loss from AIDS-related deaths (dissertation in progress), November 1993

59. Haas J, Weissman J, Cleary P, et al: Discussion of preferences for life-sustaining care by persons with AIDS: Predictors of failure in patient-physician communication. Arch Intern Med 153:1241–1248, 1993

60. Hays R, Turner H, Coates T: Social support, AIDS-related symptoms, and depression among gay men. J Consult Clin Psychol 60:463–469, 1992

61. Hecht F, Soloway B: HIV infection: A primary care approach. Reprints from AIDS Clin Care Newsletter. Publishing Division of Massachusetts Medical Society, pp 8–9, 32–40, 86.

62. Holland J, Tross S: The psychosocial and neuropsychiatric sequelae of the acquired immunodeficiency syndrome and related disorders. Ann Intern Med 103:760–764, 1985

63. Holmes V, Fernandez F, Levey J: Psychostimulant response in AIDS-related complex patients. J Clin Psychiatry 50:5–8, 1989

64. Hriso E, Kuhn T, Masdeu J, et al: Extrapyramidal symptoms due to dopamine-blocking agents in patients with AIDS encephalopathy. Am J Psychiatry 148:1558–1561, 1991

65. Irwin M, Daniels M, Bloom E, et al: Life events, depressive symptoms, and immune function. Am J Psychiatry 144:437–441, 1987

66. Jewett J, Hecht F: Preventive health care for adults with HIV infection. JAMA 269:1144–1153, 1993

67. Jimenez M, Jimenez D: Training volunteer caregivers of persons with AIDS. Social Work Health Care 1990 14:73–85, 1990, in Focus 7:7, 1992

68. Jones B, Teng E, Folstein M, et al: A new bedside test of cognition for patients with HIV infection. Ann Intern Med 119:1001–1004, 1993

69. Jones J, Dilley J: Rational suicide and HIV disease. Focus 1993, 5–6

70. Kahn D: New strategies in bipolar disorder: Part II treatment. Pract Psychiatr Behav Health 1:148–157, 1995

71. Katon W: Depression: Relationship to somatization

and chronic medical illness. Clin Psychiatry 45: 4–11, 1984

72. Katon W: Panic disorder: Epidemiology, diagnosis, and treatment in primary care. J Clin Psychiatry 47:21–27, 1986

73. Kaufmann M, Murray G, Cassem N: Use of psychostimulants in medically ill depressed patients. Psychosomatics 23:817–819, 1982

74. Kieburtz K, Zettelmaier A, Ketonen L: Manic syndrome in AIDS. Am J Psychiatry 148:1068–1070, 1991

75. Lackner J, Joseph J, Ostrow D, et al: A longitudinal study of psychological distress in a cohort of gay men. J Nerv Ment Dis 181:4–12, 1993

76. Lander J: Clinical judgments in pain management. Pain 42:15–22, 1990

77. Lebovits A, Lefkowitz M, McCarthy D, et al: The prevalence and management of pain in patients with AIDS: A review of 134 cases. Clin J Pain 5:245–248, 1989

78. Liebowitz M, Barlow D: Panic disorder: The latest on diagnosis and treatment. J Pract Psychiatr Behav Health 1:10–19, 1995

79. Lipson M: Family and reproductive issues: Disclosure within families. AIDS Clin Care 5:43–44, 1993

80. Lyketsos C, Hoover D, Guccione M, et al: Depressive symptoms as predictors of medical outcome in HIV infection. JAMA 270:1563–1567, 1993

81. MacDonald N: Suffering and dying in cancer patients: Research issues in controlling confusion, cachexia, dyspnea. In Caring for Patients at the End of Life (Special Issue). West J Med 163: 278–286, 1995

82. MacKenzie T, Popkin M: Suicide in the medical patient. Int J Psychiatry Med 17:3–22, 1987

83. Mahler J, Perry S: Assessing competency in the physically ill: Guidelines for psychiatric consultants. Hosp Community Paychiatry 39:856–861, 1988

84. McCann K, Wadsworth E: Characteristics of informal caregivers. AIDS Care 4:25–34, 1992 (reprinted in Focus 7:7, 1992)

85. McCormick TR, Conley BJ: Patients' perspectives on dying and on the care of dying patients. In Caring for Patients at the End of Life (Special Issue). West J Med 163:236–243, 1995

86. Markowitz J: Treating HIV-associated depression with psychotherapy. The AIDS Reader May/June: 95–98, 1995

87. Markowitz JC, Klerman G, Perry S: Interpersonal psychotherapy of depressed HIV-positive outpatients. Hosp Community Psychiatry 43:885–890, 1992

88. Markowitz JC, Rabkin JG, Perry SW: Treating depression in HIV-positive patients. AIDS 8:403–412, 1994

89. Martin J, Dean L: Effects of AIDS-related bereavement and HIV-related illness on psychological distress among gay men: A 7-year longitudinal study, 1985–1991. J Consult Clin Psychol 61:94–103, 1993

90. Marzuk P, Tierney H, Tardiff K, et al: Increased risk of suicide in persons with AIDS. JAMA 259: 1333–1337, 1988

91. Michels R, Marzuk P: Progress in psychiatry. N Engl J Med 329:628–637, 1993

92. Muldoon M, King N: Spirituality, health care, and bioethics. J Religion Health 34:329–349, 1995

93. Navia B, Jordan B, Price R: The AIDS dementia complex: I. Clinical features. Ann Neurol 19:517–524, 1986

94. Navia B, Price R: The acquired immunodeficiency syndrome dementia complex as the presenting sole manifestation of human immunodeficiency virus infection. Arch Neurol 44:65–69, 1987

95. Newman S, Lunn S, Harrison M: Do asymptomatic HIV-seropositive individuals show cognitive deficit? AIDS 9:1211–1220, 1995

96. Nierenberg A, Feighner J, Rudolph R, et al: Venlafaxine for treatment-resistant unipolar depression. J Clin Psychopharmacol 14:419–423, 1994

97. Olin J, Masand P: Psychostimulants for depression in hospitalized cancer patients. Psychosomatics 37: 57–62, 1996

98. Ostrow D, Grant I, Atkinson H: Assessment and management of the AIDS patient with neuropsychiatric disturbances. J Clin Psychiatry 49:14–22, 1988

99. Paton S: Stress and the informal caregiver. Focus 7: 1–4, 1992

100. Perez-Stable E, Miranda J, Munoz R, et al: Depression in medical outpatients: Underrecognition and misdiagnosis. Arch Intern Med 50:1083–1088, 1990

101. Perry S: Organic mental disorders caused by HIV: Update on early diagnosis and treatment. Am J Psychiatry 147:696–710, 1990

102. Perry S, Fishman B: Depression and HIV: How does one affect the other? JAMA 270:2609–2610, 1993

103. Perry S, Fishman B, Jacobsberg L, et al: Effectiveness of psychoeducational interventions in reducing emotional distress after human immunodeficiency virus antibody testing. Arch Gen Psychiatry 48:143–147, 1991

104. Perry S, Jacobsberg L, Fishman B, et al: Psychiatric diagnosis before serological testing for the human immunodeficiency virus. Am J Psychiatry 147: 89–93, 1990

105. Petty F: Depression and medical/surgical illness: "Who wouldn't be depressed?" Primary Care 14: 669–683, 1987

106. Potter W, Rudorfer M, Manji H: The pharmacologic treatment of depression. N Engl J Med 325: 633–642, 1991

107. Price R, Brew B: The AIDS dementia complex. J Infect Dis 158:1079–1083, 1988

108. Quill T: Doctor, I want to die. Will you help me? JAMA 270:870–873, 1993

109. Rabkin J, Gewirtz G: Depression and HIV. GMHC Treatment Issues 6:1–7, 1992

110. Rabkin J, Remien R: Depressive disorder and HIV disease: An uncommon association. Focus 10:1–6, 1995

111. Rabkin J, Remien R, Katoff L, et al: Resilience in adversity among long-term survivors of AIDS. Hosp Community Psychiatry 44:162–167, 1993

112. Rabkin J, Williams J, Remien R, et al: Depression, distress, lymphocyte subsets, and human immunodeficiency virus symptoms on two occasions in HIV-positive homosexual men. Arch Gen Psychiatry 48:111–119, 1991

113. Remen R: Spirit: Resource for healing. Noetic Sciences Review, Autumn:5–9, 1988

114. Remen R: Working in the gray zone: The dilemma of the private practitioner. Adv J Mind-Body Health 7(3):1991

115. Rundell J, Kyle K, Brown G, Thomason J: Risk factors for suicide attempts in a human immunodefi-

ciency virus screening program. Psychosomatics 33:24–27, 1992

116. Rush J: Depression in primary care: Detection, diagnosis and treatment. Am Fam Physician 47: 1776–1788, 1993

117. Sacks M, Dermatis H, Looser-Ott S, Perry S: Seroprevalence of HIV and risk factors for AIDS in psychiatric inpatients. Hosp Community Psychiatry 43: 736–737, 1992

118. Satel S, Nelson C: Stimulants in the treatment of depression: A critical overview. J Clin Psychiatry 50:241–249, 1989

119. Schmitt F, Bigley J, McKinnis R, et al: Neuropsychological outcome of zidovudine (AZT) treatment of patients with AIDS and AIDS-related complex. N Engl J Med 319:1573–1578, 1988

120. Sewell D, Jeste D, Atkinson JH, Heaton R: HIV-associated psychosis: A study of 20 cases. Am J Psychiatry 151:237–242, 1994

121. Shader R, Greenblatt D: Use of benzodiazepines in anxiety disorders. N Engl J Med 328:1398–1405, 1993

122. Smith M: Primary care and HIV disease. J Gen Intern Med 6(Suppl):S56–S62, 1991

123. Snyder S, Strain J, Wolf D: Differentiating major depression from adjustment disorder with depressed mood in the medical setting. Gen Hosp Psychiatry 12:159–168, 1990

124. Soloway B: Preparing for disability and death. AIDS Clin Care 3:76–77, 1991

125. Spiegel D, Bloom J, Kraemer H, et al: Effect of psychosocial treatment on survival of patients with metastatic breast cancer. Lancet 2:888–891, 1989

126. Spiegel D, Sands S, Koopman C: Pain and depression in patients with cancer. Cancer 74:2570–2578, 1994

127. Stoeckle J, Ronan L, Ehrlich C, et al: The uses of shadowing the doctor—and patient: On seeing and hearing their work of care. J Gen Intern Med 8:561–563, 1993

128. Swenson J, Erman M, Labelle J, et al: Extrapyramidal reactions: Neuropsychiatric mimics in patients with AIDS. Gen Hosp Psychiatry 11:248–253, 1989

129. Taylor S, Kemeny M, Aspinwall L, et al: Optimism, coping, psychological distress, and high-risk sexual behavior among men at risk for acquired immunodeficiency syndrome (AIDS). J Pers Soc Psychol 63:460–473, 1992

130. Tesar G: The agitated patient, part II: pharmacologic treatment. Hosp Community Psychiatry 44: 627–629, 1993

131. The Medical Letter: Drugs for AIDS and associated infections. 37:87–94, 1995

132. The Medical Letter: Drugs for AIDS and associated infections. 35:79–86, 1993

133. The Medical Letter: Drugs for psychiatric disorders. 33:43–50, 1991

134. The Medical Letter: Drugs that cause psychiatric symptoms. 35:65–70, 1993

135. Viederman N, Perry S: Use of a psychodynamic life narrative in the treatment of depression in the physically ill. Gen Hosp Psychiatry 3:177–185, 1980

136. Wells K, Stewart A, Hays R, et al: The functioning and well-being of depressed patients. JAMA 262: 914–919, 1989

137. White J, Darko D, Brown S, et al: Early central nervous system response to HIV infection: Sleep distortion and cognitive-motor decrements. AIDS 9: 1043–1050, 1995

138. Wolcott D, Fawzy F, Namir S: Clinical management of psychiatric disorders in HIV spectrum disease. Psychiatr Med 7:107–127, 1989

139. Wolf T, Balson P, Morse E, et al: Relationship of coping style to affective state and perceived social support in asymptomatic and symptomatic HIV-infected persons: Implications for clinical management. J Clin Psychiatry 52:171–173, 1991

140. Woods S, Tesar G, Murray G, et al: Psychostimulant treatment of depressive disorders secondary to medical illness. Clin Psychiatry 47:12–15, 1986

141. Yesavage J: Differential diagnosis between depression and dementia. Am J Med 94(Suppl 5A):23S–28S, 1993

142. Zegans L, Gerhard A, Coates T: Psychotherapies for the person with HIV disease. Psychiatr Clin North Am 17:149, 1994

143. Zislis P, Golden R, Pedersen C, et al: HIV: Psychoimmunologic and neuropsychiatric relationships. N C Med J 49:542–544, 1988

144. Zuger A: Ethical decision making in AIDS. AIDS Clin Care 2:49–52, 1990

Chapter 16

Hematologic Complications of HIV Infection

JULIE HAMBLETON

Infection with the human immunodeficiency virus (HIV) is associated with a wide spectrum of hematologic abnormalities. These abnormalities may be found at all stages of HIV disease and involve the bone marrow, cellular elements of the peripheral blood, and coagulation pathways. The cause of these abnormalities is multifactorial. A direct suppressive effect of HIV infection, ineffective hematopoiesis, infiltrative disease of the bone marrow, nutritional deficiencies, peripheral consumption secondary to splenomegaly or immune dysregulation, and drug effect all contribute to the variety of hematologic findings in these patients. Specific abnormalities in the bone marrow, peripheral blood cell lines, and coagulation complex will be reviewed here in turn.

BONE MARROW

Hematologic abnormalities in patients with HIV infection are very common.[11,43] Ineffective hematopoiesis resulting from direct suppression by HIV infection,[10,48] infiltrative disease (infectious or neoplastic), nutritional deficiencies, and drug effect have all been described.

Morphologic Features

The common morphologic features of bone marrow findings in patients with AIDS have been described.[1,8,43] Bone marrow biopsies are frequently performed to evaluate peripheral cytopenias or persistent fevers in this patient population. Most patients demonstrate normocellular marrow elements, although dyplasia has been noted, without the progression to acute leukemia. Increased numbers of plasma cells and lymphoid aggregates composed of benign-

appearing, well-differentiated lymphocytes have also been noted.[1,8,48] The myeloid-to-erythroid (M/E) ratio is generally normal in patients undergoing bone marrow biopsy. Reticulin fiber staining often reveals increased reticulin fibrosis. Abnormalities in maturation with dysmyelopoiesis (dysplasia),[18] megaloblastosis, and hemophagocytosis have also been described, whereas myeloproliferative syndromes and leukemia are not more prevalent in this patient population.[1,48]

Infiltrative disease of the bone marrow commonly contributes to the hematologic abnormalities seen in these patients. Infectious causes of infiltrative diseases include mycobacterial disease (both *Mycobacterium avium* complex and *M. tuberculosis*), fungal disease (*Histoplasma, Cryptococcus,* and *Coccidioides*), and rarely parasitic disease (*Pneumocystis* and *Leishmania*). Neoplastic infiltration is due primarily to lymphoma. Infiltration of the bone marrow by *M. avium* complex usually results in isolated anemia, whereas infiltrative disease of other causes typically manifests as pancytopenia.

Nutritional Effects

Nutritional deficiencies are not common causes of hematologic abnormalities in HIV-infected patients, although disorders of iron metabolism or iron deficiency and occult vitamin B_{12} deficiency have been described (Table 16–1). Folate deficiency is not more prevalent in this patient population. Variable reports of increased iron stores to absent iron stores have been published. Most patients have ineffective incorporation of iron into erythroid precursors, the so-called anemia of chronic disease. This leads to normal or increased iron stores on Prussian blue iron staining of the bone marrow

TABLE 16–1. SPECIAL CONSIDERATIONS IN THE APPROACH TO ANEMIA IN THE HIV-INFECTED INDIVIDUAL

Microcytosis
Consider involvement of the gastrointestinal tract with Kaposi's sarcoma, lymphoma, or infectious enteropathy (especially cytomegalovirus colitis), with resultant iron deficiency secondary to chronic blood loss

Macrocytosis
Consider:
Vitamin B_{12} or folate deficiency secondary to enteropathy with malabsorption
Hemolysis with reticulocytosis
  Drugs: dapsone, sulfa
  Autoimmunity
  Thrombotic thrombocytopenic purpura, hemolytic uremic syndrome, or disseminated intravascular coagulation (DIC) if concomitant thrombocytopenia present
  Zidovudine (AZT) drug therapy
If patient is receiving zidovudine therapy:
  Check erythropoietin level
  If <500 mU/dl, consider recombinant human erythropoietin therapy
  Evaluate vitamin B_{12} level and treat if low

Normocytic Anemia
If hemoglobin level >10 g/dl, patient exhibits no unexplained constitutional symptoms, and no other cell lines are involved, the most likely diagnosis is anemia of chronic disease secondary to HIV infection. Continued observation is advised.
If hemoglobin <10 g/dl, the patient exhibits unexplained constitutional symptoms, and other cell lines are involved, consider bone marrow infiltration
Differential Diagnosis
  Acid-fast bacillus (AFB): *Mycobacterium avium* complex or *M. tuberculosis*
  Disseminated fungal disease
    Cryptococcosis
    Histoplasmosis
    Coccidioidomycosis
  Lymphoma
Evaluation
  Blood culture for *M. avium* complex and fungus
  Cryptococcal antigen testing
  Giemsa stain of peripheral blood for histoplasmosis
  Purified protein derivative (PPD) and *Coccidioides* skin testing
  Tissue biopsy if clinically indicated
    Lymph node
    Liver
  Bone marrow biopsy
    Plastic sections for neoplasms
    Special stains and culture for AFB and fungi

biopsy. On the other hand, chronic blood loss from the gastrointestinal tract secondary to neoplastic infiltration or invasive infectious enteropathies may lead to an iron-deficient state.

The prevalence of vitamin B_{12} deficiency secondary to gastrointestinal malabsorption has been increasingly described in patients with acquired immunodeficiency syndrome (AIDS).

Low serum vitamin B_{12} levels associated with altered cobalamin transport proteins or abnormal absorption of vitamin B_{12} secondary to chronic diarrhea have been described.[12,25,42,48] Occult vitamin B_{12} deficiency may worsen the anemia associated with zidovudine therapy.[45] Therefore, it is prudent to monitor vitamin B_{12} levels periodically in patients with chronic gastrointestinal dysfunction, especially in those patients receiving zidovudine therapy.

Diagnostic Utility of Bone Marrow Biopsy

For the most part, the marrow changes in asymptomatic HIV-infected patients appear nonspecific and offer little to the clinician as a diagnostic or prognostic tool. There are, however, certain conditions for which performing bone marrow aspiration, culture, and biopsy are indicated.

HIV-infected patients with both non-Hodgkin's and Hodgkin's lymphoma frequently have marrow involvement. Marrow examination is useful not only for staging but also to assess the myeloid reserves before the initiation of cytotoxic chemotherapy. Patients with thrombocytopenia in the absence of anemia or leukopenia warrant bone marrow evaluation to ensure adequate megakaryocytes. In rare instances, diagnoses other than immune thrombocytopenic purpura may be established.

Occasionally a patient has constitutional symptoms associated with anemia and/or other cytopenias. In the absence of a revealing workup, bone marrow examination may be indicated to rule out lymphoma or underlying opportunistic infection. Evidence of Kaposi's sarcoma does not characteristically appear in the bone marrow aspirate or biopsy specimen; however, lymphomatous involvement may be found. Granulomatous disease with a positive acid-fast bacillus stain suggests *M. avium* complex or *M. tuberculosis* infection, although well-formed granulomas may not be apparent.

In a retrospective review of patients with known or suspected HIV infection, 387 bone marrow biopsy examinations were performed to evaluate the presence of opportunistic pathogens or lymphoma.[39] Disseminated fungal infections occurred in <5% of patients studied, with bone marrow examination leading to the most rapid and accurate diagnosis. Mycobacterial infection was diagnosed in 16% of patients studied. Bone marrow culture was found to be equally as sensitive for the diagnosis of disseminated mycobacterial disease as blood culture (86% versus 77% sensitivity, respectively; $p >$ 0.05). No previously undiagnosed case of lymphoma was found by bone marrow examination for cytopenias and constitutional symptoms; however, bone marrow biopsies were routinely performed for staging lymphoma.

PERIPHERAL CELL LINES

Peripheral cytopenias are common in HIV-infected individuals, and are due to either decreased production in the bone marrow or accelerated destruction in the peripheral circulation. In general, the cytopenias increase in frequency as HIV-disease progresses. Anemia, granulocytopenia, and thrombocytopenia occur in 17%, 8%, and 13%, respectively, of asymptomatic HIV-infected individuals.[59] These percentages all increase with advancing HIV disease.

Erythrocytes

Review of the peripheral blood smear in patients with HIV infection often reveals nonspecific abnormalities. Anisopoikilocytosis, often with ovalocytes and rouleaux formation, is a common finding, and increased vacuolization of peripheral monocytes may be seen.[55] Anemia is the most common hematologic abnormality noted in patients with HIV disease (see Table 16–1).[50] In patients with persistent lymphadenopathy, the development of anemia often antedates the evolution to overt AIDS. In patients with overt AIDS, anemia occurs in 66% to 85%.[48,59] The majority have chronic disease-type anemia, with low reticulocyte counts and low erythropoietin levels.[50] In such states, adequate iron stores are demonstrated in the reticuloendothelial system, but the inability to incorporate this stored iron into erythroid precursors results in a normocytic, normochromic anemia. The etiology of anemia in these patients is multifactorial and complex. Ineffective erythropoiesis may be a consequence of actual HIV infection of erythroid precursors or result from inappropriate tumor necrosis factor (TNF) release, which is an inhibitor of red blood cell (RBC) production in vitro.[14,50]

Iron deficiency with a microcytic, hypochromic anemia may result from chronic blood loss, which can result from Kaposi's sarcoma or lymphomatous involvement of the gastrointestinal tract. Thrombocytopenia with resultant occult bleeding may lead to iron deficiency.

Infiltrative disease of the bone marrow caused by *M. avium* complex is a common cause of isolated anemia, usually without concomitant decrement in the other cell lines.[16] Some of the most profound anemias, with hematocrit concentrations in the 15% to 20% range, occur in patients with mycobacterial disease. Similarly, patients with lymphoma may develop profound anemia, often with concomitant cytopenias of the other cell lines.

Infection with B19 parvovirus is increasingly recognized as a cause of intractable anemia in patients with HIV disease. Classically associated with transient aplastic crises in patients with underlying hemolytic diseases or with erythroblastosis fetalis, parvovirus selectively infects actively replicating erythroid precursors, resulting in RBC lysis and erythroid hypoplasia. Clearance of this infection is mediated by an intact humoral response. Immunocompromised patients, however, may fail to clear the infection[15,37] or maintain an adequate immunoglobulin G (IgG) antibody response.[5] Diagnosis of B19 parvovirus infection is made by serologic studies or by bone marrow examination noting giant, abnormal pronormoblasts and in situ hybridization using sequence-specific DNA probes. A course of intravenous or intramuscular immunoglobulin is the therapy of choice. Profound or symptomatic anemia should be corrected with packed RBC transfusions.

Despite the prevalence of RBC autoantibodies, antibody-mediated hemolysis is not a common cause of anemia in this patient population. Upwards of 20% to 43% of AIDS patients have a positive direct antiglobulin test (direct Coombs), but frank hemolysis is rare.[32,54] Conversely, drug-induced anemia is commonly noted. Dapsone therapy for the treatment of *Pneumocystis carinii* pneumonia or other infections can induce methemaglobinemia or hemolysis in patients with glucose-6-phosphate dehydrogenase (G6PD) deficiency, and zidovudine antiretroviral therapy results in a transfusion-dependent anemia in approximately 20% of patients.[45]

Leukocytes

HIV infection affects the lymphocyte, neutrophil, and macrophage-monocyte cell lines. Despite the hypergammaglobulinemia noted in these patients, they suffer complications from both defective cellular immunity and dysregulated humoral immunity. The hallmark of HIV infection is the progressive depletion of CD4 + lymphocytes. This decrement presumably occurs through direct viral invasion of these cells. Early in HIV infection, one may see an initial increase in the CD8 + population before a decline in the number of CD4 + cells is noted. Infection of macrophages and monocytes and the triggering of an autoimmune response are two other mechanisms by which lymphocyte depletion may occur. Normally, activated T lymphocytes and monocytes produce cytokines or growth factors necessary for stem cell growth and differentiation. Decreased production of these cytokines results from HIV invasion of these cells. For a review of the immunopathogenic mechanisms of HIV infection, refer to the review by Fauci et al.[14]

Granulocytopenia independent of drug use has been described in patients with AIDS. The most common cause appears to be ineffective granulopoiesis.[27] Antineutrophilic antibodies have been described as a possible cause of peripheral neutropenia; however, their clinical significance remains elusive.[10,30,35,48] Defects in qualitative functions of the monocyte-macrophage and granulocyte line have also been described. Defective polymorphonuclear leukocyte chemotaxis, deficient degranulating responses, inhibition of leukocyte migration, and ineffective killing have all been reported.[36,56] Similarly, monocytes exhibit a marked reduction in chemotaxis in response to stimuli.[6]

Drug-induced neutropenia is common in the HIV-infected individual.[27,45] Medications used to treat infections such as *Pneumocystis carinii* pneumonia, toxoplasmosis, and cytomegaloviral retinitis or colitis cause neutropenia. Similarly, zidovudine is also implicated as a cause of neutropenia, often necessitating dose reduction or cessation of therapy. Other dideoxynucleosides (e.g., 3TC, ddC, and ddI) and protease inhibitors are associated with less bone marrow toxicity (Table 16–2 lists the more commonly used drugs that cause neutropenia). Moreover, patients receiving chemotherapy for treatment of HIV-associated malignancies typically develop neutropenia. Irrespective of the cause of neutropenia, severe neutropenia complicated by a febrile episode should be evaluated aggressively for development of bacteremia, as in the non–HIV-infected population.[24]

TABLE 16–2. DRUGS COMMONLY USED IN TREATING PATIENTS WITH HIV INFECTION THAT CAUSE MYELOSUPPRESSION

Antiretroviral dideoxynucleosides (e.g., zidovudine [AZT])
Other antiviral agents (e.g., ganciclovir [DHPG])
Antifungal agents (e.g., flucytosine)
Sulfonamides
Dihydrofolate reductase inhibitors
   Trimetrexate
   Pyrimethamine
   Trimethoprim
Pentamidine
Antineoplastic therapy
Interferon-α

Platelets

The most common platelet abnormality found in HIV-infected patients is thrombocytopenia. In patients with HIV-related immune thrombocytopenia (ITP), platelet-associated immunoglobulin is present.[28] Other causes of HIV-related thrombocytopenia include circulating immune complexes that precipitate on the platelet surface, resulting in clearance by the reticuloendothelial system[28]; cross-reactive antibodies to platelet surface glycoproteins[3]; and direct retroviral infection of megakaryocytes.[31,60,61]

Most patients with HIV-related ITP have only minor submucosal bleeding, characterized by petechiae, ecchymoses, and occasional epistaxis. Rare patients have gastrointestinal blood loss. The majority, however, have not demonstrated life-threatening bleeding episodes. Unlike non–AIDS-related immune thrombocytopenia, mild splenomegaly may occur, especially in patients with generalized lymphadenopathy.

Laboratory findings typically reveal isolated thrombocytopenia, with a dearth of platelets seen on review of the peripheral blood smear. An increased number of megakaryocytes may be noted on examination of the bone marrow aspirate and biopsy, typical of peripheral platelet consumption.

Management of HIV-Related Thrombocytopenia

As with non–HIV-infected persons, thrombocytopenic patients with HIV infection should be evaluated for a secondary cause of their thrombocytopenia, and medications known to cause thrombocytopenia should be discontinued. For autoimmune-mediated thrombocytopenia

(ITP), steroid and immunoglobulin therapy can be initiated for those patients needing immediate restoration of their platelet counts. This may include patients who are experiencing bleeding who will be undergoing a splenectomy procedure, or in whom the platelet count is dangerously low and the treating physician wishes to raise the count immediately. The response of patients with HIV-related ITP to steroid therapy is variable, as the platelet count oftentimes falls as the steroid dose is tapered, and the risk of further immune suppression is real. Splenectomy has been a successful therapeutic intervention for patients who fail to respond to steroid therapy, and is generally not associated with greater morbidity or mortality than in patients with non–HIV-associated ITP.[40,49]

Intravenous gammaglobulin (IVIG; 400 mg/kg every day for 4 to 5 days) may be used to raise the platelet count rapidly, although transiently, lasting 2 to 3 weeks.[44] The mechanism probably is blockade of the reticuloendothelial system. The high cost and transient nature of immunoglobulin therapy limits its use to situations in which acute bleeding is occurring or as a preoperative intervention for patients undergoing splenectomy when rapid elevation of the platelet count is necessary. Although platelet transfusions generally are not indicated in patients with thrombocytopenia of immune origin, treatment with intravenous gammaglobulin before transfusion in emergency situations may improve platelet elevation.

For those patients who do not require an immediate increase in their platelet counts, the institution of antiretroviral therapy, if the patient is not yet on such therapy, may be warranted. Normalization and partial responses of platelet counts have been noted with the institution of zidovudine therapy.[41,52] Interferon-α has also been shown to be efficacious in treating patients with HIV-associated ITP in several small studies, yet may be more beneficial to those patients with less advanced HIV disease.[13,51,57] Partial responses appear to be more common than complete normalization of platelet counts, and the drug is relatively well tolerated at doses of 3 million units subcutaneously three times a week. Intravenous or intramuscular administration of anti-D immunoglobulin has been shown to benefit some Rh-positive patients who, preferably, have not had a splenectomy.[7,19,46] The presumed mechanism of this therapy is Fc receptor blockade by antibody-coated RBCs substituting for the antibody-coated platelets. Clinically significant hemolysis does not appear to complicate this approach.[7]

The nonandrogenizing testosterone danazol, initially thought to be efficacious in reversing HIV-related thrombocytopenia, has not proved so in large-scale clinical trials; less widely accepted interventions include vincristine and plasmapheresis.

Patients with isolated immune-mediated thrombocytopenia associated with HIV infection are generally the most healthy in the spectrum of HIV-infected individuals. Clinical bleeding is minimal, responses to therapeutic interventions are variable, and spontaneous remissions do occur. Thus, a viable alternative is to simply observe the patient closely and institute no therapies directed at correcting the thrombocytopenia until necessary. For those patients with evidence of CD4 + lymphocyte depletion, or high viral load, antiretroviral therapy may be beneficial.

HIV-ASSOCIATED COAGULOPATHIES

In patients with a variety of disease states such as systemic lupus erythematosus or AIDS, who are intravenous drug users, who receive certain drug therapy (i.e., chlorpromazine), and who have lymphoproliferative malignancies, a circulating inhibitor of coagulation may be noted. These so-called lupus anticoagulants are acquired antibodies, either IgG or IgM, that are directed against proteins that bind phospholipids.[47] The presence of such an inhibitor is established by the use of phospholipid-dependent coagulation assays, such as the activated partial thromboplastin time (aPTT) or Russell viper venom time (RVV), or is confirmed on enzyme-linked immunosorbent assay (ELISA), depending on the nature of the antibody.[47] Paradoxically, this "anticoagulant" is associated with in vitro prolongation of the aPTT or RVV, but clinically, is associated with increased thrombosis in the non–HIV-infected individual. In patients with HIV infection, the presence of a lupus anticoagulant does not appear to be associated with an increased incidence of thrombosis.[4] The anticoagulant may manifest during HIV-related infections, and often disappears with treatment of the infection.[48,59] If a patient has a prolonged aPTT with no history of bleeding, presence of the lupus anticoagulant should be suspected. Invasive procedures may be performed in the presence of the lupus anticoagulant without increased bleeding risk.[4]

Several reports describe thrombotic thrombocytopenic purpura (TTP) in the HIV-infected population.[29,38,53] TTP is a relatively rare disease that includes fever, neurologic abnormalities, renal abnormalities, purpura, microangiopathic hemolysis, and thrombocytopenia. The exact pathogenesis of this disease is unknown, but seems to arise from vascular injury caused by immune complexes, endotoxin, or other causes of endothelial injury. The disorder has been associated with increased platelet agglutination and abnormally large circulating von Willebrand factor complexes.

At present, it is unclear whether the occurrence of TTP in HIV-infected individuals is related to circulating immune complexes or immunoglobulin dysregulation associated with HIV disease. The mortality of this disease is high, as in the non–HIV-infected population, and therapy should include plasmapheresis and plasma transfusion.

HEMATOLOGIC CONSEQUENCES OF ANTI-HIV THERAPY

Many therapeutic interventions contribute to HIV-related hematologic disorders (see Table 16–2). Zidovudine, a thymidine analog and the most widely used drug in the care of these patients, greatly affects all three hematopoietic cell lines, and in vitro studies have demonstrated its toxicity toward myeloid and erythroid precursors.[20] As a thymidine analog, the primary action of zidovudine is termination of reverse transcriptase activity of the HIV virus. Zidovudine may also inhibit DNA polymerases, thus impairing normal hematopoiesis in the host.[45,48] Other nucleotide analogs used for antiretroviral therapy (e.g., ddC, ddI, D4T, and 3TC) and the protease inhibitors are associated with less bone marrow toxicity. In a large-scale collaborative study, all three hematopoietic cell lines were affected by zidovudine therapy: significant anemia developed in 34% of patients, and blood transfusions were required in 21%; neutropenia developed in 16% of patients; and thrombocytopenia developed in 12%.[45] Advanced HIV disease, preexisting cytopenias, and low vitamin B_{12} levels were associated with a greater risk of zidovudine-induced hematologic toxicities. Although zidovudine increases the mean corpuscular volume in most patients, bone marrow examination usually reveals hypoplasia, aplasia, or maturation arrest.[17,45,48,58] Overt megaloblastic changes are not always noted.

In general, the myelosuppression seen with

TABLE 16–3. COLONY-STIMULATING FACTORS: SUGGESTED GUIDELINES FOR USE

Justification for Use
Granulocyte-Macrophage Colony-Stimulating Factor (GM-CSF) and Granulocyte CSF (G-CSF)
Chemotherapy (per protocol guidelines)
Patients unable to sustain an absolute neutrophil count (ANC) >500 secondary to treatment with other myelosuppressive agents
Erythropoietin (EPO)
Symptomatic anemia while receiving zidovudine with EPO level <500 mU/dl
Dosing
GM-CSF and G-CSF
Initial dose, 5 µg/kg/day subcutaneously (SQ)
Titration:
    For neutropenia unresponsive to initial dose after 1 week, increase to 7.5 µg/kg/day
    If unresponsive to 7.5 µg/kg/day after 1 week, increase to 10 µg/kg/day
    If unresponsive to 10 µg/kg/day after 1 week, discontinue CSF therapy
Discontinue therapy for unresponsive neutropenia or ANC >500
Reported side effects: viral-like prodrome, fever, myalgias, and thrombocytopenia (anecdotal); these effects occur more frequently with GM-CSF than with granulocyte-CSF (G-CSF)
Erythropoietin
Initial dose, 100 µg/kg/day SQ three times each week
Obtain pretreatment EPO level, reticulocyte count, and ferritin level
Follow reticulocyte count
Patient may require iron replacement if reticulocyte count and ferritin level decrease
Injections may be slightly painful

zidovudine therapy is reversed by discontinuance of the drug,[45,58] but close observation with monitoring of blood counts is necessary. Drug trials have documented the efficacy of lower dose zidovudine therapy, which results in fewer side effects. Other drugs commonly used in treating HIV infections, including ganciclovir (DHPG), foscarnet, sulfa derivatives (used to treat toxoplasmosis or *Pneumocystis* infections), and pentamidine, also cause myelosuppression.

COLONY-STIMULATING FACTORS IN HIV DISEASE

Colony-stimulating factors (CSFs) now play an integral role in the treatment of HIV-related cytopenias (Table 16–3).[22,34] Theoretically, these agents could increase the number of target cells for HIV replication or enhance viral replication within target cells, leading to HIV disease progression.[33] In vitro studies have documented increased viral production in the presence of macrophage-CSF (M-CSF), granulocyte-macrophage CSF (GM-CSF), and interleukin-3, but not granulocyte-CSF (G-CSF).[27] Clinical studies, however, have not documented an acceleration of HIV disease caused by the use of CSFs.[21,33]

In several trials, neutropenic patients with AIDS responded to GM-CSF with a rapid increase in neutrophils and their precursors in conjunction with improved qualitative neutrophil functions,[2,23] and many chemotherapeutic trials now involve the administration of CSFs.

Human recombinant erythropoietin is oftentimes administered to HIV-infected patients with anemia secondary to zidovudine therapy. The best response is seen in patients whose endogenous erythropoietin levels are <500 mU/dl.[2,48] Individual patients with elevated erythropoietin levels may respond to such therapy, but this should be addressed on a case-by-case basis.[9] The concomitant administration of G-CSF or GM-CSF and erythropoietin may limit the hematologic toxicities of zidovudine therapy.[26]

REFERENCES

1. Abrams D, Chinn E, Lewis B: Hematologic manifestations in homosexual men with Kaposi's sarcoma. Am J Clin Pathol 81:13–18, 1984
2. Baldwin C, Gasson J, Quan S: Granulocyte-macrophage colony-stimulating factor enhances neutrophil function in acquired immunodeficiency syndrome patients. Proc Natl Acad Sci U S A 85: 2763–2766, 1988
3. Battaieb A, Fromont P, Louche F, et al: Presence of cross-reactive antibody between HIV and platelet glycoproteins in HIV-related immune thrombocytopenic purpura. Blood 80:162–169, 1992
4. Bloom E, Abrams D, Rodgers G: Lupus anticoagulant in the acquired immunodeficiency syndrome. JAMA 256:491–493, 1986
5. Bremner J, Beard B, Cohen A: Secondary infection with parvovirus B19 in an HIV-positive patient. AIDS 7:1131–1132, 1993
6. Brizzi M, Porcu P, Porteri A, et al: Haematologic abnormalities in the acquired immunodeficiency syndrome. Haematologica 75:454–463, 1990
7. Bussel J, Graziano JN, Kimberly RP, et al: Intravenous anti-D treatment of immune thrombocytopenic purpura: Analysis of efficacy, toxicity, and mechanism of effect. Blood 77(9):1884–1893, 1991
8. Castella A, Croxson T, Mildvan D: The bone marrow in AIDS: A histologic, hematologic, and microbiologic study. Am J Clin Pathol 84:425–432, 1985
9. DaCosta N, Hultin M: Effective therapy of human immunodeficiency virus-associated anemia with recombinant human erythropoietin despite high endogenous erythropoietin. Am J Hematol 36:71–72, 1991
10. Donahue R, Johnson M, Zon L: Suppression of in vitro haematopoiesis following human immunodeficiency virus infection. Nature 326:200–203, 1987
11. Doweiko J: Hematologic aspects of HIV infection. AIDS 7:753–757, 1993
12. Ehrenpreis E, Carlson SJ, Boorstein HL, et al: Malabsorption and deficiency of vitamin B12 in HIV-infected patients with chronic diarrhea. Dig Dis Sci 39(10):2159–2162, 1994
13. Fabris F, Sgarabotto D, Zanon E, et al: The effect of a single course of alpha-2B-interferon in patients with HIV-related and chronic idiopathic immune thrombocytopenia. Autoimmunity 14(3):175–179, 1993
14. Fauci A, Schnittman S, Polii G: Immunopathogenic mechanisms in human immunodeficiency virus (HIV) infection. Ann Intern Med 114:678–693, 1991
15. Frickhofen N, Abkowitz JL, Safford M, et al: Persistent B19 parvovirus infection in patients infected with HIV type 1: A treatable cause of anemia in AIDS. Ann Intern Med 113:926–933, 1990
16. Gascom P, Sathe S, Rameshwar P: Impaired erythropoiesis in the acquired immunodeficiency syndrome with disseminated *Mycobacterium avium* complex. Am J Med 94:41–48, 1993
17. Gill P, Rarick M, Brynes R: Azidothymidine associated with bone marrow failure in the acquired immunodeficiency syndrome. Ann Intern Med 107: 502–505, 1987
18. Goasguen J, Bennett J: Classification and morphologic features of the myelodysplastic syndromes. Semin Oncol 19:4–13, 1992
19. Gringeri A, Cattaneo M, Santagostino E, et al: Intramuscular anti-D immunoglobulins for home treatment of chronic immune thrombocytopenic purpura. Br J Haematol 80(3):337–340, 1992
20. Groopman J: Zidovudine intolerance. Rev Infect Dis 12(Suppl 5):S500–S506, 1990
21. Groopman J: Management of the hematologic complications of human immunodeficiency virus infection. Rev Infect Dis 12:931–937, 1990
22. Groopman J, Feder D: Hematopoietic growth factors in AIDS. Semin Oncol 19:408–414, 1992
23. Groopman J, Mitsuyasu R, DeLeo M: Effect of recombinant human granulocyte-macrophage colony-stimulating factor on myelopoiesis in the acquired immunodeficiency syndrome. N Engl J Med 317: 593–598, 1987
24. Hambleton J, Aragon T, Modin G, et al: Outcome for hospitalized patients with fever and neutropenia who are infected with the human immunodeficiency virus. Clin Infect Dis 20:363–371, 1995
25. Harriman G, Smith P, Horne M: Vitamin B12 malabsorption in patients with acquired immunodeficiency syndrome. Arch Intern Med 149:2039–2041, 1989
26. Henry D, Beall G, Benson C: Recombinant human erythropoietin in the therapy of anemia associated with HIV infection and zidovudine therapy: Overview of four clinical trials. Ann Intern Med 117: 739–748, 1992

27. Israel D, Plaisance K: Neutropenia in patients infected with human immunodeficiency virus. Clin Pharm 10:268–279, 1991

28. Karpatkin S: Immunologic thrombocytopenic purpura in HIV-seropositive homosexuals, narcotic addicts and hemophiliacs. Semin Hematol 25:219–229, 1988

29. Leaf A, Laubenstein L, Raphael B: Thrombotic thrombocytopenic purpura associated with human immunodeficiency virus type 1 infection. Ann Intern Med 109:194–197, 1988

30. Leiderman I, Greenberg M, Adelsberg B, et al: A glycoprotein inhibitor of in vitro granulopoiesis associated with AIDS. Blood 70:1267–1272, 1987

31. Louche F, Bettaieb A, Henri A, et al: Infection of megakaryocytes by HIV in seropositive patients with immune thrombocytopenic purpura. Blood 78:1697–1705, 1991

32. McGinniss M, Macher A, Rook A, et al: Red cell autoantibodies in patients with acquired immune deficiency syndrome. Transfusion 26:405–409, 1986

33. Miles S: The use of hematopoietic growth factors in HIV infection and AIDS-related malignancies. Cancer Invest 9:229–238, 1991

34. Miles S: Hematopoietic growth factors as adjuncts to antiretroviral therapy. AIDS Res Hum Retroviruses 8:1073–1079, 1992

35. Murphy P, Lane C, Fauci A, et al: Impairment of neutrophil bactericidal capacity in patients with AIDS. J Infect Dis 158:627–630, 1988

36. Murphy M, Metcalfe P, Waters A: Incidence and mechanism of neutropenia and thrombocytopenia in patients with human immunodeficiency virus infection. Br J Haematol 66:337–340, 1987

37. Naides S, Howard EJ, Swack NS, et al: Parvovirus B19 infection in HIV type 1-infected persons failing or intolerant to zidovudine therapy. J Infect Dis 168:101–105, 1993

38. Nair J, Bellevue R, Bertoni M, et al: Thrombotic thrombocytopenic purpura in patients with the acquired immunodeficiency syndrome-related complex. Ann Intern Med 109:209–212, 1988

39. Northfelt D, Mayer A, Kaplan L: The usefulness of diagnostic bone marrow examination in patients with human immunodeficiency virus (HIV) infection. J Acquir Immune Defic Syndr 4:659–666, 1991

40. Oksenhendler E, Bierling P, Chevret S, et al: Splenectomy is safe and effective in HIV-related immune thrombocytopenia. Blood 82:29–32, 1993

41. Oksenhendler E, Bierling P, Ferchal F: Zidovudine for thrombocytopenic purpura related to human immunodeficiency virus infection. Ann Intern Med 110:365–368, 1989

42. Paltiel O, Falutz J, Veilleux M, et al: Clinical correlates of subnormal vitamin B12 levels in patients infected with the human immunodeficiency virus. Am J Hematol 49(4):318–322, 1995

43. Perkocha L, Rodgers G: Hematologic aspects of human immunodeficiency virus infection: Laboratory and clinical considerations. Am J Hematol 29:94–105, 1988

44. Perret B, Baumgartner C: Workshop on immunoglobulin therapy of lymphoproliferative syndromes, mainly AIDS-related complex, and AIDS. Vox Sang 52:1–14, 1986

45. Richman D; AZT Collaborative Working Group: The toxicity of azidothymidine in the treatment of patients with AIDS and AIDS-related complex. N Engl J Med 317:192–197, 1987

46. Rossi E, Damasio E, Terragna A: HIV-related thrombocytopenia: A therapeutical update. Haematologica 76:141–149, 1991

47. Roubey RAS: Autoantibodies to phospholipid-binding plasma proteins: A new view of lupus anticoagulants and other "antiphospholipid" autoantibodies. Blood 84(9):2854–2867, 1994

48. Scadden D, Zon L, Groopman J: Pathophysiology and management of HIV-associated hematologic disorders. Blood 74:1455–1463, 1989

49. Schneider P, Abrams D, Rayner A, et al: Immunodeficiency-associated thrombocytopenic purpura: Response to splenectomy. Arch Surg 122:1175–1178, 1987

50. Spivak J, Barnes DC, Fuchs E, et al: Serum immunoreactive erythropoietin in HIV-infected patients. JAMA 261:3104–3107, 1989

51. Stellini R, Rossi G, Paraninfo G: Interferon therapy in intravenous drug users with HIV-associated idiopathic thrombocytopenic purpura. Haematologica 77:418–420, 1992

52. Swiss Group for Clinical Studies on AIDS: Zidovudine for the treatment of thrombocytopenia associated with human immunodeficiency virus. Ann Intern Med 109:718–721, 1988

53. Thompson C, Damon LE, Ries CA, et al: Thrombotic microangiopathies in the 1980s: Clinical features, response to treatment, and the impact of the HIV epidemic. Blood 80:1890–1895, 1992

54. Toy P, Reid M, Burns M: Positive direct antiglobulin test associated with hyperglobulinemia in acquired immunodeficiency syndrome. Am J Hematol 19:145, 1985

55. Treacy M, Lai L, Costello C, et al: Peripheral blood and bone marrow abnormalities in patients with HIV related disease. Br J Haematol 65:289–294, 1987

56. Valone F, Payan D, Abrams D, et al: Defective polymorphonuclear leukocyte chemotaxis in homosexual men with persistent lymph node syndrome. J Infect Dis 150:267–271, 1984

57. Vianelli N, Cantai L, Gugliotta L: Recombinant alpha interferon 2b in the therapy of HIV-related thrombocytopenia. AIDS 7:823–827, 1993

58. Walker R, Parker R, Kovacs J: Anemia and erythropoiesis in patients with the acquired immunodeficiency syndrome and Kaposi sarcoma treated with zidovudine. Ann Intern Med 108:372–376, 1988

59. Zon L, Groopman J: Hematologic manifestations of the human immune deficiency virus. Semin Hematol 25:208–218, 1988

60. Zucker-Franklin D, Seremetius S, Zheng Z: Internalization of HIV-type 1 and other retroviruses by megakaryocytes and platelets. Blood 75:1920–1923, 1990

61. Zucker-Frankli D, Termin C, Cooper M: Structural changes in the megakaryocytes of patients infected with HIV-1. Am J Pathol 134:1295–1303, 1989

Cardiovascular Complications of HIV Infection

MELVIN D. CHEITLIN

We are now halfway into the second decade of the HIV infection pandemic. Although cardiovascular involvement in patients with AIDS was recognized early in the epidemic, the incidence of cardiovascular disease specifically related to the AIDS infection is low. Pericarditis and pulmonary hypertension are well-recognized problems that require specific treatment, and these are certainly the most frequently seen clinical problems. Myocardial involvement with AIDS is clinically unusual but, despite this, much has been written about the incidence, significance, and approach to therapy in patients who have been demonstrated to have left ventricular dysfunction. There are now several prospective studies that allow an estimation of the prevalence and incidence of cardiomyopathy in AIDS patients. The etiology of the left ventricular dysfunction is still not well understood.

This chapter reviews the approach to treatment of cardiovascular disease present in patients with AIDS, both related and incidental to the AIDS infection.

CARDIOVASCULAR INVOLVEMENT IN PATIENTS WITH AIDS

Disease of the cardiovascular system can be related to the AIDS infection itself or be present in patients with AIDS and unrelated to the primary disease. Thus, pericarditis and pulmonary hypertension are probably related to the HIV disease, either from direct involvement by the HIV organism or because the patient's autoimmune defenses against opportunistic infection are weakened by the HIV disease. Conversely, infective endocarditis in intravenous drug users is common in patients both with and without HIV disease. Furthermore, coronary artery dis-

ease and congenital heart disease may be incidentally found in patients who are HIV positive. Nevertheless, the treatment of the nonrelated disease is affected by the presence of the HIV disease.

The following is a listing of the most important clinical problems seen in patients with HIV infection:

- *Pericarditis:* In my experience, this is the most frequently encountered cardiovascular clinical problem in patients with HIV disease, both with and without tamponade. There is now evidence that the presence of pericardial effusion, with or without clinical pericarditis, is a bad prognostic sign and probably occurs late in the course of the disease.
- *Pulmonary hypertension:* This is seen mostly in patients with multiple pulmonary infections, usually *Pneumocystis carinii*, but occasionally is seen in patients without preceding pulmonary infection.
- *Myocardial involvement:* The incidence of myocardial involvement depends on the way in which myocardial involvement is diagnosed.
  - In autopsy studies on consecutive patients dying with AIDS, the incidence of myocardial involvement is 15% to 50%. For the most part, this involvement is that of focal myocarditis.
  - If echocardiography is used, the incidence of abnormal wall motion varies from 12% to 41%.
  - In both autopsy and echocardiographic series, the abnormalities are found in patients who have no clinical findings of heart disease.
  - Clinical involvement of the cardiovascular system as myocarditis or cardiomyopathy is distinctly unusual.
- *Valvular abnormalities:* This includes ineffec-

tive endocarditis, almost exclusively seen in intravenous drug users, marantic endocarditis, and mitral valve prolapse.

- *Arrhythmias*
- *Venous thrombosis and pulmonary embolism*

Clinical cardiovascular disease is unusual in AIDS patients. In large autopsy series, cardiovascular disease as a cause of death is rare. Most patients die of opportunistic infection, central nervous system involvement, neoplasms, or gastrointestinal involvement.[40,42,48] The prevalence of cardiovascular disease reported in AIDS patients varies depending on whether diagnosis is based on clinical findings or more sensitive techniques, such as echocardiography or microscopic examination of the heart at autopsy. The incidence of cardiovascular disease also depends on the population of AIDS patients reported. In a series reported from New York City, where 40% to 50% of the IV drug users are HIV positive, the incidence of clinical cardiovascular disease, especially infective endocarditis, is higher than in series reported from San Francisco, where the HIV risk factor is overwhelmingly homosexuality.[20]

It is also important to recognize that reports from hospitals that do primary care for HIV-positive patients will have a lower incidence of clinical cardiovascular disease than reports from tertiary care facilities, where problem cases are referred. For these reasons, in autopsy reports of cardiovascular involvement from primary care centers, the prevalence of cardiovascular involvement is 5% to 20%.[40,42] When echocardiography and microscopic evidence of lymphocytic infiltration of the myocardium are used as an indicator for cardiovascular involvement, the prevalence of cardiovascular involvement in AIDS patients is closer to 50%.[39]

CLINICAL DIAGNOSIS AND WORKUP

The only patients with AIDS who require specific cardiovascular diagnostic evaluation are those with clinically evident cardiovascular problems. There is no therapeutic advantage to identifying patients with subclinical cardiovascular involvement and, therefore, no justification for screening of patients with electrocardiograms (ECGs) or more expensive techniques, such as echocardiography.

Symptoms of cardiovascular disease are nonspecific, and many, such as dyspnea, commonly are due to pulmonary involvement rather than cardiovascular disease. Specific signs of cardiovascular involvement, such as the presence of an enlarged cardiac silhouette on a radiograph, the development of a pericardial friction rub, the clinical picture of congestive heart failure with S_3 gallop, pulmonary edema, or the development of a pathologic systolic murmur or diastolic murmur, are all findings that should initiate a cardiovascular diagnostic workup. The coincidental occurrence of coronary artery disease, hypertensive cardiovascular disease, congenital heart disease, and myocardial disease caused by illicit drugs, such as cocaine, should also be considered.[7]

The most helpful laboratory studies are the chest radiography, an ECG, and two-dimensional transthoracic echocardiography. To evaluate valvular function or diastolic left ventricular function, Doppler echocardiography is the most useful. Whenever a question of pulmonary hypertension arises, the use of Doppler in detecting tricuspid regurgitation, found in a high proportion of normal hearts, makes it possible to estimate the pulmonary artery systolic pressure. If the velocity of the regurgitant jet by the modified Bernoulli equation is known, the systolic pressure gradient between the right ventricle and the right atrium across the tricuspid valve can be calculated. When this pressure is added to the clinically estimated central venous pressure, the systolic pressure of the pulmonary artery can be estimated with a fair degree of accuracy.[62]

For almost all patients with suspected cardiovascular involvement, these simple, noninvasive tests should suffice. Proceeding to invasive studies, such as cardiac catheterization or angiography, is rarely necessary unless indicated by the need to work up incidental problems, such as coronary heart disease.

The value of doing pericardial and myocardial biopsy to find treatable etiologies in patients with pericardial or myocardial disease is controversial. In general, the incidence of finding treatable etiologies of pericardial or myocardial disease is very low. However, if such a problem that is treatable with special therapy is found, it is obviously important.

The major argument for myocardial biopsy was that, if myocarditis was found, steroid and/or antimetabolite therapy would be indicated. Mason and colleagues have shown that steroid or antimetabolite therapy in myocarditis has no advantage over conventional medical management, eliminating the rationale for myocardial biopsy.[45]

WORKUP AND THERAPY OF SPECIFIC CARDIOVASCULAR PROBLEMS

Pericarditis and Pericardial Effusion

In autopsy series, the prevalence of pericardial involvement varies from 3%[60] to almost 37%.[44] In the experience at San Francisco General Hospital, pericardial effusion is found in about 30% of patients who have had an ECG ordered for suspicion of cardiovascular involvement. This prevalence by echocardiography is similar to that reported by Corallo et al, wherein 38% of the patients studied by echocardiography had pericardial effusion.[13]

Although clinical presentation of pericarditis with pleuritic-type chest pain and pericardial friction rub is seen, asymptomatic pericardial effusion is more common. The initial suspicion of cardiovascular disease frequently is made on finding a large cardiac silhouette on a chest radiograph. Dyspnea caused by compression of the lung by a large pericardial effusion is another common presentation of pericardial effusion.

Cardiac tamponade manifested by an enlarged cardiac silhouette, elevation of central venous pressure, pulsus paradoxis, and later tachycardia and hypotension is not uncommon. Deaths from tamponade have been reported occasionally.[56] In the experience at San Francisco General Hospital, cardiac tamponade is seen in about one third of patients with pericardial effusion,[21] which is similar to the report by Monsuez et al of 28% with or developing cardiac tamponade.[47]

The etiology of the pericardial effusion can be heart failure or pericarditis due to specific organisms, such as *Mycobacterium tuberculosis,* or to unknown pathogens, either viral infections or the HIV organism itself. Another important etiology for pericardial effusion is tumor involvement by Kaposi's sarcoma or lymphoma. Reynolds et al reported 14 AIDS patients with pericarditis in whom *M. tuberculosis* was found to be the etiology in 37%.[52] Other organisms, such as *Mycobacterium avium-intracellulare,*[61] and other pathogens, such as staphylococcus, pneumococcus, and fungi, have been reported.

Treatment of Pericarditis and Pericardial Effusion

An asymptomatic small pericardial effusion needs no therapy. If the patient has a large effusion compressing the lung or has signs of tamponade, such as an elevated central venous pressure, pericardiocentesis is indicated, with removal of fluid to reverse the hemodynamic compromise and to examine the fluid by culture and microscopic examination for possible treatable etiologies, such as *M. tuberculosis* or lymphoma. Waiting for diastolic collapse of the right atrium by echocardiography before doing a pericardiocentesis is not necessary. With a large effusion, a catheter can be introduced percutaneously into the pericardial cavity and connected to closed-drainage suction for 24 to 48 hours. Usually, there is no recurrence. If the patient has clinical pericarditis with pain and fever with a small effusion, examination of the pericardial fluid and pericardial tissue looking for a treatable etiology is possible by drainage through an open pericardiotomy, usually from a subxiphoid approach.

At San Francisco General Hospital, in 10 of 25 patients with clinical pericardial effusion or pericarditis or both, no specific etiology was found on examination of the pericardial effusion and pericardial tissue.[21] Some of the patients had lymphoma, and the pericardial effusion was thought to be related to the tumor, but in none in whom tissue or fluid was examined could evidence of a tumor be found.

The presence of pericardial effusion is probably a sign of poor prognosis. We have done a prospective study of 195 HIV-positive patients recruited as outpatients and followed with serial echocardiograms every 4 months for 3 years at San Francisco General Hospital.[26] We found an incidence of pericardial effusion of 4% per year for all infected patients and 11% per year for AIDS patients. The presence of pericardial effusion was a sign of poor prognosis, because these patients had a 6-month mortality of 64% vs 7% for similar AIDS patients without effusion. It is doubtful that the pericardial effusion is the cause of the poor prognosis, because it is rare for patients to die from pericardial tamponade. The presence of pericardial effusion in patients with AIDS is a bad prognostic sign and probably occurs late in the course of the disease.

Flum and colleagues[19] also reported that AIDS-associated pericardial effusion is a sign of grave prognosis. They reported 29 patients who had surgical "pericardial windows" for effusions; 7 (24%) were found to have a specific etiology on culture or biopsy (2 with adenocarcinoma, 3 with lymphoma, 1 with *Staphylococcus aureus,* and 1 with *M. tuberculosis*). In 94% of cases there was no change in clinical management based on the results of biopsy or culture because either the patient was receiving appropriate therapy or the therapy could not be instituted because of the underlying illness. The mortality was high: 69% at 8 weeks after the pericardial window. They concluded that pericardial windows for diagnosis provided little practical information and were justified only to relieve pericardial tamponade.

Pulmonary Hypertension

Early in the epidemic, patients were seen with ECG evidence of right ventricular hypertrophy. At autopsy, dilation of the right ventricle with normal left ventricle was described in about 15% of cases.[2,40] Himelman et al[32] reported six patients with severe pulmonary hypertension who had increased pulmonary vascular resistance on catheterization. The majority of these patients had multiple pulmonary infections, mostly *P. carinii,* although one had had no previous pneumonias. Patients with primary pulmonary hypertension have been reported.[46] At autopsy, no evidence for HIV infection in the pulmonary vascular endothelium was found by polymerase chain reaction or in situ hybridization. There were electron microscopic changes in the endothelial cells similar to those seen in patients with lupus erythematosus, and these authors postulated a sequence of injury to the endothelial cell by paracrine cytokines releasing vasoactive substances or growth factors, resulting in increased pulmonary vascular resistance. With multiple pulmonary infections, interstitial fibrosis and destruction of the capillary bed are possible causes of increased pulmonary vascular resistance. With the development of pulmonary hypertension, increased afterload on the right ventricle, right ventricular hypertrophy and dilatation, and eventually right heart failure result.

Treatment of Pulmonary Hypertension

If the patient's pulmonary hypertension and its consequences are the most important clinical problem, normalization of blood gases and treatment of underlying pulmonary infection are most important. Hypoxia, respiratory acidosis, and to a lesser degree hypercarbia are pow-

erful causes of pulmonary vasoconstriction. If hypoxia persists, supplemental low-flow oxygen can be helpful. If these measures are not successful, an empiric trial of a variety of vasodilators is indicated in an attempt to find one that will reduce pulmonary vascular resistance and increase to normal or maintain cardiac output without dropping systemic vascular resistance to the point where systemic arterial pressure drops. To do this safely, the patient must be hospitalized, and the cardiac output, pulmonary artery pressure, pulmonary vascular resistance, and systemic arterial pressure must be monitored invasively.[53] With a pulmonary arterial catheter in place, we have used the following vasodilators sequentially: 100% oxygen, nitroglycerin, hydralazine, nifedipine, lisinopril, converting enzyme inhibitors, and prostaglandin E_1. If an appropriate drug is found, it can be continued chronically. If arterial blood pressure drops, the drug must be discontinued. In our experience, finding a drug that is effective chronically is rare, and the patient with pulmonary hypertension has a very poor prognosis.

Barst and colleagues[3] have reported a 12-week study of continuous intravenous infusion of prostacyclin in patients with primary pulmonary hypertension. They achieved a 21% drop in pulmonary vascular resistance compared to a 9% rise in patients on conventional management. Even if the AIDS patients responded to prostacyclin, it is doubtful whether such a therapy would be justified in patients in the late stages of AIDS.

Myocardial Involvement

Myocardial involvement is the most controversial topic concerning cardiovascular disease in AIDS patients. The prevalence of myocardial involvement in patients with HIV disease depends on the definition. Clinical cardiomyopathy, that is, myocardial disease causing signs and symptoms including heart failure, is rare. Myocardial involvement defined as microscopic inflammatory cell myocarditis with or without any evidence of myocardial cell necrosis is found more commonly. Focal myocarditis is seen in 15% to 50% of cases in autopsy series.[2,20,40,42] What is being described is usually focal collections of inflammatory cells with or without adjacent myocardial cell necrosis. Rarely is the myocarditis diffuse, and rarely was there clinical evidence of myocardial involvement before death. When searched for diligently, pathogenic organisms, both fungal and parasitic, such as *Toxoplasma, Candida albicans,* and *Coccidioides,* can be found about a quarter to a third of the time. It is probable that opportunistic viral infections known to cause myocarditis also could be responsible for these findings. These might include Coxsackie B virus and cytomegalic inclusion disease.

Myocarditis is rarely the cause of death in these patients. Myocarditis is said to occur in the late stages of the disease in patients with a low CD4 count. When the diagnosis of myocardial involvement is made by echocardiography, on which decreased left ventricular function or a dilated left ventricle is seen, the prevalence is also high. Himelman et al[31] reported 71 patients with AIDS who had been sent for echocardiography. There were eight patients who had left ventricular dilatation or decreased contractility or both, four of whom had clinical congestive heart failure. Corallo et al[13] performed echocardiograms on 102 consecutive patients with AIDS, none with congestive heart failure, and found 41% with left ventricular hypokinesia.

Prospective studies by echocardiography are beginning to be reported. Blanchard et al[5] followed 50 patients with AIDS and found that 7 (14%) developed echocardiographic evidence of left ventricular dysfunction. When repeat echocardiograms were done, three had improved left ventricular function and four did not. All four who did not improve died within 1 year. Herskowitz et al[29] followed 59 AIDS patients with normal initial echocardiograms for 11 months and performed serial echocardiograms. Eleven patients developed left ventricular dysfunction over 725 months of follow-up, a rate of 1.5 patients per 100 patient-months. De Castro et al[16] reported serial echocardiograms on 114 HIV-positive patients, three quarters of whom were IV drug users. Of 72 AIDS patients, 16.6% had dilated cardiomyopathy and 18% had pericardial effusion. They concluded that 46% of HIV-infected patients would develop cardiovascular abnormalities as a result of opportunistic infection or malignancy.

Currie and colleagues[14] reported a prospective echocardiography survey in 296 HIV-infected adults conducted over 4 years. They found 13 (4%) with dilated cardiomyopathy. The patients with dilated cardiomyopathy had medically defined CD4 cell counts (<100/mm^3). Survival was significantly reduced in subjects with cardiomyopathy compared to those with normal hearts on echocardiography. The

excess mortality remains significant when compared only to patients with CD4 cell counts of <20/mm^3. In patients whose death was related to AIDS median survival time was 101 days in those with cardiomyopathy compared to 472 days in those with normal hearts on echocardiography. Death in the cardiomyopathy patient was most often due to AIDS related causes rather than to congestive heart failure.

At San Francisco General Hospital, we have conducted a 4-year prospective study using serial quantitative echocardiographic Doppler techniques. All patients were recruited as outpatients. There were 74 AIDS patients followed for a mean of 16.5 ± 12 months. The control populations were HIV-positive patients without disease, HIV-positive patients with AIDS-related complex, and HIV-negative gay men. Over the follow-up period, there were no differences in systolic left ventricular function (end-diastolic volume, end-systolic volume, or ejection fraction) within or among any of the groups. There were no differences between groups in the numbers of patients whose ejection fraction changed by more than 2 standard deviations during follow-up. Most of the patients with reduced left ventricular function on echocardiogram had no clinical evidence of cardiac disease, and the etiology of these changes is not obvious.

In summarizing most series of patients, the number of AIDS patients seen with clinically important cardiomyopathy not explained by known agents, such as alcohol, toxoplasmosis, hypertrophic cardiomyopathy, cocaine use, acute myocardial infarction, or drug toxicity, is small. Clinical cardiomyopathy is seen in 1% to 4% of AIDS patients.

The etiology of the changes in left ventricular function is as yet undetermined. Obviously, HIV infection (myocarditis) is a leading contender. The fact that the myocardial cell lacks the CD4 receptor argues against the possibility of direct HIV invasion of the myocardial cell. By in situ hybridization, polymerase chain reaction, and culture,[8,9,25,41] the HIV organism has been located in or near the myocardial cell. These findings have been sparse, with the HIV organism not proved to be within the myocardial cell rather than in a macrophage or endothelial cell and frequently being in tissue from patients without clinical or microscopic evidence of myocarditis. It is possible that the myocardial cell is injured by some other mechanism, allowing entrance of the HIV organism. Epstein-Barr virus has been shown to facilitate entry and replication of HIV into CD4 receptor-negative B cells.[23]

Opportunistic infections can cause myocarditis and even clinical congestive heart failure and death. Toxoplasmosis has been reported as well as myocarditis due to cytomegalovirus and Epstein-Barr virus.[1] Niedt and Schinella,[49] in a study of 56 AIDS patients, found that 77% had been infected with cytomegalovirus, 4 of whom had clinical cardiac involvement (ECG changes, arrhythmias, or congestive heart failure) and demonstrated inclusion bodies and myocarditis.

Myocardial damage can result from cytokine release from HIV-infected monocytes and lymphocytes. The cytokine acts as a paracrine substance, and the adjacent myocardial cells are affected. Ho et al[33] reported this mechanism as the etiology of neuroglia cell dysfunction in patients with AIDS. If cytokines are released into the circulation by infected macrophages and monocytes, myocardial cell dysfunction could result.[50] Circulating cytokines have been demonstrated in patients with advanced HIV infection.[38]

Another postulated mechanism for myocardial cell dysfunction is autoimmune myocarditis, which could be initiated by a change in some myocardial cell component, inducing autoimmune antibodies. Such cardiac autoantibodies have been demonstrated in AIDS patients with cardiomyopathy by Herskowitz et al,[28] but it is not clear whether the cardiac autoantibodies are the cause or the result of myocardial injury.

Although other etiologies for cardiac myocardial dysfunction, such as nutritional deficiency of both calories[22] and such microelements as selenium,[35] have been reported, the effects of both therapeutic and illicit drugs are the most likely etiology of myocardial dysfunction. Most patients with HIV infection are taking multiple drugs, some of which are known to be cardiotoxic. Reversible cardiomyopathy has been described in patients taking interleukin-2,[54] alpha$_2$-interferon,[17] and adriamycin. More recently, foscarnet[6] and high-dose ifosfamide[51] have been reported to cause severe reversible cardiomyopathy.

Herskowitz et al[30] reported decreases in left ventricular function by echocardiography in AIDS patients taking zidovudine. When zidovudine was discontinued, left ventricular dysfunction improved in some of the patients. Other drugs to which patients with HIV disease are exposed, such as cocaine and alcohol, have regularly been reported to cause cardiomyopathy.[11]

Treatment of Myocarditis, Cardiomyopathy, and Congestive Heart Failure

There is no evidence that a patient with HIV disease without clinical evidence of cardiac involvement benefits from by screening with ECG, chest radiography, or more expensive techniques, such as echocardiography or Doppler. Any abnormality found would not justify any specific treatment at that point in the patient's HIV disease.

In the patient with symptoms, cardiac involvement must be suspected and differentiated from symptoms caused by pulmonary or renal disease. The most effective way of doing this is by echocardiography. There are two reasons why echocardiography is essential in patients with congestive heart failure: (1) the etiology of the congestive heart failure may be apparent, that is, the patient may have valve disease, arteriosclerotic heart disease, or congenial heart disease; and (2) the echocardiogram allows identification of the pathophysiologic type of congestive heart failure. Most patients with heart failure have a dilated left ventricle and decreased systolic function. Some patients, especially elderly, hypertensive patients, have good left ventricular function, with diastolic dysfunction as the cause of the congestive heart failure.[55] This occurs in up to one third of cases. In these patients, the treatment is different from that of systolic dysfunction heart failure, with avoidance of inotropic agents and afterload reduction and judicious use of nitrates, diuretics, beta-blockade, and calcium channel blockers.

Patients with clinical congestive heart failure manifested by an S$_3$ gallop or pulmonary edema, or an elevated central venous pressure should have an echocardiogram. Pericardial effusion resulting in tamponade can occur as right heart failure and is treatable by pericardiocentesis. Occasionally, other reasons for congestive heart failure are found, such as a hypertrophic cardiomyopathy or cocaine or alcohol abuse, and withdrawal of these substances is essential. When the patient has clinical cardiomyopathy, Herskowitz et al have suggested a drug-free trial, with the removal of all drugs not absolutely essential.[30] The echocardiogram should be repeated in 2 weeks. If improvement has occurred, the suspected drug should be eliminated. Patients with clinical congestive heart failure are treated in the conventional way with rest, diuretics, digoxin, and afterload reduction, preferably by angiotensin-converting enzyme inhibition.

The value of myocardial biopsy is still in debate. In my experience, myocardial biopsy rarely has been useful. As long as there is no evidence that treatment with steroids or antimetabolites is effective in patients with myocarditis, the finding of focal collections of inflammatory cells on myocardial biopsy is not helpful and does not alter therapy.[45] Some authorities believe that the rare finding of a treatable cause of myocarditis is a justifiable reason for recommending myocardial biopsy in patients with congestive heart failure. However, it is difficult even at autopsy, when the entire heart is available for examination, to find organisms that are treatable, so that the few pieces of tissue obtainable by myocardial biopsy would likely miss such organisms.

The stage of the patient's HIV disease in the patient is an important factor. Patients who are late in their course of HIV disease and who develop congestive heart failure should be treated for their congestive heart failure without invasive studies. If congestive heart failure is found earlier in the course of the HIV infection and does not respond to a drug-free trial, it is clinically justifiable to attempt to find a treatable etiology by myocardial biopsy even though the chances of discovering such a treatable cause are very low.

Myocardial involvement by neoplasm is usually an incidental finding and not the cause of congestive heart failure. Kaposi's sarcoma was one of the first neoplasms to be described involving the heart.[58] At present, lymphoma, especially non-Hodgkin's lymphoma, is seen most often, and pericardial effusion is the most frequent clinical condition.[24] The tumor can invade the myocardium, causing arrhythmias, heart block, and even obstruction to blood flow, requiring surgical excision.[24,34,36] When the tumor is found, specific treatment is required.

VALVULAR ABNORMALITIES

Most valvular abnormalities in patients with AIDS are coincidental rather than related to the HIV infection. Infective endocarditis occurs almost exclusively in IV drug users and is rare in other HIV-positive patients.[15] Patients with marantic endocarditis usually are found by virtue of the fact that they have suffered a systemic embolization. Occasionally, a marantic thrombus is found incidentally on echocardiography. In these instances, the treatment is anticoagulation as long as no absolute contraindication to anticoagulation exists. Although it is conceivable that such a large, mobile vegetation could be found and surgical removal would be indicated, I have never seen such a case. Marantic endocarditis was reported frequently in the earlier autopsy series, with a prevalance of 4% to 10% of autopsied cases.[15] At present it is reported much less commonly. In Currie and colleagues' study of 110 outpatient subjects there were no patients with marantic endocarditis.[15]

Patients with valvular insufficiency resulting from infective endocarditis, frequently with the usual streptococcal or staphylococcal organism, should be treated in the same way as HIV-negative patients. Obviously, clinical judgment should be used when infective endocarditis is the last tragedy in the late course of a patient's HIV disease. In this instance, surgery should be avoided because the outcome in the near future will be determined by the HIV disease and not by the endocarditis.

Patients with mitral valve prolapse have been described who had HIV disease. These patients are usually cachectic, and the mitral valve prolapse may be secondary to the decrease in volume of the left ventricle, resulting in systolic prolapse of the mitral valve into the left atrium. In these patients, unless the mitral regurgitation is severe, no treatment is necessary. If mitral regurgitation is severe, the patient should be treated as would be an HIV-negative patient unless the patient is late in the course.

ARRHYTHMIAS AND OTHER CARDIOVASCULAR INVOLVEMENT

Arrhythmias can be seen as a result of myocarditis, pulmonary hypertension, congestive heart failure, or drug therapy. Torsade de pointes has been reported to result from both intravenous and inhaled pentamidine.[18,59]

Venous thrombosis[12] and pulmonary embolism[4] have been described in patients with AIDS. They can be a cause of pulmonary hypertension and are treated by anticoagulation.[43] AIDS patients have prothrombotic abnormalities, such as increased anticardiolipin immunoglobulin G (IgG) activity[57] and low protein S and protein C levels.[37] To evaluate patients with venous thrombosis and pulmonary embolism, a search for low protein C and protein S levels and elevated anticardiolipin IgG should be carried out, and a duplex Doppler examination for deep venous thrombosis should be performed. The treatment for venous thrombosis is anticoagulation.

INVASIVE CARDIOVASCULAR PROCEDURES IN PATIENT WITH AIDS

In the workup and treatment of the patient with HIV infection, it is necessary occasionally to consider a catheterization or cardiovascular surgery. Usually, the need for invasive techniques arises because of diseases that are occurring incidentally in the HIV-positive patient, such as congenital heart disease, coronary artery disease, or valve disease. Because health care workers fear HIV infection, there is a hesitancy to do invasive procedures where there would be no question with a similar indication in an HIV-negative patient.

The incidence of HIV infection in health care workers with no other risk factors for AIDS is very small. As of 1992, there have been 100 such health care workers who seroconverted after accidental exposure, usually a needlestick or knife wound, who were known to be HIV negative before the incident. Combining 14 prospective studies of the risk of HIV-1 infection to health care workers, there were 2042 parenteral exposures in 1948 patients.[27] The chance of seroconversion was 0.29% per exposure (95% confidence interval, 0.13% to 0.7%). There were no seroconversions from mucous membrane exposures in 688 people with 1061 mucous membrane exposures. Therefore, the risk of developing an HIV conversion from work exposure is very low, approximately 1 infection in 300 documented parenteral exposures to HIV-positive blood.

Even though the risk is low, it is nonetheless necessary to maintain vigorous discipline when performing invasive procedures in these patients. Judgment is necessary in deciding when the small risk of infection is justified by the value of the procedure to the patient. Patients in the late stages of HIV infection who have problems that ordinarily would justify catheterization or open heart surgery will not be benefited by such surgery if the prognosis is determined by the HIV disease. It is therefore unlikely that coronary or valve surgery can be justified if the goal is to prolong life when 70% of patients with AIDS die within 3 to 4 years of the diagnosis.[10] However, if patients with AIDS are on maximal medical management and still are incapacitated by the coronary or the valve disease, surgery is justifiable.

More commonly, the question arises in patients with HIV infection but no defining diagnosis of AIDS. Such patients may live 10 to 15 years before they develop the disease, which ultimately will be fatal, and they deserve evaluation and therapy, including invasive procedures, for the same indications as would be the case in an HIV-negative person.

CONCLUSION

Patients with HIV infection have serious problems with opportunistic infections, central nervous system involvement, and gastrointestinal disorders. Clinical cardiovascular involvement is unusual. The most important and treatable cardiovascular involvement is pericarditis and tamponade. The unusual patient with clinical cardiomyopathy should be recognized, evaluated by echocardiography, and treated with conventional treatment for congestive heart failure. It is rare that invasive techniques, such as catheterization or myocardial biopsy, are useful, although in the patient early in the HIV disease where clinical cardiomyopathy is the major problem, a vigorous search for treatable etiologies is justified.

REFERENCES

1. Acierno LJ: Cardiac complications in acquired immunodeficiency syndrome (AIDS): A review. J Am Coll Cardiol 13:1144–1154, 1989
2. Anderson DW, Virmani R, Reilly JM, et al: Prevalent myocarditis at necropsy in the acquired immunodeficiency syndrome. J Am Coll Cardiol 11:792–799, 1988
3. Barst RJ, Rubin LJ, Long WA, et al: A comparison of continuous intravenous epoprostenol (prostacyclin) with conventional therapy for primary pulmonary hypertension. The Primary Pulmonary Hypertension Study Group. N Engl J Med 334:296–301, 1996
4. Becker DM, Saunders TJ, Wispelwey B, Schain DC: Case report. Venous thromboembolism in AIDS. Am J Med Sci 303:395–397, 1992

5. Blanchard DG, Hagenhoff C, Chow LC, et al: Reversibility of cardiac abnormalities in human immunodeficiency virus (HIV)-infected individuals: A serial echocardiographic study. J Am Coll Cardiol 17:1270–1276, 1991

6. Brown DL, Sather S, Cheitlin MD: Reversible cardiac dysfunction associated with foscarnet therapy for cytomegalovirus esophagitis in an AIDS patient. Am Heart J 125:1439–1441, 1993

7. Brown J, King A, Francis CK: Cardiovascular effects of alcohol, cocaine, and acquired immune deficiency. Cardiovasc Clin 21:341–376, 1991

8. Calabrese LH, Proffitt MR, Yen-Lieberman B, et al: Congestive cardiomyopathy and illness related to the acquired immunodeficiency syndrome (AIDS) associated with isolation of retrovirus from myocardium. Ann Intern Med 107:691–692, 1987

9. Cenacchi G, Re MC, Furlini G, et al: Human immunodeficiency virus type 1 antigen detection in endomyocardial biopsy: An immunomorphological study. Microbiologica 13:145–149, 1990

10. Centers for Disease Control: Acquired immunodeficiency syndrome—United States update. MMWR 35:17–21, 1986

11. Chokshi SK, Moore R, Pandian NG, Isner JM: Reversible cardiomyopathy associated with cocaine intoxication. Ann Intern Med 111:1039–1040, 1989

12. Cohen JR, Lackner R, Wenig P, Pillari G: Deep venous thrombosis in patients with AIDS. NY State J Med 90:159–161, 1990

13. Corallo S, Mutinelli MR, Moroni M, et al: Echocardiography detects myocardial damage in AIDS: Prospective study in 102 patients. Eur Heart J 9:887–892, 1988

14. Currie PF, Jacob AJ, Foreman AR, et al: Heart muscle disease related to HIV infection: Prognostic implications. BMJ 309:1605–1607, 1994

15. Currie PF, Sutherland GR, Jacob AJ, et al: A review of endocarditis in acquired immunodeficiency syndrome and human immunodeficiency virus infection. Eur Heart J 16(suppl B):15–18, 1995

16. De Castro S, Migliau G, Silvestri A: Heart involvement in AIDS: A prospective study during various stages of the disease. Eur Heart J 13:1452–1459, 1992

17. Deyton LR, Walker RE, Kovacs JA, et al: Reversible cardiac dysfunction associated with interferon alfa therapy in AIDS patients with Kaposi's sarcoma. N Engl J Med 321:1246–1249, 1989

18. Engrav MB, Coodley G, Magnusson AR: Torsade de pointes after inhaled pentamidine. Ann Emerg Med 21:1403–1405, 1992

19. Flum DR, McGinn JT Jr, Tyras DH: The role of the "pericardial window" in AIDS. Chest 107:1522–1525, 1995

20. Francis CK: Cardiac involvement in AIDS. Curr Probl Cardiol 15:575–639, 1990

21. Galli FC, Cheitlin MD: Pericardial disease in AIDS: Frequency of tamponade and therapeutic and diagnostic use of pericardiocentesis. J Am Coll Cardiol 19:266A, 1992

22. Goldberg SJ, Comerci GD, Feldman L: Cardiac output and regional myocardial contraction in anorexia nervosa. J Adolescent Health Care 9:15–21, 1988

23. Goldblum N, Daefler S, Llana T, et al: Susceptibility to HIV-1 infection of a human B-lymphoblastoid cell line, DG75, transfected with subgenomic DNA fragments of Epstein-Barr virus. Dev Biol Stand 72; 309–313, 1990

24. Goldfarb A, King CL, Rosenzweig BP, et al: Cardiac lymphoma in the acquired immunodeficiency syndrome. Am Heart J 118:1340–1344, 1989

25. Grody WW, Cheng L, Lewis W: Infection of the heart by the human immunodeficiency virus. Am J Cardiol 66:203–206, 1990

26. Heidenreich PA, Eisenberg MJ, Kee LL, et al: Pericardial effusion in AIDS: Incidence and survival. Circulation 92:3229–3234, 1995

27. Henderson DK, Fahey BJ, Willy M, et al: Risk for occupational trasmission of human immunodeficiency virus type 1 (HIV-1) associated with clinical exposures: A prospective evaluation. Ann Intern Med 113:740–746, 1990

28. Herskowitz A, Ansari AA, Neumann DA, et al: Cadiomyopathy in acquired immunodeficiency syndrome: Evidence for autoimmunity (Abstract no. 1284). Circulation 80(Suppl II):II-322, 1989

29. Herskowitz A, Vlahovr D, Willoughby S, et al: Prevalence and incidence of left ventricular dysfunction in patients with human immunodeficiency virus infection. Am J Cardiol 71:955–958, 1993

30. Herskowitz A, Willoughby SB, Baughman KL, et al: Cardiomyopathy associated with antiretroviral therapy in patients with HIV infection: A report of six cases. Ann Intern Med 116:311–313, 1992

31. Himelman RB, Chung WS, Chernoff DN, et al: Cardiac manifestations of human immunodeficiency virus infection: A two-dimensional echocardiographic study. J Am Coll Cardiol 13:1030–1036, 1989

32. Himelman RB, Dohrmann M, Goodman P, et al: Severe pulmonary hypertension and cor pulmonale in the acquired immunodeficiency syndrome. Am J Cardiol 64:1396–1399, 1989

33. Ho DD, Pomerantz RJ, Kaplan JC: Pathogenesis of infection with human immunodeficiency virus. N Engl J Med 317:278–286, 1987

34. Horowitz MD, Cox MM, Neibart RM, et al: Resection of right atrial lymphoma in patients with AIDS. Int J Cardiol 34:139–142, 1992

35. Kavanaugh-McHugh AL, Ruff A, Perlman E, et al: Selenium deficiency and cardiomyopathy in acquired immunodeficiency syndrome. J Parenter Enter Nutr 15:347–349, 1991

36. Kelsey RC, Saker A, Morgan M: Cardiac lymphoma in a patient with AIDS. Ann Intern Med 115:370–371, 1991

37. Lafeuillade A, Alessi M-C, Poizot-Martin I, et al: Protein S deficiency and HIV infection (Letter). N Engl J Med 324:1220, 1991

38. Lahdevirta J, Maury CP, Teppo AM, Repo H: Elevated levels of circulating cachectin/tumor necrosis factor in patients with acquired immunodeficiency syndrome. Am J Med 85:289–291, 1988

39. Levy WS, Simon GL, Rios JC, Ross AM: Prevalence of cardiac abnormalities in human immunodeficiency virus infection. Am J Cardiol 63:86–89, 1989

40. Lewis W: AIDS: Cardiac findings from 115 autopsies. Prog Cardiovasc Dis 32:207–215, 1989

41. Lipshultz SE, Fox CH, Perez-Atayde AR, et al: Identification of human immunodeficiency virus-1 RNA and DNA in the heart of a child with cardiovascular abnormalities and congenital acquired immune deficiency syndrome: Case report. Am J Cardiol 66:246–250, 1990

42. Magno J, Margaretten W, Cheitlin M: Myocardial involvement in acquired immunodeficiency syn-

drome: Incidence in a large autopsy study (Abstract 1829). Circulation 78:II-459, 1988

43. Maliakkal R, Friedman SA, Sridhar S: Progressive pulmonary thromboembolism in association with HIV disease. NY State J Med 92:403–404, 1992

44. Marche C, Trophilme D, Mayorga R, et al: Cardiac involvement in AIDS: A pathological study (Abstract 7103). Program of the 4th International Conference on AIDS, Stockholm, p. 403, 1988

45. Mason JW, O'Connell JB, Herskowitz A, et al: A clinical trial of immunosuppressive therapy for myocarditis. The Myocarditis Treatment Trial Investigation. N Engl J Med 333:269–275, 1995

46. Mette SA, Palevsky HI, Pietra GG: Primary pulmonary hypertension in association with human immunodeficiency virus infection: A possible viral etiology for some forms of hypertensive pulmonary arteriopathy. Am Rev Respir Dis 145:1196–1200, 1992

47. Monsuez JJ, Kinney EL, Vittecoq D, et al: Comparison among acquired immune deficiency syndrome patients with and without clinical evidence of cardiac disease. Am J Cardiol 62:1311–1313, 1988

48. Moskowitz L, Hensley GT, Chan JC, Adams K: Immediate causes of death in acquired immunodeficiency syndrome. Arch Pathol Lab Med 109:735–738, 1985

49. Niedt GW, Schinella RA: Acquired immunodeficiency syndrome: Clinicopathologic study of 56 autopsies. Arch Pathol Lab Med 109:727–734, 1985

50. Parrillo JE, Burch C, Shelhamer JH, et al: A circulating myocardial depressant substance in humans with septic shock: Septic shock patients with a reduced ejection fraction have a circulating factor that depresses in vitro myocardial cell performance. J Clin Invest 76:1539–1553, 1985

51. Quezado ZM, Wilson WH, Cunnion RE, et al: High-dose ifosfamide is associated with severe, reversible cardiac dysfunction. Ann Intern Med 118:31–36, 1993

52. Reynolds M, Berger M, Hecht S, et al: Large pericardial effusions associated with the acquired immune deficiency syndrome (AIDS) (Abstract). J Am Coll Cardiol 17:221A, 1991

53. Rich S: Primary pulmonary hypertension. Prog Cardiovasc Dis 31:205–238, 1988

54. Samlowski WE, Ward JH, Craven CM, Freedman RA: Severe myocarditis following high-dose interleukin-2 administration. Arch Pathol Lab Med 113:838–841, 1989

55. Shah PM, Pai RG: Diastolic heart failure. Curr Probl Cardiol 17:787–868, 1992

56. Steigman CK, Anderson DW, Macher AM, et al: Fatal cardiac tamponade in acquired immunodeficiency syndrome with epicardial Kaposi's sarcoma. Am Heart J 116:1105–1107, 1988

57. Stimmler MM, Quismorio FP Jr, McGehee WG, et al: Anticardiolipin antibodies in acquired immunodeficiency syndrome. Arch Intern Med 149:1833–1835, 1989

58. Welch K, Finkbeiner W, Alpers CE, et al: Autopsy findings in the acquired immune deficiency syndrome. JAMA 252:1152–1159, 1984

59. Wharton JM, Demopulos PA, Goldschlager N: Torsade de pointes during administration of pentamidine isethionate. Am J Med 83:571–576, 1987

60. Wilkes MS, Fortin AH, Felix JC, et al: Value of necropsy in acquired immunodeficiency syndrome. Lancet 2:85–88, 1988

61. Woods GL, Goldsmith JC: Fatal pericarditis due to Mycobacterium avium-intracellulare in acquired immunodeficiency syndrome. Chest 95:1355–1357, 1989

62. Yock PG, Popp RL: Noninvasive estimation of right ventricular systolic pressure by Doppler ultrasound in patients with tricuspid regurgitation. Circulation 70:657–662, 1984

Chapter *18*

Endocrinologic Manifestations of HIV Infection

MORRIS SCHAMBELAN, DEBORAH E. SELLMEYER, and CARL GRUNFELD

Endocrine dysfunction can result from human immunodeficiency virus (HIV) infection, its associated opportunistic infections and malignancies, or as a complication of drugs used in the treatment of these disorders. As in any severe illness, HIV infection and its complications can also be accompanied by changes in the rate of hormone secretion and/or clearance without overt clinical manifestations. In this chapter we will attempt to distinguish those abnormalities of endocrine function that require further evaluation and possible treatment from those that merely represent the body's normal response to severe illness.

HYPOTHALAMIC-PITUITARY AXIS

Studies that have systematically evaluated pituitary functional reserve in patients with HIV infection (e.g., using gonadatropin or thyrotropin-stimulating hormones) have generally not found evidence for anterior pituitary dysfunction.[24,85,101] These findings contrast with the relatively high incidence of pathologic findings at autopsy: in 49 patients with the acquired immunodeficiency syndrome (AIDS) in whom the pituitary was specifically examined, direct infectious involvement was noted in six adenohypophyses (five by cytomegalovirus [CMV] and one by *Pneumocystis carinii*) and three neurohypophyses (two by CMV and one by *Toxoplasma gondii*).[105] A single patient has been described who had well-documented panhypopituitarism in association with cerebral toxoplasmosis; a large necrotic pituitary was noted at autopsy and toxoplasma were demonstrated in cerebral abscesses although not in the pituitary per se.[87]

Another patient with cerebral CMV infection developed hypopituitarism on a hypothalamic basis.[114]

Growth failure occurs in some children with HIV infection, but growth hormone (GH) deficiency does not appear to be common. In three boys with hemophilia, HIV infection, and short stature, peak GH levels were normal but two had low insulin-like growth factor I (IGF-I) levels.[64] Similarly, GH response to glucagon stimulation was normal and IGF-I levels were subnormal in 14 HIV-positive children with failure to thrive.[108] However, another group found subnormal IGF-I only in one malnourished child, while eight others who were less ill had normal levels.[70] A fourth study reported no differences in IGF-I levels between control, asymptomatic HIV-positive and symptomatic HIV-positive children; however, they found resistance to GH, IGF, and insulin stimulation of erythroid precursor colony formation in symptomatic HIV-infected children, suggesting a syndrome of hormone resistance.[37] A subnormal IGF-I level, in the face of an apparently normal GH level, is a common occurrence in malnutrition.[56] Thus, growth failure in children with HIV infection may be due to malnutrition rather than hypothalamic-pituitary dysfunction.

In adults, low levels of IGF-I were found in malnourished patients with HIV infection.[104] In contrast, two cohorts of AIDS patients with significant previous weight loss had normal levels of IGF-I.[73,89] When these patients were given pharmacologic doses of growth hormone, IGF-I levels were increased, although not quite to the same extent as in patients without HIV, suggesting growth hormone resistance.

257

Three groups have found normal prolactin levels in patients with AIDS.[24,39,85] However, small but statistically significant[40] or moderate[19] elevations in prolactin levels have been noted in some patients with AIDS. Concomitant drug treatment (e.g., with opiates or phenothiazines) may have contributed to the hyperprolactinemia in some cases.[19] Whether the perturbation in prolactin levels could contribute to gonadal dysfunction (see below) has not been determined.

Hyponatremia occurs commonly in patients with AIDS: at the time of admission to the hospital, one third to one half of patients with AIDS have a low serum sodium level.[1,20,115] In one report, two thirds of the hyponatremic patients were judged to be euvolemic on the basis of clinical assessment and their serum sodium level remained subnormal despite saline administration.[1] In these patients, arginine vasopressin levels were noted to be inappropriately high for the serum osmolality, a finding that is compatible with a diagnosis of the syndrome of inappropriate antidiuretic hormone secretion (SIADH). However, since more than half of this group were being treated with trimethoprim, which could have impaired sodium conservation during saline replacement,[16] it is possible that pathogenetic mechanisms other than SIADH may have contributed to the hyponatremia.

ADRENAL

Adrenal pathology, particularly CMV infection, is found commonly in patients who have died from AIDS.[2,7,11,25,65,71,97,100,124] In at least one such postmortem study, the degree of CMV involvement correlated with the degree of adrenal necrosis.[38] In most reports, the estimated loss of functioning tissue was below the level required to produce adrenal insufficiency. However, two other case reports have appeared describing adrenal insufficiency in patients with CMV and very extensive adrenalitis.[2,7] Other pathologic lesions that have been noted frequently include hemorrhage, infection with *Toxoplasma, Cryptococcus, Mycobacterium tuberculosis, Mycobacterium avium* complex, and infiltration with Kaposi's sarcoma and lymphoma.[11,38]

Glucocorticoid Hormones

Although a few initial reports of adrenal insufficiency in patients with AIDS[41,50] implied an

important clinical consequence for the frequently observed adrenal pathology, subsequent prospective studies in larger groups of patients indicate that glucocorticoid (cortisol) deficiency is relatively rare in this setting.[24,55,70,84,85,101,118] Perhaps this is not surprising in view of the functional reserve of this organ: It is generally thought that more than 90% of adrenal tissue must be destroyed before clinically significant cortisol deficiency occurs. In the most detailed examination of adrenal function in patients with HIV infection, Membrano et al[84] noted that basal levels of cortisol, rather than being low, were actually significantly greater in hospitalized patients with AIDS than in normal control subjects and that only 4 patients out of 74 had impaired glucocorticoid secretion. Notably, among the patients with impaired glucocorticoid secretion adrenocorticotropin (ACTH) levels were not elevated, suggesting an abnormality in the hypothalamic-pituitary axis rather than a primary adrenal lesion as the cause of their impaired glucocorticoid secretion. Another study reported similar increases in basal cortisol, but also ACTH levels, in 63 HIV-infected patients, 23 of whom had AIDS[118]; with one exception, these patients responded normally to stimulation with ACTH. Many other studies report normal[24,31,101] or elevated[6,17,55,84,118] basal cortisol levels.

Elevations in circulating levels of cortisol are seen frequently during severe illness, including infection.[5,27] These changes are likely due to cytokines, such as interleukin-1 (IL-1), IL-6, and tumor necrosis factor (TNF), that have been shown to directly stimulate both cortisol and ACTH secretion.[42] When cortisol secretion is increased under conditions of severe illness, the response to dynamic tests of adrenal functional reserve (using ACTH or insulin) may not be normal, yet such individuals may have normal adrenal function after recuperation.[110] Recovery from adrenal insufficiency induced by both meningiococcus and blastomycosis has also been reported.[8,94]

Although clinically significant glucocorticoid deficiency is relatively infrequent, subtle abnormalities of adrenal biosynthesis may be quite common in patients with HIV infection. For example, plasma concentrations of the products of the 17-deoxysteroid pathway (corticosterone, deoxycorticosterone, and 18-OH-deoxycorticosterone) were substantially reduced in comparison to controls both before and after ACTH stimulation, whereas cortisol (17-hydroxy pathway) secretion was normal.[84] A diminished response of 17-deoxysteroids with normal cortisol levels was also noted in children with HIV infection who underwent acute stimulation with ACTH.[92] Because the 17-deoxysteroid products are probably not functionally important at normal plasma concentrations, these findings cannot be taken as evidence of clinically significant adrenal functional impairment. Whether this altered biosynthetic pattern could represent a harbinger of subsequent impaired adrenal capacity in patients with AIDS[84] or an adaptive mechanism that preserves cortisol secretion at the expense of reduced secretion of steroids that do not appear to have biologic significance remains to be determined.

The concept of shunting of adrenal biosynthetic products toward glucocorticoids was also suggested by Villette et al,[120] who noted that levels of adrenal androgen were decreased while cortisol was increased in HIV-infected men undergoing studies of hormonal circadian variation. Because ACTH levels were significantly reduced in those patients, these authors further suggested that cortisol levels might be maintained by a nonpituitary factor. The finding of high cortisol levels with normal levels of ACTH may be due to the effects of a cytokine such as IL-1 or TNF, which directly stimulate cortisol production and could result in a secondary inhibition of ACTH secretion.[22] However, IL-1 and IL-6 may also affect the hypothalamic-pituitary axis by directly stimulating the release of corticotropin-releasing hormone by the hypothalamus or ACTH by pituitary cells.[106,126]

Several drugs that are used commonly in the treatment of patients with AIDS are known to alter adrenal function or steroid hormone metabolism. For example, ketoconazole inhibits cortisol synthesis[98] and could lead to adrenal insufficiency, particularly in patients with limited adrenal reserve. Rifampin enhances cortisol metabolism, which can result in adrenal insufficiency in patients with Addison's disease who are on maintenance glucocorticoid therapy,[67] and which could also produce adrenal failure in patients with limited adrenal reserve.[28] Megestrol acetate can reduce plasma cortisol levels, perhaps due to its intrinsic cortisol-like activity at the high doses (400 to 1200 mg/day) used to stimulate appetite.[75]

Even if relatively uncommon, the prevalence of glucocorticoid insufficiency in patients with AIDS is clearly greater than that in the general population, in which Addison's disease has been estimated to occur in 60 cases per million.[90] It seems reasonable, therefore, to test adrenal function in those patients with AIDS who have symptoms or signs consistent with the diagnosis of adrenal insufficiency. Patients with low baseline cortisol levels who fail to respond to stimulation with ACTH clearly require glucocorticoid maintenance therapy. It is more difficult to propose the appropriate treatment for those individuals with the more common finding of a normal or high basal cortisol level with minimal or no further increase in response to acute ACTH stimulation,[80] since the majority of such individuals will have a normal cortisol response to 3 days of continuous ACTH stimulation.[84] These results suggest that patients with "borderline" stimulated cortisol values may not require routine glucocorticoid maintenance therapy. On the other hand, some clinicians would give glucocorticoids to such patients at times of stress, provided that treatment is limited in duration, so that the adverse effects of prolonged steroid therapy can be avoided.

Mineralocorticoid Hormones

Mineralocorticoid hormone deficiency results in renal sodium wasting, hypotension, hyperkalemia, metabolic acidosis, and elevated levels of plasma renin activity. Despite the frequency of hyponatremia and hyperkalemia in patients with AIDS, specific studies of mineralocorticoid hormone secretion and of the functional integrity of the renin-angiotensin system in such patients are quite limited. One patient who presented with hyponatremia, hyperkalemia, and normal cortisol levels may have had an isolated deficiency of aldosterone secretion, since aldosterone levels were low normal despite hyperreninemia.[52] His cortisol reserve appeared to be subnormal in response to ACTH stimulation, however, and the apparent benefit of treatment with a mineralocorticoid (fludrocortisone) may have been due in part to concomitant administration of a glucocorticoid (hydrocortisone). However, in a more systematic study, no abnormalities in circulating renin or aldosterone levels were noted in 63 HIV-infected patients, 23 of whom had AIDS.[118] Similarly, no abnormalities in aldosterone or renin levels were reported in 74 patients with AIDS and 19 with ARC who underwent an extensive evaluation of adrenal function including direct stimulation of aldosterone secretion by the angiotensin peptide des-asp[1]-angiotensin II.[84]

The finding of low renin and aldosterone values that failed to increase normally in response to intravenously administered furosemide and assumption of an upright posture suggested the diagnosis of so-called hyporeninemic hypoaldosteronism in four patients with AIDS and unexplained hyperkalemia.[62] It should be noted, however, that these patients were taking trimethoprim-sulfamethoxazole at the time they were studied. Sulfonamides can cause interstitial nephritis,[3] a disorder associated with hyporeninemic hypoaldosteronism.[107] Alternatively, abnormalities of potassium homeostasis in patients taking trimethoprim-sulfamethoxazole may be due to the trimethoprim which, in the large doses frequently employed in the treatment of *Pneumocystis carinii* pneumonia, can block amiloride-sensitive luminal sodium channels and secondarily limit potassium secretion in distal nephron segments.[16] Transient hyperkalemia has also been reported to occur during treatment with pentamidine, a finding that was reversed on discontinuation of the agent and that was attributed to nephrotoxicity.[68]

THYROID

Autopsy series in patients dying of AIDS have reported both opportunistic infections and AIDS-related neoplasms in the thyroid gland. The relationship between these lesions and clinical abnormalities is not clear, as CMV inclusion bodies have been found in the thyroid even in the absence of significant thyroid dysfunction.[32] Inflammatory thyroiditis due to *Pneumocystis carinii* has been reported in at least 12 patients.[4,26,34,51,81,96,102,112,119] Seven patients had hypothyroidism, three had hyperthyroidism, and one had normal thyroid function. Antibodies were negative when tested and thyroid gland visualization with radionucleotide scanning was decreased. Treatment of pneumocystis reversed hyperthyroidism in two patients. Invasion of the thyroid with Kaposi's sarcoma[66,88,124] has been reported; in one case, destruction of the thyroid by Kaposi's sarcoma with resulting primary hypothyroidism has been described.[88] The thyroid can also be infected during disseminated fungal infections such as *Cryptococcus neoformans* and *Aspergillus fumigatus*.[78,79]

It is important to distinguish between abnormalities of thyroid function that are secondary to destruction of the thyroid or pituitary and those that are the result of severe illness. With thyroid/pituitary destruction, levels of thyroxine (T_4) decrease dramatically, while triiodothyronine (T_3) levels may be low or in the low normal range. With thyroidal destruction, thyroid-stimulating hormone (TSH) levels increase dramatically, whereas with pituitary disruption, TSH levels may be low or low normal. During severe systemic nonthyroidal illness, the conversion of T_4 to T_3 is impaired, resulting in decreased circulating levels of T_3 and variable levels of T_4. These changes are usually accompanied by increases in reverse T_3 (rT_3) levels. A variable but usually small increase in TSH levels may occur during the recovery from nonthyroidal illness. Such changes in thyroid hormone homeostasis are commonly referred to as the "euthyroid-sick syndrome."[13,122] Experiments studying caloric deprivation, which is accompanied by a decrease in T_3, demonstrate that replacement therapy with T_3 accelerates negative nitrogen balance.[12,35] As a consequence it is thought that decreases in T_3 during severe illness limit both protein catabolism and energy expenditure.[13,122]

Patients with AIDS show abnormalities of thyroid function tests that are similar in many respects to those in other acute and chronic illnesses; however, true hypothyroidism is rare. There are many studies of thyroid hormone levels in patients with AIDS but, while some studies have found decreased T_3 levels, others have not.[24,33,47,59,69,74,85,101,116] As a consequence, the question has been raised as to whether the failure to decrease T_3 in AIDS is inappropriate and could therefore contribute to weight loss and/or negative nitrogen balance.[74] Review of these studies indicates that, in the presence of severe illness, patients with AIDS show the appropriate decrease in serum T_3 levels.[47] For example, those patients who have active weight loss show decreased T_3 levels, whereas patients with stable weight have higher levels and show significantly decreased rT_3 levels.[47] Many of these patients with decreased T_3 levels have acute secondary infection. Indeed, when patients with *Pneumocystis carinii* pneumonia and other infections are studied, serum T_3 levels are consistently depressed.[33,47,69,74,116] Serum T_3 levels serve as a marker for the severity of illness; patients who die during admissions for those illnesses have a higher prevalence of low T_3 levels.[74,85,116]

Some changes in thyroid hormone homeostasis occur in AIDS that are not commonly found in the euthyroid-sick syndrome. The clinical importance of these changes is not yet understood, but they may influence interpretation of thyroid function. For example, the serum protein that binds thyroid hormone, thyroid binding globulin (TBG), is increased early in the course of HIV infection and AIDS.[10,47,57,69,74,93] As a consequence, total T_3 levels may underestimate the decrease in free (or active) T_3 levels. In contrast, during severe nonthyroid illness TBG can be decreased.

In patients with AIDS, particularly in the absence of secondary infection, TSH levels are elevated and TSH secretion in response to TRH is exaggerated.[47,57,93,108] Thus, patients with AIDS who are not infected and whose weight is stable may have a compensated hypothyroid state. In contrast, TSH is not elevated during the acute course of most other nonthyroidal illnesses, although there are some exceptions.[13,122]

Levels of rT_3 consistently decrease early in the course of HIV infection and AIDS even in the absence of decreased T_3 levels.[47,69,74] In contrast, during other nonthyroidal illnesses, serum rT_3 levels usually increase when conversion of T_4 to T_3 is decreased. Severely ill patients with AIDS, particularly those who are terminal, may show such increases in rT_3.[74] The functional significance of rT_3 is unknown.

Rifampin increases thyroid clearance by inducing hepatic microsomal enzymes similar to the effects on hepatic steroid metabolism. As a consequence, patients on L-thyroxine replacement treated with rifampin may require higher doses and rifampin may precipitate hypothyroidism in patients with limited pituitary or thyroid reserve.[60]

GONAD

Testicular atrophy and infections are frequent findings in patients with AIDS. In men with AIDS in whom testes were examined at autopsy, marked decrease in spermatogenesis, thickening of the tunica propria, mild to moderate interstital infiltrate, and/or fibrosis have been reported.[14,21,23] Opportunistic infections, predominantly CMV, have been noted in 25% to 31% of testes examined in the larger series reported.[14,23] Expression of HIV protein is found in the interstitium of the testes, as well as in lymphocytes in the seminiferous tubules.[23,99] Furthermore, HIV RNA can be found in testicular spermatogonia by in situ polymerase chain reaction (PCR) hybridization.[91]

Although it is difficult to interpret the functional significance of decreased testicular volume and spermatogenesis in autopsy specimens, symptomatic hypogonadism clearly occurs in patients with HIV infection.[17,19,24,72,101,120,121] Dobs et al[24] found that 28 of 42 pa-

tients with AIDS had decreased libido and 14 were impotent. Free testosterone levels were subnormal in 45% of the patients with AIDS yet, in the majority, luteinizing hormone (LH) and follicle-stimulating hormone (FSH) levels were not elevated and the response to stimulation with gonadotropin-releasing hormone was normal in all but one. These findings and similar results by Raffi et al[101] suggest that the hypogonadism is due to a functional disorder of the hypothalamus. Croxson et al,[19] who also found lower total testosterone levels in patients with AIDS, did not observe inappropriately low LH or FSH values, implying primary testicular failure rather than hypogonadotrophic hypogonadism in their patients. The discrepancy in these findings may be explained in part by the absence, within their population, of intravenous drug abusers, which were included in the patient population studied by Dobs et al.[24] Opiate abuse per se is known to cause hypogonadotropic hypogonadism.[111]

Drugs that are used commonly in the treatment of patients with AIDS may affect gonadal function. Ketoconazole is associated with decreased levels of total and free testosterone leading to oligospermia, azospermia, and gynecomastia.[98] Chemotherapy for lymphoma also commonly results in infertility.

In summary, men with AIDS tend to have an increased incidence of impotence and low testosterone levels. In women with advanced AIDS, particularly in those with severe wasting, ovarian failure, manifested clinically by amenorrhea, is commonly noted.[125]

PANCREAS

When administered intravenously in the large doses employed in the treatment of *Pneumocystis carinii* infections, pentamidine commonly causes pancreatic beta-cell toxicity resulting in acute hypoglycemia due to increased insulin secretion. If the injury to the beta cell is of sufficient magnitude, the hypoglycemic phase may be followed by beta-cell death and the development of diabetes mellitus.[9,95,113,123] Both hypoglycemia and diabetes mellitus may also occur during treatment with inhaled pentamidine.[15,63]

Megestrol acetate is used widely as an appetite stimulant in the treatment of anorexia and cachexia in AIDS. It has recently been reported that the drug can induce diabetes mellitus,[54] although the prevalence of hyperglycemia in controlled trials is low and may not exceed that seen in the placebo group. Whether this side effect is secondary to increased caloric intake or another effect of the drug (such as its intrinsic cortisol-like activity) is not yet known.

MINERAL HOMEOSTASIS

Foscarnet, which is used in the treatment of refractory CMV retinitis and mucocutaneous herpes simplex virus infections, has been reported to cause hypocalcemia, possibly by forming a complex with ionized calcium.[61] The hypocalcemia can result in potentially serious clinical sequelae. Fatal hypocalcemia has been reported when foscarnet was given together with parenteral pentamidine.[127] Hypomagnesemia, hyperphosphatemia, and hypokalemia can also occur with foscarnet treatment[36] as can nephrogenic diabetes insipidus.[29]

LIPID METABOLISM

Plasma cholesterol levels decrease early in the course of HIV infection, a finding that is sustained through the development of AIDS.[18,46,109,128] High-density lipoprotein (HDL) levels appear to decrease first and remain at the same level. Low-density lipoprotein (LDL) levels progressively decrease but, in the later stages of AIDS, very-low-density lipoprotein (VLDL) cholesterol levels increase slightly. The LDL particles are abnormally dense.[30] The causes of hypocholesterolemia have not yet been defined. In particular, the role of gastrointestinal disturbances and malabsorption is unknown.

With progression from asymptomatic HIV infection to AIDS, plasma triglyceride levels increase.[45,46,86,128] In CDC stage IV AIDS, triglycerides average twice normal. However, a subset of patients may have higher plasma triglyceride levels (>500 mg/dl), which puts them at risk for triglyceride-induced pancreatitis. The latter syndrome is of particular concern in patients taking antiretroviral therapy that also predisposes to pancreatitis (i.e. didanosine [ddI] and zalcitabine [ddC]). Patients with the higher levels of triglycerides may have underlying genetic defects in addition to the abnormalities induced by HIV infection. However, antiretroviral therapy of previously untreated patients with AIDS lowers both interferon-α and triglyceride levels.[86]

Several changes in triglyceride metabolism have been reported in AIDS that contribute to hypertriglyceridemia. First, lipoprotein lipase, the enzyme responsible for triglyceride clearance, is decreased.[46] The actual clearance of triglycerides is even more dramatically slowed.[46] Finally, the hepatic synthesis of fatty acids from other substrates is increased in patients with HIV infection and AIDS with consequent increase in newly synthesized fatty acids in the circulation.[53]

The increase in plasma triglyceride levels is highly correlated with circulating levels of interferon-α, a cytokine that appears in circulation with the onset of CDC stage IV AIDS.[46] An even stronger correlation is found between interferon-α levels and both the decreases in triglyceride clearance and the increase in fasting levels of newly synthesized fatty acids.[46,53]

THE WASTING SYNDROME IN AIDS

A variety of metabolic disturbances have been described in AIDS that could theoretically contribute to the wasting syndrome. However, recent studies indicate that such metabolic disturbances alone cannot account for the wasting syndrome. For example, an early theory linked weight loss to abnormalities in triglyceride metabolism. However, there is no correlation between the presence of hypertriglyceridemia and wasting in AIDS.[45] AIDS patients with elevated triglyceride levels frequently maintain body weight for extended periods of time.[45]

Increased resting energy expenditure (REE) is a common indication of hypermetabolism, a phenomenon that occurs in patients with sepsis and burns and was thought to cause the wasting syndrome (for review, see reference 43). It was therefore of interest to find striking elevations in REE in patients with HIV infection and AIDS.[43,48,58,59,82,83,89] REE increases very early in HIV infection even before CD4 cell counts drop,[58] presumably reflecting the host response to the virus; these findings suggest that HIV is not latent but rather contained. REE increases further with the development of AIDS, but such increases may reflect the presence of secondary infections.[48,82] Surprisingly, there was no correlation between the increase seen in REE and weight loss.[48,59]

In contrast, studies on the mechanism of wasting suggested that patients with AIDS who have active secondary infections universally show rapid weight loss, averaging 5% of body weight in 4 weeks.[48] Such patients have striking decreases in caloric intake that correlate with weight loss.[48,77] However, it should be pointed out that patients with AIDS and secondary infection maintain a high REE in the face of decreased caloric intake. These findings should be contrasted to those in non–HIV-infected patients who develop compensatory decreases in REE that limit weight loss during decreased caloric intake.[43] Patients with rapid weight loss have decreased total energy expenditure (TEE), hence in a sense are hypometabolic, but their decrease in caloric intake leaves them with a large relative energy deficit.[77] Thus, the rapid weight loss seen in AIDS with secondary infection is a product of a failed homeostatic mechanism and is a function of both decreased food intake and increased REE.

Prospective studies have confirmed that rapid weight loss is a harbinger of infection. Rapid weight loss episodes (>4 kg in <4 months) were accompanied by secondary infection 82% of the time.[76] When patients with slower weight loss (>4 kg in ≥4 months) were analyzed, 65% had gastrointestinal disease. Patients with slow weight loss may also have elevated REE, slightly lower TEE, and reduced caloric intake.[77] On the basis of these studies it is strongly recommended that the weight for each patient with HIV infection and AIDS be plotted in a graph in the patient's chart; weight loss should then prompt the clinician to look for appropriate causes.[44]

The first line of treatment for patients with AIDS and active weight loss is to find the underlying causes and treat them. However, recovery from weight loss is frequently only partial, resulting in long-term wasting.[76] As a consequence, direct therapies of the wasting syndrome are being sought. Two agents that stimulate appetite have been approved: dronabinol for AIDS-related anorexia, and megestrol acetate for AIDS-related weight loss. Megestrol acetate (at doses of 800 mg/day) leads to more weight gain, fewer significant side effects, and less drop-out from therapy. Use of these agents should be considered in patients with significant weight loss (<90% of ideal body weight), especially in the presence of anorexia. However, both agents lead to increases in weight that primarily consist of fat. Other therapies are being studied for their ability to form lean body mass, particularly muscle; these include growth hormone,[89] IGF-1,[73] and anabolic steroids.

ACKNOWLEDGMENTS

This work was supported in part by grant R90SF211 from the Universitywide AIDS Research Program and by grants DK40990, DK45833, D49448, and T32-DK07418 from the National Institutes of Health.

REFERENCES

1. Agarwal A, Soni A, Ciechanowsky M, et al: Hyponatremia in patients with acquired immunodeficiency syndrome. Nephron 53:317–321, 1989
2. Angulo JC, Lopez JI, Flores N: Lethal cytomegalovirus adrenalitis in a case of AIDS. Scand J Urolo Nephrol. 28:105–106, 1994
3. Appel GB, Neu HC: The nephrotoxicity of antimicrobial agents (third of three parts). N Engl J Med 296:784–787, 1977
4. Battan R, Mariuz P, Raviglione MC, et al: *Pneumocystis carinii* infection of the thyroid in a hypothyroid patient with AIDS: Diagnosis by fine needle aspiration biopsy. J Clin Endocrinol Metab 72:724–726, 1991
5. Beisel WR: Metabolic response to infection. In Sanford JB, Luby JP, eds. The Science and Practice of Clinical Medicine. New York, Grune & Stratton, 1981
6. Biglino A, Limone P, Forno B, et al: Altered adrenocorticotropin and cortisol response to corticotropin-releasing hormone in HIV-1 infection. Eur J Endocrinol 133:173–179, 1995
7. Bleiweis IJ, Pervez NK, Hammer GS, et al: Cytomegalovirus-induced adrenal insufficiency and associated renal cell carcinoma in AIDS. Mt Sinai J Med 53:676–679, 1986
8. Bosworth DC: Reversible adrenocortical insufficiency in fulminant meningococcemia. Arch Intern Med 139:823–824, 1979
9. Bouchard PH, Sal P, Reach G, et al: Diabetes mellitus following pentamidine induced hypoglycemia in humans. Diabetes 31:40–45, 1982
10. Bourdoux PR, DeWitt SA, Servais GM, et al: Biochemical thyroid profile in patients infected with the human immunodeficiency virus. Thyroid 1:147–149, 1991
11. Bricaire F, Marche C, Zoubi D, et al: Adrenocortical lesions and AIDS. Lancet i:881, 1988
12. Burman KD, Wartofsky L, Dinterman RE, et al: The effect of T_3 and reverse T_3 administration on muscle protein catabolism during fasting as measured by 3-methylhistidine excretion. Metabolism 8:805–813, 1979
13. Cavalieri RR: The effects of nonthyroid disease and drugs on thyroid function tests. Med Clin North Am 75:27–39, 1991

14. Chabon AB, Stenger RJ, Grabstald H: Histopathology of testis in acquired immunodeficiency syndrome. Urology 29:658–663, 1987

15. Chen JP, Braham RL, Squires KE: Diabetes after aerosolized pentamidine. Ann Intern Med 114:913–914, 1991

16. Choi MJ, Fernandez PC, Patnaik A, et al: Brief report: Trimethoprim-induced hyperkalemia in a patient with AIDS. N Engl J Med 328:703–706, 1993

17. Christeff N, Gharakhanian S, Thoble N, et al: Evidence for changes in adrenal and testicular steroids during HIV infection. JAIDS 5:841–846, 1992

18. Constans J, Pellegrin JL, Peuchant E, et al: Plasma lipids in HIV-infected patients: A prospective study in 95 patients. Eur J Clin Invest 24:416–420, 1994

19. Croxson TS, Chapman WE, Miller LK, et al: Changes in the hypothalamic-pituitary-gonadal axis in human immunodeficiency virus infected homosexual men. J Clin Endocrinol Metab 68:317–321, 1989

20. Cusano AJ, Thies HL, Siegal FP, et al: Hyponatremia in patients with acquired immunodeficiency syndrome. JAIDS 3:949–953, 1990

21. Da Silva M, Schevchuk MM, Cronin WJ, et al: Detection of HIV-related protein in testes and prostates of patients with AIDS. Am J Clin Pathol 93:196–201, 1990

22. Darling G, Goldstein DS, Stull R, et al: Tumor necrosis factor: Immune endocrine interaction. Surgery 106:1155–1160, 1989

23. De Paepe ME, Waxman M: Testicular atrophy in AIDS: A study of 57 autopsy cases. Hum Pathol 20:210–214, 1989

24. Dobs AS, Dempsy MA, Ladenson PW, Polk F: Endocrine disorders in men infected with HIV. Am J Med 84:611–616, 1988

25. Drew WL: Cytomegalovirus infection in patients with AIDS. J Infect Dis 158:449–456, 1988

26. Drucker D, Bailey D, Rotstein L: Thyroiditis as the presenting manifestation of disseminated extrapulmonary *Pneumocystis carinii* infection. J Clin Endocrinol Metab 71:1663–1665, 1990

27. Edgehl RH, Meguid MM, Aun F: The importance of the endocrine and metabolic responses to shock and trauma. Crit Care Med 5:257–263, 1977

28. Ediger SK, Isley WL: Rifampicin-induced adrenal insufficiency in the acquired immunodeficiency syndrome: Difficulties in diagnosis and treatment. Postgrad Med J 64:405–406, 1988

29. Farese RV, Schambelan M, Hollander H, et al: Nephrogenic diabetes insipidus associated with foscarnet treatment of cytomegalovirus retinitis. Ann Intern Med 112:955–956, 1990

30. Feingold KR, Krauss RM, Pang M, et al: The hypertriglyceridemia of acquired immunodeficiency syndrome is associated with an increased prevalence of low density lipoprotein subclass pattern B. J Clin Endocrinol Metab 76:1423–1427, 1993

31. Findling JW, Buggy BP, Gilson IH, et al: Longitudinal evaluation of adrenocortical function in patients infected with the human immunodeficiency virus. J Clin Endocrinol Metab 79:1091–1096, 1994

32. Frank TS, Livolsi VA, Connor AM: Cytomegalovirus infection of the thyroid in immunocompromised adults. Yale J Biol Med 60:1–8, 1987

33. Fried JC, LoPresti JS, Micon M, et al: Serum triiodothyronine values: Prognostic indicators of acute mortality due to *Pneumocystis carnii* pneumonia associated with the acquired immunodeficiency syndrome. Arch Intern Med 150:406–409, 1990

34. Gallant JE, Enriquez RE, Cohen KL, Hammers LW: *Pneumocystis carinii* thyroiditis. Am J Med 84:303–306, 1988

35. Gardner DF, Kaplan MM, Stanley CA, Utiger RD: Effect of triiodothyronine replacement on the metabolic and pituitary response to starvation. N Engl J Med 300:579–584, 1979

36. Gearhart MO, Sorg TB: Foscarnet-induced severe hypomagnesemia and other electrolyte disorders. Ann Pharmacother 27:285–288, 1993

37. Geffner ME, Yeh DY, Landaw EM, et al: *In vitro* insulin-like growth factor-1, growth hormone, and insulin resistance in symptomatic human immunodeficiency virus infected children. Pediatr Res 34:66–72, 1993

38. Glasgow BJ, Steinsapir KD, Anders K, Layfield LJ: Adrenal pathology in AIDS. Am J Clin Pathol 84:594–597, 1985

39. Gorman JM, Warne PA, Begg MD, et al: Serum prolactin levels in homosexual men and bisexual men with HIV infection. Am J Psychiatry 149:367–370, 1992

40. Graef AS, Gonzalez SS, Baca VR, et al: High serum prolactin levels in asymptomatic HIV-infected patients and in patients with acquired immunodeficiency syndrome. Clin Immun Immunopathol 72:390–393, 1994

41. Greene LW, Cole W, Greene JB, et al: Adrenal insufficiency as a complication of AIDS. Ann Intern Med 101:497–498, 1984

42. Grunfeld C, Feingold KR: The metabolic effects of tumor necrosis factor and other cytokines. Biotherapy 3:148–158, 1991

43. Grunfeld C, Feingold KR: Metabolic disturbances and wasting in the acquired immunodeficiency syndrome. N Engl J Med 327:329–337, 1992

44. Grunfeld C, Feingold KR: Body weight as essential data in the management of patients with human immunodeficiency virus infection and the acquired immunodeficiency syndrome. Am J Clin Nutr 58:317–318, 1993

45. Grunfeld C, Kotler DP, Hamadeh R, et al: Hypertriglyceridemia in the acquired immunodeficiency syndrome. Am J Med 86:27–31, 1989

46. Grunfeld C, Pang M, Doerrler W, et al: Lipids, lipoproteins, triglyceride clearance and cytokines in human immunodeficiency virus infection and the acquired immunodeficiency syndrome. J Clin Endocrinol Metab 74:1045–1052, 1992

47. Grunfeld C, Pang M, Doerrler W, et al: Indices of thyroid function and weight loss in human immunodeficiency virus infection and the acquired immunodeficiency syndrome. Metabolism 42:1270–1276, 1993

48. Grunfeld C, Pang M, Shimizu L, et al: Resting energy expenditure, caloric intake and short term weight change in human immunodeficiency virus infection and the acquired immunodeficiency syndrome. Am J Clin Nutr 55:455–460, 1992

49. Guarda LA, Luna MA, Smith JL, et al: Acquired im-

munodeficiency syndrome: Postmortem findings. Am J Clin Pathol 81:549–557, 1984

50. Guenther EE, Rabinowe SL, Van Niel A, et al: Primary Addison's disease in a patient with AIDS. Ann Intern Med 100:847–848, 1984

51. Guttler R, Singer P: *Pneumocystis carinii* thyroiditis: Case report and review of the literature. Arch Intern Med 153:393–396, 1993

52. Guy RJC, Turberg Y, Davidson RN, et al: Mineralocorticoid deficiency in HIV infection. Br Med J 298:496–497, 1989

53. Hellerstein MK, Grunfeld C, Wu K, et al: Increased de novo hepatic lipogenesis in HIV-infected humans. J Clin Endocrinol Metab 76:559–565, 1993

54. Henry K, Rathgaber S, Sullivan C, McCabe K: Diabetes mellitus induced by megestrol acetate in a patient with AIDS and cachexia. Ann Intern Med 116:53–54, 1992

55. Hilton CW, Harrington PT, Prasad C, Svec F: Adrenal insufficiency in AIDS. South Med J 81:1493–1495, 1988

56. Hintz RL, Suskind R, Amatayakul K, et al: Plasma somatomedin and growth hormone values in children with protein-calorie malnutrition. J Pediatr 92:153–156, 1978

57. Hommes MJT, Romijn J, Endert E, et al: Hypothyroid-like regulation of the pituitary-thyroid axis in stable human immunodeficiency virus infection. Metabolism 42:556–561, 1993

58. Hommes MJT, Romijn JA, Endert E, Sauerwein HP: Resting energy expenditure and substrate oxidation in human immunodeficiency virus (HIV)-infected asymptomatic men: HIV affects host metabolism in the early asymptomatic stage. Am J Clin Nutr 54:311–315, 1991

59. Hommes MJT, Romijn JA, Godfried MH, et al: Increased resting energy expenditure in HIV-infected men. Metabolism 39:1186–1190, 1990

60. Isley WL: Effect of rifampin therapy on the thyroid function tests in a hypothyroid patient on replacement L-thyroxine. Ann Intern Med 107:517–518, 1987

61. Jacobson MA, Gambertoglio JG, Aweeka FT, et al: Foscarnet-induced hypocalcaemia and effects of foscarnet on calcium metabolism. J Clin Endocrinol Metab 72:1130–1135, 1991

62. Kalin MF, Poretsky L, Seres DS, Zumoff B: Hyporeninemic hypoaldosteronism associated with AIDS. Am J Med 82:1035–1038, 1987

63. Karboski JA, Godley PJ: Inhaled pentamidine and hypoglycemia. Ann Intern Med 108:490, 1988

64. Kaufman FR, Gomperts ED: Growth failure in boys with hemophilia and HIV infection. Am J Pediatr Hematol Oncol 11:292–294, 1989

65. Klatt EC, Shibata D: Cytomegalovirus infection in the acquired immunodeficiency syndrome. Arch Pathol Lab Med 112:540–544, 1988

66. Krauth PH, Katz JF: Kaposi's sarcoma involving the thyroid in a patient with AIDS. Clin Nucl Med 12:848–849, 1987

67. Kyriazopoulou V, Parparousi O, Vagenakis AG: Rifampicin-induced adrenal crisis in addisonian patients receiving corticosteroid replacement therapy. J Clin Endocrinol Metab 59:1204–1206, 1984

68. Lachaal M, Venuto RC: Nephrotoxicity and hyperkalemia in patients with acquired immunodeficiency

69. Lambert M, Zech F, De Nayer P, et al: Elevation of serum thyroxine-binding globulin (but not of cortisol-binding globulin and sex hormone-binding globulin) associated with the progression of human immunodeficiency virus infection. Am J Med 89:748–751, 1990

70. Laue L, Pizzo PA, Butler K, Cutler GB: Growth and neuroendocrine dysfunction in children with AIDS. J Pediatr 117:541–545, 1990

71. Laulund S, Visfeldt J, Klunken L: Patho-anatomical studies of patients dying of AIDS. Acta Pathol Microbiol Immunol Scand 94:201–221, 1986

72. Lefrere JJ, Laplance JL, Vittecoq D, et al: Hypogonadism in AIDS. AIDS 2:135–136, 1988

73. Lieberman SA, Buttefield GE, Harrison D, Hoffman AR: Anabolic effects of recombinant insulin-like growth factor-I in cachectic patients with the acquired immunodeficiency syndrome. J Clin Endocrinol Metab 78:404–410, 1994

74. Lopresti JS, Fried JC, Spencer CA, Nicolof JT: Unique alterations of thyroid hormone indices in AIDS. Ann Intern Med 110:970–975, 1989

75. Loprinzi CL, Jensen MD, Jiang N-S, Schaid DJ: Effect of megestrol acetate on the human pituitary-adrenal axis. Mayo Clin Proc 67:1160–1162, 1992

76. Macallan DC, Noble C, Baldwin C, et al: Prospective analysis of patterns of weight change in stage IV human immunodeficiency virus infection. Am J Clin Nutr 58:417–424, 1993

77. Macallan DC, Noble C, Baldwin C, et al: Energy expenditure and wasting in human immunodeficiency virus infection. N Engl J Med 333:83–88, 1995

78. Mahac J, Mejatheim M, Goldsmith SJ: Gallium-67 citrate uptake in cryptococcal thyroiditis in a homosexual male. J Nucl Med Allied Sci 29:283–285, 1985

79. Martinez-Ocana JC, Romen J, Llatjos M, et al: Goiter as a manifestation of disseminated aspergillosis in a patient with AIDS. Clin Infect Dis 17:953–954, 1993

80. May ME, Carey RM: Rapid adrenocorticotropic hormone test in practice. Am J Med 79:679–683, 1985

81. McCarthy M, Coker R, Claydon E: Case report: Disseminated *Pneumocystis carinii* infection in a patient with the acquired immunodeficiency syndrome causing thyroid gland calcification and hypothyroidism. Clin Radiol 45:209–210, 1992

82. Melchior JC, Raguin G, Boulier A, et al: Resting energy expenditure in human immunodeficiency virus-infected patients: Comparison between patients with and without secondary infections. Am J Clin Nutr 57:614–619, 1993

83. Melchior JD, Salmon D, Rigaud D, et al: Resting energy expenditure is increased in stable, malnourished HIV-infected patients. Am J Clin Nutr 53:437–441, 1991

84. Membreno L, Irony I, Dere W, et al: Adrenocortical function in AIDS. J Clin Endocrinol Metab 65:482–487, 1987

85. Merenich JA, McDermott MT, Asp AA, et al: Evidence of endocrine involvement early in the course of human immunodeficiency virus infection. J Clin Endocrinol Metab 70:566–571, 1990

syndrome treated with pentamidine. Am J Med 87:260–263, 1989

86. Mildvan D, Machado SG, Wilets I, Grossberg SE: Endogenous interferon and triglyceride concentrations to assess response to zidovudine in AIDS and advanced AIDS-related complex. Lancet 339: 453–456, 1992

87. Milligan SA, Katz MS, Craven PC, et al: Toxoplasmosis presenting as panhypopituitarism in a patient with AIDS. Am J Med 77:760–764, 1984

88. Mollison LC, Mijch A, McBride G, Dwyer B: Hypothyroidism due to destruction of the thyroid by Kaposi's sarcoma. Rev Infect Dis 13:826–827, 1991

89. Mulligan K, Grunfeld C, Hellerstein MK, et al: Anabolic effects of recombinant human growth hormone in patients with wasting associated with human immunodeficiency virus infection. J Clin Endocrinol Metab 77:956–962, 1993

90. Nerup J: Addison's disease—a review of some clinical, pathological and immunological features. Dan Med Bull 21:201–217, 1974

91. Nuovo GJ, Becker J, Simsir A, et al: HIV-1 nucleic acids localize to the spermatogonia and their progeny. A study by polymerase chain reaction in situ hybridization. Am J Pathol 144:1142–1148, 1994

92. Oberfield SE, Kairam R, Bakshi S, et al: Steroid response to adrenocorticotropin stimulation in children with human immunodeficiency virus infection. J Clin Endocrinol Metab 70:578–581, 1990

93. Olivieri A, Sorcini M, Fazzini C, et al: Thyroid hypofunction related with the progression of human immunodeficiency virus infection. J Endocrinol Invest 16:407–413, 1993

94. Osa SR, Peterson RE, Roberts RB: Recovery of adrenal reserve following treatment of disseminated South American blastomycosis. Am J Med 71: 298–301, 1981

95. Osei K, Falko JM, Nelson KP, Stephens R: Diabetogenic effect of pentamidine: In vitro and in vivo studies in a patient with malignant insulinoma. Am J Med 77:41–46, 1984

96. Patel A, Snowden D, Kemp R, et al: Pneumocystis thyroiditis. Med J Aust 156:136–137, 1992

97. Pillay D, Lipman MCI, Lee CA, et al: A clinico-pathological audit of opportunistic viral infections in HIV-infected patients. AIDS 7:969–974, 1993

98. Pont A, Graybill JR, Craven PC, et al: High dose ketoconazole therapy and adrenal and testicular function in humans. Arch Intern Med 144:2150–2153, 1984

99. Pudney J, Anderson D: Orchitis and human immunodeficiency virus type 1 infected cells in reproductive tissues from men with the acquired immunodeficiency syndrome. Am J Pathol 139:149–160, 1991

100. Pulakhandam U, Dincsoy HP: Cytomegaloviral adrenalitis and insufficiency in AIDS. Am J Clin Pathol 93:651–656, 1990

101. Raffi F, Brisseau J-M, Plachon B, et al: Endocrine function in 98 HIV-infected patients: A prospective study. AIDS 5:729–733, 1991

102. Ragni MV, Dekker A, De Rubertis FR, et al: *Pneumocystis carinii* infection presenting as necrotizing thyroiditis and hypothyroidism. Am J Clin Pathol 95: 489–493, 1991

103. Reichert CM, O'Leary TJ, Levens DL, et al: Autopsy pathology in AIDS. Am J Pathol 112:357–382, 1983

104. Salbe AD, Kotler DP, Wang J, et al: Predictive value of IGF₁ concentration in HIV-infected patients. Clin Res 39:385A, 1991

105. Sano T, Kovacs K, Scheithauer BW, et al: Pituitary pathology in acquired immunodeficiency syndrome. Arch Pathol Lab Med 113:1066–1070, 1989

106. Sapolsky R, Rivier C, Yamamoto G, et al: Interleukin-1 stimulates the secretion of hypothalamic corticotropin releasing factor. Science 238:522–524, 1987

107. Schambelan M, Sebastian A, Biglieri EG: Prevalance, pathogenesis, and functional significance of aldosterone deficiency in hyperkalemic patients with chronic renal insufficiency. Kidney Int 17:89–101, 1980

108. Schwartz LJ, St Louis Y, Wu R, et al: Endocrine function in children with human immunodeficiency virus infection. Am J Dis Child 145:330–333, 1991

109. Shor-Posner G, Basit A, Lu Y, et al: Hypocholesterolemia is associated with immune dysfunction in early human immunodeficiency virus-1 infection. Am J Med 94:515–519, 1993

110. Sibbald WJ, Short A, Cohen MP, Wilson RF: Variations in adrenocortical responsiveness during severe bacterial infections. Ann Surg 186:29–33, 1977

111. Smith CG, Asch RH: Drug abuse and reproduction. Fertil Steril 48:355, 1987

112. Spitzer RD, Chan JC, Marks JB, et al: Case report: Hypothyroidism due to *Pneumocystis carinii* thyroiditis in a patient with acquired immunodeficiency syndrome. Am J Med Sci 302:98–100, 1991

113. Stahl-Bayliss CM, Kalman CM, Laskin OL: Pentamidine induced hypoglycemia in patients with the acquired immunodeficiency syndrome. Clin Pharmacol Ther 39:271–275, 1986

114. Sullivan WM, Kelley GG, O'Connor PG, et al: Hypopituitarism associated with a hypothalamic CMV infection in a patient with AIDS. Am J Med 92: 221–223, 1992

115. Tang WW, Kaptein EM, Feinstein EI, Massry SG: Hyponatremia in hospitalized patients with the acquired immunodeficiency syndrome (AIDS) and the AIDS-related complex. Am J Med 94:169–174, 1993

116. Tang WW, Kaptein EM: Thyroid hormone levels in AIDS or ARC. West J Med 151:627–631, 1989

117. Tapper ML, Rotterdam HZ, Lerner CW, et al: Adrenal necrosis in AIDS. Ann Intern Med 100: 239–241, 1984

118. Verges B, Chavanet P, Desgres J, et al: Adrenal function in HIV infected patients. Acta Endocrinol 121:633–637, 1989

119. Vijayakumar V, Bekerman C, Blend MJ, et al: Role of Ga-67 citrate in imaging extrapulmonary pneumocystis in HIV positive patients. Clin Nucl Med 18:337–338, 1993

120. Villette JM, Bourin P, Doinel C, et al: Circadian variations in plasma levels of hypophyseal, adrenocortical and testicular hormones in men infected with human immunodeficiency virus. J Clin Endocrinol Metab 70:572–577, 1990

121. Wagner G, Rabkin JG, Rabkin R: Illness stage, concurrent medications, and other correlates of low testosterone in men with HIV illness. J

Acquir Immun Syndr Hum Retrovirol 8:204–207, 1995

122. Wartofsky L, Burman KD: Alterations in thyroid function in patients with systemic illness: The "euthyroid sick syndrome." Endocr Rev 3:164–217, 1982

123. Waskin H, Stehr-Green JK, Helmick CG, Sattler FR: Risk factors for hypoglycemia associated with pentamidine therapy for *Pneumocystis* pneumonia. JAMA 260:345–347, 1988

124. Welch K, Finkbeiner W, Alpers CE, et al: Autopsy findings in the acquired immune deficiency syndrome. JAMA 252:1152–1159, 1984

125. Widy-Wirski R, Berkely S, Downing R, et al: Evaluation of the WHO clinical case definition of AIDS in Uganda. JAMA 260:3186–3289, 1985

126. Woloski BMRNJ, Smith EM, Meyer WJ III, et al: Corticotropin-releasing activity of monokines. Science 230:1035–1037, 1985

127. Youle MS, Clarbour J, Gazzard B: Severe hypocalcaemia in AIDS patients treated with foscarnet and pentamidine. Lancet i:1455–1456, 1988

128. Zangerle R, Sarcletti M, Gallati H, et al: Decreased plasma concentrations of HDL cholesterol in HIV-infected individuals are associated with immune activation. JAIDS 7:1149–1156, 1994

Chapter 19

Renal Complications
of HIV Infection

MICHAEL H. HUMPHREYS

Renal manifestations of human immunodeficiency virus (HIV) infection can be grouped into three major categories. Certain fluid, electrolyte, and acid–base abnormalities have been observed with frequency in HIV-infected patients. Acute renal failure can also occur in acquired immunodeficiency syndrome (AIDS) patients and is often a manifestation of drug nephrotoxicity. Finally, chronic renal failure progressing to end-stage renal disease has also been observed with a high frequency in some centers. These renal manifestations all occur almost exclusively in patients with symptomatic AIDS.

FLUID, ELECTROLYTE, AND ACID–BASE ABNORMALITIES

Hyponatremia

A number of electrolyte disturbances are seen frequently in HIV-infected patients.[19] The most common of these is hyponatremia, which has been reported in as many as 20% to 56% of hospitalized patients with AIDS[1,12,15,29,35,38] and has also been identified in outpatients.[12] The basis for the hyponatremia is variable. The largest single cause is volume depletion resulting from extrarenal fluid losses (usually from diarrhea), and in most of these cases, the restoration of normal extracellular fluid volume is accompanied by correction of the hyponatremia.[1,12,29,35,38] A smaller number of patients develop hyponatremia in the absence of any evidence of hypovolemia; these patients have the characteristic findings of the syndrome of inappropriate secretion of antidiuretic hormone (SIADH). Plasma ADH concentration, when measured in some such patients, has been inappropriately elevated for the degree of hypona-

tremia and hypoosmolaility, lending strong support for this mechanism underlying the hyponatremia.[1] Patients with symptomatic AIDS frequently present with opportunistic infections of the lungs and central nervous system; such infections are known to stimulate excessive release of ADH to produce SIADH. In a few patients, evidence of adrenal insufficiency accompanies the hyponatremia, and treatment with glucocorticoid hormone improves the serum sodium concentration.[1,12,38] AIDS patients have a high incidence of adrenal abnormalities (see Chapter 18).

Whatever its cause, the development of hyponatremia in an HIV-infected patient is a sign of poor prognosis, since survival is much shorter than in patients with similar diagnoses who are not hyponatremic.[12,35,38]

Hyperkalemia

Attention has recently focused on the occurrence of hyperkalemia in symptomatic AIDS patients usually undergoing treatment for opportunistic infection.[19] Hyperkalemia can develop in patients being treated with high doses of trimethoprim, usually on the order of 20 mg/kg/day,[10,17,21,37] and has been attributed to impaired secretion of potassium in the collecting duct. Trimethoprim shares structural similarity with the potassium-sparing diuretic triamterene, and, at the high doses used for treatment of *Pneumocystis* infections, prevents normal tubular potassium secretion, thereby causing the hyperkalemia.[10,37] It has been suggested that hyperchloremic metabolic acidosis may accompany the hyperkalemia in some patients.[21] Hyperkalemia may also result from pentamidine nephrotoxicity; when this occurs, azotemia is also present.[26] In each of these settings, the hyperkalemia will resolve after cessation of the drug.

Metabolic Acidosis

Although patients with AIDS may present with a variety of simple and mixed acid–base disorders, it has only recently become appreciated that they may also develop lactic acidosis.[9,16] One well-documented case suggested that the cause of the excess lactate production was a "mitochondrial myopathy" caused by interruption of normal mitochondrial respiration in skeletal muscle by zidovudine.[16] However, not all case reports were of patients who received this drug.[9] Recognition of this entity rests with a severe metabolic acidosis with an increased anion gap; blood lactate levels, when measured, have been >5, and frequently >10 mmol/liter.[9,16] No form of treatment has been uniformly successful, and survival is shortened in these patients.[9]

ACUTE RENAL FAILURE

HIV-infected patients are also subject to the development of acute renal failure.[30] Drug nephrotoxicity is the basis in many cases, so this complication occurs almost exclusively in patients with symptomatic AIDS. The two major types of acute renal failure are ischemic, related to severe hypovolemia from fluid losses, and nephrotoxic, following administration of one or more agents used in the diagnosis and treatment of AIDS complications.[30,36] Ischemic acute renal failure is recognized by the clinical findings of hypovolemia, oliguria, rapidly evolving azotemia, the presence of brown granular casts in the urinary sediment, and a high (>1%) fractional excretion of sodium (FE_{Na}). Nephrotoxic acute renal failure may be nonoliguric or oliguric; although the FE_{Na} is often greater than 1%, it may in some cases be less. A list of some potentially nephrotoxic agents used in AIDS patients is presented in Table 19–1. Renal function generally recovers once the inciting agent has been discontinued, although hemodialytic support may be necessary occasionally. Recovery is also the rule in patients with ischemic acute renal failure.

CHRONIC RENAL DISEASE

Although HIV-infected patients may develop virtually any form of parenchymal renal dis-

TABLE 19–1. NEPHROTOXIC DRUGS USED IN THE TREATMENT OF AIDS PATIENTS

Known nephrotoxicity
  Amphotericin B
  Acyclovir
  Aminoglycosides
  Dapsone (rare)
  Foscarnet
  Pentamidine
  Rifampin
Potential for nephrotoxicity
  Sulfamethoxazole
  Sulfadiazine
Drugs requiring dose adjustment in renal insufficiency
  Acyclovir
  Ethambutol
  Fluconazole
  Ganciclovir
  Pyrazinamide
  Zidovudine

ease,[14,27] attention has focused on renal lesions thought possibly to relate specifically to the infection. Two main types of glomerular involvement leading to proteinuria and the nephrotic syndrome have been described.[18] In one, immune complex deposition in glomeruli leads to a proliferative glomerulonephritis and renal insufficiency. Kimmel and associates[22] described four such patients in whom circulating immune complexes containing HIV antigen were present; renal biopsy revealed proliferative glomerulonephritis, and eluates of biopsy tissue revealed the same types of complexes in renal tissue after polymerase chain reaction (PCR) amplification. This same group had earlier reported two other HIV-infected patients with IgA nephropathy who also had circulating IgA immune complexes with HIV antigens[23]; eluates of renal biopsy tissue again revealed the presence of HIV *gag* and *env* sequences.[23] Thus, deposition in glomeruli of immune complexes containing viral antigens may result in proliferative glomerulonephritis. These complexes may arise from trapping of circulating complexes or from in situ complex formation to viral antigens in renal tissue. Another form of immune-mediated renal disease may occur in HIV-positive patients coinfected with hepatitis C virus (HCV). HCV infection is associated with the development of membranoproliferative glomerulonephritis (MPGN), often accompanied by cryoglobulinemia.[20] Coinfection of HCV with HIV can also lead to the occurrence of MPGN.[32]

A different form of glomerular disease in HIV-infected patients has been described more frequently.[18] Often called HIV-associated nephropathy, its histologic characteristics are those of focal and segmental glomerulosclerosis (FSGS) with interstitial inflammation and fibrosis and tubular dilatation and atrophy; indeed, these characteristics have been regarded as so distinctive as to constitute a specific pathologic entity.[11,13] It has been reported primarily from centers in urban areas of the east and west coasts of the United States; worldwide, over 90% of reported cases have occurred in people of African descent, with a high preponderance of males.[5] Clinically, it is characterized by high-grade proteinuria, usually in the nephrotic range (>3.5 g/day), normal or large kidneys with increased echodensity on diagnostic ultrasound, and renal insufficiency that rapidly progresses in weeks to months to end-stage renal disease; noteworthy is the rarity of hypertension and peripheral edema in these patients despite the severity of the renal failure and proteinuria.[5,6,8] Although usually diagnosed in patients with AIDS, it has been the initial manifestation of HIV infection in a small number of cases. Initially thought to be highly associated with injection drug use, this mode of HIV transmission is involved in less than half the cases,[7] and the occurrence of this lesion in infants and children with AIDS from vertical HIV transmission[34] indicates that drug use is not necessary for its development.

The pathogenesis of this form of renal involvement in HIV infection is not clear. HIV DNA can be demonstrated in microdissected segments and infiltrating cells of renal biopsy tissue of such patients,[22] and may be linked to the pathologic process, although viral DNA was also identified in the tissue of patients without any renal disease.[22] Mice transgenic for a noninfective HIV construct express viral DNA in kidney tissue, and also develop FSGS.[25] A recent preliminary report indicates that HIV is a potent stimulator of transforming growth factor-β,[4] a cytokine strongly implicated in the development of fibrosis. Activation of this cytokine could well be the basis for the extensive interstitial fibrosis and glomerular sclerosis that are the hallmarks of HIV-associated nephropathy.[18] Future research should clarify the cause of FSGS in HIV-infected patients.

At the present time, there is no proven therapy of either proliferative glomerulonephritis or FSGS in patients with HIV infection. A small series of patients with HIV-associated FSGS responded to steroid treatment,[33] and two other patients with other renal lesions have also responded to prednisone therapy.[2,24] A prospective, randomized multicenter trial of prednisone in HIV-associated FSGS is now under way. Data suggesting improvement with zidovudine[28] are not impressive, and it must be expected that patients will progress to end-stage renal disease. Patients with MPGN due to HCV infection may respond to treatment with interferon-α,[20] but there is as yet no experience with this agent in patients coinfected with HIV. Decisions about dialysis treatment must be made on an individual basis. Initial reports indicated that AIDS patients treated with hemodialysis had a very short survival time,[5,30] an observation that raised the question of whether dialysis should even be offered. However, overall improvement in AIDS management, and earlier diagnosis of HIV-associated renal disease, has led to an improvement in the poor initial results, and other patients will do well on continuous ambulatory peritoneal dialysis. There is general agreement that transplantation is not an option for these patients. Renal failure complicates the management of HIV-related complications, since many of the agents used are nephrotoxic, or are renally eliminated, requiring dosage reduction.[3]

REFERENCES

1. Agarwal A, Soni A, Ciechanowsky M, et al: Hyponatremia in patients with the acquired immunodeficiency syndrome. Nephron 53:317–321, 1989
2. Appel RG, Neill J: A steroid-responsive nephrotic syndrome in a patient with human immunodeficiency virus (HIV) infection. Ann Intern Med 113:892–895, 1990
3. Berns JS, Cohen RM, Stumacher RJ, Rudnick MR: Renal aspects of therapy for human immunodeficiency virus and associated opportunistic infections. J Am Soc Nephrol 1:1061–1080, 1991
4. Border W, Yamamoto T, Noble N, et al: HIV-associated nephropathy is linked to TGF-β and matrix protein expression in human kidney (Abstract). J Am Soc Nephrol 4:675, 1993
5. Bourgoignie JJ, Meneses R, Ortiz C, et al: The clinical spectrum of renal disease associated with human immunodeficiency virus. Am J Kidney Dis 12:131–137, 1988
6. Bourgoignie JJ, Meneses R, Pardo V: The nephropathy related to acquired immune deficiency syndrome. Adv Nephrol 17:113–126, 1988
7. Bourgoignie JJ, Pardo V: The nephropathology in human immunodeficiency virus (HIV-1) infection. Kidney Int 40:S19–S23, 1991
8. Carbone L, D'Agati V, Cheng JT, Appel GB: Course

and prognosis of human immunodeficiency virus-associated nephropathy. Am J Med 87:389–395, 1989

9. Chattha G, Arieff AI, Cummings C, Tierney LM Jr: Lactic acidosis complicating the acquired immunodeficiency syndrome. Ann Intern Med 118:37–39, 1993

10. Choi MJ, Fernandez PC, Patnaik A, et al: Brief report: Trimethoprim-induced hyperkalemia in a patient with AIDS. N Engl J Med 328:703–706, 1993

11. Cohen AH, Nast CC: HIV-associated nephropathy. A unique combined glomerular, tubular, and interstitial lesion. Mod Pathol 1:87–97, 1988

12. Cusano AJ, Thies HL, Siegal FP, et al: Hyponatremia in patients with acquired immune deficiency syndrome. J Acquir Immune Defic Syndr 3:949–953, 1990

13. D'Agati V, Suh JI, Carbone L, et al: Pathology of HIV-associated nephropathy: A detailed morphologic and comparative study. Kidney Int 35:1358–1370, 1989

14. Gardenswartz MH, Lerner CW, Seligson GR, et al: Renal disease in patients with AIDS: A clinicopathologic study. Clin Nephrol 21:197–204, 1984

15. Glassock RJ, Cohen AH, Danovitch G, Parsa KP: Human immunodeficiency virus (HIV) infection and the kidney. Ann Intern Med 112:35–49, 1990

16. Gopinath R, Hutcheon M, Cheema-Dhadli S, Halperin M: Chronic lactic acidosis in a patient with acquired immunodeficiency syndrome and mitochondrial myopathy: Biochemical studies. J Am Soc Nephrol 3:1212–1219, 1992

17. Greenberg S, Reiser IW, Chou SY, Porush JG: Trimethoprim-sulfamethoxazole induces reversible hyperkalemia. Ann Intern Med 119:291–295, 1993

18. Humphreys MH: Human immunodeficiency virus-associated glomerulosclerosis. Kidney Int 48:311–320, 1995

19. Humphreys MH, Schoenfeld P: Electrolyte, acid-base, and endocrine disturbances in patients with HIV infection. In Kimmel PL, Berns JS, eds. Contemporary Issues in Nephrology. 29. Renal and Urologic Aspects of HIV infection. New York, Churchill Livingstone, 1995, pp 27–40

20. Johnson RJ, Gretch DR, Yamabe H, et al: Membranoproliferative glomerlonephritis associated with hepatitis C virus infection. N Engl J Med 328:465–470, 1993

21. Kalin MF, Poretsky L, Seres DS, Zumoff B: Hyporeninemic hypoaldosteronism associated with acquired immune deficiency syndrome. Am J Med 82:1035–1038, 1987

22. Kimmel PL, Ferreira-Centeno A, Farkas-Szallasi T, et al: Viral DNA in microdissected renal biopsy tissue from HIV infected patients with nephrotic syndrome. Kidney Int 43:1347–1352, 1993

23. Kimmel PL, Phillips TM, Ferreira-Centeno A, et al: Brief report: Idiotypic IgA nephropathy in patients with human immunodeficiency virus infection. N Engl J Med 327:702–706, 1992

24. Kimmel PL, Phillips TM, Ferreira-Centeno A, et al: HIV-associated immune-mediated renal disease. Kidney Int 44:1327–1340, 1993

25. Kopp JB, Klotman ME, Adler SH, et al: Progressive glomerulosclerosis and enhanced renal accumulation of basement membrane components in mice transgenic for human immunodeficiency virus type 1 genes. Proc Natl Acad Sci U S A 89:1577–1581, 1992

26. Lachaal M, Venuto RC: Nephrotoxicity and hyperkalemia in patients with acquired immunodeficiency syndrome treated with pentamidine. Am J Med 87:260–263, 1989

27. Mazbar SA, Schoenfeld PY, Humphreys MH: Renal involvement in patients infected with HIV: Experience at San Francisco General Hospital. Kidney Int 37:1325–1332, 1990

28. Michel C, Dosquet P, Ronco P, et al: Nephropathy associated with infection by human immunodeficiency virus: A report on 11 cases including 6 treated with zidovudine. Nephron 62:434–440, 1992

29. Peter SA: Electrolyte disorders and renal dysfunction in acquired immunodeficiency syndrome patients. J Natl Med Assoc 83:889–891, 1991

30. Rao TKS, Berns JS: Acute renal failure in patients with HIV infection. In Kimmel PL, Berns JS, eds. Contemporary Issues in Nephrology. 29. Renal and Urologic Aspects of HIV Infection. New York, Churchill Livingstone, 1995, pp 41–57

31. Rao TKS, Friedman EA, Nicastri AD: The types of renal disease in the acquired immunodeficiency syndrome. N Engl J Med 316:1062–1068, 1987

32. Rodriguez RA, Khakmahd OK, Balkovetz DF, et al: Membranoproliferative glomerulonephritis (MPGN) associated with cryoglobulinemia in patients coinfected with the human immunodeficiency virus (HIV) and the hepatitis V virus (HCV) (Abstract). J Am Soc Nephrol 6:431, 1995

33. Smith, C, Pawar R, Carey JT, et al: Effect of corticosteroid therapy on human immunodeficiency virus associated nephropathy. Am J Med 97:145–151, 1994

34. Strauss J, Abitbol C, Zilleruelo G, et al: Renal disease in children with the acquired immunodeficiency syndrome. N Engl J Med 321:625–630, 1989

35. Tang WW, Kaptein EM, Feinstein EI, Massry SG: Hyponatremia in hospitalized patients with the acquired immunodeficiency syndrome (AIDS) and the AIDS-related complex. Am J Med 94:169–174, 1993

36. Valeri A, Neusy AJ: Acute and chronic renal disease in hospitalized AIDS patients. Clin Nephrol 35:110–118, 1991

37. Velazquez H, Perazella MA, Wright FS, Ellison DH: Renal mechanism of trimethoprim-induced hyperkalemia. Ann Intern Med 119:296–301, 1993

38. Vitting KE, Gardenswartz MH, Zabetakis PM: Frequency of hyponatremia and nonosmolar vasopressin release in the acquired immunodeficiency syndrome. JAMA 263:973–978, 1990

Section III

Specific Infections and Malignant Conditions

Chapter 20

Pneumocystis carinii
Pneumonia

JOHN D. STANSELL and LAURENCE HUANG

Pneumocystis carinii increasingly has become recognized as a cause of disease among immunocompromised populations since its discovery nearly 90 years ago.[16] An organism of relatively low virulence, *P. carinii* poses no significant health threat to immunocompetent persons. However, *P. carinii* is a major source of suffering and death in persons with impaired host immunity due to malnutrition, neoplasia, organ transplant, or human immunodeficiency virus (HIV) infection. Prior to the 1980s, the number of *P. carinii* pneumonia cases diagnosed in the United States each year was small. Since 1981, this number has exploded, paralleling the rise of symptomatic HIV infection. Indeed, the occurrence of *P. carinii* pneumonia in clusters of homosexual men and injection drug users in 1981 was the harbinger of the current acquired immunodeficiency syndrome (AIDS) epidemic.[44,82] While *P. carinii* pneumonia accounted for nearly two thirds of AIDS-index diagnoses early in the epidemic,[95] recent data suggest a reduction in this proportion as a result of widespread primary *P. carinii* prophylaxis use.[13,14] Moreover, improved management of acute *P. carinii* pneumonia and routine use of secondary *P. carinii* prophylaxis have resulted in improved treatment outcomes and longer life expectancy for those persons at risk for the disease.

Although many gaps in our knowledge of *P. carinii* persist, we have gained significant knowledge about susceptibility, diagnosis, treatment, and prevention of this disease over the 15 years of the AIDS epidemic. This chapter will focus upon the current state of knowledge and emerging concepts about *P. carinii* pneumonia in HIV-infected persons.

MICROBIOLOGY

The inability to culture *P. carinii* outside of immunocompromised animal models has se-verely hampered our understanding of this organism. The lack of a reliable in vitro culture method has made drug development and epidemiologic study difficult. Furthermore, a definitive environmental reservoir for the organism has never been identified and the inability to observe the life cycle of the organism has led to much misunderstanding.

In 1909, Chagas described *P. carinii* in the lungs of trypanosome-infected guinea pigs and believed it to be a new trypanosome.[16] Despite recognition as being unique from trypanosomes, the misconception that *P. carinii* was a protozoan persisted for 80 years after its discovery based on the organism's morphology, inability to grow on fungal media, and susceptibility to antiprotozoal agents. In 1970, ultrastructural studies noting that *P. carinii* lacked organelles characteristic of protozoa while possessing features suggestive of fungi began to cast doubt upon the protozoal classification.[155] In 1988, two independent groups presented evidence from 18S ribosomal RNA homology studies that strongly indicated the organism was a fungus.[27,145] Since these first reports, a watershed of studies have corroborated the assignment of *P. carinii* to the fungal kingdom. Sequence analysis of genes encoding dihydrofolate reductase,[24] thymidylate synthase,[25] actin,[33] tubulin,[23] ATPase,[84] as well as mitochondrial gene sequences[114] all incontrovertibly link *P. carinii* to the fungi. Although the exact phylogenetic lineage is still undetermined, recent reviews place *P. carinii* among the ascomycetes.[26]

P. carinii is a unicellular eukaryote that reproduces by both sexual and asexual means and has several distinct stages to its life cycle.[125] The trophozoite, the predominant intrapulmonary form, is 3 to 5 μm in size and avidly adheres to type 1 pneumocytes. This adhesion may facilitate absorption of nutrients directly through the alveolar-capillary membrane. Large trophozoites likely undergo asexual binary fission to produce small, haploid trophs that subsequently mature to large, diploid trophozoites. The fusion of two haploid trophs, or gemetic cells, may initiate the sexual reproduction of the organism, sporogenesis, or encystment. The parent cell, which resembles a large trophozoite, becomes round and smooth, and develops a thick cell wall. Within the mature cyst, eight haploid intracytoplasmic bodies or spores develop. These spores, which are indistinguishable from trophozoites, are released from a rupture in the cell wall. The collapsed cysts, which resemble crescents, are readily observed on silver-stained clinical specimens from *P. carinii*–infected persons (Color Plate IC).

EPIDEMIOLOGY AND TRANSMISSION

P. carinii can be found in the lungs of many mammalian species including human, mouse, rat, ferret, pig, horse, and rabbit. Morphologically, these organisms are indistinguishable and, based on the widespread presence of the organism among commonly encountered animals, it might be tempting to consider human *P. carinii* infection a zoonosis. However, evidence is clear from immunologic and genetic studies that these organisms are not identical. Examination of DNA homology of highly conserved portions of the gene encoding mitochondrial ribosomal RNA has demonstrated significant divergence among all species.[136,160] Examination of the chromosomes from each mammalian species reveals unique species karyotypes.[164] Analysis of genetic divergence of the gene coding for the major surface glycoprotein (MSG) of *P. carinii* suggests organisms infecting different mammalian species are genetically distinct and that *P. carinii* is host-species-specific.[162] Transmission studies further document this species specificity. Although transmission of *P. carinii* can be achieved between animals of the same species,[59] attempts to transmit *P. carinii* infection between separate, distinct species have failed.[162] Thus, it is unlikely that animals are the environmental reservoir for *P. carinii* transmittal to man.

Transmittal of *P. carinii* is likely to require inhalation of the infectious unit. Studies by Hughes documented that immunocompromised germ-free rats maintained in sterile environments did not develop *P. carinii* pneumonia.[58] Similarly, immunocompromised animals maintained in isolators and fed unsterilized food and water or lung tissue from infected animals did not develop the disease.[59] Conversely, even limited exposure of germ-free severe combined immunodeficiency (SCID) mice to ambient air or infected animals resulted in the transmittal of the disease.[139] These studies indicate that de novo infection results from inhalation of airborne organisms. Moreover, air samples obtained from both laboratory and rural settings have demonstrated human *P. carinii* genetic material when subjected to polymerase chain reaction (PCR).[159,162]

Several serologic studies have demonstrated that most humans develop an antibody response to specific *P. carinii* antigens by 4 years of age.[88,108,112] This seroconversion occurs worldwide, attesting to the ubiquitous nature of *Pneumocystis*.[137] It also attests to the asymptomatic nature of primary infection in immunocompetent persons. Because of the widespread exposure to *P. carinii* and subsequent development of disease only in the setting of immunocompromise, it has been theorized that *P. carinii* organisms lay dormant in the immunocompetent host and *P. carinii* pneumonia occurs as a result of reactivation at a time of progressive immunocompromise. However, recent studies involving sensitive molecular probes failed to identify resident *P. carinii* genetic material in the lungs of immunocompetent persons. Peters and colleagues searched with PCR probes for *P. carinii* genetic material in the homogenized postmortem lungs of 15 immunocompetent persons with negative results.[110] Similarly, others failed to identify *P. carinii* in immunocompetent persons by monoclonal antibody staining of fixed lung specimens[89] or by PCR probes of bronchoalveolar lavage fluid.[161]

The situation is quite different in immunocompromised persons, however. Several studies have now identified *P. carinii* genetic material in sputum, bronchoalveolar lavage fluid, and blood of persons with immunocompromising conditions, specifically, organ transplantation or HIV infection.[28,30,75,78,147] Despite the presence of *P. carinii* in these immunocompromised individuals, many of them did not have clinical symptoms that would suggest pneumonia, nor did they progress to clinical *P. carinii* pneumonia thereafter.[75] This suggests that long periods of asymptomatic colonization may precede recognizable respiratory disease in immunocompromised persons. In addition, the clearance of *pneumocystis* organisms from the lungs of immunocompromised persons who have been treated for *P. carinii* pneumonia may be slow or may not occur at all. Vargas et al.[154] have recently looked at the persistence of organisms in the lungs of steroid treated rats after specific treatment for the infection and subsequent withdrawal of immunocompromising drugs. These investigators found organisms persisting for 1 year in a significant number of study animals.[154] It is conceivable that, in the face of progressive immunologic decline, AIDS patients even with clinical resolution of respiratory illness and subsequent use of secondary *P. carinii* prophylaxis, may not completely eradicate *P. carinii* from their lungs.

These findings beg the question of whether person-to-person transmission of *P. carinii* occurs. Early reports of disease due to *P. carinii* were clusters of pneumonia among malnourished children[35] or among children hospitalized for treatment of malignant disease.[109,124] *P. carinii* colonization in a seemingly immunocompetent person exposed to *P. carinii*–infected animals has been described.[144] In a multicenter, observational study of the pulmonary complications of HIV infection, two HIV-seronegative control subjects who had exposure to patients with *P. carinii* pneumonia, were subsequently found to harbor *P. carinii* in induced sputum and bronchoalveolar lavage fluid specimens. Neither of these subjects had clinical evidence of pulmonary disease at the time of discovery or over the course of the study (J.D. Stansell, unpublished observations). Finally, serum titers of antibodies directed against *P. carinii* have been found to be elevated among health care workers who care for AIDS patients.[74] These results call into question whether infection control measures, especially respiratory isolation, are warranted for persons with *P. carinii* pneumonia. Recommendations await further research.

HOST DEFENSES

The natural host defenses and immunologic responses that both protect humans from *P. carinii* and modify the expression of disease in immunocompromised persons are incompletely understood. Although cell-mediated immunity appears to play the decisive role in protection from *P. carinii*, studies indicate that humoral immunity also appears to be important in the host's ability to avoid infection or recover from *P. carinii* pneumonia. Patients with seemingly pure B-lymphocyte dysfunction or pure T-lymphocyte dysfunction or both are at risk for developing *P. carinii* pneumonia.

Early studies indicated that immunization and significant serum antibody titers against *P. carinii* were inadequate to protect rats subjected to corticosteroid immunosuppression from *P. carinii* pneumonia. A recent study, however, demonstrates near complete protection of mice immunized against *P. carinii,* and then subsequently administered intratracheal organisms and selectively depleted of their CD4 lymphocytes by administration of monoclonal antibodies directed against CD4 or Thy-1 epitopes.[48] Not only were *P. carinii* organisms absent on microscopy at days 10 and 19 of the study, but they were undetectable by PCR probe as well. This study suggests a major role for humoral immunity in protection from *P. carinii* infection.

Studies illustrate that passively administered antibodies to *P. carinii* can modulate the burden of organisms in immunodeficient animal models with *P. carinii* pneumonia.[38] Analogously, B cells in addition to T cells are necessary for resolution of *P. carinii* pneumonia in immunodeficient rodents.[50] Similar results are obtained using SCID mice that spontaneously develop *P. carinii* infection.[122] This study also documented an improvement in survival by greater than threefold in mice treated with hyperimmune serum. How humoral immunity exerts its effect upon *P. carinii* pneumonia is uncertain, but opsonization, complement-mediated organism lysis, and interference with cell adhesion have all been postulated as possible mechanisms. Confirmation awaits further research.

Cell-mediated immunity appears to occupy the pivotal role in prevention and control of *P. carinii* infection. Shellito and colleagues demonstrated that conventional BALB/c rats could be rendered susceptible to *P. carinii* pneumonia by administration of monoclonal antibodies directed against CD4 lymphocytes.[135] SCID mice, which develop *P. carinii* pneumonia spontaneously from their environment, can be protected from *P. carinii* by administration of CD4 lymphocytes from immunocompetent donors.[49] Moreover, administration of anti-CD4 monoclonal antibody to these mice eliminates the protective effect. Similar studies in SCID mice have shown that CD4 lymphocytes, but not CD8 lymphocytes, play a vital role in control of *P. carinii.*[121] A recent study suggests a role for the major surface glycoprotein in eliciting the cellular immune response. In this study, CD4 lymphocytes incubated with the glycoprotein had a salutary effect upon *P. carinii* pneumonia in rats.[148] Although CD4 lymphocytes are clearly essential for the control of *P. carinii*, the manner in which these cells exert their effect and their interaction with other effector cells are largely unknown. The CD4 lymphocyte, through secretion of cytokines, particularly interferon-γ and interleukin-2, orchestrates much of cell-mediated immunity and, possibly, humoral immunity. CD4 lymphopenia and disruption of cytokine activity are hallmarks of HIV disease.

PATHOPHYSIOLOGY

Overwhelmingly, *P. carinii* infection is a pulmonary process. Once inhaled, the infective form of *P. carinii*, the precise identity of which is unknown, establishes residence in the alveolus. There, the organism attaches itself to alveolar type 1 cells through bridges of cellular fibronectin and surface glycoproteins.[116,117] Although the organism tightly interdigitates with the type 1 cell, there is no fusion of the cellular membranes. Attachment may facilitate nutrient access directly from the alveolar-capillary bed and appears necessary for organism replication.

It is clear from the prolonged immunosuppression required to induce *P. carinii* pneumonia in animal models and the indolent onset of respiratory symptoms in AIDS patients that *P. carinii* replicates at a relatively slow pace. Eventually, however, large numbers of organisms inhabit the alveoli and alveolar-capillary permeability increases abnormally. Microscopic examination of lung tissue at this time will reveal alveoli filled with foamy, vaculated, eosinophilic exudates. This exudate consists of *P. carinii* organisms, degenerative cell membranes, surfactant, and host proteins.[163,166] There is a paucity of inflammatory cells present. There is a disruption of surfactant production by type II cells with a fall in phospholipid production.[163] Rarely, organisms may invade the interstitium, and interstitial fibrosis may follow successful treatment of severe cases. Subsequently, the alveolar epithelial surface degenerates. Subepithelial blebs form, filled with fluid that has traversed the alveolar-capillary membrane due to disrupted permeability. Ultimately, the epithelial cells are lost with denudation of the basement membrane. This presents a clinical picture not unlike the diffuse alveolar damage seen with adult respiratory distress syndrome (ARDS). Lung volumes, lung compliance, and the diffusing capacity for carbon monoxide (DL$_{CO}$) are severely reduced. The resulting functional abnormality in patients with *P. carinii* pneumonia is impairment of gas exchange. Poor distribution of inspired air into alveoli that are partially or completely filled with parasites and inflammatory debris leads to ventilation-

perfusion mismatch or frank right-to-left shunt. The result is progressive dyspnea and hypoxemia and, ultimately, respiratory failure.

RISK FACTORS FOR *PNEUMOCYSTIS CARINII* PNEUMONIA

Two major prospective, observational cohort studies have sought to answer the question of who is at risk for *P. carinii* pneumonia. The first, the Multicenter AIDS Cohort Study (MACS), determined a markedly increased risk for *P. carinii* pneumonia among participants with CD4 lymphocyte counts <200 cells/μl who were not receiving *P. carinii* prophylaxis.[111] These HIV-infected persons had a nearly fivefold greater risk of developing *P. carinii* pneumonia compared to HIV-infected persons who had never had a CD4 lymphocyte count <200 cells/μl. The presence of fever and oral thrush also independently influenced the risk of progression to *P. carinii* pneumonia. The results of this study led directly to the publication of the 1989 Centers for Disease Control recommendations for the use of prophylaxis against *P. carinii* in HIV-infected persons.[12] Unfortunately, a number of factors limited the generalizability of the MACS data: (1) the cohort was entirely composed of homosexual men; (2) there was often a broad interval between CD4 lymphocyte count determination and *P. carinii* pneumonia diagnosis; and (3) data were censored for any AIDS-defining illness.

In contrast, the Pulmonary Complications of HIV Infection Study was designed to define the types and frequency of lung disorders and the course and outcomes of these disorders in a population that closely approximated the demographics of the AIDS epidemic in 1990.[118] The study cohort included 775 homosexual/bisexual men, 253 injection drug–using men and women, and 54 women who acquired HIV infection through heterosexual contact. There were 968 HIV-seropositive men and 151 HIV-seropositive women enrolled in the study. Whites comprised 69% of the cohort, blacks 23%, and Hispanics and Asians 8%. The cohort was followed for a mean of 52 months and CD4 lymphocyte counts were tightly clustered around a *P. carinii* pneumonia diagnosis. The median time from CD4 lymphocyte count determination to diagnosis was 26 days. Data were censored only for first-episode *P. carinii* pneumonia; other opportunistic infections or malignancies did not preclude inclusion. Ninety-five per cent of *P. carinii* pneumonia cases occurred in individuals with a CD4 lymphocyte count <200 cells/μl and 79% of subjects had a CD4 lymphocyte count <100 cells/μl.[141] The median CD4 lymphocyte count at the time of *P. carinii* pneumonia diagnosis was 29 cells/μl. Persons with baseline CD4 lymphocyte counts in the range of 100 to 200 cells/μl had a rate of 5.95 cases per 100 persons years for developing *P. carinii* pneumonia, irrespective of *P. carinii* prophylaxis use. The rate dramatically increased to 11.13 cases per 100 person-years for persons with baseline CD4 lymphocyte counts <100 cells/μl. Univariate analysis revealed fever and/or night sweats >2 weeks' duration, oral thrush, or unintentional weight loss to significantly increase risk of *P. carinii* pneumonia.

CLINICAL PRESENTATION

Data from the Pulmonary Complications of HIV Infection Study confirm that *P. carinii* pneumonia rarely presents without respiratory symptoms. In this study, subjects underwent a complete history and physical examination, laboratory testing including CD4/CD8 lymphocyte count measurement, chest radiography, and pulmonary function testing at 3- to 6-month intervals in order to identify subclinical opportunistic infections.[118] Despite this intense effort, no diagnoses of *P. carinii* pneumonia were established in asymptomatic subjects.[72,73,134] Furthermore, respiratory illnesses, including *P. carinii* pneumonia, were preceded by respiratory symptoms—cough and/or shortness of breath. Nonspecific constitutional symptoms such as fever, night sweats, fatigue, or weight loss, while associated with increased risk for developing *P. carinii* pneumonia, were not associated with identifiable lung diseases in the absence of respiratory symptoms.

Unlike persons immunocompromised for reasons other than HIV, HIV-infected persons usually have a prolonged prodromal illness associated with *P. carinii* pneumonia. One study found nearly 1 month of constitutional symptoms prior to presentation in most HIV-infected patients.[70] However, the tempo of the illness varies from one patient to the next. Moreover, in assessing the HIV-infected patient with respiratory complaints, an understanding of that patient's baseline status is important. In the Pulmonary Complications of HIV Infection Study, 90% of the subjects had respiratory complaints at some time during the study and over two thirds had complained of a cough during a study visit. For many of these subjects, their re-

spiratory symptoms were secondary to chronic conditions rather than acute infection.

P. carinii pneumonia commonly presents with fever and slowly progressive dyspnea on exertion. The onset of nonproductive cough frequently follows this protracted prodrome. Profound fatigue usually presents in concert with respiratory symptoms. Pleuritic chest pain can accompany either *P. carinii* or pyogenic pneumonia. The rapid onset of spiking fevers and/or rigors is uncommon and distinguishes *P. carinii* from pyogenic infection. Cough productive of purulent sputum indicates a pyogenic infection or coinfection. Persons presenting with a cough productive of purulent sputum should undergo an evaluation for an alternate etiology, receive several days of antibacterial therapy, and then be reassessed. If the suspicion for *P. carinii* pneumonia remains high after treatment for pyogenic infection, then an evaluation for *P. carinii* pneumonia should be undertaken.

On physical examination, a temperature >38.5°C, tachypnea, and the stigmata of immunosuppression such as thrush, oral hairy leukoplakia, onychomycoses, or Kaposi's sarcoma are frequently encountered. Auscultation and percussion of the lungs is often normal. Occasionally, fine basilar rales may be encountered on auscultation. Findings of focal lung consolidation are unusual for *P. carinii* pneumonia and should prompt an evaluation for an alternate or at least a coexisting etiology.

Laboratory data reflect the underlying HIV infection rather than infection with *P. carinii*. One laboratory test frequently elevated in patients with *P. carinii* pneumonia is the serum lactate dehydrogenase (LDH). Published studies report the sensitivity of an elevated serum LDH for *P. carinii* pneumonia to be in the range of 83% to 100%.[37,46,65–67,77,120,167] Proper interpretation of a serum LDH, however, requires consideration of a number of factors. First, the serum LDH is nonspecific for *P. carinii* pneumonia and elevations result from many pulmonary and nonpulmonary etiologies. Next, patients with *P. carinii* pneumonia may have a normal or minimally elevated serum LDH and there is significant overlap between the serum LDH values in patients with *P. carinii* pneumonia and in those with other pulmonary diseases. Third, most of the published studies consisted of hospitalized patients with *P. carinii* pneumonia, some of who were critically ill and on mechanical ventilation. The study that reported the lowest sensitivity of an elevated serum LDH for *P. carinii* pneumonia (83%) consisted of ambulatory outpatients presenting to an urgent care clinic,[67] suggesting that severity of disease and the patient population studied may affect the sensitivity of the serum LDH for *P. carinii* pneumonia. Finally, many of the studies occurred at a time when *P. carinii* prophylaxis was not in routine use and perhaps the presentation of disease was more severe. One study that measured the serum LDH in patients who developed *P. carinii* pneumonia despite receiving aerosolized pentamidine prophylaxis reported a sensitivity of an elevated serum LDH for *P. carinii* pneumonia of 82%.[86]

Despite these diagnostic limitations, the serum LDH often has value in assessing prognosis and response to therapy. Multiple studies have shown a strong correlation between the degree of serum LDH elevation and survival.[2,29,37,66,77,167] A high serum LDH value or a rising serum LDH while on *P. carinii* treatment correlates with a worse prognosis, a failure of therapy, and increased mortality, whereas a low serum LDH value or a declining serum LDH on *P. carinii* treatment correlates with a better prognosis, a response to therapy, and decreased mortality.

The chest radiograph is the cornerstone of the evaluation of an HIV-infected patient with suspected *P. carinii* pneumonia. Similar to the serum LDH, however, the degree of radiographic abnormality seen depends on the severity of disease and the population studied. *P. carinii* pneumonia most commonly presents with bilateral, symmetric reticular or granular opacities.[17,21,36,146] Thin-walled, air-containing cysts or pneumatoceles are an increasingly common finding[128] and seem to be associated with prolonged, indolent disease and perhaps choice of prophylaxis (Fig. 20–1). Pneumatoceles may be present at the time of diagnosis or may develop while on therapy. These pneumatoceles are often multiple in number, can be quite large (Fig. 20–2), and may predispose patients to pneumothorax (Fig. 20–3). However, pneumothorax may occur spontaneously in the absence of demonstrable pneumatoceles.[42,87] Focal infiltrates, lobar consolidation, or nodules with or without cavitation are occasionally seen.[68] Apical disease mimicking tuberculosis has been associated with aerosolized pentamidine prophylaxis,[15,64] although a similar presentation also occurs in patients receiving other forms of *P. carinii* prophylaxis or no preventive therapy. In our experience, intrathoracic adenopathy and pleural effusions are rarely due to *P. carinii*

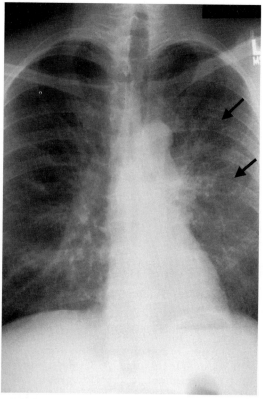

FIGURE 20–1. Posteroanterior chest radiograph of an HIV-infected patient with *Pneumocystis carinii* pneumonia revealing the characteristic bilateral reticular and granular infiltrates as well as two pneumatoceles (*arrows*). (From Huang L, Stansell JD: AIDS and the Lung. Med Clin North Am 80(4):775–801, 1996, with permission.)

pneumonia. These radiographic findings should prompt a search for an alternate or at least a coexisting process such as tuberculosis, fungal pneumonia, or pulmonary Kaposi's sarcoma.

P. carinii pneumonia may present with a normal chest radiograph. Published studies report the incidence of *P. carinii* pneumonia presenting with a normal chest radiograph to be in the range of 0% to 39%.[17,21,36,106,146] In our experience, *P. carinii* pneumonia presents with a normal chest radiograph in fewer than 10% of cases.

Unfortunately, there are few studies on the resolution or diminution of respiratory signs/symptoms and radiographic abnormalities in successfully treated *P. carinii* pneumonia. In our experience, just as the onset of *P. carinii* pneumonia may be indolent, the resolution from disease may be slow. Fever, tachypnea, and oxygen requirements may persist for several days to a week or more, even with successful therapy. Often the first indication of therapeutic success is the patient's subjective feeling of recovery and the observation that the patient can take a deeper breath. The pace of weaning from supplemental oxygen is not only dependent on the severity of disease but also on the antecedent pulmonary function. Persons with severe disease or *P. carinii* pneumonia superimposed on chronic lung disease will experience a protracted requirement for supplemental oxygen.

The chest radiograph may worsen during the first week of treatment despite clinical improvement. Usually, chest radiographic abnormalities improve over the course of a week to several weeks. However, chest radiographs occasionally have persistent abnormalities weeks to months after successful treatment. Similarly, the single-breath DLco usually improves to a plateau over several weeks but rarely returns to predisease values. Occasionally, severe inflammation with resulting fibrosis results in a clinical picture similar to advanced restrictive lung disease with markedly reduced lung volumes, decreased lung compliance, and severe reductions in the

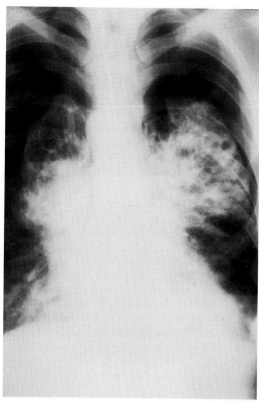

FIGURE 20–3. Posteroanterior chest radiograph of an HIV-infected patient with *Pneumocystis carinii* pneumonia presenting with bilateral pneumothoraces.

DLco. Individuals with these conditions may remain pulmonary cripples throughout the remainder of their lives.

COMPLICATIONS

Hypoxemia and Respiratory Failure

Moderate to severe *P. carinii* pneumonia is characterized by disruption of the alveolar epithelial surface and perturbation of the forces that govern the movement of gases and fluids across the alveolar-capillary interface. Cellular debris sloughed from the alveolar epithelium and fluid leaked across the denuded alveolar-capillary membrane accumulate in the alveolar space as a consequence of *P. carinii* infection. Gas exchange is impaired, pulmonary shunt fraction increases, and hypoxemia results. In severe cases of *P. carinii* pneumonia, this pathophysiologic process is similar to ARDS. Even less fulminant cases are often accompanied by a

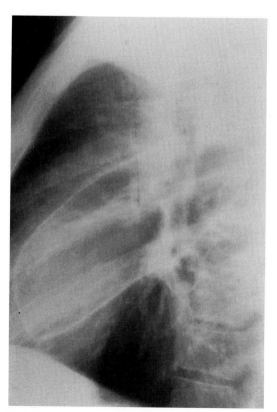

FIGURE 20–2. Lateral chest radiograph of an HIV-infected patient demonstrating a large pneumatocele.

"treatment effect." In these cases, the initiation of therapy is accompanied by a deterioration in gas exchange and worsening hypoxemia 3 to 5 days into therapy. One hypothesis for this deterioration is that the dead or dying *P. carinii* organisms elicit an inflammatory reaction that furthers the injury to the alveolar-capillary membrane. In patients with moderate to severe *P. carinii* pneumonia, this deterioration may be sufficient to cause respiratory failure and the need for ventilatory assistance. The routine use of adjuvant corticosteroids in moderate to severe disease has significantly decreased the need for mechanical ventilation. However, the exact mechanism by which corticosteroids protect the lung from this "treatment effect" is unclear. One hypothesis is that corticosteroids may blunt the inflammatory reaction resulting from antipneumocystis treatment and thereby protect the pulmonary parenchyma from accelerated injury.

The recognition that impairment of hydrostatic forces across the alveolar-capillary membrane results from active *P. carinii* infection prompted a reexamination of fluid therapy. The parsimonious use of colloids and crystalloids reduces the risk of overhydration and alveolar flooding. In patients who require ventilatory assistance, the judicious use of positive end-expiratory pressure may significantly improve oxygenation. However, the risk of pneumothorax and bronchopleural fistula (BPF) formation versus the potential for improvement in oxygenation and survival must always be balanced. Alternative ventilation techniques, such as high-frequency ventilation, have not been shown to improve survival.

The prognosis for patients with *P. carinii* pneumonia requiring mechanical ventilation has improved and deteriorated over the course of the epidemic. From 1981 to 1985, only 14% of persons with *P. carinii* pneumonia admitted to an intensive care unit (ICU) at San Francisco General Hospital (SFGH) for ventilatory support survived the hospitalization.[157] From 1986 to 1988, survival improved to nearly 40%.[158] The reasons for this improvement are not entirely obvious but are probably multifactorial. Clearly, greater experience with caring for such patients played a role. In addition, more patients received adjunctive corticosteroids compared to the previous era. More careful screening of candidates for ICU admission and ventilatory support may have also been a factor. A recent report suggests that the prognosis for patients with *P. carinii* pneumonia requiring mechanical ventilation has again deteriorated.[156] Wachter and colleagues report that overall survival for 37 patients admitted to an ICU at SFGH for ventilatory support from 1989 to 1991 was 24%. Predictors of poor outcome were low CD4 lymphocyte count on admission and development of pneumothorax during mechanical ventilation.

Pneumothorax

The emergence of bullous lung disease and spontaneous pneumothorax demonstrated the tissue destructive potential of *P. carinii*. As inflammation persists and tissue necrosis proceeds, air spaces may enlarge to form frank bullae. These bullae possess an active margin of inflammation that serves as the growth front. As the bullae enlarge, they may impinge upon the subpleural space. As a result of necrosis or air trapping, bullae may rupture into the pleural cavity. Small pneumothoraces may not require tube thoracostomy and can resolve without active intervention. However, careful observation is always warranted, for progressive enlargement is common. Unfortunately, we have seen several life-threatening or fatal tension pneumothoraces due to failure to vent seemingly clinically insignificant pneumothoraces. Certainly, immediate venting is required for all pneumothoraces that impair hemodynamic or respiratory function.[142]

The goal of chest tube placement is full expansion of the lung. However, this may not be attainable depending on the duration that the lung has been collapsed and the degree of lung compliance lost. Frequently, the use of tube thoracostomy to expand the lung will entrain a constant flow of air through a BPF. Various interventions have been used to produce closure of a BPF. Most have been unqualified failures. At SFGH, we generally have a conservative approach toward management of a BPF. Treatment of the underlying pneumonia, withdrawal, if possible, of adjuvant corticosteroids or mechanical ventilation, and patience are the hallmarks of BPF management at this institution. If the lungs remain expanded for brief periods off suction, pleural sclerosis may be attempted. The installation of tetracycline, bleomycin, or talc into the pleural space incites pleural inflammation and, subsequently, adhesion of the pleural surfaces. If successful, pleural sclerosis may prevent further pneumothoraces. If only partially successful, the partially adhered pleural surfaces may prevent tension pneumothorax. Thoracoscopy with stapling has been performed with success for rare patients in whom no alternatives existed. However, this procedure can only be performed in those patients able to tolerate the procedure who have a single BPF amenable to surgical closure. As a last resort, a patient may be discharged with a chest tube in place connected to a one-way valve. Unfortunately, our experience with Heimlich valves has been dismal. Blockage due to pleural secretions, tension pneumothorax, and infection are frequent complications seen with one-way valve therapy.[142]

Chronic Airway Disease

Much as we were slow to note the tissue destructive effects of *P. carinii*, we have been slow to appreciate the chronic airway disease that develops as a consequence of *P. carinii* pneumonia. Patients recovered from *P. carinii* pneumonia may display symptoms suggestive of chronic bronchitis such as a chronic, often debilitating, cough productive of clear sputum. These unfortunate patients frequently become colonized with hospital-acquired bacterial pathogens that are difficult or impossible to eradicate; as a result, pyogenic infections are common. In time, the cycles of infection and progressive airway destruction may produce frank bronchiectasis.[52] The vicious cycle of infection, treatment with broad-spectrum antibiotics, selection of increasingly resistant organisms, particularly *Pseudomonas* sp., and recurrent pneumonia is a common scenario among patients with advanced HIV disease and a history of *P. carinii* pneumonia.

Extrapulmonary Disease

Virtually all cases of *P. carinii* infection involve only the lungs, although the organism's ability to disseminate in rare patients has been recognized for many years. Recent advances in detection by substrate amplification have affirmed the presence of *P. carinii* organisms in the blood.[78] One review related disseminated *P. carinii* infection to inhaled chemoprophylaxis with aerosolized pentamidine; extrapulmonary disease is generally not seen in patients receiving systemic chemoprophylaxis with trimethoprim-sulfamethoxazole (TMP/SMX) or dapsone.[100] Reported sites of dissemination include the lymph nodes, spleen, liver, bone marrow, skin, thyroid, choroid of the eye, adrenal gland, ear, peritoneum, intestine, meninges, and pancreas.[100] Although the relation between aerosolized pentamidine and extrapulmonary pneumocytosis has not been proven, the association is compelling. At SFGH, extrapulmonary *P. carinii* has virtually disappeared with the shift to systemic *P. carinii* prophylaxis. However, clinicians should always consider extrapulmonary *P. carinii* in the differential diagnosis of any febrile HIV-infected patient who is receiving aerosolized pentamidine or other, inadequate, *P. carinii* prophylaxis.

DIAGNOSIS

At SFGH, we have used a diagnostic algorithm for suspected *P. carinii* pneumonia with success (Fig. 20–4). Patients with a clinical presentation suggestive of *P. carinii* pneumonia and a compatible chest radiograph undergo a diagnostic procedure (sputum induction) for microbiologic identification of *P. carinii*. Patients with a suggestive clinical presentation but a normal or unchanged chest radiograph undergo pulmonary function testing. On pulmonary function testing, patients with *P. carinii* pneumonia often display restrictive pulmonary physiology with decreased lung volumes and increased air flows. However, a more sensitive indicator of alveolar-capillary block,[129] and hence *P. carinii* pneumonia, is a decrease in the DLCO.[18,53] Recent data report that the sensitivity of a decreased DLCO (defined as <75% of the predicted value, corrected for hemoglobin) for *P. carinii* is 90% in symptomatic patients with normal or unchanged chest radiographs.[55] Moreover, the combination of a normal or unchanged chest radiograph and a DLCO >75% predicted virtually rules out the possibility of *P. carinii* pneumonia.[55] Thus, we recommend that these patients either be clinically observed without further evaluation or treatment for *P. carinii* or be evaluated/treated for another process. Although a decreased DLCO is a sensitive test for *P. carinii*, it lacks specificity. Therefore, patients with suspected *P. carinii* pneumonia who have a decreased DLCO still undergo a diagnostic procedure for microbiologic identification of *P. carinii*.

The low specificity of a decreased DLCO for *P. carinii* led us to evaluate alternative diagnostic tests. *P. carinii* pneumonia has a characteristic

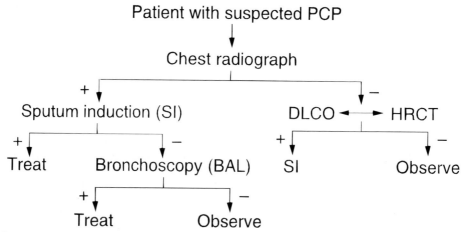

FIGURE 20–4. San Francisco General Hospital diagnostic algorithm for the evaluation of patients with suspected *Pneumocystis carinii* pneumonia (PCP). DLCO, single-breath diffusing capacity for carbon monoxide; HRCT, high-resolution computed tomograph of the chest; BAL, bronchoalveolar lavage. (From Huang L, Stansell JD: AIDS and the Lung. Med Clin North Am 80(4):775–801, 1996, with permission.)

appearance on high-resolution computed tomography (HRCT) of the chest–that is, patchy areas of ground-glass attenuation through which vessels are seen and a background of interlobular septal thickening[5,94,123] (Fig. 20–5). We studied HRCT in persons with suspected *P. carinii* pneumonia but a normal, unchanged, or equivocal chest radiograph (J. Gruden, manuscript in press). In this study, no patient with suspected *P. carinii* pneumonia; a normal, unchanged, or equivocal chest radiograph; and an HRCT without ground-glass opacities had a diagnosis of *P. carinii* pneumonia established either on bronchoscopy or after 60 days of clinical follow-up. Unfortunately, similar to a decreased DLCO, an HRCT with ground-glass

opacities lacks specificity for *P. carinii* and persons with suspected *P. carinii* pneumonia who have these findings on HRCT must undergo a diagnostic procedure for microbiologic identification of *P. carinii*. Whether HRCT will supplant the DLCO in the diagnostic algorithm for suspected *P. carinii* pneumonia awaits further analysis.

Gallium scanning is a highly sensitive but nonspecific test for *P. carinii*. In addition, the test suffers from relatively high cost, time delays in obtaining the imaging, and the baseline mild to moderate gallium uptake in the lungs of HIV-infected persons without active pulmonary infection. In our opinion, these factors, combined with the availability and sensitivity of both

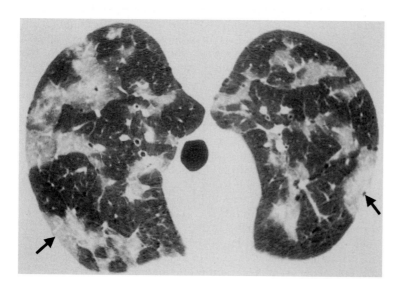

FIGURE 20–5. High-resolution computed tomograph of the chest of an HIV-infected patient with *Pneumocystis carinii* pneumonia and a normal chest radiograph revealing the characteristic patchy areas of ground glass opacities (*arrows*). (From Huang L, Stansell JD: AIDS and the Lung. Med Clin North Am 80(4):775–801, 1996, with permission.)

pulmonary function testing and HRCT scanning, render the test rarely useful in diagnosing *P. carinii* pneumonia.

Although cough productive of clear-white sputum is a frequent presenting complaint in patients with *P. carinii* pneumonia, expectorated sputum is rarely suitable for microscopic evaluation. Similarly, purulent sputum, whether spontaneously produced or induced, is inadequate for *P. carinii* examination. Cells and cellular debris in such specimens make identification of *P. carinii* organisms virtually impossible. Patients in whom there is high suspicion of *P. carinii* pneumonia who have a purulent sputum specimen should be treated with a course of antibiotics and possibly *P. carinii* therapy first. If the diagnosis remains in question, then a sputum induction should be obtained after the respiratory secretions have cleared.

Induction of nonpurulent sputum is a simple, inexpensive, and effective means of diagnosing *P. carinii* pneumonia.[6,71,97,103,113,168] After the patient cleanses the oral cavity with a soft brush and normal saline, a deep sputum specimen is induced by the inhalation of hypertonic (3%) saline. The sample is then digested, centrifuged, plated, and stained.[97] Modified Giemsa, toluidine blue O, or Gomori methenamine silver stain can be used to identify *P. carinii* organisms. Newer direct and indirect fluorescent antibody techniques have improved the sensitivity for induced sputum examination.[71,98] At SFGH, the sensitivity of induced sputum examination for *P. carinii* has been consistently between 74% and 83%.[54,97] However, this range of sensitivities is not high enough to confidently exclude a diagnosis of *P. carinii* pneumonia if a negative result is obtained and, therefore, further diagnostic testing is necessary.

In cases of suspected *P. carinii* pneumonia in which induced sputum examination is negative for *P. carinii* and other pathogens, a fiberoptic bronchoscopy with bronchoalveolar lavage (BAL) should be performed. Bronchoscopy with BAL fluid examination is sensitive for *P. carinii*.[11,41,104,107] In contrast to a negative induced sputum examination, a negative BAL fluid examination for *P. carinii* may be sufficient to rule out a diagnosis of *P. carinii* pneumonia. A review at SFGH of 100 HIV-infected patients with suspected *P. carinii* pneumonia who had a negative BAL fluid examination for *P. carinii* and had no *P. carinii* therapy identified two cases of subsequent *P. carinii* pneumonia within 60 days of the initial negative evaluation (one

case after 46 days, the other after 51 days).[54] Thus, a negative BAL fluid examination for *P. carinii* may obviate the need for more invasive procedures (i.e., transbronchial biopsy). However, in populations of HIV-infected persons with a high background incidence of *Mycobacterium tuberculosis* infection, the diagnosis of tuberculosis may be enhanced by the use of transbronchial biopsy.

The coordinated effort of a number of services is vital to the optimal use of our diagnostic algorithm. First, clinicians initiate an evaluation and refer those patients with suspected *P. carinii* pneumonia for sputum induction. Next, the Pulmonary Service screens all requests for sputum induction. The Pulmonary Service denies approximately 25% to 30% of all requests (in which case recommendations for further evaluation or treatment are provided). Those patients for whom the request is approved undergo sputum induction the same day as the screening. Third, a pulmonary laboratory technician closely supervises all patients undergoing sputum induction in order to obtain a good specimen. Finally, one of two microbiology technicians processes all specimens for *P. carinii* and reviews each slide with a microbiologist. In our opinion, these factors combine to permit the pursuit of definitive diagnoses of *P. carinii* pneumonia preferable to empiric therapy.

Is empiric *P. carinii* pneumonia therapy a viable option?[3,4,90,153] Certainly, there are a host of pressures upon clinicians today that make empiric *P. carinii* pneumonia therapy attractive. However, empiric therapy should be approached with caution and appropriate patients should be selected carefully. A number of criteria should be met before empiric therapy is begun (Table 20–1). First, the patient must be at risk for *P. carinii* pneumonia, usually on the basis of a CD4 lymphocyte count <200 cells/μl or a prior history of *P. carinii* pneumonia. Next, the patient should not be on *P. carinii* prophylaxis, especially TMP/SMX. Since the development of *P. carinii* pneumonia while on this combination is infrequent, clinicians who are presented with such a patient should make every effort to find an alternate diagnosis before embarking on a course of empiric therapy. Third, the patient should have a clinical and radiographic presentation strongly suggestive of *P. carinii* pneumonia. The presence of atypical features should prompt a consideration of alternate diagnoses. Furthermore, the patient

TABLE 20–1. CRITERIA FOR EMPIRIC _PNEUMOCYSTIS CARINII_ PNEUMONIA THERAPY

Patient is at risk for _P. carinii_ pneumonia.
  CD4 lymphocyte count <200 cells/μl
  History of prior _P. carinii_ pneumonia
Patient is not receiving _P. carinii_ pneumonia prophylaxis (especially TMP/SMX)
Patient has a clinical presentation suggestive of _P. carinii_ pneumonia
  History of dyspnea on exertion and/or nonproductive cough
  Chest radiograph reveals bilateral interstitial infiltrates
  No evidence of another infectious process
Patient has mild disease
  Room air Pao_2 >70 mm Hg, alveolar–arterial oxygen difference <35 mm Hg
Patient is reliable
Patient is compliant with medications
Patient can tolerate oral medications
  No complaints of nausea, vomiting, or diarrhea
  No previous adverse reactions to proposed _P. carinii_ pneumonia therapy
Patient is at low risk for tuberculosis, histoplasmosis, coccidioidomycosis, or other infection likely to mimic _P. carinii_ pneumonia
Sputum induction is unavailable or its sensitivity for _P. carinii_ is low
Careful follow-up is available

should have mild disease. The potential consequences of a missed or delayed diagnosis in a patient with severe respiratory dysfunction argue strongly for the pursuit of a definitive diagnosis in most, if not all, cases. Next, the patient should be reliable, compliant with medications, able to tolerate the proposed therapy (without nausea/vomiting, diarrhea, or a history of previous adverse drug reactions to that therapy), able to recognize the early progression of symptoms, and willing to return for follow-up visits. In patients fulfilling these criteria, empiric therapy may be a suitable alternative to invasive diagnostic procedures. However, if there is clinical progression or even a slow clinical response to empiric therapy, then diagnostic tests and procedures should be pursued.[83]

TREATMENT

At the time the first cases of AIDS-related _P. carinii_ pneumonia were recognized, two drugs, TMP/SMX and pentamidine isethionate, were available for treatment. Indeed, it was the sudden increase in requests for pentamidine that alerted the Centers for Disease Control to a possible new epidemic. Unfortunately, both drugs show a high frequency of adverse reactions and

poor tolerability.[43,81,143] Accordingly, a concerted effort has been made to identify and develop new treatment regimens that are free of serious side effects or at least do not have overlapping toxicity. These efforts have met with mixed success. Currently, several choices are available for treatment of _P. carinii_ pneumonia (Tables 20–2 and 20–3).

Trimethoprim/Sulfamethoxazole

TMP/SMX remains the drug of choice for the treatment of _P. carinii_ pneumonia. No other drug or drug combination has been shown to be superior to TMP/SMX in efficacy.[57,69,85,126, 131,132,149,151,165] TMP and SMX both act to inhibit key enzymatic steps in folate metabolism. TMP inhibits dihydrofolate reductase (DHFR) preventing the synthesis of tetrahydrofolate from dihydrofolate, while SMX acts upon dihydropteroate synthase (DHPS) to prevent the conversion of _para_-aminobenzoate to dihydrofolic acid. Although TMP alone has no demonstrable antipneumocystis activity, when combined with SMX, it produces a synergistic inhibition of _P. carinii_. Significantly, neither of these two agents is the most avid enzyme inhibitor in their class. Pyrimethamine, trimetrexate (TMTX), and methotrexate are orders of magnitude more inhibitory for DHFR than TMP, whereas many sulfones and sulfonamides show greater inhibition of DHPS than SMX. However, TMP/SMX benefits from its availability as a single-combination medication, excellent bioavailability, similar half-lives, and two decades of clinical use. Moreover, utilizing the rat model, Hughes and colleagues have recently demonstrated the combination of TMP and SMX to be the most potent inhibitor of _P. carinii_ among commonly used medications.[62]

In 1978, Hughes and colleagues documented the efficacy of TMP/SMX in children with cancer and established the dose of the combination of 20 mg/kg/day of the TMP component.[60] Subsequent studies in AIDS patients sought to match this established dose in comparative trials. Wharton and colleagues studied 40 patients with their first episode of _P. carinii_ pneumonia in a prospective, randomized trial of TMP/SMX at a dose of 20 mg/kg/day versus pentamidine at a dose of 4 mg/kg/day.[165] Of 20 patients treated with TMP/SMX, 75% survived past the 21-day treatment period but 10% required a switch to pentamidine due to treatment failure and 50% due to adverse drug reac-

TABLE 20–2. TREATMENT OPTIONS FOR MODERATE TO SEVERE *P. CARINII* PNEUMONIA

Treatment Regimen	Dose(s), Route, Frequency	Side Effect(s)
Trimethoprim (TMP)/ sulfamethoxazole (SMX)	15 mg/kg (TMP), IV, divided every 6–8 hr*	Rash†, fever, N/V, ↑liver function tests, ↑K⁺, neutropenia
Pentamidine isethionate	3–4 mg/kg, IV, once daily	Nephrotoxicity, ↑K⁺, ↓Ca²⁺/Mg²⁺, ↑amylase, ↓↑glucose‡
Trimetrexate plus leucovorin ± dapsone§	45 mg/m², IV, once daily, plus 20 mg/m², PO, every 6 hr ± 100 mg, PO, once daily	Neutropenia, thrombocytopenia, rash, fever, ↑liver function tests, hemolytic anemia (check G6PD level), methemoglobinemia
Clindamycin plus primaquine	1800 mg, IV, divided every 6–8 hr plus 30 mg (base), PO, once daily	Rash, N/V, diarrhea, hemolytic anemia (check G6PD), methemoglobinemia

* TMP/SMX is dispensed as a fixed-combination.

† Mild rash that does not cause bullous skin lesions and does not involve mucous membranes can often be treated with antihistamines first and should not necessarily result in discontinuation of drug.

‡ Avoid other nephrotoxic agents (nonsteroidal antiinflammatory agents, aminoglycosides, foscarnet, amphotericin B). Risk of hypotension can be minimized if infusion is given over a 2- to 3-hr period.

§ A study is in progress comparing TMP/SMX to trimetrexate/dapsone (plus leucovorin).

N/V, nausea and vomiting; G6PD, glucose-6-phosphate dehydrogenase.

tions. Klein and co-workers studied 160 patients with moderate to severe *P. carinii* pneumonia in a prospective, randomized trial of TMP/SMX at a dose of 20 mg/kg/day versus pentamidine at a dose of 4 mg/kg/day.[69] Of 92 patients randomized to TMP/SMX, 67% survived but only 24% were able to successfully complete treatment, with 42% failing due to disease progression, and 34% failing due to drug toxicity. Similarly, Sattler and colleagues studied 215 patients with moderate to severe disease in a prospective, randomized trial of TMTX at a dose of 45 mg/m²/day (plus leucovorin) versus TMP/SMX at a dose of 20 mg/kg/day.[132] Among those treated with TMP/SMX, 88% survived off respiratory support at day 21 of therapy, while 20% failed TMP/SMX due to lack of efficacy and 28% required discontinuation due to drug toxicity. Of note, all of these studies antedated the routine use of adjunctive corticosteroids.

In 1988, Sattler and colleagues published the results of a prospective, noncrossover trial of TMP/SMX versus pentamidine in 70 patients.[131] Rather than using a fixed dose of TMP/SMX, dosing was adjusted to maintain a TMP serum level of 5 to 8 μg/ml. The average dose received by those assigned to TMP/SMX was 12 mg/kg/day. Despite this dose reduction, 86% of TMP/SMX-treated patients survived and were without respiratory support at the end of treatment. As a result of this study, TMP/SMX at a dose of 15 mg/kg/day of the TMP component has become the widely accepted dose. Unfortunately, few trials have utilized this dose in comparing therapies for moderate to severe *P. carinii* pneumonia. A randomized trial of TMP/SMX versus clindamycin/primaquine had a mixed population of mild and severe disease, oral and intravenous therapy, and inconsistent steroid use. However, dosing TMP/SMX at 15

TABLE 20–3. TREATMENT OPTIONS FOR MILD TO MODERATE *P. CARINII* PNEUMONIA

Treatment Regimen	Dose(s), Route, Frequency	Side Effect(s)
Trimethoprim(TMP)/ sulfamethoxazole (SMX)	15 mg/kg (TMP), PO, divided every 6–8 hr	See Table 20–2
Clindamycin plus primaquine	1800 mg, PO, divided every 6–8 hr plus 30 mg (base), PO, once daily	See Table 20–2
Trimethoprim plus dapsone	15 mg/kg, PO, divided every 6–8 hr plus 100 mg, PO, once daily	Rash, N/V, hemolytic anemia, (check G6PD level), methemoglobinemia
Atovaquone	750 mg, PO (suspension), twice daily	Rash, GI (N/V/diarrhea); well tolerated but poorly absorbed, especially in patients with diarrhea
Pentamidine isethionate	3–4 mg/kg, IV, once daily	See Table 20–2
Trimetrexate plus leucovorin ± dapsone	45 mg/m², IV, once daily plus 20 mg/m², PO, every 6 hrs ± 100 mg, PO, once daily	See Table 20–2

N/V, nausea and vomiting; GI, gastrointestinal; GGPD, glucose-6-phosphate dehydrogenase.

to 20 mg/kg/day resulted in successful outcomes in 91% and dose-limiting toxicity in only 20%.[149,151]

The best current insight into the efficacy and tolerability of TMP/SMX comes from trials of oral therapy for mild to moderate *P. carinii* pneumonia. In these studies, 320 mg TMP and 1600 mg SMX (two DS tablets) given orally three times daily (tid) approximates the 15 mg/kg/day intravenous dosing schedule. In a prospective, randomized trial of 322 patients with mild to moderate *P. carinii* pneumonia who received TMP/SMX at a dose of 320 mg TMP and 1600 mg SMX tid versus atovaquone tablets at a dose of 750 mg tid, 7% of the 146 evaluable persons assigned to TMP/SMX failed due to lack of therapeutic efficacy and 20% failed due to treatment-limiting adverse reactions.[57] Similar results were obtained in the recently completed AIDS Clinical Trials Group (ACTG) 108 study examining the efficacy and safety of three orally available combinations for the treatment of mild to moderate *P. carinii* pneumonia (320 mg TMP and 1600 mg SMX tid versus TMP 300 mg tid plus dapsone 100 mg daily versus clindamycin 600 mg tid with primaquine base 30 mg daily).[126] Overall, 54% of participants completed therapy on the assigned drug, with 50% of those randomized to TMP/SMX completing 3 weeks of assigned treatment. Of patients randomized to TMP/SMX, 9% experienced clinical disease progression on or before day 21 necessitating alternative therapy and 36% had dose-limiting toxicity.

The commonly encountered toxicities associated with TMP/SMX include rash, drug fever, nausea, vomiting, liver function abnormalities, hyperkalemia, and bone marrow suppression, particularly neutropenia (Table 20–2).[43,45] Typically, these toxicities manifest within the first 8 to 12 days of therapy but may develop at any point during treatment.[126] Adverse drug reactions often can be attributed to elevated drug levels of TMP, SMX, or both,[57,134] suggesting that monitoring drug levels or dose-reducing medications may ameliorate drug toxicity.

Over the course of the HIV epidemic, clinicians have grown increasingly comfortable with managing non–life-threatening drug toxicity due to TMP/SMX. The routine use of antihistamines to treat rash and antiemetics to treat the gastrointestinal complaints has allowed patients to remain on TMP/SMX treatment. The use of granulocyte colony-stimulating factor (G-CSF) and erythropoietin may influence the course of

drug-induced cytopenias; however, the role these expensive modalities will play has yet to be determined. Attempts to ameliorate myelosuppression with coadministration of folinic acid have failed to define any beneficial effect. To the contrary, results would indicate a deleterious effect on outcome of *P. carinii* treatment with an increased risk of therapeutic failure and death among persons receiving such adjunctive therapy.

Pentamidine

Traditionally, pentamidine has been the second-line agent for the treatment of *P. carinii* pneumonia. Typically, clinicians turn to this agent when patients become intolerant of or fail to respond to TMP/SMX. Unfortunately, pentamidine is associated with frequent, severe and, oftentimes, permanent toxicities. Today, alternatives to pentamidine are available for the treatment of patients intolerant or unresponsive to TMP/SMX and a strategy of using pentamidine as a second-line agent must be reexamined.

Pentamidine isethionate is an aromatic diamine with an uncertain mechanism of action against *P. carinii*. Despite its long use in the treatment of *P. carinii* pneumonia, relatively little is known about the pharmacokinetics and pharmacodynamics of this drug. Studies indicate a large volume of distribution and a long elimination half-life.[19] The drug appears to be preferentially concentrated in certain major organs, particularly the kidneys, and probably requires several days to reach a therapeutic concentration in the lungs.[143]

Several clinical trials examined the efficacy and toxicity of pentamidine at a dose of 4 mg/kg/day compared to TMP/SMX.[69,131,165] In 20 patients with a first episode of *P. carinii* pneumonia, 95% of patients treated with pentamidine survived past the 21-day treatment period but only 45% actually completed therapy on pentamidine.[165] In 68 patients with moderate to severe *P. carinii* pneumonia, 74% of patients randomized to receive pentamidine survived, but only 35% were able to successfully complete treatment, with 40% failing due to disease progression, and 25% failing due to drug toxicity.[69] Neither of these studies found any significant difference between pentamidine and TMP/SMX in terms of survival, therapeutic failure, or adverse effects.

In a randomized, noncrossover trial involving

70 patients with moderate to severe disease, pentamidine was considerably less effective than TMP/SMX.[131] Only 61% of persons assigned to treatment with pentamidine at a dose of 4 mg/kg/day survived off respiratory support to day 21 of therapy compared with 86% of persons assigned to TMP/SMX (95% CI for the difference in response, 5% to 45%; $p = 0.03$). Although the dose of pentamidine was adjusted 30% to 50% for rising serum creatinine, nephrotoxicity occurred in 64%, hypotension in 27%, and hypoglycemia in 21% of pentamidine-treated patients. Finally, a small trial to evaluate an attenuated dose (3.2 ± 0.9 mg/kg/day) of pentamidine in the treatment of mild to moderate *P. carinii* pneumonia found successful outcomes in 81% with major adverse drug reactions occurring in 14% and minor reactions in 38%.[20]

The major toxicities related to pentamidine administration are renal and pancreatic (Table 20–2). The exact mechanism of nephrotoxicity is incompletely understood. However, special caution must be used to avoid administering pentamidine with other potentially nephrotoxic drugs such as aminoglycosides, nonsteroidal antiinflammatory agents, foscarnet, or amphotericin B. Hypoglycemia results from direct toxicity to pancreatic islet cells and may presage frank diabetes mellitus. Occurring an average of 8 days into therapy, these toxicities appear to depend upon the cumulative dose. A 5-year retrospective review of the incidence of pentamidine-related adverse drug reactions at SFGH in patients who received at least 5 days of pentamidine therapy found a 72% incidence of treatment-limiting toxicity. Renal toxicity occurred in 49%, hypoglycemia in 24%, and pancreatitis in 9% of pentamidine-treated patients.[102]

Clindamycin/Primaquine

The combination of the lincosamide antibiotic clindamycin (600 to 900 mg every 6 to 8 hours) with the dihydrofolate reductase inhibitor primaquine (15 to 30 mg/day) has gained widespread acceptance and use against all degrees of severity of *P. carinii* pneumonia. Neither drug has activity against *P. carinii* by itself, but animal models confirm the activity of the combination.[119] Unfortunately, rigorous, standardized trials of this combination are largely lacking. Various doses, dosing schedules, and drug formulations have been investigated in a variety of disease severities.[7,8,69,101,126,150,151] The combination was effective in all but 2 of 28 episodes of *P. carinii* pneumonia (25 patients, 17 of whom had been unresponsive or intolerant to conventional treatment and 8 of whom were being treated for the first time).[150] In a noncomparative, open-label study of 36 patients with mild to moderate *P. carinii* pneumonia and in a similar study of 60 patients, a 92% rate of successful treatment and a 13% incidence of dose-limiting toxicities was found with clindamycin (900 mg every 8 hours intravenously or 450 mg every 6 hours orally) and primaquine (30 mg/day base).[7,8]

A randomized, blinded trial in 65 patients with *P. carinii* pneumonia found virtually identical efficacy using clindamycin plus 15 mg/day of primaquine compared to TMP/SMX.[149] Rash was the most common side effect, occurring in 60% of patients, and gastrointestinal upset was the most common side effect seen with TMP/SMX. A recent update confirmed the above findings in a cohort of over 100 patients.[151] ACTG 108 offers the best insight into the use of oral clindamycin 600 mg every 8 hours plus primaquine 30 mg/day, versus TMP/SMX or TMP/dapsone.[126] Of the 64 persons with mild to moderate *P. carinii* pneumonia assigned to clindamycin/primaquine, 52% completed 3 weeks of therapy on the study drug combination, 7% experienced clinical disease progression on or before day 21 of therapy, and 33% had dose-limiting toxicity. No statistical differences in efficacy or toxicity were found between any of the three treatment arms. Unfortunately, this study lacked adequate power to find a difference in efficacy but could detect a 25% difference in adverse drug events. Virtually all of the adverse drug events occurred during the first 2 weeks of therapy. Among persons receiving clindamycin/primaquine, rash was the most frequently encountered dose-limiting toxicity, occurring in 21%. Cytopenias occurred in 12%, gastrointestinal intolerance in 3%, and elevations in liver enzymes in 2%. Drug fever accounted for <2% of dose-limiting drug reactions in the clindamycin/primaquine group.

Primaquine and clindamycin are strong oxidants and are relatively contraindicated in persons with glucose-6-phosphate dehydrogenase (G6PD) deficiency (Table 20–3). Methemoglobinemia is also a potential dose-limiting toxicity, although modest levels of methemoglobin (<15%) can be found in most primaquine-treated patients and only a few will require treatment with reducing agents or alternative therapy.

Trimetrexate

Trimetrexate (TMTX) is a highly lipophilic folate antagonist structurally related to methotrexate. The drug readily diffuses across cell membranes and inhibits DHFR 1500 times more potently than TMP.[1] TMTX's affinity for DHFR and the potential for interruption of folate metabolism is so great that folinic acid (leucovorin) must be given with TMTX. Herein lies the mechanism of action of TMTX/folinic acid. Folinic acid, a hydrophilic compound, requires active transport across cell membranes. Mammalian cells possess such an active transport system, whereas *P. carinii* apparently lacks such a system. Therefore, human cells are protected from the antifolate effects of TMTX by the administration of folinic acid, whereas *P. carinii* cannot accumulate folinic acid and therefore is fully susceptible to the folate inhibitory effects of the drug. The long half-life of the drug (8 to 10 hours) permits once-a-day dosing. The drug is principally metabolized by the liver and the glucuronide or sulfate salt excreted by the kidney.

An open-label, nonrandomized trial of TMTX (30 mg/m^2/day)/folinic acid (20 mg/kg every 6 hours) alone or in combination with sulfadiazine (1 g every 6 hours) enrolled 49 patients and stratified them by intolerance to or disease progression on TMP/SMX.[1] Eighty-eight per cent of the patients with a history of intolerance to sulfonamide treated with TMTX/folinic acid as initial treatment were alive and receiving no respiratory support 2 weeks after completion of therapy. In those treated with TMTX/folinic acid because of disease progression on or intolerance to initial treatment with TMP/SMX, 69% survived. Among those initially treated with TMTX/folinic acid plus sulfadiazine, 77% survived. Initial enthusiasm was somewhat tempered by a 60% relapse rate in the 3 months following completion of therapy in the group receiving TMTX/folinic acid as initial therapy. The relapse rate was 6% among those receiving TMTX/folinic acid/sulfadiazine and 0% among those receiving TMTX/folinic acid for salvage therapy. However, this study was performed prior to the routine use of secondary *P. carinii* prophylaxis. TMTX was well tolerated, with neutropenia and thrombocytopenia being the most common dose-limiting toxicity. A TMTX

dose of 45 mg/m^2/day with a folinic acid dose of 80 mg/m^2/day was later established as the optimum dose for treatment of *P. carinii* pneumonia.[130]

The clearest insight into monotherapy with TMTX/folinic acid for *P. carinii* pneumonia is ACTG 029/031.[132] ACTG 029/031 was a randomized, double-blind multicenter trial comparing TMTX at a dose of 45 mg/m^2/day plus folinic acid at a dose of 20 mg/m^2 every 6 hours to TMP/SMX at a dose of 20 mg/kg/day in patients with moderate to severe *P. carinii* pneumonia. Since the trial began accrual prior to the National Institutes of Health–University of California (NIH-UC) Expert Panel Consensus statement recommendations for steroid use in *P. carinii* pneumonia, use of adjunctive corticosteroids was not permitted. Study end-points were mortality at day 21 of therapy and clinical response at days 10 and 21. Two hundred fifteen patients were enrolled and maintained in the double-blind portion of the trial until day 10. At that point, patients were assessed as "responders" or "failures." Responders progressed into the open-label phase of the trial comparing oral TMP/SMX to continued intravenous TMTX/folinic acid while "failures" were offered alternative therapy. By day 10 of therapy, the failure rate was 16% in the TMP/SMX group and 27% in the TMTX/folinic acid group ($p = 0.064$). By day 21, 20% of TMP/SMX patients and 38% of TMTX/folinic acid patients were considered clinical failures ($p = 0.008$). Similarly, there was a trend toward improved survival at day 21 with TMP/SMX compared to TMTX/folinic acid. These differences in mortality were significant by day 49 of therapy, 16% versus 31% ($p = 0.028$). Relapse occurred in 13% of the TMTX treatment group and none of the TMP/SMX treatment group during days 21 through 49. However, dose-limiting toxicity was much more common in the TMP/SMX treatment group with 29% experiencing toxicity-related discontinuations. Only 10% of TMTX/folinic acid treatment group had similar dose-limiting toxicity. The most common side effects encountered were hepatitis (13% TMP/SMX versus 4% TMTX), gastrointestinal intolerance (7% TMP/SMX versus 1% TMTX), and cytopenias (13% TMP/SMX versus 4% TMTX). These results confirmed that although effective in the treatment of moderate to severe *P. carinii* pneumonia, TMTX/folinic acid as monotherapy is not as effective as TMP/SMX. Similar results were obtained when single-agent dapsone was evaluated for treatment of *P. carinii*.[127] However, both of these agents have activity against *P. carinii* and would be an attractive combination due to efficacy and toxicity profiles. A small, phase 1 trial of TMTX at a dose of 45 mg/m^2/day, folinic acid at a dose of 80 mg/m^2/day plus dapsone at a dose of 100 mg/day compared to TMP/SMX at a dose of 15 mg/kg/day in moderate to severe *P. carinii* pneumonia has been completed (J.D. Stansell, unpublished data). All patients received adjunctive corticosteroids at recommended doses. Fifteen patients were randomized to receive TMTX/folinic acid/dapsone and five patients to TMP/SMX. Twelve of 15 (80%) TMTX/folinic acid/dapsone patients and three of five (60%) TMP/SMX patients were responders at day 21. There were two episodes of grade III/IV toxicity among the TMTX/folinic acid/dapsone treatment group and four episodes among the TMP/SMX group. No patient who successfully completed either therapy relapsed during the month following therapy. These data suggest TMTX/folinic acid plus dapsone may be clinically useful against *P. carinii*. Where the combination fits in the armamentarium awaits further large-scale clinical trials.

Trimethoprim/Dapsone

Because oral TMP/SMX is poorly tolerated, alternative oral combinations have been sought for the treatment of mild *P. carinii* pneumonia. One of the first combinations to receive widespread attention was TMP plus the sulfone antibiotic, dapsone. Dapsone is a powerful DHPS inhibitor that has been used successfully to treat murine *P. carinii*.[63] Although dapsone had an unacceptably high rate of treatment failure when used alone,[127] the combination of dapsone plus TMP (dapsone 100 mg/day plus TMP 20 mg/kg/day) was an effective *P. carinii* pneumonia treatment in an open-label, pilot study of 15 patients at SFGH.[76] Two patients in this small trial experienced dose-limiting toxicity. A subsequent prospective, randomized clinical trial compared the safety and efficacy of TMP at a dose of 20 mg/kg/day plus dapsone at a dose of 100 mg/day with TMP/SMX at a dose of 20 mg/kg/day in 60 patients with mild to moderate *P. carinii* pneumonia.[85] Disease progression occurred in 2 of 30 patients assigned to TMP/dapsone compared to 3 of 30 assigned to TMP/SMX ($p \geq 0.3$). Fifty-seven per cent of the TMP/SMX-treated patients encountered dose-limiting toxicity compared to 30% of the

TMP/dapsone-treated group ($p < 0.025$). The major toxicities with TMP/dapsone were rash and gastrointestinal complaints.

ACTG 108 examined oral TMP/dapsone in a comparative trial with oral TMP/SMX and clindamycin/primaquine. Fifty-nine patients with mild to moderate *P. carinii* pneumonia were randomized to TMP at a dose of 300 mg tid plus dapsone at a dose of 100 mg/day. Sixty per cent of patients on TMP/dapsone completed 21 days of therapy on assigned therapy and 12% experienced disease progression on or before day 21 of therapy compared to 9% of TMP/SMX- and 7% of clindamycin/primaquine-treated patients ($p = 0.7$). There were no differences in death at day 81 between the treatment arms. Twenty-four per cent of patients assigned to TMP/dapsone experienced dose-limiting toxicity compared to 36% of TMP/SMX-treated patients and 33% of clindamycin/primaquine-treated patients. The most frequent dose-limiting adverse drug reactions were rash (10%), nausea and vomiting (8.5%), neutropenia (3%), and diarrhea (3%). Finally, a quality-of-life instrument indicated a trend toward better quality-of-life outcomes with TMP/dapsone compared to the other two study arms at completion of therapy. This study, as in earlier studies, demonstrates TMP/dapsone to be effective and well-tolerated treatment for mild to moderate *P. carinii* pneumonia.

Atovaquone

Atovaquone, an oral hydroxynapthoquinone, inhibits electron transport in the mitochondrial oxidation-reduction pathway of *P. carinii*. Complicating the use of this medication has been its poor bioavailability, particularly when coupled with chronic diarrhea, although the introduction of a suspension product has somewhat ameliorated concern about achieving adequate serum drug levels. The medication has been evaluated for the treatment of mild to moderate *P. carinii* pneumonia in both open-label and randomized comparison clinical trials.[22,31,57] In 34 patients with mild to moderate disease (mean room air Pao$_2$ = 78 mm Hg) treated with several dosages of single-agent atovaquone, treatment was discontinued in four patients for toxicity (rash and drug fever in two patients each) and in five patients for disease progression.[31] Seven (26%) of the 27 successfully treated patients experienced recurrent *P. carinii* pneumonia within 6 months despite secondary *P. carinii* prophylaxis. Outcomes did not appear to be dose related. A prospective, randomized trial of atovaquone tablets at a dose of 750 mg tid versus TMP/SMX at a dose of 320 mg TMP plus 1600 mg SMX tid in 322 patients with mild to moderate *P. carinii* pneumonia found that treatment failed in 20% of 138 evaluable persons assigned to atovaquone due to lack of therapeutic efficacy compared with 7% of the TMP/SMX group (*p* = 0.002); treatment failed in 7% due to treatment-limiting adverse reactions compared with 20% for the TMP/SMX group (*p* = 0.001).[57] The most common treatment-limiting adverse effects seen in the atovaquone group were rash (4%) and liver dysfunction (3%). There were 11 deaths in the atovaquone arm compared to a single death in the TMP/SMX arm within 4 weeks of completion of therapy (*p* = 0.003). These deaths and therapeutic failures on the atovaquone arm were highly correlated with the presence of diarrhea at entry into the study. A similar randomized, open-label trial has compared atovaquone tablets at a dose of 750 mg every 8 hours to pentamidine at a dose of 4 mg/kg/day in patients with a history of intolerance to TMP/SMX.[22] As in the previous study, atovaquone was less effective (29% disease progression for atovaquone versus 17% for pentamidine; *p* = 0.18) but better tolerated (4% dose-limiting toxicity compared to 36% for pentamidine; *p* < 0.001). The mortality rate was similar in both groups (nine deaths) but is generally believed to be unacceptably high compared to other treatment regimens. These studies and continued concerns about the adequacy of drug levels achieved in AIDS patients lends uncertainty about the role of atovaquone (especially as a single agent) in the treatment of HIV-associated *P. carinii* pneumonia. Certainly, at present, this medication cannot be viewed as a first- or second-line agent.

Aerosolized Pentamidine

Two small, open-label trials and a large, double-blind comparative trial with TMP/SMX at a dose of 15 mg/kg/day have shown inhaled pentamidine to be an inferior treatment for *P. carinii* pneumonia.[20,93,138] Significantly higher rates of recrudescence of symptoms and relapse of *P. carinii* pneumonia were found in patients treated with inhaled pentamidine at a dose of 600 mg/day compared to those receiving parenteral pentamidine at a dose of 3 mg/kg/day.[20]

Similarly, treatment failure was significantly higher (55%) with inhaled pentamidine compared to parenteral pentamidine at a dose of 4 mg/kg/day (0%).[138] ACTG 040[93] examined the efficacy of aerosolized pentamidine 600 mg/day versus TMP/SMX at a dose of 15 mg/kg/day in 367 patients with an alveolar–arterial oxygen difference <55 mm Hg. This study documented a significantly higher rate of treatment failure, more protracted recovery, and more frequent relapse among the aerosolized pentamidine-treated group. These studies overwhelmingly affirm the limited, if any, role for aerosolized pentamidine in the treatment of *P. carinii* pneumonia.

Adjuvant Corticosteroid Therapy

Despite the availability of effective antipneumocystis drugs, the mortality rate of *P. carinii* pneumonia remains appreciable. The majority of these deaths are caused by progressive lung disease that culminates in intractable hypoxemic respiratory failure. A frequent clinical observation is that worsening often takes place suddenly 3 to 5 days after beginning antipneumocystis therapy, even in patients whose disease had been slowly progressive. Several trials have now documented the usefulness of adjunctive corticosteroids in mitigating the sudden deterioration in gas exchange seen several days into standard treatment. Four clinical trials now support the use of corticosteroids in moderate to severe *P. carinii* pneumonia.[10,34,92,99] An early deterioration in oxygen saturation occurred in 8 of 19 placebo-treated patients compared to 1 of 18 steroid-treated patients.[92] In the largest study, corticosteroids significantly decreased the early deterioration in gas exchange.[10] These investigators further demonstrated that patients with the most severe disease benefitted the most. In the most severely ill cohort studied, adjunctive corticosteroids significantly ameliorated respiratory failure and death.[34] Based on these conclusive studies, the NIH-UC Expert Panel for Corticosteroids as Adjunctive Therapy for Pneumocystis Pneumonia (1990) concluded that such therapy "can clearly reduce the likelihood of death, respiratory failure, or deterioration of oxygenation in patients with moderate-to-severe pneumocystis pneumonia."[96] The panel further recommended that adjunctive corticosteroids be used in adults or adolescents (children >13 years old) with documented or suspected *P. carinii* pneumonia if they are hypoxic, as defined by an arterial PO_2 of ≤ 70 mm Hg or an alveolar–arterial PO_2 difference ≥ 35 mm Hg. Adjunctive corticosteroids, either oral prednisone or intravenous methylprednisolone, should be started when specific antipneumocystis treatment is begun; a delay in the administration of corticosteroids may nullify their effectiveness. There is no reason why these drugs cannot be used along with antipneumocystis treatment in patients who meet the indications while diagnostic efforts are underway. But if no diagnosis or some other diagnosis is made, the need for corticosteroids must be carefully reevaluated.

DIAGNOSTIC APPROACH TO CLINICAL FAILURE OF *PNEUMOCYSTIS CARINII* PNEUMONIA THERAPY

When a patient being treated appropriately for *P. carinii* pneumonia either fails to clinically improve or worsens, a number of factors should be considered (Table 20–4). First, how was the original diagnosis of *P. carinii* established? If the

TABLE 20–4. DIAGNOSTIC APPROACH TO CLINICAL FAILURE OF *P. CARINII* PNEUMONIA THERAPY

Review diagnosis:
  How was the initial diagnosis of *P. carinii* pneumonia established?
    Induced sputum? Bronchoscopy? Empiric?
  Was there a concurrent process initially?
    Review microbiology results and cultures
  Has another process supervened?
    Repeat diagnostic tests (i.e., chest radiograph)
Review treatment:
  Is the patient receiving the best *P. carinii* pneumonia treatment?
  Is the patient receiving adjuvant corticosteroids?
  Is the dose of the medication correct?
  Does the patient have nausea/vomiting or diarrhea?
    Switch to intravenous therapy
  Allow adequate time for initial therapy to work (usually 5–8 days)
Consider further evaluation:
  Consider bronchoscopy
    If initial diagnosis of *P. carinii* pneumonia was obtained from induced sputum examination, bronchoscopy may provide higher yield for other infections or may provide a diagnosis of pulmonary Kaposi's sarcoma
    If initial diagnosis of *P. carinii* pneumonia was obtained from BAL examination, repeat bronchoscopy may provide evidence for new infection
    If initial diagnosis of *P. carinii* pneumonia was empiric, bronchoscopy may confirm diagnosis or provide alternate diagnosis

patient was empirically diagnosed, then strong consideration should be given to pursuing a definitive diagnosis. If the patient had a microbiologic diagnosis of *P. carinii,* then a review of the microbiology results may reveal a coexistent infection or raise the specter of a coexistent infection such as to warrant further investigation. If the patient had a diagnosis of *P. carinii* pneumonia based on induced sputum examination and is known to have mucocutaneous Kaposi's sarcoma, then bronchoscopy may provide a diagnosis of pulmonary Kaposi's sarcoma. Unless an answer is readily found, diagnostic tests such as the chest radiograph should be repeated to evaluate for a supervening process. Concurrent with these considerations, a review of the patient's *P. carinii* therapy should consider whether the patient is receiving the "best" treatment option, whether adjuvant corticosteroids are warranted, and whether the patient has nausea/vomiting or diarrhea such that a switch to an intravenous route is prudent. As described earlier, patients with *P. carinii* pneumonia may have slow resolution of their disease, and it may be several days to a week or more until their clinical status improves. If a patient fails to improve after this time period or if the patient progressively deteriorates, then an evaluation for an alternate process is recommended and a switch in *P. carinii* therapy may be indicated.

PROPHYLAXIS

The definition of when an HIV-infected person is at significant risk for developing *P. carinii* pneumonia and the validation of effective preventive therapies have done more to improve the quantity and quality of life of AIDS patients than any other intervention. Multiple studies convincingly document the benefit of prophylaxis over placebo in preventing *P. carinii* pneumonia and extending life.[32,39,56,91] The risk of developing first-episode *P. carinii* pneumonia increases with declining CD4 lymphocyte count or the advent of constitutional symptoms.[111] HIV-infected persons whose CD4 lymphocyte counts decline <100 cells/μl have nearly an order of magnitude greater risk of developing *P. carinii* pneumonia compared to persons with CD4 lymphocyte counts between 200 and 400 cells/μl. HIV-infected persons who have experienced an episode of *P. carinii* pneumonia risk a 35% chance of recurrent disease at 6 months

TABLE 20–5. PRIMARY AND SECONDARY PROPHYLAXIS OPTIONS FOR *P. CARINII*

Prophylaxis Regimen	Dose(s), Route, Frequency	Comments
Trimethoprim (TMP)/sulfamethoxazole (SMX)*	DS tablet, PO, once daily DS tablet, PO, thrice weekly SS tablet, PO, once daily	Also effective prophylaxis against toxoplasmosis and many bacterial pathogens
Dapsone	100 mg, PO, once daily	
Aerosolized pentamidine	300 mg, via Respirgard II nebulizer, every 4 weeks	Risk of extrapulmonary *P. carinii* infection
Dapsone plus Pyrimethamine	100 mg, PO, once daily plus 25 mg, PO, thrice weekly	
Atovaquone†		

* TMP/SMX is dispensed as a fixed-combination (single strength [SS] tablet = TMP 80 mg/SMX 400 mg, double-strength [DS] tablet = TMP 160 mg/SMX 800 mg).

† Studies are underway comparing atovaquone to dapsone and to aerosolized pentamidine for *P. carinii* prophylaxis.

and a 60% chance of recurrence at 1 year if prophylaxis is not provided.

TMP/SMX, dapsone with or without pyrimethamine, and aerosolized pentamidine are the three agents most commonly used to prevent *P. carinii* pneumonia (Table 20–5).[9,80] Many studies compared these drugs at different dosages and dosing intervals for primary and secondary prophylaxis. What emerges from these studies is that all of these drugs and combinations have advantages and disadvantages. Nevertheless, none has been shown to be superior to TMP/SMX for prevention of *P. carinii* pneumonia. This fact is best illustrated by two large studies—one of primary prophylaxis and one of secondary prophylaxis.

ACTG 081 was an open-label, randomized trial that evaluated the effectiveness of three treatment strategies in preventing first-episode *P. carinii* pneumonia in HIV-infected persons with CD4 lymphocyte counts <200 cells/μl.[9] The study arms were TMP/SMX (one double-strength tablet bid), dapsone (50 mg bid), or aerosolized pentamidine (300 mg once per month). Persons experiencing drug intolerance were assigned to an alternative therapy in a predefined manner. In 842 patients who underwent a median follow-up of 39 months, there were 137 reported cases of *P. carinii* pneumonia. The estimated 36-month risk of *P. carinii* pneumonia was 18%, 17%, and 21% (p = NS), respectively, for TMP/SMX, dapsone, and aerosolized pentamidine. However, for persons with a CD4 lymphocyte count <100 cells/μl at study entry, the risk was 33% for aerosolized pentamidine compared to 19% for TMP/SMX and 22% for dapsone (p = 0.04). Moreover, an "as-treated" analysis revealed that only 4 of the 34 patients in the TMP/SMX arm who developed

P. carinii pneumonia did so while actually receiving the drug, whereas 37 of the 38 treatment failures occurring in the aerosolized pentamidine arm and 21 of the 34 treatment failures in the dapsone arm occurred "on therapy." Thus, the oral regimens appear to be superior for *P. carinii* prophylaxis. Unfortunately, only 21% of the TMP/SMX group and 25% of the dapsone group completed the study on their originally assigned drug compared to 88% of the aerosolized pentamidine group. Twenty-eight per cent of the TMP/SMX group and 33% of the dapsone group required dose reduction only during the course of the study. This study clearly demonstrates the advantage of systemic therapy, particularly TMP/SMX, over inhalation therapy in preventing *P. carinii* pneumonia. Other studies found similar benefits to TMP/SMX prophylaxis strategies at either attenuated doses[133] or different dosing intervals.[79,115] The bottom line is that TMP/SMX at any dose from 80 to 320 mg TMP per day given at least three times weekly is the first-line choice for primary *P. carinii* pneumonia prophylaxis for the markedly immunocompromised patient. Alternatives include other systemic therapies, usually dapsone with or without pyrimethamine, but also clindamycin/primaquine, clindamycin/pyrimethamine, and combinations with the extended-spectrum macrolides, azithromycin and clarithromycin.[40,51,61] Recent studies by Hughes suggest that most of the prophylactic benefit from TMP/SMX may be achieved by using SMX alone.[61] Aerosolized pentamidine should be considered for possible use in the less immunocompromised patient but clearly lacks the efficacy of systemic therapy in persons with a CD4 lymphocyte count <100 cells/μl. Trials comparing the efficacy of atovaquone suspension versus dapsone and aerosolized pentamidine in TMP/SMX-intolerant patients are underway.

Similar findings document the superiority of TMP/SMX for secondary *P. carinii* prophylaxis (maintenance therapy) of AIDS patients after an initial episode of *P. carinii* pneumonia. In 310 AIDS patients who had recently recovered from *P. carinii* pneumonia, patients were randomized to receive either TMP/SMX (one double-strength tablet daily) or aerosolized pentamidine (300 mg via nebulizer once per month).[47] All patients received zidovudine and the median follow-up was 17.4 months. There were 14 (11.4%) *P. carinii* recurrences among 154 patients assigned to the TMP/SMX arm versus 36 (27.6%) recurrences among the pentamidine-treated group (*p* < 0.001). By an intent-to-treat analysis, the risk of recurrence was 3.25 times higher for the pentamidine-treatment group. In fact, only four of the participants who received TMP/SMX for more than 3 weeks and tolerated the drug actually developed recurrent

disease. In contrast, all of the *P. carinii* pneumonia recurrences in the aerosolized pentamidine-treatment group occurred while the patients were on drug. As expected, aerosolized pentamidine was the better tolerated of the two regimens. Only 4% of the pentamidine-treatment group required crossover compared to 27% of the TMP/SMX group. These data establish the primacy of TMP/SMX for secondary *P. carinii* prophylaxis in AIDS patients. Unfortunately, there are few data on the role of other systemic antibiotics in secondary *P. carinii* prophylaxis. What information exists suggests activity of weekly dapsone or dapsone/pyrimethamine comparable to aerosolized pentamidine.[47,105,140,152] No study has looked at dapsone with or without pyrimethamine given daily for the prevention of recurrent *P. carinii* pneumonia. Certainly, the first choice to prevent recurrent *P. carinii* pneumonia, as with primary *P. carinii* prophylaxis, should always be systemic antibiotics. Aerosolized pentamidine should be considered only in those patients intolerant of all systemic options.

REFERENCES

1. Allegra CJ, Chabner BA, Tuazon CU, et al: Trimetrexate for the treatment of *Pneumocystis carinii* pneumonia in patients with the acquired immunodeficiency syndrome. N Engl J Med 317:978–985, 1987
2. Antinori A, Maiuro G, Pallavicini F, et al: Prognostic factors of early fatal outcome and long-term survival in patients with *Pneumocystis carinii* pneumonia and acquired immunodeficiency syndrome. Eur J Epidemiol 9:183–189, 1993
3. Beck EJ, French PD, Helbert MH, et al: Empirically treated *Pneumocystis carinii* pneumonia in London, 1983–1989. Int J STD AIDS 3:285–287, 1992
4. Bennett CL, Horner RD, Weinstein RA, et al: Empirically treated *Pneumocystis carinii* pneumonia in Los Angeles, Chicago, and Miami: 1987–1990. J Infect Dis 172:312–315, 1995
5. Bergin CJ, Wirth RL, Berry GJ, et al: *Pneumocystis carinii* pneumonia: CT and HRCT observations. J Comput Assist Tomogr 14:756–759, 1990
6. Bigby TD, Margolskee D, Curtis JL, et al: The usefulness of induced sputum in the diagnosis of *Pneumocystis carinii* pneumonia in patients with the acquired immunodeficiency syndrome. Am Rev Respir Dis 133:515–518, 1986
7. Black JR, Feinberg J, Murphy RL, et al: Clindamycin and primaquine as primary treatment for mild and moderately severe *Pneumocystis carinii* pneumonia in patients with AIDS. Eur J Clin Microbiol Infect Dis 10:204–207, 1991
8. Black JR, Feinberg J, Murphy RL, et al: Clindamycin and primaquine therapy for mild-to-moderate episodes of *Pneumocystis carinii* pneumonia in patients

with AIDS: AIDS Clinical Trials Group 044. Clin Infect Dis 18:905–913, 1994
9. Bozzette SA, Finkelstein DM, Spector SA, et al: A randomized trial of three antipneumocystis agents in patients with advanced human immunodeficiency virus infection. NIAID AIDS Clinical Trials Group. N Engl J Med 332:693–699, 1995
10. Bozzette SA, Sattler FR, Chiu J, et al: A controlled trial of early adjunctive treatment with corticosteroids for *Pneumocystis carinii* pneumonia in the acquired immunodeficiency syndrome. California Collaborative Treatment Group. N Engl J Med 323:1451–1457, 1990
11. Broaddus C, Dake MD, Stulbarg MS, et al: Bronchoalveolar lavage and transbronchial biopsy for the diagnosis of pulmonary infections in the acquired immunodeficiency syndrome. Ann Intern Med 102:747–752, 1985
12. Centers for Disease Control: Recommendations for prophylaxis against *Pneumocystis carinii* pneumonia for adults and adolescents infected with human immunodeficiency virus. MMWR 41 (RR-4):1–11, 1992
13. Centers for Disease Control: HIV/AIDS Surveillance Report, No 5, 1994
14. Centers for Disease Control: HIV/AIDS Surveillance Report, No 6, 1994
15. Chaffey MH, Klein JS, Gamsu G, et al: Radiographic distribution of *Pneumocystis carinii* pneumonia in patients with AIDS treated with prophylactic inhaled pentamidine. Radiology 175:715–719, 1990
16. Chagas C: Novo trypanomiazaea humana. Ueber eine neve trypanosomiasis de menschen. Mem Inst Oswaldo Cruz 1:159–218, 1909

17. Cohen BA, Pomeranz S, Rabinowitz JG, et al: Pulmonary complications of AIDS: Radiologic features. AJR Am J Roentgenol 143:115–122, 1984

18. Coleman DL, Dodek PM, Golden JA, et al: Correlation between serial pulmonary function tests and fiberoptic bronchoscopy in patients with *Pneumocystis carinii* pneumonia and the acquired immune deficiency syndrome. Am Rev Respir Dis 129:491–493, 1984

19. Conte J Jr: Pharmacokinetics of intravenous pentamidine in patients with normal renal function or receiving hemodialysis. J Infect Dis 163:169–175, 1991

20. Conte J Jr, Chernoff D, Feigal D Jr, et al: Intravenous or inhaled pentamidine for treating *Pneumocystis carinii* pneumonia in AIDS. A randomized trial. Ann Intern Med 113:203–209, 1990

21. DeLorenzo LJ, Huang CT, Maguire GP, et al: Roentgenographic patterns of *Pneumocystis carinii* pneumonia in 104 patients with AIDS. Chest 91:323–327, 1987

22. Dohn MN, Weinberg WG, Torres RA, et al: Oral atovaquone compared with intravenous pentamidine for *Pneumocystis carinii* pneumonia in patients with AIDS. Atovaquone Study Group. Ann Intern Med 121:174–180, 1994

23. Dyer M, Volpe F, Delves CJ, et al: Cloning and sequence of a beta-tubulin cDNA from *Pneumocystis carinii:* Possible implications for drug therapy. Mol Microbiol 6:991–1001, 1992

24. Edman JC, Edman U, Cao M, et al: Isolation and expression of the *Pneumocystis carinii* dihydrofolate reductase gene. Proc Natl Acad Sci U S A 86:8625–8629, 1989

25. Edman U, Edman JC, Lundgren B, et al: Isolation and expression of the *Pneumocystis carinii* thymidylate synthase gene. Proc Natl Acad Sci U S A 86:6503–6507, 1989

26. Edman JC, Sogin ML: Molecular phylogeny of *Pneumocystis carinii.* In Walzer PD, eds. *Pneumocystis carinii* Pneumonia. New York, Marcel Dekker, Inc, vol. 69, 1994, pp 91–105

27. Edman JC, Kovacs JA, Masur H, et al: Ribosomal RNA sequence shows *Pneumocystis carinii* to be a member of the fungi. Nature 334:519–522, 1988

28. Eisen D, Ross BC, Fairbairn J, et al: Comparison of *Pneumocystis carinii* detection by toluidine blue O staining, direct immunofluorescence and DNA amplification in sputum specimens from HIV positive patients. Pathology 26:198–200, 1994

29. el-Sadr W, Simberkoff MS: Survival and prognostic factors in severe *Pneumocystis carinii* pneumonia requiring mechanical ventilation. Am Rev Respir Dis 137:1264–1267, 1988

30. Evans R, Joss AW, Pennington TH, et al: The use of a nested polymerase chain reaction for detecting *Pneumocystis carinii* from lung and blood in rat and human infection. J Med Microbiol 42:209–213, 1995

31. Falloon J, Kovacs J, Hughes W, et al: A preliminary evaluation of 566C80 for the treatment of *Pneumocystis* pneumonia in patients with the acquired immunodeficiency syndrome. N Engl J Med 325:1534–1538, 1991

32. Fischl MA, Dickinson GM, La Voie L: Safety and efficacy of sulfamethoxazole and trimethoprim chemoprophylaxis for *Pneumocystis carinii* pneumonia in AIDS. JAMA 259:1185–1189, 1988

33. Fletcher LD, McDowell JM, Tidwell RR, et al: Structure, expression and phylogenetic analysis of the gene encoding actin I in *Pneumocystis carinii.* Genetics 137:743–750, 1994

34. Gagnon S, Boota AM, Fischl MA, et al: Corticosteroids as adjunctive therapy for severe *Pneumocystis carinii* pneumonia in the acquired immunodeficiency syndrome. A double-blind, placebo-controlled trial. N Engl J Med 323:1444–1450, 1990

35. Gajdusek D: *Pneumocystis carinii*—etiologic agent of interstitial plasma cell pneumonia of premature and young infants. Pediatrics 19:543–565, 1957

36. Gamsu G, Hecht ST, Birnberg FA, et al: *Pneumocystis carinii* pneumonia in homosexual men. AJR Am J Roentgenol 139:647–651, 1982

37. Garay SM, Greene J: Prognostic indicators in the initial presentation of *Pneumocystis carinii* pneumonia. Chest 95:769–772, 1989

38. Gigliotti F, Hughes WT: Passive immunoprophylaxis with specific monoclonal antibody confers partial protection against *Pneumocystis carinii* pneumonitis in animal models. J Clin Invest 81:1666–1668, 1988

39. Girard PM, Landman R, Gaudebout C, et al: Prevention of *Pneumocystis carinii* pneumonia relapse by pentamidine aerosol in zidovudine-treated AIDS patients. Lancet 1:1348–1353, 1989

40. Girard PM, Landman R, Gaudebout C, et al: Dapsone-pyrimethamine compared with aerosolized pentamidine as primary prophylaxis against *Pneumocystis carinii* pneumonia and toxoplasmosis in HIV infection. The PRIO Study Group. N Engl J Med 328:1514–1520, 1993

41. Golden JA, Hollander H, Stulbarg MS, et al: Bronchoalveolar lavage as the exclusive diagnostic modality for *Pneumocystis carinii* pneumonia. A prospective study among patients with acquired immunodeficiency syndrome. Chest 90:18–22, 1986

42. Goodman PC, Daley C, Minagi H: Spontaneous pneumothorax in AIDS patients with *Pneumocystis carinii* pneumonia. AJR Am J Roentgenol 147:29–31, 1986

43. Gordin FM, Simon GL, Wofsy CB, et al: Adverse reactions to trimethoprim-sulfamethoxazole in patients with the acquired immunodeficiency syndrome. Ann Intern Med 100:495–499, 1984

44. Gottlieb MS, Schroff R, Schanker HM, et al: *Pneumocystis carinii* pneumonia and mucosal candidiasis in previously healthy homosexual men: Evidence of a new acquired cellular immunodeficiency. N Engl J Med 305:1425–1431, 1981

45. Greenberg S, Reiser IW, Chou SY, et al: Trimethoprim-sulfamethoxazole induces reversible hyperkalemia. Ann Intern Med 119:291–295, 1993

46. Grover SA, Coupal L, Suissa S, et al: The clinical utility of serum lactate dehydrogenase in diagnosing *pneumocystis carinii* pneumonia among hospitalized AIDS patients. Clin Invest Med 15:309–317, 1992

47. Hardy WD, Feinberg J, Finkelstein DM, et al: A controlled trial of trimethoprim-sulfamethoxazole or aerosolized pentamidine for secondary prophylaxis of *Pneumocystis carinii* pneumonia in patients with the acquired immunodeficiency syndrome. AIDS Clinical Trials Group Protocol 021. N Engl J Med 327:1842–1848, 1992

48. Harmsen AG, Chen W, Gigliotti F: Active immunity

to *Pneumocystis carinii* reinfection in T-cell-depleted mice. Infect Immun 63:2391–2395, 1995

49. Harmsen AG, Stankiewicz M: Requirement for CD4+ cells in resistance to *Pneumocystis carinii* pneumonia in mice. J Exp Med 172:937–945, 1990

50. Harmsen AG, Stankiewicz M: T cells are not sufficient for resistance to *Pneumocystis carinii* pneumonia in mice. J Protozool 38:44S–45S, 1991

51. Heald A, Flepp M, Chave JP, et al: Treatment for cerebral toxoplasmosis protects against *Pneumocystis carinii* pneumonia in patients with AIDS. The Swiss HIV Cohort Study. Ann Intern Med 115:760–763, 1991

52. Holmes AH, Trotman-Dickenson B, Edwards A, et al: Bronchiectasis in HIV disease. Q J Med 85:875–882, 1992

53. Hopewell PC, Luce JM: Pulmonary involvement in the acquired immunodeficiency syndrome. Chest 87:104–112, 1985

54. Huang L, Hecht FM, Stansell JD, et al: Suspected *Pneumocystis carinii* pneumonia with a negative induced sputum examination. Is early bronchoscopy useful? Am J Respir Crit Care Med 151:1866–1871, 1995

55. Huang L, Stansell JD, Osmond D, et al: Utility of diffusing capacity (DLco) measurement in subjects with suspected *P. carinii* pneumonia (PCP) and a normal chest radiograph (CXR). Am J Respir Crit Care Med 151:A797, 1995

56. Hirschel B, Lazzarin A, Chopard P, et al: A controlled study of inhaled pentamidine for primary prevention of *Pneumocystis carinii* pneumonia. N Engl J Med 324:1079–1083, 1991

57. Hughes W, Leoung G, Kramer F, et al: Comparison of atovaquone (566C80) with trimethoprim-sulfamethoxazole to treat *Pneumocystis carinii* pneumonia in patients with AIDS. N Engl J Med 328:1521–1527, 1993

58. Hughes WT: Natural mode of acquisition for de novo infection with *Pneumocystis carinii*. J Infect Dis 145:842–848, 1982

59. Hughes WT, Bartley DL, Smith BM: A natural source of infection due to *Pneumocystis carinii*. J Infect Dis 147:595, 1983

60. Hughes WT, Feldman S, Chaudhary SC, et al: Comparison of pentamidine isethionate and trimethoprim-sulfamethoxazole in the treatment of *Pneumocystis carinii* pneumonia. J Pediatr 92:436–440, 1978

61. Hughes WT, Killmar J: Efficacy of sulfonamides alone in prophylaxis for *Pneumocystis carinii* pneumonia. Third Conference on Retroviruses and Opportunistic Infections. Washington, DC, 1996

62. Hughes WT, Killmar JT, Oz HS: Relative potency of 10 drugs with anti–*Pneumocystis carinii* activity in an animal model. J Infect Dis 170:906–911, 1994

63. Hughes WT, Smith BL: Efficacy of diaminodiphenylsulfone and other drugs in murine *Pneumocystis carinii* pneumonitis. Antimicrob Agents Chemother 26:436–440, 1984

64. Jules-Elysee KM, Stover DE, Zaman MB, et al: Aerosolized pentamidine: Effect on diagnosis and presentation of *Pneumocystis carinii* pneumonia. Ann Intern Med 112:750–7, 1990

65. Kagawa FT, Kirsch CM, Yenokida GG, et al: Serum lactate dehydrogenase activity in patients with AIDS and *Pneumocystis carinii* pneumonia. An adjunct to diagnosis. Chest 94:1031–1033, 1988

66. Kales CP, Murren JR, Torres RA, et al: Early predictors of in-hospital mortality for *Pneumocystis carinii* pneumonia in the acquired immunodeficiency syndrome. Arch Intern Med 147:1413–1417, 1987

67. Katz MH, Baron RB, Grady D: Risk stratification of ambulatory patients suspected of *Pneumocystis* pneumonia. Arch Intern Med 151:105–110, 1991

68. Kennedy CA, Goetz MB: Atypical roentgenographic manifestations of *Pneumocystis carinii* pneumonia. Arch Intern Med 152:1390–1398, 1992

69. Klein NC, Duncanson FP, Lenox TH, et al: Trimethoprim-sulfamethoxazole versus pentamidine for *Pneumocystis carinii* pneumonia in AIDS patients: Results of a large prospective randomized treatment trial. AIDS 6:301–305, 1992

70. Kovacs JA, Hiemenz JW, Macher AM, et al: *Pneumocystis carinii* pneumonia: A comparison between patients with the acquired immunodeficiency syndrome and patients with other immunodeficiencies. Ann Intern Med 100:663–671, 1984

71. Kovacs JA, Ng VL, Masur H, et al: Diagnosis of *Pneumocystis carinii* pneumonia: Improved detection in sputum with use of monoclonal antibodies. N Engl J Med 318:589–593, 1988

72. Kvale PA, Hansen NI, Markowitz N, et al: Routine analysis of induced sputum is not an effective strategy for screening persons infected with human immunodeficiency virus for *Mycobacterium tuberculosis* or *Pneumocystis carinii*. Pulmonary Complications of HIV Infection Study Group. Clin Infect Dis 19:410–416, 1994

73. Kvale PA, Rosen MJ, Hopewell PC, et al: A decline in the pulmonary diffusing capacity does not indicate opportunistic lung disease in asymptomatic persons infected with the human immunodeficiency virus. Pulmonary Complications of HIV Infection Study Group. Am Rev Respir Dis 148:390–395, 1993

74. Leigh TR, Millett MJ, Jameson B, et al: Serum titres of *Pneumocystis carinii* antibody in health care workers caring for patients with AIDS. Thorax 48:619–621, 1993

75. Leigh TR, Wakefield AE, Peters SE, et al: Comparison of DNA amplification and immunofluorescence for detecting *Pneumocystis carinii* in patients receiving immunosuppressive therapy. Transplantation 54:468–470, 1992

76. Leoung GS, Mills J, Hopewell PC, et al: Dapsone-trimethoprim for *Pneumocystis carinii* pneumonia in the acquired immunodeficiency syndrome. Ann Intern Med 105:45–48, 1986

77. Lipman ML, Goldstein E: Serum lactic dehydrogenase predicts mortality in patients with AIDS and *Pneumocystis* pneumonia. West J Med 149:486–487, 1988

78. Lipschik GY, Gill VJ, Lundgren JD, et al: Improved diagnosis of *Pneumocystis carinii* infection by polymerase chain reaction on induced sputum and blood. Lancet 340:203–206, 1992

79. Mallolas J, Zamora L, Gatell JM, et al: Primary prophylaxis for *Pneumocystis carinii* pneumonia: A randomized trial comparing cotrimoxazole, aerosolized pentamidine and dapsone plus pyrimethamine. AIDS 7:59–64, 1993

80. Martin MA, Cox PH, Beck K, et al: A comparison of the effectiveness of three regimens in the prevention of *Pneumocystis carinii* pneumonia in human

immunodeficiency virus-infected patients [see comments]. Arch Intern Med 152:523–528, 1992

81. Masur H, Lane HC, Kovacs JA, et al: NIH conference. *Pneumocystis* pneumonia: From bench to clinic. Ann Intern Med 111:813–826, 1989

82. Masur H, Michelis MA, Greene JB, et al: An outbreak of community-acquired *Pneumocystis carinii* pneumonia: Initial manifestation of cellular immune dysfunction. N Engl J Med 305:1431–1438, 1981

83. Masur H, Shelhamer J: Empiric outpatient management of HIV-related pneumonia: Economical or unwise? Ann Intern Med 111:451–453, 1996

84. Meade JC, Stringer JR: Cloning and characterization of an ATPase gene from *Pneumocystis carinii* which closely resembles fungal H + ATPases. J Eukaryot Microbiol 42:298–307, 1995

85. Medina I, Mills J, Leoung G, et al: Oral therapy for *Pneumocystis carinii* pneumonia in the acquired immunodeficiency syndrome. A controlled trial of trimethoprim-sulfamethoxazole versus trimethoprim-dapsone. N Engl J Med 323:776–782, 1990

86. Meeker DP, Matysik GA, Stelmach K, et al: Diagnostic utility of lactate dehydrogenase levels in patients receiving aerosolized pentamidine. Chest 104: 386–388, 1993

87. Metersky ML, Colt HG, Olson LK, et al: AIDS-related spontaneous pneumothorax. Risk factors and treatment. Chest 108:946–951, 1995

88. Meuwissen J, Tauber I, Leeuwenberg A, et al: Parasitologic and serologic observations of infection with *Pneumocystis* in humans. J Infect Dis 136: 43–49, 1977

89. Millard PR, Heryet AR: Observations favouring *Pneumocystis carinii* pneumonia as a primary infection: A monoclonal antibody study on paraffin sections. J Pathol 154:365–370, 1988

90. Miller RF, Millar AB, Weller IV, et al: Empirical treatment without bronchoscopy for *Pneumocystis carinii* pneumonia in the acquired immunodeficiency syndrome. Thorax 44:559–564, 1989

91. Montaner JS, Lawson LM, Gervais A, et al: Aerosol pentamidine for secondary prophylaxis of AIDS-related *Pneumocystis carinii* pneumonia. A randomized, placebo-controlled study. Ann Intern Med 114:948–953, 1991

92. Montaner JS, Lawson LM, Levitt N, et al: Corticosteroids prevent early deterioration in patients with moderately severe *Pneumocystis carinii* pneumonia and the acquired immunodeficiency syndrome (AIDS). Ann Intern Med 113:14–20, 1990

93. Montgomery AB, Feigal D Jr, Sattler F, et al: Pentamidine aerosol versus trimethoprim-sulfamethoxazole for *Pneumocystis carinii* in acquired immune deficiency syndrome. Am J Respir Crit Care Med 151:1068–1074, 1995

94. Moskovic E, Miller R, Pearson M: High resolution computed tomography of *Pneumocystis carinii* pneumonia in AIDS. Clin Radiol 42:239–243, 1990

95. Murray JF, Felton CP, Garay SM, et al: Pulmonary complications of the acquired immunodeficiency syndrome. Report of a National Heart, Lung, and Blood Institute workshop. N Engl J Med 310: 1682–1688, 1984

96. National Institutes of Health-University of California Expert Panel: Consensus statement on the use of corticosteroids as adjunctive therapy for severe *Pneumocystis carinii* pneumonia in the acquired im-

munodeficiency syndrome. N Engl J Med 323: 1500–1504, 1990

97. Ng VL, Gartner I, Weymouth LA, et al: The use of mucolysed induced sputum for the identification of pulmonary pathogens associated with human immunodeficiency virus infection. Arch Pathol Lab Med 113:488–493, 1989

98. Ng VL, Yajko DM, McPhaul LW, et al: Evaluation of an indirect fluorescent-antibody stain for detection of *Pneumocystis carinii* in respiratory specimens. J Clin Microbiol 28:975–979, 1990

99. Nielsen TL, Eeftinck Schattenkerk JK, Jensen BN, et al: Adjunctive corticosteroid therapy for *Pneumocystis carinii* pneumonia in AIDS: A randomized European multicenter open label study. J Acquir Immune Defic Syndr 5:726–731, 1992

100. Northfelt DW, Clement MJ, Safrin S: Extrapulmonary pneumocystosis: Clinical features in human immunodeficiency virus infection. Medicine 69: 392–398, 1990

101. Noskin GA, Murphy RL, Black JR, et al: Salvage therapy with clindamycin/primaquine for *Pneumocystis carinii* pneumonia. Clin Infect Dis 14:183–188, 1992

102. O'Brien JG, Dong BJ, Coleman RL, et al: Five year retrospective review of the risk factors associated with adverse drug reactions in patients with HIV treated with intravenous pentamidine for *Pneumocystis carinii* pneumonia. 35th Interscience Conference on Antimicrobial Agents and Chemotherapy. San Francisco, CA, 1995

103. O'Brien RF, Quinn JL, Miyahara BT, et al: Diagnosis of *Pneumocystis carinii* pneumonia by induced sputum in a city with moderate incidence of AIDS. Chest 95:136–138, 1989

104. Ognibene FP, Shelhamer J, Gill V, et al: The diagnosis of *Pneumocystis carinii* pneumonia in patients with the acquired immunodeficiency syndrome using subsegmental bronchoalveolar lavage. Am Rev Respir Dis 129:929–932, 1984

105. Opravil M, Hirschel B, Lazzarin A, et al: Once-weekly administration of dapsone/pyrimethamine vs. aerosolized pentamidine as combined prophylaxis for *Pneumocystis carinii* pneumonia and toxoplasmic encephalitis in human immunodeficiency virus-infected patients. Clin Infect Dis 20:531–541, 1995

106. Opravil M, Marincek B, Fuchs WA, et al: Shortcomings of chest radiography in detecting *Pneumocystis carinii* pneumonia. J Acquir Immune Defic Syndr 7:39–45, 1994

107. Orenstein M, Webber CA, Cash M, et al: Value of bronchoalveolar lavage in the diagnosis of pulmonary infection in acquired immune deficiency syndrome. Thorax 41:345–349, 1986

108. Peglow SL, Smulian AG, Linke MJ, et al: Serologic responses to *Pneumocystis carinii* in health and disease. J Infect Dis 161:296, 1990

109. Perera DR, Western KA, Johnson HD, et al: *Pneumocystis carinii* pneumonia in a hospital for children. JAMA 214:1074–1078, 1970

110. Peters SE, Wakefield AE, Sinclair K, et al: A search for *Pneumocystis carinii* in post-mortem lungs by DNA amplification. J Pathol 166:195–198, 1992

111. Phair J, Munoz A, Detels R, et al: The risk of *Pneumocystis carinii* pneumonia among men infected with human immunodeficiency virus type 1. Multicen-

ter AIDS Cohort Study Group. N Engl J Med 322: 161–165, 1990

112. Pifer LL, Hughes WT, Stagno S, et al: *Pneumocystis carinii* infection: Evidence for a high prevalence in normal and immunosuppressed children. Pediatrics 61:35–41, 1978

113. Pitchenik AE, Ganjei P, Torres A, et al: Sputum examination for the diagnosis of *Pneumocystis carinii* pneumonia in the acquired immunodeficiency syndrome. Am Rev Respir Dis 133:226–229, 1986

114. Pixley FJ, Wakefield AE, Banerji S, et al: Mitochondrial gene sequences show fungal homology for *Pneumocystis carinii*. Mol Microbiol 5:1347–1351, 1991

115. Podzamczer D, Santin M, Jimenez J, et al: Thrice-weekly cotrimoxazole is better than weekly dapsone-pyrimethamine for the primary prevention of *Pneumocystis carinii* pneumonia in HIV-infected patients. AIDS 7:501–506, 1993

116. Pottratz ST, Martin W: Role of fibronectin in *Pneumocystis carinii* attachment to cultured lung cells. J Clin Invest 85:351–356, 1990

117. Pottratz ST, Paulsrud J, Smith JS, et al: *Pneumocystis carinii* attachment to cultured lung cells by pneumocystis gp 120, a fibronectin binding protein. J Clin Invest 88:403–407, 1991

118. The Pulmonary Complications of HIV Infection Study Group: Design of a prospective study of the pulmonary complications of human immunodeficiency virus infection. J Clin Epidemiol 46: 497–507, 1993

119. Queener SF, Bartlett MS, Richardson JD, et al: Activity of clindamycin with primaquine against *Pneumocystis carinii* in vitro and in vivo. Antimicrob Agents Chemother 32:807–813, 1988

120. Quist J, Hill AR: Serum lactate dehydrogenase (LDH) in *Pneumocystis carinii* pneumonia, tuberculosis, and bacterial pneumonia. Chest 108: 415–418, 1995

121. Roths JB, Sidman CL: Both immunity and hyperresponsiveness to *Pneumocystis carinii* result from transfer of CD4+ but not CD8+ T cells into severe combined immunodeficiency mice. J Clin Invest 90:673–678, 1992

122. Roths JB, Sidman CL: Single and combined humoral and cell-mediated immunotherapy of *Pneumocystis carinii* pneumonia in immunodeficient SCID mice. Infect Immun 61:1641–1649, 1993

123. Rotondo A, Guidi G, Catalano O, et al: High resolution computed tomography (HRCT) of pulmonary infections in AIDS patients. Rays 19:208–215, 1994

124. Ruebush TK, Weinstein RA, Baehner RL, et al: An outbreak of *Pneumocystis* pneumonia in children with acute lymphocytic leukemia. Am J Dis Child 132:143–148, 1978

125. Ruffolo JJ: *Pneumocystis carinii* cell structure. In Walzer PD, ed. *Pneumocystis carinii* Pneumonia. New York, Marcel Dekker, Inc, vol 69, 1994, pp 25–43

126. Safrin S, Finkelstein DM, Feinberg J, et al: A double-blind, randomized comparison of oral trimethoprim-sulfamethoxazole, dapsone-trimethoprim, and clindamycin-primaquine for treatment of mild-to-moderate *Pneumocystis carinii* pneumonia in patients with AIDS. Ann Intern Med 124: 792–802, 1996

127. Safrin S, Sattler FR, Lee BL, et al: Dapsone as a single agent is suboptimal therapy for *Pneumocystis carinii* pneumonia. J Acquir Immune Defic Syndr 4: 244–249, 1991

128. Sandhu JS, Goodman PC: Pulmonary cysts associated with *Pneumocystis carinii* pneumonia in patients with AIDS. Radiology 173:33–35, 1989

129. Sankary RM, Turner J, Lipavsky A, et al: Alveolar-capillary block in patients with AIDS and *Pneumocystis carinii* pneumonia. Am Rev Respir Dis 137: 443–449, 1988

130. Sattler FR, Allegra CJ, Verdegem TD, et al: Trimetrexate-leucovorin dosage evaluation study for treatment of *Pneumocystis carinii* pneumonia. J Infect Dis 161:91–96, 1990

131. Sattler FR, Cowan R, Nielsen DM, et al: Trimethoprim-sulfamethoxazole compared with pentamidine for treatment of *Pneumocystis carinii* pneumonia in the acquired immunodeficiency syndrome. A prospective, noncrossover study. Ann Intern Med 109:280–287, 1988

132. Sattler FR, Frame P, Davis R, et al: Trimetrexate with leucovorin versus trimethoprim-sulfamethoxazole for moderate to severe episodes of *Pneumocystis carinii* pneumonia in patients with AIDS: A prospective, controlled multicenter investigation of the AIDS Clinical Trials Group Protocol 029/031. J Infect Dis 170:165–172, 1994

133. Schneider MM, Hoepelman AI, Eeftinck Schattenkerk JK, et al: A controlled trial of aerosolized pentamidine or trimethoprim-sulfamethoxazole as primary prophylaxis against *Pneumocystis carinii* pneumonia in patients with human immunodeficiency virus infection. The Dutch AIDS Treatment Group. N Engl J Med 327:1836–1841, 1992

134. Schneider RF, Hansen NI, Rosen MJ, et al: Lack of usefulness of radiographic screening for pulmonary disease in asymptomatic HIV-infected adults. Pulmonary Complications of HIV Infection Study Group. Arch Intern Med 156:191–195, 1996

135. Shellito J, Suzara VV, Blumenfeld W, et al: A new model of *Pneumocystis carinii* infection in mice selectively depleted of helper T lymphocytes. J Clin Invest 85:1686–1693, 1990

136. Sinclair K, Wakefield AE, Banerji S, et al: *Pneumocystis carinii* organisms derived from rat and human hosts are genetically distinct. Mol Biochem Parasitol 45:183–184, 1991

137. Smulian AG, Sullivan DW, Linke MJ, et al: Geographic variation in the humoral response to *Pneumocystis carinii*. J Infect Dis 167:1243–1247, 1993

138. Soo Hoo GW, Mohsenifar Z, Meyer RD: Inhaled or intravenous pentamidine therapy for *Pneumocystis carinii* pneumonia in AIDS. A randomized trial. Ann Intern Med 113:195–202, 1990

139. Soulez B, Palluault F, Cesbron JY, et al: Introduction of *Pneumocystis carinii* in a colony of SCID mice. J Protozool 38:123S–125S, 1991

140. Slavin MA, Hoy JF, Stewart K, et al: Oral dapsone versus nebulized pentamidine for *Pneumocystis carinii* pneumonia prophylaxis: An open randomized prospective trial to assess efficacy and haematological toxicity. AIDS 6:1169–1174, 1992

141. Stansell JD, Charlebois E, Turner J, et al: Baseline and time variable predictors of *Pneumocystis carinii* pneumonia (PCP) in HIV-infected persons: Results of the Pulmonary Complications of HIV Infection Study. Am J Respir Crit Care Med 149: A977, 1994

142. Stansell JD, Hopewell PC: *Pneumocystis carinii* Pneumonia: Risk factors, clinical presentation, and natural history. In Sattler FR, Walzer PD, eds. *Pneumocystis carinii*. London, Bailliere Tindall, vol 2, 1995, pp 449–460

143. Stein DS, Stevens RC: Treatment-associated toxicities: Incidence and mechanisms. In Sattler FR, Walzer PD, eds. *Pneumocystis carinii*. London, Bailliere Tindall, vol 2, 1995, pp 505–530

144. Stiller RA, Paradis IL, Dauber JH: Subclinical pneumonitis due to *Pneumocystis carinii* in a young adult with elevated antibody titers to Epstein-Barr virus. J Infect Dis 166:926–930, 1992

145. Stringer SL, Stringer JR, Blase MA, et al: *Pneumocystis carinii*: Sequence from ribosomal RNA implies a close relationship with fungi. Exp Parasitol 68: 450–461, 1989

146. Suster B, Akerman M, Orenstein M, et al: Pulmonary manifestations of AIDS: Review of 106 episodes. Radiology 161:87–93, 1986

147. Tamburrini E, Mencarini P, De Luca A, et al: Diagnosis of *Pneumocystis carinii* pneumonia: Specificity and sensitivity of polymerase chain reaction in comparison with immunofluorescence in bronchoalveolar lavage specimens. J Med Microbiol 38: 449–453, 1993

148. Theus SA, Andrews RP, Steele P, et al: Adoptive transfer of lymphocytes sensitized to the major surface glycoprotein of *Pneumocystis carinii* confers protection in the rat. J Clin Invest 95:2587–2593, 1995

149. Toma E, Fournier S, Dumont M, et al: Clindamycin/primaquine versus trimethoprim-sulfamethoxazole as primary therapy for *Pneumocystis carinii* pneumonia in AIDS: A randomized, double-blind pilot trial. Clin Infect Dis 17:178–184, 1993

150. Toma E, Fournier S, Poisson M, et al: Clindamycin with primaquine for *Pneumocystis carinii* pneumonia. Lancet 1:1046–1048, 1989

151. Toma E, Raboud J, Thorne A, et al: Clindamycin-primaquine versus trimethoprim-sulfamethoxazole for PCP in AIDS. 35th Interscience Conference on Antimicrobial Agents and Chemotherapy. San Francisco, CA 1995

152. Torres RA, Barr M, Thorn M, et al: Randomized trial of dapsone and aerosolized pentamidine for the prophylaxis of *Pneumocystis carinii* pneumonia and toxoplasmic encephalitis. Am J Med 95:573–583, 1993

153. Tu JV, Biem HJ, Detsky AS: Bronchoscopy versus empirical therapy in HIV-infected patients with presumptive *Pneumocystis carinii* pneumonia. A decision analysis. Am Rev Respir Dis 148:370–377, 1993

154. Vargas SL, Hughes WT, Wakefield AE, et al: Limited persistence in and subsequent elimination of *Pneumocystis carinii* from the lungs after *P. carinii* pneumonia. J Infect Dis 172:506–510, 1995

155. Vavra J, Kucera K: *Pneumocystis carinii*: Its ultrastructure and ultrastructural affinities. J Protozool 17: 463–483, 1970

156. Wachter RM, Luce JM, Safrin S, et al: Cost and outcome of intensive care for patients with AIDS, *Pneumocystis carinii* pneumonia, and severe respiratory failure. JAMA 273:230–235, 1995

157. Wachter RM, Luce JM, Turner J, et al: Intensive care of patients with the acquired immunodeficiency syndrome. Outcome and changing patterns of utilization. Am Rev Respir Dis 134:891–896, 1986

158. Wachter RM, Russi MB, Bloch DA, et al: *Pneumocystis carinii* pneumonia and respiratory failure in AIDS: Improved outcomes and increased use of intensive care units. Am Rev Respir Dis 143:251, 1991

159. Wakefield AE, Fritscher CC, Malin AS, et al: Genetic diversity in human-derived *Pneumocystis carinii* isolates from four geographical locations shown by analysis of mitochondrial rRNA gene sequences. J Clin Microbiol 32:2959–2961, 1994

160. Wakefield AE, Peters SE, Banerji S, et al: *Pneumocystis carinii* shows DNA homology with the ustomycetous red yeast fungi. Mol Microbiol 6:1903–1911, 1992

161. Wakefield AE, Pixley FJ, Banerji S, et al: Detection of *Pneumocystis carinii* with DNA amplification. Lancet 336:451–453, 1990

162. Wakefield GA: Re-examination of epidemiological concepts. In Sattler FR, Walzer PD, eds. *Pneumocystis carinii*. London, Bailliere Tindall, vol 2, 1995, pp 431–448

163. Walzer PD: Pathogenic Mechanisms. In Walzer PD, ed. *Pneumocystis carinii* Pneumonia. New York, Marcel Dekker, Inc, vol 69, 1994, pp 251–265

164. Weinberg GA, Durant PJ: Genetic diversity of *Pneumocystis carinii* derived from infected rats, mice, ferrets, and cell cultures. J Eukaryot Microbiol 41: 223–228, 1994

165. Wharton JM, Coleman DL, Wofsy CB, et al: Trimethoprim-sulfamethoxazole or pentamidine for *Pneumocystis carinii* pneumonia in the acquired immunodeficiency syndrome. A prospective randomized trial. Ann Intern Med 105:37–44, 1986

166. Yoneda K, Walzer PD: Attachment of *Pneumocystis carinii* to type I alveolar cells studied by freeze-fracture electron microscopy. Infect Immun 40: 812–815, 1983

167. Zaman MK, White DA: Serum lactate dehydrogenase levels and *Pneumocystis carinii* pneumonia. Diagnostic and prognostic significance. Am Rev Respir Dis 137:796–800, 1988

168. Zaman MK, Wooten OJ, Suprahmanya B, et al: Rapid noninvasive diagnosis of *Pneumocystis carinii* from induced liquefied sputum. Ann Intern Med 109: 7–10, 1988

Chapter 21

Disseminated *Mycobacterium avium* Complex and Other Bacterial Infections

MARK A. JACOBSON

DISSEMINATED *MYCOBACTERIUM AVIUM* COMPLEX INFECTIONS IN AIDS

Epidemiology and Pathogenesis

Disseminated *Mycobacterium avium* complex (MAC) infection is emerging as one of the most important opportunistic infectious complications of the acquired immunodeficiency syndrome (AIDS). The association of disseminated MAC infection with AIDS was recognized early in the human immunodeficiency syndrome (HIV) epidemic[17,38] (disseminated MAC infection had been reported only rarely in patients without HIV disease[23]). Among patients with HIV, disseminated MAC infection has occurred almost exclusively in patients with advanced AIDS, essentially only in patients with <50 CD4 lymphocytes/μl.[11,19,42] According to Centers for Disease Control statistics, disseminated MAC was reported as an index AIDS diagnosis in only 5.3% of AIDS cases between 1981 and 1987.[24] However, in a large retrospective series from this same time period involving 366 AIDS patients, this opportunistic infection was diagnosed during the course of illness in 18%; the attack rate may have been even higher, since 53% of 79 autopsies in this series showed evidence of disseminated MAC.[20] More recent prospective natural history studies suggest that one third to one half of AIDS patients might develop disseminated MAC infection in the absence of any MAC-specific antimicrobial prophylaxis. Among patients with advanced HIV disease who had serial blood specimens cultured for mycobacteria over a median 1-year period, the 2-year actuarial incidence of MAC mycobacteremia was approximately 40%.[42] Also,

in a subcohort analysis of 844 men with AIDS in the Multicenter AIDS Cohort Study, 33.4% of those who received early *Pneumocystis carinii* prophylaxis subsequently developed disseminated MAC infection.[21]

MAC is a ubiquitous soil and water saprophyte. The source of MAC invasion in AIDS patients may be gastrointestinal or respiratory. The presence of large clusters of mycobacteria within macrophages of the small bowel lamina propria suggests that the bowel might be the portal of entry. However, respiratory isolation of MAC also frequently precedes disseminated infection, suggesting MAC infection may begin in the lungs as well.[28] It is still unknown whether disseminated MAC infection results from new environmental acquisition of the organism or reactivation of quiescent, endogenous mycobacteria after severe immunosuppression has occurred, although most data points toward the former.

In AIDS, the key host defect allowing dissemination of MAC may be macrophage dysfunction. MAC is able to survive within macrophages unless intracellular killing mechanisms (defective in AIDS) are activated. Also, lymphokines present in abnormally low levels in AIDS, such as tumor necrosis factor, interferon-γ, and interleukin-2, may play an important role in the diminished host defense against MAC.

In AIDS, MAC causes high-grade, widely disseminated infection. Nearly all AIDS patients with invasive MAC infection (as opposed to stool, urine, or respiratory secretion colonization) have had positive mycobacterial blood cultures.[20] In the majority of those autopsied, MAC also could be isolated from spleen, lymph nodes (Color Plate I*D*), liver, lung, adrenals, colon, kidney, and bone marrow. The magnitude of mycobacteremia can range from 1 to 10^4 colony-forming units (cfu) per milliliter of blood.[57] At autopsy, bone marrow, spleen, lymph nodes, and liver have yielded up to 1010 cfu/g of tissue.[57] Histopathologic studies of involved organs typically have shown absent or poorly formed granulomas and acid-fast bacteria within macrophages.[17]

Clinical Manifestations

Because most AIDS patients with disseminated MAC infection have other concomitant infections or neoplasms, and because MAC appears to result in little histopathologic evidence of inflammatory response or tissue destruction, the relationship between constitutional symptoms, organ dysfunction, and MAC infection has been uncertain. Nevertheless, several large retrospective studies strongly suggest a negative effect of disseminated MAC infection on mortality and morbidity in AIDS. Horsburgh et al noted a median 4-month survival among 39 patients with untreated disseminated MAC infection compared to 11 months among 39 controls matched for absolute CD4 lymphocyte count, prior AIDS status, history of antiretroviral therapy, history of *Pneumocystis carinii* pneumonia (PCP) prophylaxis, and year of diagnosis ($p < 0.0001$).[22] At San Francisco General Hospital, we have examined the association between disseminated MAC infection and survival after index PCP diagnosis.[28] Among 137 consecutive patients who had a sterile body site cultured for mycobacteria within 3 months of their first AIDS-defining episode of PCP, median survival was significantly shorter in those with disseminated MAC infection than in those with negative cultures (107 versus 275 days; $p < 0.01$), even after controlling for age, absolute lymphocyte count, and hemoglobin concentration. We have also examined the association between disseminated MAC infection and blood transfusion requirements.[30] Between July 1, 1987, and June 30, 1988, blood specimens from 574 patients were submitted to our mycobacteriology laboratory for culture. Among the AIDS/ARC patients transfused during the same time period, patients with a positive blood culture for MAC had a relative risk of 5.23 ($p < 0.001$) for receiving packed red blood cell (PRBC) transfusions compared to patients whose blood submitted for mycobacterial culture was negative, thus confirming an association between disseminated MAC infection and increased morbidity in AIDS.

There are four clinical syndromes, often overlapping, that have been associated anecdotally with disseminated MAC infection. The characteristics of these syndromes are summarized in Table 21–1. In a prospective natural history study of MAC bacteremia underway at San Francisco General Hospital, we have interviewed patients regarding symptoms and evaluated laboratory test results at the time of diagnostic evaluation for disseminated MAC infection.[7] We have observed that, among patients with <50 CD4 lymphocytes/μl, a history of fever for >30 days, a hemocrit <30%, or a serum albumin level <3.0 g/dl are all sensitive predictors of MAC bacteremia. However, neither severe fatigue, diarrhea, weight loss, neutropenia, nor thrombocytopenia discriminated between those who were subsequently found to be blood culture positive or negative for MAC.

Since 1987, there have been increasing numbers of cases in which AIDS patients receiving antiretroviral therapy with zidovudine have developed localized visceral or cutaneous MAC abscesses without mycobacteremia.[1,44] Unlike disseminated infection (see below), these lesions have responded remarkably well to drainage and antimycobacterial therapy. These case series have led to speculation that improved immune function resulting from zidovudine therapy was responsible for localization of infection.

Diagnosis

Special blood culture techniques for isolating mycobacteria, such as the broth-based BACTEC

TABLE 21–1. CLINICAL SYNDROMES ASSOCIATED WITH DISSEMINATED MAC INFECTION IN AIDS

Systemic
Fever, malaise, weight loss, often associated with anemia, neutropenia
Gastrointestinal
Chronic diarrhea and abdominal pain (MAC invasion of colon often observed at autopsy)
Chronic malabsorption (Whipple's-like histopathologic changes in small intestine often observed at autopsy)
Extrabiliary obstructive jaundice secondary to periportal lymphadenopathy

Data from Greene JB, Sidhu GS, Lewin S, et al: *Mycobacterium avium-intracellulare:* A cause of disseminated life-threatening infection in homosexuals and drug abusers. Ann Intern Med 97:539–546, 1982.

system or agar-based Dupont Isolator system, appear to be the most sensitive methods for diagnosing disseminated MAC infection.[61] With these techniques, the sensitivity approaches 100%. Specific DNA probes for MAC have recently become available; these probes make it possible to differentiate MAC from other mycobacteria within hours when there is sufficient mycobacterial growth in broth or agar.[13] Time to culture positivity ranges from 5 to 51 days. It is uncommon for blood cultures to be negative when there is a positive histologic diagnosis from lymph node, liver, or bone marrow biopsies. However, one advantage of biopsied specimens is that stains may demonstrate acid-fast bacteria (AFB) or granuloma weeks before blood cultures turn positive.

The clinical significance of MAC isolated from sputum or stool remains controversial. In our prospective natural history study, we have found that only two thirds of patients with negative blood cultures but positive stool or sputum cultures for MAC subsequently developed disseminated MAC infection.[6] Therefore, at this time, neither stool nor sputum culture can be recommended as a screening test to identify patients likely to develop MAC bacteremia.

Therapy

MAC is resistant to all standard antituberculous drugs (except ethambutol) at concentrations achievable in plasma. Yet, half or more of MAC strains can be inhibited by achievable concentrations of rifabutin, rifampin, clofazimine, cycloserine, amikacin, ethionamide, ethambutol, azithromycin, clarithromycin, ciprofloxacin, or sparfloxacin (Table 21–2).[14,15,26,58–61] Unfortunately, drug levels necessary to kill MAC in vitro (minimum bactericidal concentration) have been 8 to >32 times that of inhibitory levels.[59] Whereas combinations of antimycobacterial agents have shown in vitro inhibitory synergism, bactericidal synergism has been more difficult to demonstrate.[58,59] In addition, for in vivo killing, drugs must penetrate macrophages as well as the MAC cell wall. Nevertheless, in animal models of disseminated MAC infection, both single and combination antimycobacterial regimens have reduced mycobacterial colony counts by several logs and improved survival.[14,25,36]

Results of several sequential trials reported by the California Collaborative Treatment Group (CCTG) highlight the caution needed when in-

TABLE 21–2. DRUGS CAPABLE OF INHIBITING MOST MAC STRAINS AT CONCENTRATIONS ACHIEVABLE IN PLASMA

Rifabutin
Cycloserine
Rifampin
Ethambutol
Azithromycin
Sparfloxacin
Clofazimine
Amikacin
Ciprofloxacin
Ethionamide
Clarithromycin

terpreting results of treatment trials that have no control arm. In 1990, this group reported striking microbiologic and clinical effects in previously untreated patients with disseminated MAC who were given a combination regimen that included intravenous amikacin and oral rifampin, ethambutol, and ciprofloxacin.[8] Given the modest results that had previously been reported with oral antimycobacterial agents, many drew the conclusion from this uncontrolled trial that the amikacin was primarily responsible for the efficacy of this regimen. Subsequently, the CCTG reported similar microbiologic and clinical results in another similarly designed uncontrolled trial in which intravenous amikacin was replaced by oral clofazimine.[35] More data regarding the clinical utility of intravenous amikacin are now available from a controlled trial conducted by the NIAID-sponsored AIDS Clinical Trials Group (ACTG) in which 72 patients with previously untreated disseminated MAC were all given a combination oral regimen of rifampin, ethambutol, ciprofloxacin, and clofazimine and were also randomized to receive or not receive additional intravenous amikacin.[45] In this controlled trial, there were no significant differences in microbiologic or clinical outcomes, demonstrating that the cost, inconvenience, and risk of toxicity of intravenous amikacin is unlikely to translate into a significant clinical benefit for patients with disseminated MAC.

Data on in vivo microbiologic efficacy against MAC have been most impressive with the new macrolides, in particular clarithromycin. A multicenter, randomized, placebo-controlled, dose-ranging trial of clarithromycin monotherapy in patients with previously untreated disseminated MAC reported a median decrease of >2 log in blood MAC colony-forming units—a more potent microbiologic effect than reported in any earlier treatment trials.[5] This microbiologic effect was accompanied by significant clinical improvement according to an analysis of symptoms and quality-of-life indices. However, a globally beneficial dose–response effect was not observed. Unacceptably high gastrointestinal toxicity occurred at the 2000-mg bid dose. Although the 1000-mg bid dose had greater microbiologic efficacy than the 500-gm bid dose, there was actually a trend toward increased mortality in the former group (13 versus 3 deaths while on study in the 1000- and 500-mg dosing arms, respectively).[5] However, when the survival analysis was controlled for differences in baseline characteristics expected to influence survival such as Karnofsky performance score, survival did not significantly differ between these two dosing arms. Not surprisingly, drug resistance emerged after 2 to 3 months of monotherapy in this trial, affecting approximately half of patients in all dosing arms. Hence, although there is a growing consensus that the currently optimal agent for disseminated MAC therapy is a macrolide such as clarithromycin, it is clear that the macrolide must be combined with other antimycobacterial agents in an attempt to prevent or at least delay emergence of resistance, which is almost certain to be associated with clinical deterioration.

Azithromycin is another effective macrolide for MAC treatment.[62] In a similarly designed trial of azithromycin monotherapy, patients with newly diagnosed positive MAC blood cultures were randomized to receive either 600 or 1200 mg/day of azithromycin. At 6 weeks, approximately half of blood cultures were sterile in both groups; the mean reduction in mycobacteremia was 2.0 and 1.55 log, respectively ($p > 0.05$).[2] Antimycobacterial efficacy was therefore similar to that of clarithromycin monotherapy. Also, as with clarithromycin, there was increased gastrointestinal intolerance with the higher dose.

Nonmacrolide antimycobacterial agents have been evaluated in several randomized, controlled trials. In a small placebo-controlled trial, patients with newly diagnosed, previously untreated disseminated MAC infection were randomized to receive a combination of rifampin (600 mg/day), ethambutol (25 mg/kg/day), and ciprofloxacin (750 mg/day) or matching placebo. After 8 weeks on study, MAC colony-forming units in blood had decreased by >1 log in four of nine treated patients versus none of ten placebo recipients and had increased by >1 log in one and seven patients, respectively ($p =$

0.006).[32] A significant reduction was observed in the number of days of fever experienced by patients assigned to active drug, even after controlling for use of antipyretic agents such as ibuprofen.

In order to determine which of the orally bioavailable nonmacrolide antimycobacterial agents might be the most potent in vivo, the CCTG conducted a randomized, controlled trial in which patients with previously untreated disseminated MAC were assigned to receive a 4-week regimen of rifampin, ethambutol, or clofazimine monotherapy.[34] In this trial, only ethambutol resulted in a statistically significant reduction in blood MAC colony-forming units, suggesting that ethambutol might be the most potent of these three antimycobacterial agents.

Recent data regarding rifabutin treatment for disseminated MAC have also been particularly promising. Interestingly, when rifabutin was evaluated in the 1980s as a treatment for MAC at doses of 100 to 300 mg/day, it was found to be ineffective. In a recent randomized, blind, placebo-controlled trial in which patients with newly diagnosed disseminated MAC were assigned to receive clofazimine/ethambutol or clofazimine/ethambutol/rifabutin (600 mg/day), approximately half of the patients receiving the rifabutin-containing regimen had a >2-log decrease in blood MAC colony-forming units or sterilization of the blood compared with none of those receiving only clofazimine/ethambutol.[54] The long-term clinical benefit of combination regimens that include both macrolide and nonmacrolide agents for treatment of disseminated MAC has been confirmed recently in a randomized multicenter trial conducted by the Canadian MAC Study Group in which 187 evaluable patients with MAC mycobacteremia were randomized to receive a regimen of clarithromycin 1000 mg bid, rifabutin 600 mg qd, and ethambutol 15 mg/kg/day versus ciprofloxacin 750 mg bid, rifampin 600 mg qd, clofazimine 100 mg qd, and ethambutol 15 mg/kg/day. The in vivo quantitative antimycobacterial effect was significantly better with the macrolide-containing regimen, as was median survival (8.7 versus 5.2 months; $p < 0.001$).[49]

Nonetheless, the composition of the optimal treatment regimen for disseminated MAC is still unclear. Certainly, a macrolide such as clarithromycin or azithromycin should be used. Evidence from a recent trial examining several clarithromycin-containing combination regimens suggests that clofazimine compares

TABLE 21–3. AN EMPIRIC REGIMEN FOR THE TREATMENT OF DISSEMINATED *M. AVIUM* COMPLEX INFECTION

Clarithromycin 500 mg PO bid (alternatively azithromycin 500 or 600 mg PO qd)
PLUS, one or more of the following agents:
1. Ethambutol 15–25 mg/kg qd
2. Rifabutin 450–600 mg PO qd
3. Clofazimine 100–200 mg PO qd
4. Ciprofloxacin 750 mg PO qd or bid

poorly to ethambutol as a second drug added to clarithromycin.[10] Table 21–3 summarizes what are currently considered to be the best options for the treatment of disseminated MAC.[39] A macrolide such as clarithromycin or azithromycin should be combined with at least one other agent, and the regimen should be continued indefinitely because mycobacteremia is likely to recur or worsen if treatment is discontinued. The best available data from clinical trials points to ethambutol (at a dose of 15 to 25 mg/kg/day) and rifabutin (at a dose of 450 to 600 mg/day) as being the best options to choose from when adding a second agent to the macrolide. It is not known whether adding more than one of these agents to the macrolide is beneficial. New multicenter clinical trials are underway to answer this question.

Finally, in HIV-infected patients, it may be difficult to distinguish tuberculosis from MAC disease. Therefore, an antituberculous regimen should be instituted whenever acid-fast bacteria are demonstrated (and cannot yet be differentiated between MAC and *M. tuberculosis*) in a specimen from a patient with HIV infection and clinical evidence of mycobacterial disease.[40]

Prophylaxis

Since 40% of patients with advanced HIV disease are likely to develop disseminated MAC, it makes sense to develop a strategy for preventing this disease in patients at risk. Since there are few specific, clearly defined risk factors for developing disseminated MAC disease, other than a low CD4 lymphocyte count, any prophylactic strategy has to be applied to the entire population at risk (i.e., those patients with <50 CD4 cells/μl).

Results of combined analysis of two randomized, placebo-controlled trials of rifabutin prophylaxis, conducted in over 1000 patients with advanced HIV disease, demonstrated that prophylactic rifabutin, at a dose of 300 mg/day, reduced the incidence of mycobacteremia by half.[43] Patients who received rifabutin and subsequently developed mycobacteremia had blood MAC isolates that retained susceptibility to rifabutin. However, neither trial alone, nor the combined analysis, demonstrated that rifabutin significantly reduced mortality. Although a combined analysis of both trials revealed an increased incidence of fever, fatigue, anemia, alkaline phosphatase elevations, and hospitalizations in patients who received placebo compared with those who received rifabutin, patients assigned to placebo in these trials tended to have lower absolute CD4 counts, which may have accounted for some of the greater morbidity.

Preliminary data are also now available from a placebo-controlled study in which 682 patients with advanced HIV disease were randomized to receive either clarithromycin 500 mg or placebo bid. During a median 9-month follow-up, only 5% of clarithromycin-assigned patients versus 15% of placebo-assigned patients developed mycobacteremia ($p < 0.001$).[46] More importantly, median survival was significantly longer for clarithromycin than for placebo-assigned patients (>700 versus 573 days). However, among the clarithromycin-assigned patients who did develop disseminated MAC infection, 58% had mycobacteremia with MAC isolates that were highly resistant to clarithromycin (minimum inhibitory concentration [MIC] >512 μg/ml).

Based on these data, a Public Health Service Task Force has recommended lifetime prophylaxis with rifabutin (or clarithromycin) for all HIV-infected patients with <100 CD4 cells/μl.[39] The Task Force also noted that clinicians must carefully weigh the potential benefits of MAC prophylaxis against the potential for toxicity (primarily rash, neutropenia, and gastrointestinal intolerance) and drug interactions and the possibility that addition of another drug to the medical regimen of patients with advanced HIV disease may affect their compliance with other prescribed medications. Because these concerns are generally applicable to most patients with <100 CD4 cells/μl, there remains substantial uncertainty about the ultimate role of MAC prophylaxis in the overall care of patients with late-stage HIV disease. One exception in which there may be more certainty is when a patient upon whom a workup is being performed for pulmonary tuberculosis is found to have respiratory MAC colonization. Although sputum screening is neither sensitive nor specific for disseminated MAC, a positive sputum culture for MAC in a patient with advanced HIV disease has a 65% positive predictive value for subsequent disseminated MAC occurring within the next year.[28] In such a case, aggressive prophylaxis is warranted.

OTHER ATYPICAL MYCOBACTERIAL INFECTIONS IN AIDS

Disseminated infections caused by *M. kansasii, M. gordonae, M. fortuitum, M. chelonei, M. haemophilum, M. marinum, M. genavense,* and *M. xenopi* also have been reported in patients with AIDS.[3,12,24,37,47] These cases generally have had clinical presentations similar to that of MAC infection and pathologic evidence of pulmonary, intestinal, liver, and bone marrow involvement. In vitro sensitivity of isolates to standard antituberculous drugs has been variable.[12,29,47] *M. kansasii* has been the most frequently reported of these other atypical mycobacteria, with disseminated infection present at the time of the index AIDS diagnosis in 0.2% of patients.[24] Response to antimycobacterial therapy was poor in one small series of AIDS patients with disseminated *M. kansasii* infection.[51] However, there are reports of complete clinical resolution of pulmonary *M. kansasii* infection in AIDS patients treated with antituberculous therapy.[29,37] Generally, these AIDS-associated *M. kansasii* isolates have been sensitive to rifampin and ethambutol and resistant to isoniazid. Given the frequent sensitivity of other atypical mycobacteria to one or more standard antituberculous drugs, multidrug therapy tailored to in vitro sensitivities is indicated for AIDS patients with non-MAC atypical mycobacterial infection. Of note, many of these other atypical mycobacterial strains are susceptible to clarithromycin or azithromycin.

OTHER BACTERIAL INFECTIONS ASSOCIATED WITH HIV DISEASE

HIV-infected patients, especially those with advanced disease, have increased susceptibility to systemic bacterial infections, in particular encapsulated organisms (*Streptococcus pneumoniae* and *Haemophilus influenzae*), *Staphylococcus aureus,* and enteric gram-negative bacilli.[9,27,33]

TABLE 21–4. MECHANISMS BY WHICH PATIENTS WITH HIV DISEASE MAY HAVE INCREASED SUSCEPTIBILITY TO BACTERIAL PATHOGENS

B-cell dysfunction (diminished IgG subclass capsule-specific antibodies)
Decreased CD4-mediated antibody-dependent cellular cytoxicity
Decreased local mucosal IgA production
Impaired neutrophil chemotaxis and killing
Impaired complement activation
Diminished liver/spleen macrophage clearance of opsonized bacteria

From Janoff EN, Breiman RF, Daley CL, Hopewell PC: Pneumococcal disease during HIV infection. Ann Intern Med 117:314–324, 1992, with permission.

These bacterial pathogens are often the immediate cause of death in AIDS patients and cause considerable morbidity. Mechanisms by which patients with HIV disease may have increased susceptibility to bacterial pathogens are summarized in Table 21–4.[33]

Pneumococcus

Invasive pneumococcal disease is the most common serious bacterial infection affecting patients with HIV disease.[4] Population-based studies suggest pneumococcal pneumonia and bacteremia, respectively, occur 10 and 100 times more frequently in patients with AIDS than in an age-matched population.[33] Also, recurrent disease occurs more commonly among HIV-infected patients than in controls with invasive pneumococcal disease. Recently, disturbing reports of nosocomially acquired pneumococcal disease in HIV-infected patients have been noted.[33] Increasing reports of penicillin-resistant pneumococcus in the United States are also worrisome. The clinical presentation of pneumococcal pneumonia in patients with HIV disease is similar to that in non-HIV patients with community-acquired pneumococcal pneumonia, although bacteremia and diffuse interstitial infiltrates are more common.[33] Generally, a 10- to 14-day course of antibiotics (parenteral, then oral) is recommended for invasive pneumococcal disease. If a patient fails to improve rapidly, penicillin-resistant infection should be considered. Because of the high incidence and recurrence rate of invasive pneumococcal disease in patients with advanced HIV disease, there may be a role for chronic antibiotic prophylaxis. Although randomized trials specifically addressing the efficacy of pneumococcal antibiotic prophylaxis have not been conducted, results from one *Pneumocystis carinii* prophylaxis trial showed that patients randomized to receive trimethoprim-sulfamethoxazole (TMP/SMX) had a significantly lower rate of serious bacterial infections than those randomized to receive aerosolized pentamidine prophylaxis.[18] Although the pneumococcal vaccine has been recommended by many experts as an immunization prophylaxis strategy for patients with HIV disease, so far, no data have demonstrated the clinical efficacy of this vaccine, and individual vaccine failures have been described,[33] as has a transient increase in peripheral blood HIV viral load after immunization.

Haemophilus Influenzae

Haemophilus species are the second most common cause of HIV-associated bacterial pneumonias.[4] The clinical presentation often involves diffuse interstitial infiltrates and bacteremia. Although the *Haemophilus influenzae* type B vaccine has been recommended for patients with HIV disease, there are no clinical data supporting its efficacy. Also, many *H. influenzae* isolates from patients with AIDS are nontypeable.[4,52]

Staphylococcus Aureus

S. aureus is a common cause of HIV-related bacteremia and soft tissue bacterial infection.[27] Invasive *S. aureus* infection is often nosocomially acquired and associated with intravenous catheter use. Among HIV-infected patients with *S. aureus* bacteremia, late metastatic complications occur more commonly than in non–HIV-infected historical controls.[27] It has been hypothesized that the increased frequency of *S. aureus* skin and nasal carriage observed in patients with HIV disease may be important in the pathogenesis of this serious bacterial infection.[27] Given the increased risk of late metastatic infection with *S. aureus* bacteremia, a minimum of 10 days of parenteral antistaphylococcal therapy is indicated.

Pseudomonas Aeruginosa

Invasive *P. aeruginosa* infection has recently received increased attention as a complication of late-stage HIV disease. Several retrospective series describe an increasing incidence of bacteremia, pneumonia, sinusitis, and soft tissue and bone infections caused by this organism, primarily in patients with <100 CD4 cells/μl.[9,16,55,56] In some series, absolute neutropenia or chronic use of agents with antibacterial

activity, such as TMP/SMX, were risk factors for invasive *P. aeruginosa* infection.

Salmonella

Salmonella bacteremia was a commonly reported AIDS-defining opportunistic infection in the 1980s, often associated with clinical symptoms and signs of gastroenteritis. Relapses were common, sometimes even with appropriate antibiotic suppressive therapy. Salmonella bacteremia is now uncommon and relapses are unusual in patients receiving >400 mg/day of zidovudine. This decrease in incidence has been attributed to the antibacterial activity of zidovudine and TMP/SMX, which are frequently administered chronically to patients with AIDS. Ciprofloxacin is now considered to be the optimal therapy for AIDS-related salmonella bacteremia.[48]

Management of Bacterial Pneumonia

Pneumonia is the most common bacterial cause of morbidity and mortality among HIV-infected patients. Although the choice of antimicrobial therapy ideally should be guided by rapid identification of a specific pathogen, in reality, the infecting organism is often unknown at the time that therapy is instituted for community-acquired pneumonia, and often may not be identified over the course of treatment. Empiric antibiotic therapy must therefore be based on other considerations.

We recently completed a retrospective study designed to determine the microbiologic characteristics (including antibiotic susceptibility) of community-acquired bacterial pneumonia in patients with or known to be at high risk for HIV disease.[4] Two hundred sixteen consecutive patients admitted to San Francisco General Hospital meeting a case definition of community-acquired bacterial pneumonia were studied. One or more etiologic pathogens were definitively identified in 75% of cases. *S. pneumoniae*, *Haemophilus* species, *S. aureus*, and gram-negative bacilli (in that order) were the pathogens most frequently identified. In patients who had a bacteriologic diagnosis made, 18.6%, 6.8%, 4.3%, and 0% had pneumonia caused by pathogens resistant to ampicillin, cefuroxime, TMP/SMX, or ceftazidime, respectively. Presenting clinical characteristics did not consistently define a subset of patients at lower risk for resistance.

Based on these data, in the absence of a diagnostic sputum Gram's stain, and pending definitive microbiologic diagnosis, initial empiric therapy for HIV-related community-acquired bacterial pneumonia probably should be a second- or third-generation cephalosporin, or possibly TMP/SMX.

Management of Sinusitis

Bacterial sinusitis is a common complication of advanced HIV disease and can be difficult to treat.[16,55,63] Patients with CD4 counts <200/μl are particularly prone to developing chronic sinusitis involving multiple sinuses. Etiologic pathogens for chronic sinusitis include streptococcal, haemophilus, and staphylococcal species and *P. aeruginosa*.[16,55,63] Antimicrobial therapy should target these organisms. Some specialists also recommend inhaled corticosteroids and/or mucolytic agents such as guaifenesin. Patients who do not respond to an empiric course of antibiotic therapy within 2 to 3 weeks should be referred to an otolaryngologist for sinus aspiration in order to make a definitive microbiologic diagnosis.

Neutropenia and the Risk of Bacterial Infection

Neutropenia is common in advanced HIV disease (half of AIDS patients have absolute neutrophil counts <1500 cells/μl, even in the absence of myelosuppressive drug exposure,

opportunistic infections, or neoplasms), but profound neutropenia (absolute neutrophil count <100 cells/μl) is uncommon. Serious bacterial infections have been associated with chemotherapy-induced neutropenia in cancer patients, but not with antiviral therapy–induced neutropenia in patients with advanced HIV disease. Studies of zidovudine treatment document increased bacterial infection rates with absolute neutrophil counts <500 cells/μl but not with counts in the range of 500 to 1000 compared to higher counts.[50] A recently published, well-controlled retrospective study of 118 HIV patients with absolute neutrophil counts <1000 cells/μl and 118 nonneutropenic patients matched by CD4 count reported no significant association between neutropenia and either bacteremia, pneumonia, endocarditis, or enterocolitis.[41] However, for all infections combined, the adjusted odds ratios were 5.1 (95% CI 1.6 to 16.0) and 6.5 (95% CI 0.7 to 60.0) for absolute neutrophil counts <1000 and <500 cells/μl, respectively, and bacterial infection. Trials with ganciclovir and foscarnet therapy suggest central line infections are not related to absolute neutrophil count.[53] Therefore, on the basis of currently available data, it appears that absolute neutrophil counts <1000 cells/μl may confer an increased risk of bacterial infection. With absolute neutrophil counts <500 cells/μl, concomitant myelosuppressive medications must be dose-modified or adjunctive myeloid colony-stimulating factor therapy coadministered in order to continue administering drugs with known myelosuppressive toxicity. Of note, AIDS patients with severe myelosuppressive drug-induced neutropenia (<500 cells/μl) do generally respond to adjunctive treatment with granulocyte colony-stimulating factor.[31]

REFERENCES

1. Barbaro DJ, Orcutt VL, Coldiron BM: *Mycobacterium avium-Mycobacterium intracellulare* infection limited to the skin and lymph nodes in patients with AIDS. Rev Infect Dis 11:625–628, 1989

2. Berry A, Koletar S, Williams D: Azithromycin therapy for disseminated *Mycobacterium avium-intercellulare* in AIDS patients (Abstract 292). First National Conference on Human Retroviruses, Washington, DC, 1993

3. Bottger EC, Teske A, Kirschner P, et al: Disseminated *Mycobacterium genavense* infection in patients with AIDS. Lancet 340:76–80, 1992

4. Burack JH, Hahn JA, Saint-Maurice D, Jacobson MA: Microbiology of community-acquired bacterial pneumonia in persons with and at risk for HIV-1

infection: Implications for rational empiric antibiotic therapy. Arch Intern Med 154:2589–2596, 1994

5. Chaisson RE, Benson C, Dube M, et al: Clarithromycin therapy for bacteremic *Mycobacterium avium* complex disease. Ann Intern Med 121:905–911, 1994

6. Chin DP, Hopewell PC, Yajko DM, et al: *Mycobacterium avium* complex in the respiratory or gastrointestinal tract and the risk of *M. avium* complex bacteremia in patients with the human immunodeficiency virus. J Infect Dis 169:289–295, 1994

7. Chin DP, Reingold AL, Horsburgh CR Jr, et al: Predicting *Mycobacterium avium* complex bacteremia in patients with the human immunodeficiency virus: A prospectively validated model. Clin Infect Dis 19:668–674, 1994

8. Chiu J, Nussbaum J, Bozzette S, et al: Treatment of

disseminated *Mycobacterium avium* complex infection in AIDS with amikacin, ethambutol, rifampin, and ciprofloxacin. Ann Intern Med 113:358–361, 1990

9. Dropulic LK, Leslie JM, Eldred LJ, et al: Clinical manifestations and risk factors of *Pseudomonas aeruginosa* infection in patients with AIDS. J Infect Dis 171: 930–937, 1995

10. Dube MP, Sattler F, Torriani F, et al: A randomized study of clarithromycin plus clofazimine, with or without ethambutol, for treatment and prevention of relapse of disseminated MAC (DMAC) in AIDS (Abstract I201). 35th Interscience Conference on Antimicrobial Agents and Chemotherapy, San Francisco, CA, 1995

11. Ellner JJ, Goldberger MJ, Parenti DM: *Mycobacterium avium* infection and AIDS: Therapeutic dilemma in rapid evolution. J Infect Dis 163:1326–1335, 1991

12. Eng RHK, Forrester C, Smith SM, et al: *Mycobacterium xenopi* infection in a patient with acquired immunodeficiency syndrome. Chest 86:145–147, 1984

13. Evans KD, Nakasone AS, Sutherland PA, et al: Identification of *Mycobacterium tuberculosis* and *Mycobacterium avium-M. intracellulare* directly from primary BACTEC cultures by using acridinium-ester labelled DNA probes. J Clin Microbiol 30:2427–2431, 1992

14. Fernandes PB, Hardy DJ, McDaniel D, et al: In vitro and in vivo activities of clarithromycin against *Mycobacterium avium*. Antimicrob Agents Chemother 33: 1531–1534, 1989

15. Gangadharam PRJ, Kesavalu L, Rao PNR, et al: Activity of amikacin against *Mycobacterium avium* complex under simulated in vivo conditions. Antimicrob Agents Chemother 32:886–889, 1988

16. Godofsky EW, Zinreich J, Armstrong M, et al: Sinusitis in HIV-infected patients: A clinical and radiographic review. Am J Med 93:163–170, 1992

17. Greene JB, Sidhu GS, Lewin S, et al: *Mycobacterium avium-intracellulare:* A cause of disseminated life-threatening infection in homosexuals and drug abusers. Ann Intern Med 97:539–546, 1982

18. Hardy WD, Feinberg J, Finkelstein DM, et al: A controlled trial of trimethoprim-sulfamethoxazole or aerosolized pentamidine for secondary prophylaxis of *Pneumocystis carinii* pneumonia in patients with the acquired immunodeficiency syndrome. N Engl J Med 327:1842–1848, 1992

19. Havlik JA, Horsburgh CR, Metchock B, et al: Disseminated *Mycobacterium avium* complex infection: Clinical identification and epidemiologic trends. J Infect Dis 165:577–580, 1992

20. Hawkins CC, Gold JWM, Whimbey E, et al: *Mycobacterium avium* complex infections in patients with the acquired immunodeficiency syndrome. Ann Intern Med 105:184–188, 1986

21. Hoover DR, Saah A, Bacellar H, et al: Clinical manifestations of AIDS in the era of *Pneumocystis* prophylaxis. N Engl J Med 329:1922–1926, 1993

22. Horsburgh CR, Havlik JA, Ellis DA, et al: Survival of patients with acquired immune deficiency syndrome and disseminated *Mycobacterium avium* complex infection with and without antimycobacterial chemotherapy. Am Rev Respir Dis 144:557–559, 1991

23. Horsburgh CR, Mason UG, Farhi DC, et al: Disseminated infection with *Mycobacterium avium-intracellulare*. Medicine 64:36–48, 1985

24. Horsburgh CR, Selik RM: The epidemiology of disseminated nontuberculosis mycobacterial infection in the acquired immunodeficiency syndrome (AIDS). Am Rev Respir Dis 139:4–7, 1989

25. Inderlied CB, Kolonoski PT, Wu M, et al: Amikacin, ciprofloxacin, and imipenem treatment for disseminated *Mycobacterium avium* complex infection of beige mice. Antimicrob Agents Chemother 33: 176–180, 1989

26. Inderlied CB, Kolonoski PT, Wu M, et al: In vitro and in vivo activity of azithromycin (CP 62,993) against the *Mycobacterium avium* complex. J Infect Dis 159: 994–997, 1989

27. Jacobson MA, Gellermann H, Chambers H: *Staphyloccus aureus* bacteremia and recurrent staphyloccal infection in patients with acquired immunodeficiency syndrome and AIDS-related complex. Am J Med 85:172–176, 1988

28. Jacobson MA, Hopewell PC, Yajko DM, et al: Natural history of disseminated *Mycobacterium avium* complex infection in AIDS. J Infect Dis 164:994–998, 1991

29. Jacobson MA, Isenberg WM: *Mycobacterium kansasii* diffuse pulmonary infection in a patient with acquired immune deficiency syndrome. Am J Clin Pathol 91: 236–238, 1989

30. Jacobson MA, Peiperl L, Volberding PA, et al: Red blood cell transfusion therapy for anemia in patients with AIDS and ARC: Incidence associated factors, and outcome. Transfusion 30:133–137, 1990

31. Jacobson MA, Stanley HD, Heard SE: Ganciclovir with recombinant methionyl human granulocyte colony-stimulating factor for treatment of cytomegalovirus disease in AIDS patients (Letter). AIDS 6: 515–516, 1992

32. Jacobson MA, Yajko DM, Northfelt D, et al: Randomized, placebo-controlled trial of rifampin, ethambutol, and ciprofloxacin for AIDS patients with disseminated *Mycobacterium avium* complex infection. J Infect Dis 168:112–119, 1993

33. Janoff EN, Breiman RF, Daley CL, Hopewell PC: Pneumococcal disease during HIV infection. Ann Intern Med 117:314–324, 1992

34. Kemper C, Havlir D, Haghighat D, et al: The individual microbiologic effect of three antimycobacterial agents, clofazimine, ethambutol, and rifampin, on *Mycobacterium avium* complex bacteremia in patients with AIDS. J Infect Dis 170:157–164, 1994

35. Kemper CA, Meng TC, Nussbaum J, et al: Treatment of *Mycobacterium avium* complex bacteremia in AIDS with a four-drug oral regimen. Ann Intern Med 116: 466–472, 1992

36. Kolonoski PT, Wu M, Petrofsky ML, et al: Combination of amikacin, azithromycin and clofazimine for the treatment of disseminated *Mycobacterium avium* complex infection in beige mice (Abstract 1323). 29th International Conference on Antimicrobial Agents & Chemotherapy, Houston, 1989

37. Levine B, Chaisson RE: *Mycobacterium kansasii:* A cause of treatable pulmonary disease associated with advanced human immunodeficiency virus (HIV) infection. Ann Intern Med 114:861–868, 1991

38. Macher AM, Kovacs JA, Gill V, et al: Bacteremia due to *Mycobacterium avium-intracellulare* in the acquired immunodeficiency syndrome. Ann Intern Med 99: 782–785, 1983

39. Masur H, and the Public Health Service Task Force on Prophylaxis and Therapy for *Mycobacterium avium*

Complex: Special report: Recommendations on prophylaxis and therapy for disseminated *Mycobacterium avium* complex disease in patients infected with the human immunodeficiency virus. N Engl J Med 329:898–904, 1993

40. Morbidity and Mortality Weekly Report. Tuberculosis and human immunodeficiency virus infection: Recommendations of the Advisory Committee for the Elimination of Tuberculosis (ACET). 38:236–250, 1989

41. Moore R, Keruly J, Chaisson R: Neutropenia and bacterial infection in acquired immunodeficiency syndrome. Arch Intern Med 155:1965–1970, 1995

42. Nightingale SD, Byrd LT, Southern PM, et al: Incidence of *Mycobacterium avium-intracellulare* complex bacteremia in human immunodeficiency virus-positive patients. J Infect Dis 165:1082–1085, 1992

43. Nightingale SD, Cameron DW, Gordin FM, et al: Two controlled trials of rifabutin prophylaxis against *Mycobacterium avium* complex infection in AIDS. N Engl J Med 329:828–833, 1993

44. Packer SJ, Cesario T, Williams JH: *Mycobacterium avium* complex infection presenting as endobronchial lesions in immunosuppressed patients. Ann Intern Med 109:389–393, 1988

45. Parenti D, Ellner J, Hafner R, et al: A phase II/III trial of rifampin (RIF), ciprofloxacin (CIPRO), clofazimine (CLOF), ethambutol (ETH), + amikacin (AK) in the treatment (RX) of disseminated *Mycobacterium avium* (MA) infection in HIV-infected individuals (PTS) (Abstract 6). Second National Conference Human Retroviruses and Related Infections, Washington, DC, 1995

46. Pierce M, Crampton S, Henry D, et al: The effect of MAC and its prevention on survival in patients with advanced HIV infection (Abstract LB-18). 35th Interscience Conference on Antimicrobial Agents and Chemotherapy, San Francisco, CA, 1995

47. Rogers PL, Walker RE, Lane HC, et al: Disseminated *Mycobacterium haemophilum* infection in two patients with the acquired immunodeficiency syndrome. Am J Med 84:640–642, 1988

48. Schürmann D, Eljaschewitsch J, Sandfort J, et al: Efficacy of ciprofloxacin in treating AIDS-related bacteremic nontyphoidal salmonella infection (Abstract WS-B08-3). IX International Conference on AIDS, 1993. Berlin, Germany, 1993

49. Shafran SD, Singer J, Phillips P, The Canadian MAC Study Group: The Canadian randomized open-label trial of combination therapy for MAC bacteremia: final results (Abstract LB-20). 35th Interscience Conference on Antimicrobial Agents and Chemotherapy, San Francisco, CA, 1995

50. Shaunak S, Bartlett JA: Zidovudine-induced neutropenia: Are we too cautious? Lancet 2:91–92, 1989

51. Sherer R, Sable R, Sonnenberg M, et al: Disseminated infection with *Mycobacterium kansasii* in the acquired immunodeficiency syndrome. Ann Intern Med 105:710–712, 1986

52. Steinhart R, Reingold AL, Taylor F, et al: Invasive *Haemophilus influenzae* infections in men with HIV infection. JAMA 268:3350–3352, 1992

53. Studies of Ocular Complications of AIDS Research Group: Mortality in patients with the acquired immunodeficiency syndrome treated with either foscarnet or ganciclovir for cytomegalovirus retinitis. N Engl J Med 326:213–220, 1992

54. Sullam P, Gordin F, Wynne B, the Rifabutin Treatment Group: Efficacy of rifabutin in the treatment of disseminated infection due to *Mycobacterium avium* complex. Clin Infect Dis 19:84–86, 1994

55. Thompson C, Salvato P, Stroud S, Hasheeve D: Etiology of acute sinusitis in HIV infection (Abstract WS-B08-6). IX International Conference on AIDS, Berlin, Germany, 1993

56. Velmahos V, Alcid D: *Pseudomonas aeruginosa* bacteremia (PAB) in patients with AIDS: characterization of blood isolates and clinical features (Abstract 1078). 32nd Interscience Conference on Antimicrobial Agents and Chemotherapy, Anaheim, CA, 1992

57. Wong B, Edwards FF, Kiehn TE, et al: Continuous high-grade *Mycobacterium avium-intracellulare* bacteremia in patients with the acquired immune deficiency syndrome. Am J Med 78:35–40, 1985

58. Yajko DM, Kirihara J, Sanders C, et al: Antimicrobial synergism against *Mycobacterium avium* complex strains isolated from patients with acquired immune deficiency syndrome. Antimicrob Agents Chemother 32:1392–1395, 1988

59. Yajko DM, Nassos PS, Hadley WK: Therapeutic implications of inhibition versus killing of *Mycobacterium avium* complex by antimicrobial agents. Antimicrob Agents Chemother 31:117–120, 1987

60. Yajko DM, Sanders CA, Nassos PS, Hadley WK: In vitro susceptibility of *Mycobacterium avium* complex to the new fluoroquinolone sparfloxacin (CI-978; AT-4140) and comparison with ciprofloxacin. Antimicrob Agents Chemother 34:2442–2444, 1990

61. Young LS: *Mycobacterium avium* complex infection. J Infect Dis 157:863–867, 1988

62. Young LS, Wiviott L, Wu M, et al: Azithromycin for treatment of *Mycobacterium avium-intracellulare* complex infection in patients with AIDS. Lancet 338:1107–1109, 1991

63. Zurlo JJ, Feuerstein IM, Lebovics R, Lane HC: Sinusitis in HIV-1 infection. Am J Med 93:157–162, 1992

Chapter 22

Tuberculosis in Persons with Human Immunodeficiency Virus Infection

PHILIP C. HOPEWELL

Although tuberculosis was mentioned in early reports of the acquired immunodeficiency syndrome (AIDS), it was several years before this disorder received significant public or scientific attention.[66,70,71] Now, both because of increasing numbers of cases and because of outbreaks of disease caused by multiple-drug-resistant (MDR) organisms, tuberculosis is recognized as an important contemporary clinical and public health problem. The resurgence of tuberculosis cannot be accounted for entirely by the epidemic of human immunodeficiency virus (HIV) infection, although the HIV epidemic clearly is a major factor. In addition to the biologic phenomenon of HIV infection, socioeconomic conditions, such as homelessness, substance abuse, and increasing numbers of persons in institutions are playing an important role.[85] Moreover, because of the deterioration of the public health infrastructure, many communities are not equipped to manage either the increasing number of tuberculosis cases or the shifting epidemiologic and clinical features of the disease.[10,74] Additionally, the inattention of the scientific community to tuberculosis has resulted in there being few new tools with which to meet the increasing challenge of tuberculosis.[84] Although this review will focus on the interactions between *Mycobacterium tuberculosis* and HIV, it must be recognized that the problems of tuberculosis control relate to a much broader context.

The importance of the interaction between *M. tuberculosis* and HIV infection relates to at least five factors: (1) there is a high prevalence of tuberculosis in certain HIV-infected groups; (2) tuberculosis is probably the only HIV-related infection that is transmitted from person to person whether or not the exposed person is HIV-infected; (3) if diagnosed promptly and treated appropriately, tuberculosis has a high likelihood of being cured[44,67,82]; (4) tuberculosis can be prevented in HIV-infected populations;[65] and (5) data from several sources suggest that tuberculosis may accelerate the course of HIV disease.[92,94,95]

INCIDENCE OF TUBERCULOSIS AMONG PERSONS WITH HIV INFECTION

Several studies have examined the frequency with which tuberculosis develops in persons who are infected with both HIV and *M. tuberculosis*. In a prospective study of a group of HIV-seropositive and -seronegative intravenous drug users in New York City,[76] 7 (14%) of 49 HIV-seropositive subjects who had been known previously to have positive (≥5-mm induration) tuberculin skin test reactions and one anergic (defined by failure to react to tuberculin and seven additional intradermal antigens) patient developed tuberculosis in a 2-year period. This was the equivalent of 7.9 cases per 100 person-years of observation. These observations suggest that seven and perhaps all eight patients who developed tuberculosis had had preexisting tuberculous infection, indicating that endogenous reactivation was the dominant if not the only pathogenetic mechanism for developing tuberculosis. Of additional concern was the observation that 11% and 13% of the seropositive and seronegative subjects, respectively, developed positive tuberculin skin tests during the period of the study. If this observation is truly indicative of new infections, it suggests that there was a large number of infectious cases within the population.

A subsequent report on that same cohort found that the incidence of tuberculosis was 6.6 cases per 100 person-years in HIV-infected study subjects who were anergic compared with 9.7 cases among those who were tuberculin-positive.[77] It could be assumed that in a population with a high prevalence of tuberculin reactors, a negative tuberculin skin test in an HIV-infected person would likely be a false-negative and that failure to react to the other antigens was a marker for severe immune compromise. Thus, such persons would be expected to have a high rate of tuberculosis. It would not be expected that this high risk of tuberculosis would apply to anergic persons from groups in which the prevalence of tuberculin reactivity (tuberculous infection) is low. This has been the observation in a large cohort of HIV-infected persons followed prospectively. In this group, the incidence of tuberculosis among anergic subjects was 0.69 per 100 person-years, whereas among tuberculin-positive persons, the incidence was 2.23 per 100 person-years (Pulmonary Complications of HIV Infection Study Group, personal communication).

A prospective study of a group of urban women of childbearing age in Kigali, Rwanda, found that the incidence of tuberculosis was approximately 2.5% per year.[1] In comparison with HIV-negative women, the risk ratio for tuberculosis among the HIV-positive women was 22.9. Among the HIV-positive women, having had a positive tuberculin skin test was associated with a significantly increased risk of tuberculosis but the risk ratio was only 3, and 9 of 17 patients with tuberculosis had negative tuberculin tests, perhaps as a result of anergy.

In a prospective study conducted in 23 hospital infectious disease units in Italy,[4] the 12-month rate of tuberculosis among 2760 HIV-infected subjects was 2.2%. Among subjects with positive (≥ 5 mm) tuberculin tests, the 12-month incidence was 4.5%, whereas among persons who were anergic (failed to respond to seven intradermal antigens) the incidence was 2.9%. The cohort from which these data were derived consisted largely (72%) of injecting drug users.

The rate of tuberculosis in injecting drug users has been prospectively determined in a cohort from Baltimore,[41] where the overall annual rate of tuberculosis of 0.22% was substantially lower than the rate reported from Italy.[4]

There are at least four factors that influence the rate of tuberculosis among cohorts of persons with HIV infection. The first of these factors is the prevalence of latent infection with *M. tuberculosis* in the population from which the cohort was drawn. Second is the likelihood of exposure of cohort members to persons with infectious tuberculosis. This tends to parallel the prevalence of tuberculous infection in the population the cohort represents. The third factor is the severity of immune compromise among cohort members and, thus, their likelihood of developing tuberculosis if infected with the organism. Finally, the use of isoniazid preventive therapy by cohort members will have an important effect in reducing the incidence of tuberculosis.

Variations among these factors probably account for the differences in reported rates of tuberculosis in different cohorts. For example, cohorts consisting largely of middle class homosexual/bisexual men or hemophiliacs would be expected to have low rates of tuberculosis, whereas cohorts of injecting drug users living in inner cities would have high rates. Thus, tuberculosis incidence data reported for one cohort may not apply to other groups, and there is no single figure that accurately defines the risk of tuberculosis in persons with HIV infection.

PREVALENCE OF HIV INFECTION AMONG PATIENTS WITH TUBERCULOSIS

Several prospective studies in urban tuberculosis clinics have measured the prevalence of HIV infection among patients with tuberculosis. In Miami, 31% of 71 consecutive tuberculosis patients were HIV-infected.[69] In Seattle, 23% of non-Asian adults were infected with HIV.[61] In San Francisco, 28% of non-Asian tuberculosis patients between 15 and 55 years of age were HIV-seropositive.[91]

Beginning in 1988, a systematic nationwide sampling of HIV infection prevalence was undertaken by the Centers for Disease Control (CDC) in 14 urban tuberculosis clinics.[64] The median seropositivity rate in 4301 persons with or suspected of having tuberculosis was 3.4%. The rates varied widely (from 0% to 46%) among clinics. The highest rate was reported from New York City (46%) followed by Newark (34%), Boston (27%), Miami (24%), and Baltimore (13%). In 1990, the survey was expanded to 24 clinics in 16 cities and the median HIV

TABLE 22–1. ESTIMATE OF NUMBERS OF PERSONS, 15 TO 49 YEARS OF AGE, INFECTED WITH BOTH HIV AND *MYCOBACTERIUM TUBERCULOSIS*: 1992

WHO Region	Millions HIV infected	Tb Infected	Millions Dual Infection
Africa	6.50	48%	3.12 (78)§
Americas*	1.00	30%	0.30 (7.5)
Eastern Mediterranean	0.05	23%	0.11 (0.3)
Southeast Asia, and western Pacific†	1.02	40%	0.41 (10.2)
Europe and others‡	<u>1.55</u>	<u>11%</u>	<u>0.17</u> (4.2)
TOTAL	10.12	34%	4.01

* Excludes USA and Canada.
† Excludes Japan, Australia, New Zealand.
‡ USA, Canada, Japan, Australia, New Zealand.
§ Figures in parentheses are percentage of total.
From Raviglione MC, Narain JP, Kochi A: HIV-associated tuberculosis in developing countries: Clinical features, diagnosis and treatment. Bull WHO 70:515–526, 1992, with permission.

seropositivity rate was 7.5%.[63] In 1991, 33 clinics in 20 cities reported a median seropositivity rate of 9.5%. Trend data are available for 13 large urban areas in which surveys were conducted each year. The overall seroprevalence rate in these areas was 13% in 1989, 18% in 1990, and 21% in 1991. Between 1989 and 1991, HIV seroprevalence among males increased from 15% to 28% among Hispanics, 24% to 40% among African-Americans, and 12% to 20% among whites. Among Asians, the HIV seroprevalence was less than 1% throughout the period. Extrapolating from these data and from tuberculosis case rates, Onorato and associates[63] estimated approximately 2000 tuberculosis patients between 15 and 54 years of age were infected with HIV in the 13 areas participating in the study.

Data from developing countries indicate a substantial rate of HIV infection among patients with tuberculosis.[22,27,37,38,53,56,62,73,86] The World Health Organization[73] has estimated that worldwide there are probably approximately 4 million persons who are infected with both *M. tuberculosis* and HIV, nearly 80% of these being in Africa (Table 22–1). A summary of various studies[27] indicated that the prevalence of HIV infection among tuberculosis patients in sub-Saharan African countries ranged from 20% to 67%. Most of these reports have originated from urban areas. Whether or not the data are representative of the respective countries as a whole is not known.

IMPACT OF HIV INFECTION ON THE INCIDENCE OF TUBERCULOSIS

The full impact of HIV infection on the epidemiology of tuberculosis has not been defined either in the United States or abroad. Inferential information suggests, however, that the influence may be substantial. Data from the CDC[11] indicated that in the United States between 1985 and 1992 there were at least 50,000 cases of tuberculosis in excess of what would have been predicted based on the rate of decline in cases between 1953 and 1984. Although these additional cases were not proven to be attributable to HIV infection, the largest increases occurred in the areas with the highest prevalence of HIV infection. Fortunately, considerable effort has led to a decrease in tuberculosis case rates in 1993 and 1994.[12] Continued attention will be required, however, to maintain these reductions.

Country-wide data tend to underestimate the effects of HIV infection on the incidence of tuberculosis in certain parts of the United States. Perhaps the most profound effects have occurred in New York City.[10] Between 1984 and 1991 the tuberculosis case rate increased from 19.9 to 36 per 100,000 population, an 81% rise.[10,17] The increase in case rates was even more dramatic in central Harlem, where in 1989 the rate reached 169 per 100,000 persons, quite similar to case rates in eastern and central Africa.[10] In 1979 the rate in this area was 50.9 per 100,000.

In some areas of the country, although overall rates of tuberculosis have not changed dramatically, the main risk groups for the disease have changed. For example, in San Francisco during the early 1990s there was a shift away from foreign-born Asians toward U.S.-born African-Americans and whites. This shift was especially evident among persons in whom tuberculosis appears to have developed as a result of recent infection, as determined by restriction fragment length polymorphism (RFLP) analysis.[81]

Globally, the epidemic of HIV infection has had an enormous impact on the incidence of tuberculosis. In countries such as Tanzania, where a successful tuberculosis control program had been established, case rates have nearly doubled. As noted previously, the World Health Organization[73] estimates that approximately 4 million persons are infected with both *M. tuberculosis* and HIV. Although, currently, most of these dually infected persons are in Africa, in Asia there are many more persons infected with *M. tuberculosis,* and HIV infection is increasing rapidly. It is anticipated that, ultimately, HIV infection will have its greatest impact on the incidence of tuberculosis in Asia.

INFLUENCE OF HIV INFECTION ON THE PATHOGENESIS OF TUBERCULOSIS

Tuberculosis can develop either by direct progression from recently acquired infection or by reactivation of latent infection. In areas of low prevalence of tuberculosis, it is generally thought that most cases arise from latent infections, because few new infections are occurring.[23,88] However, because HIV impairs the ability to contain new tuberculous infection, the risk of rapid progression is much greater among persons with HIV infection, thus, an increasing number of cases may be occurring via this sequence. In addition, as the number of new cases providing more sources of infection increases, there will be more transmission of infection and, therefore, more opportunity for direct progression to occur. Under these circumstances, the epidemiology of tuberculosis in some parts of the United States may evolve to resemble that of developing countries in which there is a high prevalence of the disease.

Cell-mediated immunity is the predominant mechanism by which a contained tuberculous infection is kept quiescent.[26] Because of the effect HIV infection has on cell-mediated immunity, the likelihood of reactivation of latent tuberculous infection leading to clinical tuberculosis is greatly increased. For this reason persons who previously had been infected with *M. tuberculosis* are at considerably increased risk of developing tuberculosis after being infected with HIV.

In the normal host, once the cell-mediated immune response to infection with *M. tuberculosis* develops, there is a low likelihood that new exogenous infection will be acquired.[87] How-

ever, reinfection has been documented in persons without evident immune compromise.[59] Because of the immune defect induced by HIV, a person who has been previously infected with *M. tuberculosis* may still be much more vulnerable to new infection. Reinfection with drug-resistant organisms has been demonstrated by RFLP analysis among persons being treated for tuberculosis.[83] Thus, reinfection in persons with HIV infection may account for "relapses" after successful completion of antituberculosis therapy and also is a mechanism by which multidrug resistance can develop.

It has been speculated that HIV-infected patients are more likely to acquire tuberculous infection when exposed to *M. tuberculosis.*[25] Although this concept is unsubstantiated, it has been clearly demonstrated that once an HIV-infected person becomes infected with *M. tuberculosis,* the infection can progress very rapidly to cause clinical disease.[25,28] In situations where groups of HIV-infected persons are exposed to a patient with infectious tuberculosis, explosive outbreaks of tuberculosis may occur. For example, in a residential care facility for HIV-infected persons in San Francisco, tuberculosis occurred within 120 days in 11 of 31 (35%) residents exposed to a person with infectious tuberculosis.[25] The use of RFLP analysis confirmed that tuberculosis was caused by the same strain of *M. tuberculosis* in all 11 of the culture-positive patients. This pathogenetic sequence is undoubtedly responsible for the explosive outbreaks of tuberculosis caused by multiple-drug-resistant organisms that have occurred in several areas of the country.[50]

Presumably because of the pathogenicity of *M. tuberculosis,* tuberculosis tends to occur relatively early in the course of HIV infection. This is attested to by the findings of several groups that HIV-seropositive patients with tuberculosis tend to have CD4 lymphocyte counts higher than patients with other "opportunistic" infections such as *Pneumocystis carinii* pneumonia.[91,78] For example, in a study of 17 patients,[91] tuberculosis was the initial manifestation of HIV infection in all but two patients, and the median CD4 lymphocyte count was 354/μl.

DIAGNOSIS OF TUBERCULOUS INFECTION AND TUBERCULOSIS IN HIV-INFECTED PATIENTS

Tuberculin Skin Testing and Anergy Testing

As would be expected, the tuberculin skin test commonly shows little or no reaction in persons with advanced HIV infection. However, in earlier stages of the infection, reactivity may be maintained. The ability to respond to tuberculin is an indicator of the status of cell-mediated immunity that in turn is an indicator of the stage of HIV infection.

The prevalence of positive (≥5-mm induration) tuberculin skin tests decreased progressively as the CD4 cell count decreased in one study.[57] The relationship between CD4 cell count and the prevalence of tuberculin reactions is shown in Figure 22–1A. In addition, the rate of reactivity to mumps and candida skin test antigens was related to the CD4 count. Stated conversely, the prevalence of anergy increased with decreasing CD4 counts as shown in Figure 22–1B. It should be noted, however, that the prevalence of anergy was 42% among

non–HIV-infected injecting drug users and 12% among homosexual bisexual men. This finding indicates the elusive nature of the definition and physiologic implications of "anergy" and suggests that this finding should not weigh heavily in clinical decision-making.

Because of the frequency of blunted skin test responses, or anergy, it is recommended by the American Thoracic Society and the CDC that a reaction of ≥5-mm induration to 5 tuberculin units of purified protein derivative be regarded as indicative of tuberculous infection in HIV-infected persons.[3,16] The implications of using 5 mm as the cutoff for defining tuberculous infection have not been determined. One study found that a 5-mm cutoff for determining tuberculin positivity probably underestimated the rates of tuberculous infection and recom-

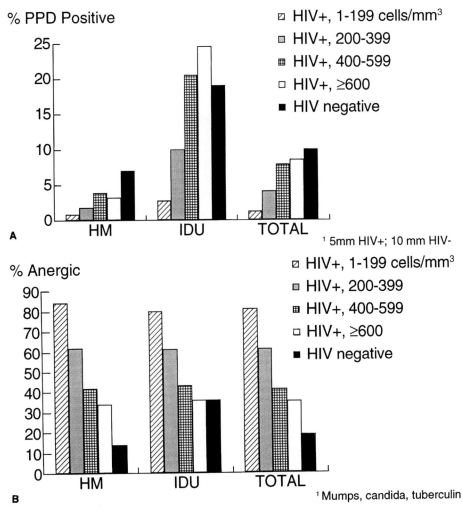

FIGURE 22–1. *A*, Tuberculin reactions in HIV infection (5 mm HIV+; 10 mm HIV−). *B*, Skin test anergy (mumps, *Candida*, tuberculin) in HIV infection. HM, homosexual men; IDU, injecting drug user.

mended a 2-mm cutoff.[42] The practicality of using such a small reaction size to define infection would appear to impose significant limitations on its use, however.[46] The validity of a 5-mm cutoff is suggested by the finding that the risk of tuberculosis is substantially increased in persons with reaction sizes ≥5 mm compared with the risk in persons with a 1- to 5-mm reaction (Pulmonary Complications of HIV Infection Study, personal communication).

Anergy testing has been recommended to determine if a negative tuberculin test is the result of immunosuppression or is truly negative, as well as to provide information as to the stage of HIV disease.[15] The antigens used include those made from candida organisms, mumps virus, and tetanus toxoid to which it is assumed that persons with intact cell-mediated immunity will respond. As noted previously, anergy may be found among persons who have no identifiable immunosuppression, thus limiting the clinical applicability of anergy testing. Moreover, in a group of patients tested at yearly intervals with tuberculin, mumps, and candida antigens, 31% of those who were "anergic" initially developed a positive reaction on follow-up testing.[19] In addition, nearly 39% of subjects who were initially tuberculin-positive and became tuberculin-negative on subsequent testing (false-negative) had positive reactions to mumps antigen at the same time as the false-negative tuberculin test.

Clinical Features of Tuberculosis

The clinical manifestations of tuberculosis occurring in patients with HIV infection vary considerably, depending on the severity of the immunosuppression.[6,18,27,43,49,54,66,70,71,78,90,91] Presumably because of the virulence of *M. tuberculosis*, tuberculosis may occur early in the course of HIV infection. In most series the majority of tuberculosis diagnoses have preceded the identification of another AIDS-defining disease. A substantial number of patients are defined as having AIDS because of a diagnosis of tuberculosis, and in a smaller number, tuberculosis appears after an AIDS diagnosis.

It has been shown that the earlier tuberculosis develops, the more "usual" is its clinical presentation, whereas the later it occurs, the more atypical are its features.[49] Clinical reports have emphasized that tuberculosis in advanced HIV infection is frequently disseminated, has unusual radiographic manifestations, and nonreactive tuberculin skin tests. Lymph node involvement, including intrathoracic adenopathy, has been described frequently. A retrospective analysis that correlated the manifestations of tuberculosis with CD4 lymphocyte counts in patients with HIV infection reported a clear association between low CD4 cell counts and an increased frequency of extrapulmonary tuberculosis, positive blood cultures for *M. tuberculosis*, and intrathoracic adenopathy on chest radiograms.[49] Conversely, pleural effusions were more frequent in persons with CD4 cell counts ≥200/μl.

A variety of unusual manifestations of tuberculosis have been noted in HIV-infected patients. These include central nervous system involvement with brain abscesses, tuberculomas, and meningitis[8,34,90]; bone (including vertebral) disease[55,90]; as well as pericarditis[24,90] gastric tuberculosis,[9] tuberculous peritonitis,[5] and scrotal tuberculosis.[89] In addition, *M. tuberculosis* has been cultured from blood as well as bone marrow.[49,58,75,79]

Despite the increased frequency of unusual forms of tuberculosis in persons with HIV infection, standard pulmonary disease tends to predominate in most series.[49,61,76,91]

Radiographic Findings

The atypical findings on chest radiographs of HIV-infected patients who have tuberculosis have received considerable emphasis. In retrospective studies, features that are not regarded as "typical" for pulmonary tuberculosis have been the norm.[18,72] Lower lung zone or diffuse infiltrations commonly have been observed rather than the usual upper lobe involvement. Cavitation has been unusual and intrathoracic adenopathy, an unusual finding in immunocompetent adults with tuberculosis, has been relatively frequent.[49]

In a prospective study by Theuer and colleagues,[91] the radiographic findings in patients with HIV infection were not distinguishable from those in patients who were HIV-seronegative. The findings included typical upper lobe infiltration, often with cavitation. A greater prevalence of atypical findings was noted in another prospective study.[69] These findings included a higher frequency of adenopathy, diffuse or lower lobe infiltration, and a lower frequency of cavitation compared with HIV-seronegative patients.

An evaluation of the radiographic course of treated pulmonary tuberculosis in persons with HIV infection[80] found that, in general, there was rapid improvement with little residual scarring after completion of therapy. Of note was the fact that all eight patients who had radiographic worsening had new superimposed diseases.

Bacteriologic and Histologic Examinations

Most reported series indicate that the prevalence of positive sputum smears and cultures in patients with pulmonary tuberculosis is approximately the same in HIV-infected and -noninfected persons, although this finding has not been universal.[62,69,91] In some instances, sputum induction or bronchoscopic procedures have been necessary to diagnose pulmonary tuberculosis. Specimens from any site of abnormality in patients with or suspected of having HIV infection should be examined for mycobacteria by smear and culture. Potential high-yield sources include lymph nodes, bone marrow, urine, and blood. In general, any acid-fast organism identified in any specimen should be regarded as being *M. tuberculosis* until proven otherwise. Such a policy will result in prompt initiation of appropriate therapy for tuberculosis and evaluation of persons in contact with the new case. With traditional methods using solid opaque media, detection of growth and speciation of mycobacteria requires 6 to 10 weeks. Radiometric culture techniques and the use of DNA probes for identification of *M. tuberculosis* and *M. avium* complex can shorten this procedure to 7 to 10 days, thereby adding greatly to the speed and efficiency of tuberculosis control measures.[39] The use of the polymerase chain reaction (PCR) for identification of *M. tuberculosis* should result in much more rapid diagnoses.[21,31,35] However, the applicability of PCR-based diagnostic tests is not yet established in day-to-day clinical use. To date, most studies have found that PCR-based methods are not more sensitive than culture.[20] Nevertheless, because of their rapidity and specificity, PCR-based methods will be a very useful adjunct in microbiologic evaluations.

In patients with more advanced HIV infection, mycobacterial infection does not produce classic granulomas. However, because tuberculosis tends to occur when HIV disease is less advanced, the ability to form granulomas may be intact. Thus, the finding of granulomas either in tissue sections or in cytologic preparations from needle aspiration biopsies should be interpreted as being more consistent with tuberculosis than nontuberculous mycobacterial disease.

TREATMENT

Most reported series of patients with tuberculosis and HIV infection demonstrate a good response to antituberculosis treatment when regimens containing isoniazid and rifampin are used.[18,43,54,69–71,82,90,91] However, in the series reported by Sunderam and co-workers[90] there were three patients who did not respond to treatment and had progressive disease. A case report from the same institution described a recurrence of tuberculosis at an extrapulmonary site (scrotal) after apparently successful treatment for pulmonary disease.[89] These reports have led to expressions of concern regarding the adequacy of current standard 6-month therapy.[47] There is now, however, substantial information indicating that treatment regimens that include isoniazid and rifampin for a full 6 months supplemented by ethambutol (or streptomycin) and pyrazinamide are as effective in HIV-infected patients with tuberculosis as those without HIV infection. However, in a study in Zaire, prolonging isoniazid and rifampin administration for an additional 6 months resulted in a lower relapse rate compared with the results in a group given placebo. Of note was the fact that the HIV-uninfected control group had the same relapse rate as the HIV-infected control group.[67]

In a prospective study comparing the outcome of therapy in HIV-infected and -noninfected patients in Haiti,[44] the treatment regimen consisted of isoniazid, rifampin, pyrazinamide, and ethambutol given three times weekly for 2 months, followed by isoniazid and rifampin three times weekly for 4 months. Although the death rate from nontuberculosis causes was greater among the HIV-infected group, rates of treatment failure and relapse were not different between HIV-seropositive patients and those who were not infected.

Current recommendations state that for adult patients with HIV infection, treatment for tuberculosis should include isoniazid 300 mg/day, rifampin 600 mg/day (450 mg/day for persons weighing <50 kg), pyrazinamide 20 to 30 mg/kg/day and ethambutol 15 mg/kg/day during the first 2 months of therapy; isoniazid and rifampin should be continued for at least another 4 months, making the total duration of therapy at least 6 months.[2] For patients judged to be potentially noncompliant, therapy should be given under direct observation. This can be facilitated by twice-weekly drug administration after an initial phase of daily treatment.

For patients with pulmonary tuberculosis, response to therapy should be determined by bacteriologic examination of sputum as well as by clinical and radiographic examinations. In patients with less accessible sites of disease, generally, only clinical and radiographic evaluations can be used to determine the response. It should be kept in mind that worsening clinical and radiographic findings may be caused by other HIV-related diseases. There is probably less of a margin for error (i.e., missed doses) in patients with HIV infection; thus, the threshold for prolonging therapy should be lower. If there is a period of noncompliance or if the disease responds more slowly than would be expected, treatment should be prolonged. Overall, however, it is probably more important to supervise closely a regimen of 6 months than to give a longer regimen with a lesser degree of supervision. Patients who cannot take isoniazid *and* rifampin together should be treated for a minimum of 18 months, usually with isoniazid *or* rifampin and ethambutol plus pyrazinamide in the initial phase. This recommendation also applies to patients with tuberculosis caused by organisms that are resistant to isoniazid *or* rifampin.

It appears that the rate of adverse reactions to antituberculosis drugs is greater in persons with HIV infection, although this has not been a uniform finding.[44,82] For this reason patients with HIV infection should be followed closely with appropriate laboratory and clinical monitoring. There has been no systematic evaluation of possible interactions of antituberculosis drugs with antiretroviral agents. The potential for increased toxicity should, however, be kept in mind. The antifungal agents ketoconazole and fluconazole both have interactions with isoniazid and rifampin resulting in reduction in serum concentrations of the antifungal agents.[32,52] In addition, ketoconazole interferes with the absorption of rifampin.[32] Impaired absorption of antituberculosis drugs may also occur in patients with HIV infection, presumably as a consequence of gastrointestinal disease. For this reason, if the response to treatment is suboptimal, serum drug concentrations should be measured.[68]

Because of the potential modifications of treatment regimens for patients with HIV infec-

tion, HIV antibody testing is desirable and should be offered to all patients with new diagnoses of tuberculosis.

TUBERCULOSIS CAUSED BY MULTIPLE-DRUG-RESISTANT ORGANISMS

Explosive outbreaks of tuberculosis caused by MDR organisms (usually resistant to at least both isoniazid and rifampin) were described in the early 1990s.[30,33,50] These outbreaks took place in hospitals and clinics and have predominantly involved HIV-infected patients.[7,14] Health care workers, both HIV-seropositive and negative, were infected. Substantial epidemiologic and laboratory (RFLP analysis) data indicated that transmission of the resistant *M. tuberculosis* took place in the health care facility. These outbreaks were characterized by very high case fatality rates, ranging from 72% to 89% after median times of 4 to 16 weeks. Also noteworthy were the relatively high rates of tuberculin skin test conversions among health care workers exposed to these patients.

There are at least three major factors that led to these outbreaks. The first was a relatively high prevalence of multiple drug resistance in the community at large and particularly in the groups that, in some areas, are most likely to be HIV-infected.[36] This high prevalence of drug resistance, which was a predictable outcome of the lack of attention and resources devoted to tuberculosis during at least the 1970s and 1980s, provided a reservoir of MDR organisms. Second is the effect of HIV on the host response to tuberculous infection. Recently acquired infection with *M. tuberculosis* in an HIV-infected person may progress very rapidly to cause clinical disease, which in turn is capable of being transmitted.[25,28] If the organism causing disease in the index patient is MDR, all of the secondary infections will be caused by MDR organisms. The third factor relates to the fact that tuberculosis in HIV-infected persons may not be so easily recognizable as in persons with a normal immune status. For that reason, the disease may go undiagnosed, perhaps in a hospital or clinic environment, for a relatively prolonged period of time.[51] During this time, unless adequate infection control measures are applied presumptively, the patient will be capable of transmitting the infection. Moreover, even if the disease is diagnosed it may not be appreciated for several weeks that the organisms are MDR because of the time required for standard techniques to identify drug resistance.

An additional important factor that contributed to the spread of MDR organisms was the lack of effective environmental controls for airborne infections in many health care facilities.[60] Even if the disease is recognized, the isolation measures applied may not be effective; consequently, transmission may occur within the facility. Because of concern with the ability of ventilation alone to provide adequate environmental control, consideration should be given to the use of ultraviolet light irradiation and filtration of ambient air.

Prompt recognition and treatment of tuberculosis caused by MDR organisms presents considerable difficulty. First, the organism must be recognized to be drug resistant. With radiometric techniques and direct inoculation of drug-containing media for every specimen, resistance patterns could be known in 7 to 10 days. However, this is a very inefficient approach and could quickly overload a laboratory. A more efficient approach would be to screen for resistance to one agent, probably rifampin, and infer multiple drug resistance if there is resistance to rifampin. If this were applied only to specimens in which acid-fast organisms are seen on smear, potential transmission of MDR organisms could be greatly reduced. A more traditional system would be to perform direct susceptibility testing on specimens that are positive for acid-fast organisms on microscopy and to do indirect testing on specimens that are smear-negative, culture-positive. By this last method, using radiometric techniques, a result would not be obtained for 14 to 21 days. If the traditional solid media and indirect testing were done, identification of resistant organisms would require 8 to 12 weeks. Under current circumstances in many areas in the United States, such delays are not acceptable.

Because of the possible delays, in areas where there is a high prevalence of tuberculosis caused by resistant organisms, empiric therapy based on endemic resistance patterns may be necessary. Such therapy should be based on knowledge of the prevailing patterns of resistance. Once the drug susceptibility results are known, regimens can be appropriately tailored. *Always,* at least two agents to which the organisms are thought to be susceptible should be used. In some instances, this may entail use of agents such as the fluorquinolones and ami-

kacin that are not yet approved as antituberculosis drugs. Table 22–2 lists possible regimens that may be used for MDR tuberculosis.[48] It should be noted that the newer macrolide antimicrobial agents that are effective against *M. avium* complex do not have significant activity against *M. tuberculosis.*[48] Treatment regimens for patients with MDR tuberculosis have not been well studied and, because of the large number of potential combinations, probably will never be subjected to prospective trials. Experience from the National Jewish Center reported by Goble and associates[40] has shown that the overall rate of cure among patients with MDR tuberculosis who were not immunocompromised was 56%.

PREVENTION

The effectiveness of isoniazid preventive therapy in persons infected with both HIV and *M. tuberculosis* has been substantiated in two reports. In a study conducted in Haiti,[65] administration of isoniazid 300 mg/day for 12 months significantly decreased the incidence of tuberculosis compared with placebo. Among newly identified HIV-infected persons who were without symptoms, rates of tuberculosis were 2.2 per 100 person-years for those given isoniazid compared with 7.5 per 100 person-years in subjects given placebo. This benefit was confined to subjects who had positive tuberculin skin test reactions. Subjects with positive tuberculin tests who were given placebo had an incidence of tuberculosis of 10 per 100 person-years compared with 1.7 per 100 person-years in those given placebo. The rates in tuberculin-negative subjects (including those who were anergic) were 5.7 and 3.2 per 100 person-years for the placebo- and isoniazid-treated groups, respectively, a difference that was not statistically significant. In addition to the benefit in preventing tuberculosis, it was observed that the group treated with isoniazid had a slower rate of progression to AIDS and also a lower risk of death. Again, this benefit was found only in the tuberculin-positive group. Earlier preliminary data from a prospective controlled trial in Zambia also showed substantial protection with isoniazid.[93]

In view of these data, tuberculin testing should be performed as a routine part of management for patients with HIV infection. Patients with reactions of ≥5 mm to 5 tuberculin units of purified protein derivative should be

TABLE 22-2. POTENTIAL REGIMENS FOR PATIENTS WITH TUBERCULOSIS WITH VARIOUS PATTERNS OF DRUG RESISTANCE

Resistance	Suggested Regimen	Duration of Therapy	Comments
Isoniazid, streptomycin, and pyrazinamide	Rifampin Pyrazinamide Ethambutol Amikacin*	6 to 9 mo	Anticipate 100% response rate and 5% relapse rate
Isoniazid and ethambutol (± streptomycin)	Rifampin Pyrazinamide Ofloxacin or ciprofloxacin Amikacin*	6 to 12 mo	Efficacy should be comparable to above regimen
Isoniazid and rifampin (± streptomycin)	Pyrazinamide Ethambutol Ofloxacin or ciprofloxacin Amikacin*	18 to 24 mo	Consider surgery
Isoniazid, rifampin, and ethambutol (± streptomycin)	Pyrazinamide Ofloxacin or ciprofloxacin Amikacin* Plus 2†	24 mo after conversion	Consider surgery
Isoniazid, rifampin, and pyrazinamide (± streptomycin)	Ethambutol Ofloxacin or ciprofloxacin Amikacin* Plus 2†	24 mo after conversion	Consider surgery
Isoniazid, rifampin, pyrazinamide, and ethambutol (± streptomycin)	Ofloxacin or ciprofloxacin Plus 3† Amikacin*	24 mo after conversion	Surgery, if possible

* If there is resistance to amikacin, kanamycin, and streptomycin, capreomycin is a good alternative. Injectable agents are usually continued for 4 to 6 months if toxicity does not intervene. All the injectable drugs are given daily (or twice or thrice weekly) and may be administered intravenously or intramuscularly.

† Potential agents from which to choose: ethionamide, cycloserine, or aminosalicylic acid. Others that are potentially useful but of unproved utility include clofazimine and amoxicillin/clavulanate. Clarithromycin, azithromycin, and rifabutin are unlikely to be active (see text).

From Iseman MDR: Treatment of multi-drug-resistant tuberculosis. N Engl J Med 329:784–791, 1993, with permission.

considered to have tuberculous infection and be offered preventive therapy. Treatment for 12 months is recommended for patients with HIV infection.[16] There are no data that suggest treatment for more than 12 months confers additional protection. Rifampin should be used as preventive therapy in persons exposed to and presumably infected with isoniazid-resistant organisms, although there are no data to support this recommendation. Recommendations for preventive therapy in persons thought to be infected with organisms resistant to isoniazid and rifampin are difficult to formulate. The use of experimental regimens such as pyrazinamide and a fluoroquinolone may be the only option.[48]

In HIV-infected persons exposed to a person with infectious tuberculosis, preventive therapy should be given regardless of the results of tuberculin skin testing. For this reason, it is important to know the HIV status of close contacts of newly discovered cases. Moreover, as opposed to the recommendations that apply in non–HIV-infected close contacts, repeated courses of preventive therapy should be given if there are subsequent exposures.

INFECTION CONTROL

As noted in the introduction, tuberculosis is the only common HIV-associated infection that can be transmitted from person to person, including persons who are not HIV-infected. For this reason, it is extremely important that tuberculosis be taken into account in applying infection control measures in persons with HIV infection. In patients who are being evaluated because of respiratory symptoms and/or findings, respiratory precautions should be applied until tuberculosis is excluded. Sputum induction and bronchoscopy should be performed in areas with adequate ventilation, with the exhausted air not being recirculated to other parts of the building. Similar considerations should apply to areas in which aerosol penta-midine is administered. Transmission of tuberculosis infection has occurred in a poorly ventilated clinic where aerosol pentamidine prophylaxis for *P. carinii* pneumonia was being administered to two patients whose sputum contained *M. tuberculosis*.[13] Guidelines for the prevention of nosocomial transmission of *M. tuberculosis* have been developed by the CDC.[29]

Because of the potentially severe consequences of new tuberculous infections in immunocompromised patients, it is prudent to be cautious in patients with tuberculosis who will be in contact with HIV-infected persons. In most patients who are being treated effectively, because of the decrease in the number of bacilli present in sputum and a decrease in the frequency of coughing, infectivity is reduced by more than 99% within 2 weeks of beginning treatment.[45] Even with a reduction of this magnitude, sputum smears may still show acid-fast bacilli. To be even more confident that infectiousness is extremely low, precautions may continue to be applied until sputum smears are negative. In most instances, however, 2 weeks of therapy is sufficient, assuming the organisms are susceptible to the agents given.

NECESSARY CHANGES IN APPROACHES TO TUBERCULOSIS CONTROL

Infection with HIV has caused a dramatic change in the natural history of tuberculosis. No longer can it be assumed that only approximately one third of close contacts of new cases will be infected as has been generally true in the United States. As noted previously, there is inferential evidence that HIV-infected persons are more likely to acquire infection with *M. tuberculosis* than is the general population.[28] Perhaps of more importance, it is quite clear that an HIV-infected person who acquires a new infection with *M. tuberculosis* is much more likely to progress rapidly to have clinical tuberculosis.[25,28] As a consequence of the rapid progression, case fatality rates for tuberculosis are much higher than in nonimmunocompromised patients, with the vast majority of fatalities occurring before treatment is started or in the first month of therapy.[82] Contributing to the higher case fatality rates is the occurrence of tuberculosis caused by MDR organisms. Su-

perimposed on these changes in the nature of the disease is the fact that the HIV-infected patients in whom tuberculosis is of greater likelihood are also more difficult to maintain on a regular treatment regimen. Thus, because there is less of a "margin of safety" in treating patients with HIV infection, labor-intensive schemes such as directly observed therapy are commonly needed.

It is clear from the major points covered in this review that basic tuberculosis control measures must be applied more quickly and with greater intensity in order to be effective. Specific applications of the principles discussed can be summarized as follows:

1. At least in hospitals and clinics providing care for HIV-infected persons, rapid radiometric means of detecting growth of mycobacteria should be used and DNA probes or other rapid techniques should be used for speciation of organisms. If such technology is not available in a given institution, strong consideration should be given to using another laboratory in which they are available.

2. Sensitivity testing of organisms isolated should be performed as quickly as possible using techniques described above.

3. Screening investigations of persons in contact with a new case of tuberculosis should be initiated immediately upon identification of a presumed (positive smear) or confirmed case. The contact interview should be performed by a person who has some familiarity with the lifestyle of the new patient in order to identify unsuspected settings in which transmission of *M. tuberculosis* may have occurred. All contacts identified should be evaluated promptly. If it is thought that either the case or his or her contacts are at risk of HIV infection, the contact should be asked his or her HIV status or be advised to have the test performed. If the contact is known or thought to be at risk of being HIV-infected, decisions about preventive therapy should not be based on skin test results; rather, preventive therapy should be given to contacts regardless of the skin test results after active tuberculosis has been excluded. Preventive therapy for persons suspected of having been infected with drug-resistant organisms should be based on prevailing sensitivity patterns.

If it is suspected or known that the contact is HIV-infected, careful questioning regarding possible symptoms of tuberculosis should be undertaken and the patient should have a thorough physical examination and chest film to exclude current tuberculosis.

4. HIV-infected patients with tuberculosis should be treated initially with isoniazid, rifampin, ethambutol, and pyrazinamide. The last two drugs can be discontinued after 2 months. The duration of therapy generally should be 6 months. Because compliance is the most important determinant of outcome, directly observed therapy is the preferable treatment scheme. As with the contact investigation, supervision of therapy is best done by a health care worker familiar with the patient's lifestyle.

If there are problems with compliance or if the response to therapy, judged clinically, radiographically, or bacteriologically, is suboptimal, therapy should be prolonged. It should be kept in mind, however, that apparent treatment failure or relapse may be caused by another HIV-related disease, not necessarily tuberculosis.

If drug resistance is known or proven, appropriate regimens that are based on prevailing community susceptibility patterns or measured sensitivities should be used. In these situations, more prolonged therapy is necessary.

5. Management of persons with HIV infection should include tuberculin testing, preferably before the CD4 cell count has declined markedly. All persons with HIV infection and positive tuberculin skin tests should be treated with isoniazid for 12 months after active tuberculosis has been excluded.

6. Appropriate infection control measures must be rigorously applied. This includes accurate assessment of the adequacy of ventilation and, in some instances, utilization of ultraviolet light and ambient air filtration.

REFERENCES

1. Allen S, Batungwanayo J, Kerlikowski K, et al: Prevalence of tuberculosis in HIV-infected urban Rwandan women. Am Rev Respir Dis 146:1439–1444, 1992

2. American Thoracic Society/Centers for Disease Control: Treatment and prevention of tuberculosis in adults and children. Am J Respir Crit Care Med 149:1359–1374, 1994

3. American Thoracic Society: Control of tuberculosis in the United States. Am Rev Respir Dis 146:1623–1633, 1992

4. Antonucci G, Girardi E, Raviglione MC et al: Risk factors for tuberculosis in HIV-infected persons: A prospective cohort study. JAMA 274:143–148, 1995

5. Barnes P, Leedom J, Radin DR, Chandrasoma P: An unusual case of tuberculous peritonitis in a man with AIDS. West J Med 144:467–469, 1986

6. Batungwanayo J, Taelman H, Dhote R, et al: Pulmonary tuberculosis in Kigali, Rwanda: Impact of human immunodeficiency virus infection on clinical and radiographic presentation. Am Rev Respir Dis 146:53–56, 1992

7. Beck-Sagué C, Dooley SW, Hutton MD, et al: Hospital outbreak of multidrug-resistant *Mycobacterium tuberculosis* infections: Factors in transmission to staff and HIV-infected patients. JAMA 268:1280–1286, 1992

8. Bishburg E, Sunderam G, Reichman LB, Kapila R: Central nervous system tuberculosis with the acquired immunodeficiency syndrome and its related complex. Ann Intern Med 105:210–213, 1986

9. Brody JM, Miller DK, Zeman RK, et al: Gastric tuberculosis: A manifestation of acquired immunodeficiency syndrome. Radiology 159:347–348, 1986

10. Brudney K, Dobkin J: Resurgent tuberculosis in New York City. Am Rev Respir Dis 144:745–749, 1991

11. Centers for Disease Control: Cases of specified notifiable diseases—United States. MMWR 39:944, 1992

12. Centers for Disease Control: Tuberculosis morbidity—United States, 1994. MMWR 44:387, 1995

13. Centers for Disease Control: *Mycobacterium tuberculosis* transmission in a health clinic—Florida. MMWR 38:256, 1989

14. Centers for Disease Control: Nosocomial transmission of multidrug resistant tuberculosis among HIV-infected patients. MMWR 40:585–591, 1991

15. Centers for Disease Control: Purified protein derivative PPD—tuberculin anergy and HIV infection: Guideline for anergy testing and management of persons at risk of tuberculosis. MMWR 40 (Suppl RR-5):27–33, 1991

16. Centers for Disease Control: Tuberculosis and human immunodeficiency virus infection: Recommendation of the Advisory Committee for Elimination of Tuberculosis. MMWR 38:236–250, 1989

17. Centers for Disease Control: Tuberculosis statistics in the United States. U.S. Department of Health and Human Services, 1991

18. Chaisson RE, Schecter GF, Theuer CP, et al: Tuberculosis in patients with the acquired immunodeficiency syndrome. Am Rev Respir Dis 136:570–574, 1987

19. Chin DP, Osmond D, Page-Shafer K, et al: Reliability of anergy skin testing in persons with HIV infection. Am J Respir Crit Care Med 153:1982–1984, 1996

20. Chin DP, Yajko DM, Hadley WK, et al: Clinical utility of a commercial test based on the polymerase chain reaction for detecting *Mycobacterium tuberculosis* in respiratory specimens. Am J Respir Crit Care Med 151:1872–1877, 1995

21. Clarridge JE III, Shawar RM, Shinnick TM, Plikaytis BB: Large-scale use of polymerase chain reaction

for detection of *Mycobacterium tuberculosis* in a routine mycobacteriology laboratory. J Clin Microbiol 31:2049–2056, 1993

22. Colebunders RL, Ryder RW, Nylambi N, et al: HIV infection in patients with tuberculosis in Kinshasa, Zaire. Am Rev Respir Dis 135:1082–1085, 1989

23. Comstock GW: Epidemiology of tuberculosis. Am Rev Respir Dis 125:8–15, 1982

24. D'Cruz IA, Sengupta EE, Abrahams C, et al: Cardiac involvement, including tuberculosis pericardial effusion, complicating acquired immune deficiency syndrome. Am Heart J 112:1100–1102, 1986

25. Daley CL, Small PM, Schecter GF, et al: An outbreak of tuberculosis with accelerated progression among persons infected with human immunodeficiency virus: An analysis using restriction-fragment—length polymorphisms. N Engl J Med 326:231–235, 1992

26. Daniel TM, Ellner JJ: Immunology of tuberculosis. In Reichman LB, Hershfield ES, eds. Tuberculosis: A Comprehensive International Approach. New York, Marcel Dekker, Inc, 1993, pp 75–101

27. De Cock KM, Soro, B, Coulibaly IM, Lucas SB: Tuberculosis and HIV infection in sub-saharan Africa. JAMA 268:1581–1587, 1992

28. DiPerri G, Danzi MC, DeChecci G, et al: Nosocomial epidemic of active tuberculosis among HIV-infected patients. Lancet 2:1502–1504, 1989

29. Dooley SW Jr, Castro KG, Hutton MD, et al: Guidelines for preventing transmission of tuberculosis in health care settings with special focus on HIV-related issues. MMWR 39 (RR-17):1–29, 1990

30. Edlin BR, Tokars JI, Grieco MH, et al: An outbreak of multiple-drug resistant tuberculosis among hospitalized patients with the acquired immunodeficiency syndrome. N Engl J Med 326:514–521, 1992

31. Eisenach KD, Sifford MD, Cave MD, et al: Detection of *Mycobacterium tuberculosis* in sputum samples using a polymerase chain reaction. Am Rev Respir Dis 144:1160–1163, 1991

32. Englehard D, Stutman HR, Mark MI: Interaction of ketoconazole with rifampin and isoniazid. N Engl J Med 311:1681–1683, 1989

33. Fischl MA, Daikos GL, Uttamchandani RB, et al: Clinical presentation and outcome of patients with HIV infection and tuberculosis caused by multiple-drug-resistant bacilli. Ann Intern Med 117:184–190, 1992

34. Fischl MA, Pitchenik AE, Spira TJ: Tuberculosis brain abscess and toxoplasma encephalitis in a patients with the acquired immunodeficiency syndrome. JAMA 253:3428–3430, 1985

35. Forbes BA, Hicks KES: Direct detection of *Mycobacterium tuberculosis* in respiratory specimens in a clinical laboratory by polymerase chain reaction. J Clin Microbiol 31:1688–1694, 1993

36. Frieden TR, Sterling T, Pablos-Mendez A, et al: The emergence of drug-resistant tuberculosis in New York City. N Engl J Med 328:521–526, 1993

37. Garcia ML: Increasing trends of tuberculosis and HIV/AIDS in Mexico (Abstract MB2441). Seventh International Conference on AIDS, Florence, 1991, p 292

38. Gilks CF, Brindle RJ, Otieno LS: Extrapulmonary and disseminated tuberculosis in HIV seropositive patients presenting to the acute medical services in Nairobi. AIDS 4:981–985, 1990

39. Glassroth J: Diagnosis of tuberculosis. In Reichman LB, Hershfield ES, eds. Tuberculosis: A Comprehensive International Approach. New York, Marcel Dekker, Inc, 1993, pp 149–165

40. Goble M, Iseman MD, Madsen LA, et al: Treatment of 171 patients with pulmonary tuberculosis resistant to isoniazid and rifampin. N Engl J Med 328:527–532, 1993

41. Graham NMH, Cohn S, Galai N, et al: Incidence of mycobacterial infection and disease in HIV⁺ and HIV⁻ IDUs (Abstract PO-B07-1154). Ninth International Conference on AIDS, Berlin, 1993, p 328

42. Graham NMH, Nelson KE, Solomon L, et al: Prevalence of tuberculin positivity and skin test anergy in HIV-1–seropositive and –seronegative intravenous drug users. JAMA 267:369–373, 1992

43. Handwerger S, Mildvan D, Senie R, McKinley FW: Tuberculosis and the acquired immunodeficiency syndrome at a New York City hospital: 1978–1985. Chest 91:176–180, 1987

44. Holt E, Cantave M, Johnson M, et al: Efficacy of supervised, intermittent, short-course therapy of tuberculosis in HIV infection (Abstract WS-B09-4). Ninth International Conference on AIDS, Berlin, 1993

45. Hopewell PC: Factors influencing transmission and infectivity of *Mycobacterium tuberculosis:* Implications for clinical and public health management. In Sande MA, Hudson LD, Root RK, eds. Respiratory Infections. New York, Churchill Livingstone, 1986, pp 191–216

46. Huebner RE, Villarino ME, Snider DE Jr: Tuberculin skin testing and the HIV epidemic. JAMA 267:409–410, 1992

47. Iseman MDR: Is standard chemotherapy adequate in tuberculosis patients infected with the HIV? Am Rev Respir Dis 136:1326, 1987

48. Iseman MDR: Treatment of multidrug-resistant tuberculosis. N Engl J Med 329:784–791, 1993

49. Jones BE, Young SMM, Antoniskis D, et al: Relationship of the manifestations of tuberculosis to CD4 cell counts in patients with human immunodeficiency virus infection. Am Rev Respir Dis 148:1292–1297, 1993

50. Kent JH: The epidemiology of multidrug-resistant tuberculosis in the United States. Med Clin North Am 77:1391–1409, 1993

51. Kramer F, Modilevsky T, Waliany AR, et al: Delayed diagnosis of tuberculosis in patients with human immunodeficiency virus infection. Am J Med 89:451–456, 1990

52. Lazar JD, Wilner KD: Drug interactions with fluconazole. Rev Infect Dis 12:5327–5333, 1990

53. Long R, Scalcini M, Manfreda J, et al: Impact of human immunodeficiency virus type 1 on tuberculosis in rural Haiti. Am Rev Respir Dis 143:69–73, 1991

54. Louie E, Rice LB, Holzman RS: Tuberculosis in non-Haitian patients with acquired immunodeficiency syndrome. Chest 90:542–545, 1986

55. Mallolas J, Gatell JM, Rovira M, et al: Vertebral arch tuberculosis in two human immunodeficiency virus-seropositive heroin addicts. Arch Intern Med 48:1125–1127, 1988

56. Mann J, Snider DE, Francis H, et al: Association between HTLV-III/LAV infection and tuberculosis in Zaire. JAMA 256:346, 1986

57. Markowitz N, Hansen NI, Wilcosky TC, et al: Tuberculin and anergy testing in HIV-seropositive and HIV-seronegative persons. Ann Intern Med 119:185–193, 1993

58. Modilevsky T, Sattler FR, Barnes PF: Mycobacterial disease in patients with human immunodeficiency virus infection. Arch Intern Med 149:2201–2205, 1989

59. Nardell E, McInnis B, Thomas B, Weidhaus S: Exogenous reinfection with tuberculosis in a shelter for the homeless. N Engl J Med 315:1570–1575, 1986

60. Nardell EA: Environmental control of tuberculosis. Med Clin North Am 77:1315–1334, 1993

61. Nolan CM, Heckbert S, Elarth A: Case-control study of the association between human immunodeficiency virus infection and tuberculosis (Abstract 4620). San Francisco, Fourth International Conference on AIDS, 1988

62. Nunn P, Gicheka R, Hages S, et al: Cross-sectional survey of HIV infection among patients with tuberculosis in Nairobi, Keyna. Tuberc Lung Dis 73:45–51, 1992

63. Onorato I, McCombs S, Morgan WM, McCray E: HIV infection in patients attending tuberculosis (TB) clinics, United States, 1988–1991 (Abstract WS-C18-6). Ninth International Conference on AIDS, Berlin, 1993, p 99

64. Onorato IM, McCray E, Field Services Branch: Prevalence of human immunodeficiency virus infection among patients attending tuberculosis clinics in the United States. J Infect Dis 165:87–92, 1992

65. Pape JW, Jean SS, Ho JL, et al: Effect of isoniazid prophylaxis on incidence of active tuberculosis and progression of HIV infection. Lancet 342:268–272, 1993

66. Pape JW, Liautaud B, Thomas F, et al: Characteristics of the acquired immunodeficiency syndrome (AIDS) in Haiti. N Engl J Med 309:945–950, 1983

67. Parriens JH, St. Louis ME, Mukadi YB, et al: Pulmonary tuberculosis in HIV-infected patients in Zaire: A controlled trial of treatment for either 6 or 12 months. N Engl J Med 332:779–784, 1995

68. Peloquin CA: Antituberculosis drugs: Pharmacokinetics. In Heifets LB, ed. Drug Susceptibility in the Chemotherapy of Mycobacterial Infection. CRC Press, Boca Raton, 1991, pp 59–88

69. Pitchenik AE, Burr J, Suarez M, et al: Human T-cell lymphotropic virus-III (HTLV-III) seropositivity and related disease among 71 consecutive patients in whom tuberculosis was diagnosed. Am Rev Respir Dis 135:875–879, 1987

70. Pitchenik AE, Cole C, Russell BW, et al: Tuberculosis, atypical mycobacteriosis, and the acquired immunodeficiency syndrome among Haitian and non-Haitian patients in South Florida. Ann Intern Med 101:641–645, 1984

71. Pitchenik AE, Fischl MA, Dickinson GM, et al: Opportunistic infections and Kaposi's sarcoma among Haitians: Evidence of a new acquired immunodeficiency state. Ann Intern Med 98:277–284, 1983

72. Pitchenik AE, Rubinson HA: The radiographic appearance of tuberculosis in patients with the acquired immunodeficiency syndrome (AIDS) and pre-AIDS. Am Rev Respir Dis 131:393–396, 1985

73. Raviglione MC, Narain JP, Kochi A: HIV-associated tuberculosis in developing countries: Clinical features, diagnosis, and treatment. Bull WHO 70:515–526, 1992

74. Reichman LB: The "U"-shaped curve of concern. Am Rev Respir Dis 144:741–742, 1991

75. Saltzman BR, Motyl MR, Friedland GH, et al: *Mycobac-*

76. Selwyn PA, Hartel D, Lewis VA, et al: A prospective study of the risk of tuberculosis among intravenous drug users with human immunodeficiency virus infection. N Engl J Med 320:545–550, 1989

77. Selwyn PA, Sckell BM, Alcabes P, et al: High risk of active tuberculosis in HIV-infected drug users with cutaneous anergy. JAMA 268:504–509, 1992

78. Shafer RW, Chirgwin KD, Glatt AE, et al: HIV prevalence, immunosuppression, and drug resistance in patients with tuberculosis in an area endemic for AIDS. AIDS 5:399–405, 1991

79. Shafer RW, Goldberg R, Sierra M, Glatt AE: Frequency of *Mycobacterium tuberculosis* bacteremia in patients with tuberculosis in an area endemic for AIDS. Am Rev Respir Dis 140:1611–1613, 1989

80. Small PM, Hopewell PC, Schecter GF, et al: Evolution of chest radiographs in treated patients with pulmonary tuberculosis and HIV infection. J Thorac Imaging 9:74, 1995

81. Small PM, Hopewell PC, Singh SP, et al: The contemporary urban epidemiology of tuberculosis in San Francisco: A population-based study using conventional and molecular methods. N Engl J Med 330:1703–1709, 1994

82. Small PM, Schecter GF, Goodman PC, et al: Treatment of tuberculosis in patients with advanced human immunodeficiency virus infection. N Engl J Med 324:289–294, 1991

83. Small PM, Shafer RW, Hopewell PC, et al: Exogenous reinfection with multidrug-resistant *Mycobacterium tuberculosis* in patients with advanced HIV infection. N Engl J Med 328:1137–1144, 1993

84. Snider DE Jr, Good RC: Research needs. In Reichman LB, Hershfield ES, eds. Tuberculosis: A Comprehensive International Approach. New York, Marcel Dekker, Inc, 1993, pp 721–734

85. Snider DE Jr, Roper WL: The new tuberculosis. N Engl J Med 326:703–705, 1992

86. Standaert B, Niragira F, Kadende P, Piot P: The association of tuberculosis and HIV infection in Burundi. AIDS Res Hum Retroviruses 5:247–251, 1989

87. Stead WW: Pathogenesis of the sporadic case of tuberculosis. N Engl J Med 277:1008–1012, 1967

88. Styblo K, Salomão MA: National tuberculosis control programs. In Reichman LB, Hershfield ES, eds. Tuberculosis: A Comprehensive International Approach. New York, Marcel Dekker, Inc, 1993, pp 573–600

89. Sunderam G, Mangura BT, Lombardo JM, Reichman LB: Failure of "optimal" four-drug short-course tuberculosis chemotherapy in a compliant patient with human immunodeficiency virus. Am Rev Respir Dis 136:1475–1478, 1987

90. Sunderam G, McDonald RJ, Maniatis T, et al: Tuberculosis as a manifestation of the acquired immunodeficiency syndrome (AIDS). JAMA 256:362–366, 1986

91. Theuer CP, Hopewell PC, Elias D, et al: Human immunodeficiency virus infection in tuberculosis patients. J Infect Dis 162:8–12, 1990

92. Toossi Z, Sierra-Madero JG, Blinkhorn RA, et al: Enhanced susceptibility of blood monocytes from patients with pulmonary tuberculosis to productive infection with human immunodeficiency virus type 1. J Exp Med 177:1511–1516, 1993

93. Wadhawan D, Mwansa N, Tembo G, Perine PL: Isonia-

zid prophylaxis among patients with HIV-1 infections (Abstract ThB 510). Sixth International Conference on AIDS, San Francisco, 1990, p 249

94. Wallis RS, Vjecha M, Amir-Tahmasseb M, et al: Influence of tuberculosis on HIV: Enhanced cytokine expression and elevated B2 microglobulin in HIV-1 associated tuberculosis. J Infect Dis 167:43, 1992

95. Whalen C, Horsburgh CR, Hom D, et al: Accelerated course of human immunodeficiency virus infection after tuberculosis. Am J Respir Crit Care Med 151: 129–135, 1995

Chapter 23

Cryptococcosis and Other Fungal Infections (Histoplasmosis, Coccidioidomycosis)

MICHAEL S. SAAG

Systemic fungal infections generally are late manifestations in HIV disease. Overall, cryptococcal infection is the most common systemic fungal infection in HIV-infected patients. However, in certain endemic regions, histoplasmosis or coccidioidomycosis is the most prevalent mycotic disorder. Although these diseases occur in normal (non–HIV-infected) hosts, among HIV-infected patients they tend to occur when the CD4 count is less than 200/mm³. Recent advances in the treatment of systemic fungal infections have substantially reduced both morbidity and mortality of these disorders. Newer diagnostic techniques along with heightened awareness on the part of clinicians have led to more rapid and accurate diagnosis. This chapter reviews the approach to diagnosis and management of cryptococcosis, histoplasmosis, and coccidioidomycosis, the three most commonly occurring systemic mycoses in HIV-infected patients.

CRYPTOCOCCUS

Microbiology

Cryptococcus neoformans is a round or oval yeast (4 to 6 μm in diameter), surrounded by a capsule that can be up to 30 μm thick. The organism grows quite readily on fungal or bacterial culture media and usually is detectable within a week after inoculation, although in some circumstances up to 4 weeks is required for growth. Therefore, clinical cultures should be maintained for a minimum of 2 weeks, and preferably 4 weeks, when *C. neoformans* disease is suspected. The organism is differentiated from other pathogenic yeasts based on its growth characteristics. The organism grows well at 37°C, does not form pseudomycelia on cornmeal or rice-Tween agar, and hydrolyzes urea, a property that allows rapid presumptive identification.[43]

On the basis of antigenic differences in the capsule, biochemical use of nutrients, and distinct DNA base sequences, four serotypes (A, B, C, and D) of *Cryptococcus* have been delineated. Serotypes A and D are classified as *C. neoformans* var. *neoformans*, and serotypes B and C are classified as *C. neoformans* var. *gattii*.[63] *C. neoformans* var. *neoformans* is the major cause of cryptococcal disease worldwide. Serotype A is the most common serotype infecting AIDS patients.[38,47] For reasons that are not clearly understood, *C. neoformans* var. *gattii* tends to infect immunocompetent hosts.[39,48] This subtype is found in certain geographic areas, including southern California, Africa, Australia, and Southeast Asia. Interestingly, even within these geographic areas, *C. neoformans* var. *gattii* does not appear to cause disease in HIV-infected patients.[48,51]

Epidemiology

Before the AIDS epidemic, cryptococcal infection occurred in a small number of immunocompetent patients but most often in patients with a compromised immune system. The most frequently affected patients were those with lymphoma, diabetics, transplant recipients, or patients requiring chronic steroid therapy.[14] In the AIDS era, cryptococcal disease is the fourth most common cause of serious opportunistic infection after *Pneumocystis carinii* pneumonia, cytomegalovirus, and myobacterial disease.[6] Disease caused by *C. neoformans* occurs in 6% to 10% of HIV-infected patients. Among those individuals who develop cryptococcal disease, it is the initial AIDS-defining illness in 40% to 45%.[7,8,13,16,27,66] At the present time, it is the third most common central nervous system (CNS) disorder in AIDS patients, behind toxoplasmosis and CNS lymphoma.

C. neoformans infection is acquired from the environment. The organism, most likely in an unencapsulated form, is inhaled into the lungs and deposited in the small airways. Once there, yeast multiply and compress the surrounding tissue but, remarkably, cause little damage. This pulmonary infection is often asymptomatic. Indeed, in 85% to 95% of patients with cryptococcal meningitis, no evidence of pneumonitis is present.[7,8] As suggested by these data, the organism has a strong propensity for dissemination to the CNS but also may involve skin, bone, and the genitourinary tract.

Clinical Manifestations

The onset of cryptococcal disease usually is insidious. The median time between the onset of symptoms and the diagnosis of cryptococcal disease is 30 days.[7,8,13] Diagnosis often is delayed by the waxing and waning course of the disease and the absence of specific symptoms. These nonspecific symptoms consist of a prolonged febrile prodrome that is indistinguishable from that of other opportunistic infections. The most common symptoms, in addition to fever, are headache and malaise.[7,8,13,53] A listing of common symptoms is presented in Table 23–1.

The incidence of extraneural cryptococcal disease in AIDS patients ranges between 20% and 60%.[7,8,16,27] Despite the lung being the portal of entry, evidence of pulmonary disease symptoms is present in only 20% to 30% of cases. Other sites of extraneural involvement include the joints, oral cavity, pericardium, myocardium, skin, mediastinum, and genitourinary tract, which is believed to provide a sanctuary for *C. neoformans* that may lead to recurring disease.[28]

The physical examination in patients with cryptococcal disease is also nonspecific. In the series by Chuck and Sande, 56% of patients were febrile, although less than one third had nuchal rigidity or other focal neurologic deficits.[7] Altered mental status, which is the most important predictor of poor outcome of patients with cryptococcal disease, is present in 20% to 30% of patients. Papilledema is seen in less than 10% of patients. Raised, sometimes umbilicated, skin lesions are reported in 3% to 10% of patients with cryptococcal meningitis. These lesions may resemble those caused by *Molluscum contagiosum* and occasionally have been misdiagnosed as Kaposi's sarcoma.

Diagnosis

The gold standard diagnostic test for cryptococcal meningitis is a positive cerebrospinal fluid (CSF) culture for *C. neoformans*. Therefore, a lumbar puncture is imperative in any individual with suspected cryptococcal meningitis. This procedure is diagnostic but may be therapeutic as well (see Management of Increased Intracranial Pressure). Although controversial, most clinicians will perform an imaging study, such as a computed tomography or magnetic resonance imaging scan, before performing a lumbar puncture in any HIV-infected patient with headache and fever. The rationale supporting this approach is that many space-occupying disease processes, such as CNS toxoplasmosis (Chapter 24) and CNS lymphoma (Chapter 28), may cause similar symptoms. The most common findings noted on brain imaging studies are cerebral atrophy and ventricular enlargement.[7,8,34] On rare occasion, mass lesions caused by *C. neoformans* (cryptococcomas) may be identified.[34] In some patients, especially in those with elevated CSF pressure, the ventricles are normal to small in size, with some evidence of generalized cerebral edema (Fig. 23–1). Assuming there is no evidence of obstructive hydrocephalus, these patients may benefit from serial spinal taps to help relieve the symptoms of elevated intracranial pressure.

After an occult mass lesion has been ruled out, a lumbar puncture should be performed. In patients with non–AIDS-associated cryptococcal meningitis, the most common CSF findings include an elevated opening pressure (>200 mm H_2O), elevated CSF white blood cell count (>20/mm^3), hypoglycorrhachia (<50% of serum glucose level), elevated CSF protein (>50 mg/dl), and a negative India ink preparation (60% to 70% will be negative) (Table

TABLE 23–1. CLINICAL MANAGEMENT OF CRYPTOCOCCAL MENINGITIS IN NON-AIDS AND AIDS PATIENTS*

	Non-AIDS	AIDS				
	43	65	7	8	42	53
Clinical						
Headache	87	81	73	67	92	89
Fever	60	88	65	62	78	75
Nausea and vomiting	53	†	42	1	8	
Altered mental status	52	19	28		27	21
Stiff neck	50	31	22		37	44
Visual disturbances	33				30	29
Cranial nerve palsies	32				6	
Papilledema	28				6	8
Ataxia	26				10	
Seizures	15	8	4	9		
Aphasia	10					
Malaise		38	76			
Photophobia		19	18		6	
Laboratory						
CSF abnormal						
WBC ($>20/mm^3$)	97	31	21	13		
Glucose ($<60\%$ of serum level)	75	65	24	17		
Protein (>45 mg/dl)	90	61	55	35		
India ink positive	60	72	74	88	77	83
Opening pressure abnormal (>200 mm H_2O)	65	62	66			
Serology						
CSF antigen positive	>90	92	91	93	99	99
Serum antigen positive	50	95	99	93	99	99
Abnormal Head CT		31	29	19		

* Given as percent of patients.
† Items without entries were not reported by investigators.
Modified with permission from Lapidus W, Saag M: Cryptococcal meningitis. In Johnson S, Johnson FN, series eds, Powderly WB, Van't Wout JW, consultant eds. The Antifungal Agents: Fluconazole. Lancashire, England, Marius Press, 1992, p 137.

23–1).[14,43] In contrast, up to 50% of patients with AIDS-associated cryptococcal meningitis have no or minimal abnormalities of their CSF formula.[7,8,66] However, the opening pressure may be elevated (>200 mm H_2O) in over 70% of the patients. Low CSF white blood cell counts ($<20/mm^3$) not only are common but also are associated with a worse prognosis.[42,53] Fortunately, in light of the normal CSF findings in most patients, there are more sensitive and specific tests for cryptococcal disease. The India ink preparation is positive in 74% to 88% of patients with cryptococcal meningitis.[7,8,42,53] Using this technique, *C. neoformans* is visible as round cells 4 to 6 μm in diameter surrounded by the characteristic thick polysaccharide capsule (Fig. 23–2). It is quite important to clearly

identify the organism within the capsule because false-positive tests have been reported as a result of an artifact. The frequency of inaccurate readings is minimized through the use of experienced technicians who are familiar with proper interpretation of the results. Even when a true-positive test is reported, the findings must be confirmed with a CSF cryptococcal antigen (CRAG) test or, ideally, a CSF fungal culture.

CRAG testing of blood and CSF is a reliable and relatively rapid diagnostic technique. Sensitivity of the CRAG test is 93% to 99% in patients with culture-proven cryptococcal meningitis.[7,8] In non–HIV-infected patients, the median CSF titer is between 1:16 and 1:32.[14] In contrast, the median CSF antigen titer in HIV-infected

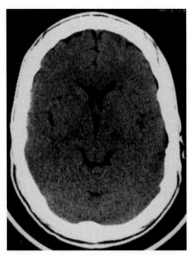

FIGURE 23–1. Representative CT scan from a patient with acute AIDS-associated cryptococcal meningitis, altered mental status, and elevated intracranial pressure (>550 mm H_2O). The paradoxical finding of normal to small-sized ventricles and absence of radiologic hydrocephalus is typical of cryptococcus meningitis. (Reprinted with permission from Ennis DM, Saag MS: Cryptococcal meningitis in AIDS. Hosp Pract 28:101, 1993.)

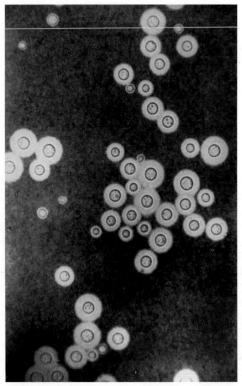

FIGURE 23–2. India ink preparation of CSF demonstrating *C. neoformans* organisms, several of which are budding. The circular organism is encased within a thick polysaccharide capsule. (Courtesy of Dr. Kathleen E. Squires.)

patients is 1:1024. On occasion, CSF titers can exceed 1:1 million. Serum CRAG tests are positive in over 99% of patients with *C. neoformans* disease. In patients with AIDS-associated cryptococcal meningitis, the serum antigen tests usually are one tube dilution higher than the CSF antigen test. The serum cryptococcal antigen test is used occasionally as a screening test for an HIV-infected patient with headache and fever. A negative test result reduces the likelihood of cryptococcal disease, whereas a positive test necessitates further evaluation with a CSF workup. Routine screening of patients with the serum CRAG test is controversial but currently is not recommended. Unfortunately, the serum CRAG is also not helpful in following patients with proven cryptococcal disease.[35] Specifically, the serum CRAG is not capable of detecting patients who are about to relapse or to assess the initial response to acute therapy. False-positive CRAG tests have been noted in patients with positive rheumatoid factor, although current techniques have largely eliminated this problem. Patients with *Trichosporon beigelii* infection may also have false-positive CRAG results.[31] *T. beigelii* infections, however, are quite uncommon. False-positive titers usually do not exceed a 1:8 dilution. Conversely, some patients with cryptococcal infection may have false-negative CRAG tests. Such results may reflect scarce or poorly encapsulated organisms, or, conversely, the number of organisms may be so large that crosslinking is impaired. This so-called prozone phenomenon may be overcome by ensuring that the tests are performed using an adequate number of dilutions.[23]

A definitive diagnosis of cryptococcal disease requires culturing the organism from body fluids or tissue. CSF fungal cultures require a minimum of 2 ml to obtain maximum sensitivity. By definition, up to 100% of cases of cryptococcal meningitis have positive CSF fungal cultures. In contrast, blood cultures are positive in only one third of patients without AIDS. However, 66% to 80% of patients with AIDS will have positive blood cultures for *C. neoformans*.[14,42]

In patients with extraneural cryptococcal disease, tissue examination can lead to a presumptive diagnosis of cryptococcosis. *C. neoformans* organisms are readily identified using methenamine silver, mucicarmine, and periodic acid–Schiff stains. Gram's stain of tissue is generally unreliable in detecting *C. neoformans* organisms.

Prognosis

Left untreated, cryptococcal meningitis is a fatal disorder. Even with aggressive intervention, the mortality among non-AIDS patients with combination amphotericin B and flucytosine therapy is reported to be as high as 30%, depending on underlying disease.[12-14] Previously, the reported mortality of acute cryptococcal meningitis in patients with AIDS was between 17% and 20%.[42] However, a recent study has demonstrated a mortality rate of 6% with aggressive therapy (see below).[53] Many studies have evaluated factors associated with treatment failure and mortality in both AIDS and non-AIDS patients. In both populations, the most important baseline prognostic factor is mental status at the time of presentation. Individuals with altered sensorium have a much worse prognosis than those who are awake and alert.[14,42] High fungal burden, as demonstrated by high CRAG titers, positive India ink test, and the presence of extraneural cryptococcal disease, also is associated with poor outcome.[14,42] Elevated intracranial pressure has been shown to be an important factor in morbidity and mortality.[53]

Treatment

Antifungal Agents

Amphotericin B (AMB) is a polyene antimicrobial agent that possesses a broad range of antifungal activity. Its fungicidal activity is due principally to the binding of ergosterol in the fungal membrane, resulting in increased membrane permeability, leakage of cellular components, and resultant cell death. The drug is very poorly absorbed when administered orally (necessitating intravenous administration), has a very high volume of distribution, and is believed to be deposited in fatty tissues throughout the body. However, AMB penetrates into CSF very poorly.

The principal limitation of AMB is its toxicity profile. Virtually all patients who receive more than 4 weeks of the drug will experience some degree of reversible renal insufficiency. During acute administration, fever, rigors, headache, and thrombophlebitis have been reported. Chronic administration results in electrolyte abnormalities, most notably hypokalemia and hypomagnesemia. Strategies to reduce the toxicity of AMB include slow administration of drug (over 4 to 6 hours), the addition of heparin (1000 U/500 ml) to reduce the incidence of

thrombophlebitis, premedication with antipyretics (acetaminophen, diphenhydramine, or both), premedication with meperidine in patients who have experienced severe rigors, and aggressive replacement of electrolytes as needed. Some investigators have attempted to modify the toxicity of AMB by modifying its formulation. Lipid complex formulations (AMB lipid complex) and liposomal preparations of amphotericin have been evaluated in clinical trials, with modest success.[9,21,45] The advantage of these formulations is that they allow higher doses (up to 3 to 5 mg/kg) of parent drug to be administered. However, preliminary studies reveal success rates that are similar to the use of AMB alone, although the toxicity does seem to be less.

Flucytosine (5-FC) is a pyrimidine derivative similar in structure to 5-fluorouracil (5-FU). When administered to susceptible fungi, 5-FC is converted to 5-FU and inhibits thymidylate synthetase, a vital enzyme needed for DNA synthesis. 5-FC has a very favorable pharmacokinetic profile, including complete absorption from the gastrointestinal tract when administered orally, a satisfactory half-life of 3 to 4 hours, and very little hepatic metabolism (the drug is excreted virtually unchanged by the kidney). Most importantly, 5-FC reaches high concentrations in the CSF, usually on the order of 70% to 90% of the serum levels. The principal toxicities of 5-FC occur primarily in organ systems that have rapidly dividing cells, namely the bone marrow (leukopenia), gastrointestinal tract (nausea, vomiting, and diarrhea), and skin (rash). Optimally, drug levels should be obtained whenever 5-FC is used to minimize toxicity and maximize effectiveness. The levels should be above 50 μg/ml and below 100 μg/ml.

In the late 1970s and through the 1980s, other oral agents were identified that possessed broad-spectrum antifungal activity (reviewed in ref. 41). The first of these agents is *ketoconazole,* an imidazole derivative with in vitro activity against *Histoplasma capsulatum, Blastomyces dermatitidis, Candida* species, and to a lesser degree, *C. neoformans.* The drug is metabolized predominantly by the liver, requires an acidic environment for absorption, penetrates the CSF poorly, and is highly protein bound. Concomitant administration of ketoconazole with rifampin or rifampin derivatives, dilantin, or carbamazepine results in negligible serum levels because of increased metabolism of drug. Drug absorption is dramatically impaired in an alkaline gastric environment created by histamine$_2$ (H$_2$) blockers or antacids. Nausea and vomiting are the principal dose-related toxicities. Less commonly, hepatic dysfunction or alteration of steroidogenesis has been noted.

Fluconazole, a bistriazole, was the second oral azole agent approved for use in the United States. The pharmacokinetic properties of fluconazole are strikingly different from those of ketoconazole. Fluconazole is well absorbed from the gastrointestinal tract (oral bioavailability 70% to 80%) and is able to achieve adequate serum levels even when exposed in an alkaline gastric environment. The drug is excreted predominantly via the kidney and undergoes minimal metabolism by the liver. Most importantly with regard to cryptococcal disease, fluconazole penetrates well into the CSF, achieving concentrations of 60% to 80% of serum concentrations. The most common side effects are gastrointestinal in nature, although skin rash has been reported in up to 3% of patients taking the drug. Rare instances of Stevens-Johnson syndrome have been reported. Fluconazole is active against *C. neoformans,* most *Candida* species, *H. capsulatum,* and *B. dermatitidis* but has little activity against *Aspergillus* species or certain *Candida* species (e.g., *C. krusei*).

Itraconazole is the most recently approved oral antifungal agent in the United States. Although itraconazole is a triazole, its pharmacologic properties are more like those of ketoconazole than those of fluconazole. Like ketoconazole, itraconazole requires an acidic gastric environment for absorption, is metabolized by the liver, and has similar drug interactions with rifampin-like derivatives, dilantin, carbamazepine, H$_2$ blockers, and antacids. Itraconazole is more potent than ketoconazole on a milligram per milligram basis and is better tolerated. The drug demonstrates in vitro activity against *H. capsulatum, B. dermatitidis, C. neoformans, Candida* species, and *Aspergillus* species. Despite its poor penetration into CSF, animal studies demonstrate significant cure rates in murine cryptococcal meningitis models.

Acute Therapy

The treatment of non–AIDS-associated cryptococcal meningitis consists of AMB (dose 0.5 mg/kg/day) plus 5-FC (150 mg/kg/day in four divided doses) given over 6 weeks. This regimen became firmly established around the same time that the AIDS epidemic was first identified. As a result, the original studies of AIDS-associated cryptococcal meningitis consisted of regimens containing AMB plus 5-FC.[27,66] Although

some centers had fairly good success with this regimen, other centers reported much higher toxicity profiles, especially with the 5-FC component of the regimen, than was noted in non-AIDS patients.[3,7]

Several studies have addressed the role of AMB with or without 5-FC as well as the newer triazole agents in the treatment of AIDS-associated cryptococcal meningitis (Table 23-2). In 1985, Kovacs et al reported success in 10 of 24 patients (42%) treated with either AMB alone (0.4 to 0.6 mg/kg/day) or AMB plus 5-FC (150 mg/kg/day).[27] Nine of the patients in this study died, two patients relapsed after successfully completing initial therapy, and three patients had persistently positive cultures at the end of therapy (quiescent disease). In 1986, Zuger et al published a report documenting a successful outcome in 75% of patients (18 of 24) treated with AMB with or without 5-FC.[66] In 1989, a retrospective study by Chuck and Sande reported a 79% 6-week survival rate among 89 patients with cryptococcal meningitis.[7] However, the 6-month survival rate was only 38% for those receiving AMB alone compared to 52% for those receiving AMB plus 5-FC. Of note, 53% of the patients receiving 5-FC had their drug discontinued because of toxicities, predominantly cytopenias. Drug levels were not followed routinely in this patient population. In a small study by Larsen et al in 1990, 6 of 6 patients treated with AMB (0.7 mg/kg/day for the first 2 weeks) plus 5-FC (150 mg/kg/day) converted their cultures to negative with minimal toxicity.[29] These data, along with historical data reported by Armstrong, suggest that higher doses of AMB (0.7 to 0.8 mg/kg/day) are required for optimal management of AIDS-associ-

TABLE 23-2. OUTCOME OF PRIMARY THERAPY OF CRYPTOCOCCAL MENINGITIS IN AIDS PATIENTS

Reference	Treatment Success	
	AMB ± 5-FC	Fluconazole
Kovacs et al[27]	10/24 (42%)	
Zuger et al[65]	18/24 (75%)	
Dismukes et al[14]		11/15 (73%)
Stern et al[49]		4/5 (80%)
Larsen et al[29]	6/6 (100%)	6/14 (43%)
Saag et al[42]	25/63 (40%)	44/131 (34%)

Reprinted with permission from Lapidus W, Saag M: Cryptococcal meningitis. In Johnson S, Johnson FN, series eds., Powderly WB, Van't Wout JW, consultant eds. The Antifungal Agents: Fluconazole. Lancashire, England, Marius Press, 1992, p 145.

ated cryptococcal meningitis.[3] Moreover, to minimize toxicity, 5-FC levels should be obtained routinely in patients receiving this drug, especially at higher doses (150 mg/kg/day).

Early pilot studies of oral fluconazole therapy indicated high response rates, although some discrepancies are noted between studies. Stern et al successfully treated four of five AIDS patients who had cryptococcal meningitis with fluconazole (50 to 200 mg/day), including two patients who had previously failed AMB therapy.[49] In contrast to the high success rate in the Stern study, Larsen et al noted clinical and mycologic success in only 6 of 14 patients (43%) treated with fluconazole (400 mg/day).[29] In that study, among five patients with less severe disease, four experienced CSF culture conversion from positive to negative. Although side effects were much less common in the fluconazole-treated group than the AMB plus 5-FC group, the investigators concluded that the AMB plus 5-FC regimen should be used initially to treat the majority of acute cryptococcal infections in AIDS patients.

In 1992, the National Institute of Allergy and Infectious Diseases Mycoses Study Group (MSG) and AIDS Clinical Trials Group (ACTG), in conjunction with Pfizer Central Research, reported the results of a large study of AIDS-associated cryptococcal meningitis.[42] The phase II/III study evaluated 194 patients assigned to receive fluconazole (200 mg/day) or AMB (median dose 0.5 mg/kg/day), randomized on a 2:1 (fluconazole/AMB) basis. Only 9 of 63 AMB recipients received concomitant 5-FC. In this study, successful improvement was defined as two negative CSF cultures within a 10-week time period in association with clinical improvement. With this criterion, 25 of 63 AMB patients (40%) and 44 of 131 patients receiving fluconazole (34%) were treated successfully. A remarkable number of patients in each group, 26% receiving fluconazole and 27% receiving AMB, had so-called quiescent disease, defined as clinical improvement but persistently positive CSF cultures at the end of therapy. Although overall survival was similar for the two groups (86% of AMB vs 82% fluconazole), a higher proportion of patients receiving fluconazole died within the first 2 weeks of therapy (19 of 24 compared to 5 of 9 for AMB). In addition, although the overall mycologic success rate was not different between the two groups, patients receiving AMB tended to have their cultures convert to negative more rapidly than those receiving fluconazole (Fig. 23–3).

Based on these results, another large study, ACTG 159/MSG 17, was initiated that evaluated the use of higher dose AMB (0.7 to 0.8 mg/kg) during the first 2 weeks of therapy, followed by fluconazole (400 mg/day) vs itraconazole (200 mg twice daily) for the rest of acute therapy (8 to 10 weeks). Before this study, itraconazole had been evaluated in over 50 HIV-infected patients with cryptococcal disease. In a study by Denning et al, among 29 evaluable patients with cryptococcal meningitis, 14 patients (48%) had a complete response, 6 patients (21%) responded initially and then relapsed, and in 9 patients (31%), therapy failed.[11]

ACTG 159/MSG 17 accrued 408 patients over 3 years. No statistical difference was noted between those patients who received AMB plus 5-FC and those who received AMB alone (60% vs 51% of patients achieved culture-negative status at 2 weeks, $p = 0.06$). After an additional 8 weeks of treatment, culture negative status was achieved in 72% of fluconazole recipients compared to 60% of those receiving itraconazole.[53] However, clinical improvement as determined by absence of fever, headache, or meningismus was observed in 70% of itraconazole recipients versus 68% of fluconazole recipients. No difference in survival was noted between any treatment group. Overall mortality at 10 weeks was 6%, substantially lower than that observed in previous studies.

A novel approach using fluconazole in combination with flucytosine has been evaluated by the California Collaborative Treatment Group.[24] The results of this study reveal a mycologic success rate of 75% and a clinical success rate of 63%. Among the 32 patients treated with this regimen, 4 patients (13%) died during the study. Although the results of the study are promising, they are tempered by the high frequency of toxicity noted, principally as a result of the flucytosine component. Over 60% of patients experienced some degree of toxicity that required alteration in dosage, and 28% required discontinuation of study medication. Further evaluation of this approach is warranted before it can be recommended as a treatment option in clinical practice (Table 23–3).

Management of Increased Intracranial Pressure

Increased intracranial pressure (ICP), usually in the form of communicating hydrocephalus, is a frequent and potentially life-threaten-

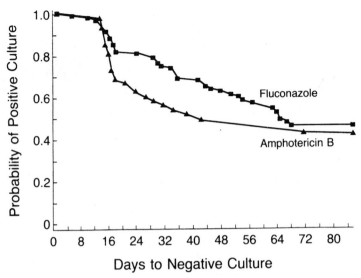

FIGURE 23–3. Kaplan-Meier estimates of the length of time to the first negative CSF culture, according to treatment group. (Reprinted with permission from Saag MS, Powderly WG, Cloud GA, et al: Comparison of amphotericin B with fluconazole in the treatment of acute AIDS-associated cryptococcal meningitis. N Engl J Med 326:86, 1992.)

ing complication of acute cryptococcal meningitis.[25] Although the cause of increased pressure has not been evaluated systematically, most authorities hypothesize that decreased absorption of CSF via the arachnoid villi is responsible, most likely resulting from impairment of the absorptive mechanism by capsular polysaccharide by-products or the yeasts themselves.[10] Other proposed mechanisms include cryptococcal-induced vasculitis, microscopic intra-

TABLE 23–3. RECOMMENDED TREATMENT OF AIDS-ASSOCIATED CRYPTOCOCCAL MENINGITIS

Acute Therapy

Amphotericin B (0.7–0.8 mg/kg/d) for 2 weeks (minimum) with or without 5-flucytosine (100 mg/kg/d in 4 divided doses)*; followed by
Fluconazole 400 mg by mouth daily for 8–10 weeks
  (Alternative: Itraconazole† 200 mg by mouth twice daily)

Maintenance Therapy

Fluconazole 200 mg by mouth daily
Alternative: Itraconazole† 200 mg by mouth twice daily
              or
          Amphotericin B (1 mg/kg) IV one or two times
          per week

Primary Prophylaxis

Not recommended (see text)

* Must adjust dose for renal insufficiency; ideally drug levels should be monitored in all patients receiving 5-FC.
† Used if patient cannot tolerate fluconazole.

cerebral abscesses with resultant parenchymal edema, or a combination of all of these effects. A peculiar aspect of the clinical picture of increased ICP is the lack of radiologic evidence of hydrocephalus per se. Indeed, the majority of patients with high CSF pressures have normal to small-sized ventricles (Fig. 23–1). A possible explanation for this phenomenon is equalization of pressures within cranial structures via transependymal flow of CSF from the subarachnoid space into cerebral tissue. An alternative explanation proposes the simultaneous existence of cerebral edema and resistance of outflow, resulting in equalization of CSF pressure with the edematous pressure within the brain tissue itself.

Elevated pressures (greater than 200 mm H_2O) are reported in over two thirds of patients with cryptococcal meningitis. Although the contribution of increased ICP to mortality, especially within the first 2 weeks, is unclear, many investigators believe it plays a critical role in the morbidity and mortality of the disease.[17] Anecdotal experience from a number of investigators indicates reduction in mortality even among high-risk patients when careful attention is paid to management of ICP.

In the absence of obstructive hydrocephalus, serial lumbar punctures provide the best mechanism of relieving the complications of ICP. Ten to 20 ml of spinal fluid can be removed safely at each tap. However, the true therapeutic benefit is most likely due to puncture defects in the dura, with persistent CSF leakage over time. Remarkably, patients with symptomatic elevation of CSF pressure often will experience prompt relief of symptoms (such as headache, nausea, and vomiting) within 30 minutes of the spinal tap and often will request repeat taps when they experience recurrent symptoms. Unfortunately, a systematic evaluation of the effect of aggressive CSF pressure management has not been performed. In the large study ACTG 159/MSG 17, opening pressures were measured in over 60% of patients, and the modes of pressure management were documented. The lower overall mortality (6%) in this study appears to be related to several factors, but the causal relationship of more aggressive pressure management with this outcome remains to be established.

On occasion, serial lumbar punctures are not sufficient to control the symptoms of increased ICP. In those instances, placement of a lumbar drain or ventriculostomy may be of acute benefit. However, placement of a ventricular-peritoneal shunt often is required in this setting to achieve long-term control of symptoms. The use of other measures to control increased ICP, such as acetazolamide or corticosteroids, remains controversial and cannot be recommended for use on a routine basis.

In summary, increased ICP ultimately may prove to be one of the most important predictors of outcome in patients with cryptococcal meningitis. In the setting of AIDS-associated cryptococcal disease, where the usual measurements of the spinal fluid formula (such as CSF glucose, protein, and white blood cell count) are within normal limits, ICP determination often becomes the most important measurement evaluated and should be obtained every time a spinal tap is performed.

Maintenance Therapy

Even after successful treatment of acute cryptococcal meningitis, 50% to 70% of patients will experience recurrent disease within 1 year if no maintenance therapy is administered.[7,8,66] This contrasts with the 12% to 25% relapse rate reported among non–HIV-infected patients.[43] Zuger et al reported no relapses among seven patients treated with weekly amphotericin B after successful initial treatment, compared to a relapse rate of 50% (four of eight patients) among patients receiving maintenance therapy over a 6-month period.[66] Chuck and Sande reported, in their retrospective review of cases at

San Francisco General Hospital, a relapse rate of 27% (7 of 26 patients) among those who did not receive maintenance therapy compared to 16% (6 of 37 patients) of those who received either ketoconazole or AMB maintenance therapy.[7] Clark et al reported a 38% relapse rate (three of eight patients) among those receiving no maintenance therapy vs a 7% rate (2 of 27 patients) among those who received AMB maintenance therapy.[8] Two separate fluconazole maintenance therapy pilot studies each reported 7% relapse rates (1 of 14 patients in a study by Stern et al[49] and 1 of 15 patients in a study by Sugar and Saunders[50]). A larger placebo-controlled study conducted by the California Collaborative Treatment Group reported a relapse rate of 15% (4 of 27 patients) in the placebo group compared to no relapses among the 34 patients receiving fluconazole therapy (100 to 200 mg/day).[4]

In a large definitive study conducted by the ACTG and the MSG, daily therapy with fluconazole (200 mg/day) was superior to AMB (1 mg/kg/week) as maintenance therapy for AIDS patients who had been treated sucessfully for acute cryptococcal meningitis.[37] Of 189 evaluable patients, 14 of 78 patients (18%) receiving AMB relapsed compared to 2 of 111 patients (2%) assigned to the fluconazole group. Kaplan-Meier estimates of relapse-free survival demonstrated a 27% difference between the two groups. Therapy-related side effects and bacterial infections were both more common in the AMB group. The study drug was discontinued because of severe toxicities in 12 patients assigned to AMB vs 6 patients assigned to fluconazole.

Based on this study, along with pilot data from previous studies, fluconazole (200 mg/day) is considered the treatment of choice as maintenance therapy for preventing relapse of cryptococcal meningitis in HIV-infected patients. The use of other triazoles, most notably itraconazole, remains a secondary choice. In a recently completed head-to-head study of itraconazole vs fluconazole conducted by the MSG (MSG 25), fluconazole was superior in preventing relapse of cryptococcal disease.[40] The study, which evaluated 107 patients who had been successfully treated for cryptococcal meningitis, was terminated based on a recommendation by an independent Data and Safety Monitoring Board, which noted a disproportionate number of relapses in one of the two study arms. A total of 15 relapses was observed, with 13 of 55 itraconazole recipients experiencing relapse of disease compared to 2 of 52 fluconazole recipients. Of note, a multivariate analysis of factors predicting the likelihood of relapse, the lack of use of 5-FC during initial acute therapy (the first 2 weeks) was *more* predictive of relapse than any other factor (relative risk 5.88, $p = 0.09$), including use of itraconazole as maintenance therapy (relative risk 4.32, $p = 0.06$). Along with the results from ACTG 159/MSG 17.

HISTOPLASMOSIS

Epidemiology and Pathogenesis

Histoplasmosis is endemic in the central and south central regions of the United States. The endemic area also extends along the river basins north into the Canadian provinces of Quebec and Ontario and south into Mexico, Central America, and South America. In the southern region of the United States, the endemic area extends to Alabama in the east and southwest Texas in the west, including the San Antonio area. Certain cities, most notably Indianapolis, Indiana, and Kansas City, Missouri, are high-incidence areas of histoplasmosis. In these hyperendemic areas, histoplasmosis has been reported to be the second or third most common opportunistic infection among HIV patients at various times.[20,44,56]

As with other systemic fungal infections, initial primary infection occurs in the lung after inhalation of arthroconidia, which are rapidly converted into the yeast phase at body temperature. The yeast are phagocytized by reticuloendothelial (RE) cells within the lung, where they continue to multiply. After the infection is well established, the organism disseminates through the body, initially within regional lymph nodes and ultimately within target organs. Two to 3 weeks after the initial infection, specific T-cell–mediated immunity is established, and the infected RE cells are better able to kill the intracellular organisms. In a normal host, the infection is usually brought under control, and the patient does not develop any further clinical manifestations. When the immune system is weakened, however, the initial infection may not be brought under control, and progressive disseminated disease ensues. In the case of an individual with a remote history of histoplasmosis who becomes immunosuppressed, reactivation disease in the form of disseminated histoplasmosis may occur. Patients at highest risk of disseminated histoplasmosis are those with defective T-cell–mediated immunity, such as patients with advanced HIV infection.

Although quite uncommon in an immunologically intact individual, progressive disseminated histoplasmosis (PDH) is the most common form of disease among AIDS patients. In nonendemic areas, PDH most likely represents reactivation disease.[20,26] However, in endemic areas, especially hyperendemic areas, PDH appears to represent disseminated primary infection, although firm epidemiologic data supporting this concept are lacking. Within endemic areas, histoplasmosis represents 5% of the opportunistic infections among AIDS patients. However, in hyperendemic areas, the incidence is as high as 25%.[56] Among these patients who develop histoplasmosis, it is the initial AIDS-defining illness in 50% to 75% of cases.

Clinical Manifestations

Disseminated histoplasmosis is generally a disease of more advanced stages of HIV infection. The median CD4 cell count at the time of diagnosis is $50/mm^3$.[56] Fever, weight loss, and other constitutional signs are present in over 95% of patients with PDH.[44,56] Respiratory complaints are the most common localizing symptoms, occurring in 50% to 60% of patients. Hepatosplenomegaly is noted in 20% to 40% of patients, lymphadenopathy in 20%, and skin or mucosal involvement in 2% to 5% of patients. Importantly, neurologic manifestations are reported in 18% to 20% of histoplasmosis cases.[2,55] This may take the form of meningitis or cerebritis. Approximately 10% of patients have a septicemic picture, characterized by high fever, hypotension, and on occasion, adult respiratory distress syndrome.[56] On rare occasions, histoplasmosis may occur as retinitis, pericarditis, prostatitis, pancreatitis, pleuritis, or colitis.

Routine laboratory test results are generally nonspecific. Peripheral white blood cell counts are similar to those of other patients with advanced HIV infection. Alkaline phosphatase and gamma-glutamyltransferase elevations are seen commonly, especially in those patients with PDH and hepatic involvement. Erythrocyte sedimentation rates are generally elevated. Chest radiographs are abnormal in up to 60% of patients.[56] The most common radiographic abnormality is diffuse infiltration, usually described as an interstitial pattern but possibly also a reticulonodular or alveolar pattern. Interestingly, mediastinal lymphadenopathy is distinctly uncommon in AIDS patients with PDH, occurring in only 3% to 5% of cases described in the literature. Nodular calcification in either the lung or mediastinal lymph nodes is reported in less than 3% of cases.

Diagnosis

Owing to the nonspecific symptoms of disseminated histoplasmosis, the disease may be difficult to diagnose. This is especially true in nonendemic areas, where clinicians may not consider the diagnosis or pathologists may be unaccustomed to identifying *H. capsulatum* in tissue specimens. Fortunately, several techniques have been identified that aid in the diagnosis of histoplasmosis.

The gold standard is a positive culture of the organism from peripheral blood or tissue specimens. The application of lysis-centrifugation blood culture techniques has greatly enhanced the reliability of blood cultures in the diagnosis of disseminated histoplasmosis.[56] Unfortunately, even with lysis-centrifugation systems, the diagnosis can take up to 2 to 3 weeks for confirmation. In experienced hands, this technique is positive in 85% to 95% of patients with disseminated histoplasmosis. Culture of tissues is less sensitive, although still an important means of establishing the diagnosis (Table 23–4).

Histopathologic evaluation of tissues is more rapid than culture and establishes the diagnosis in up to 50% of patients. The most accessible site to biopsy for histopathologic evaluation is the bone marrow. The organism usually can be identified within macrophages, and identification is readily enhanced through the use of special stains, such as methenamine silver (Color Plate II*D*). Other tissues, such as lymph node, liver, and skin, and bronchoalveolar lavage fluid, may yield a diagnosis in individuals with abnormal findings in these organ systems.

Standard serodiagnostic studies, which detect the presence of antibodies against *Histoplasma* antigens, are positive in the majority of patients. The immunodiffusion test usually reveals the presence of an M-band, but the more specific H-band is usually absent. Complement fixation serologic tests are reactive in 75% of patients with disseminated histoplasmosis. Unfortunately, the presence of antibodies does not indicate whether the patient is experiencing an active infection with histoplasmosis or simply has been infected in the past.

During the 1980s, Wheat et al established a diagnostic histoplasma antigen test (Table 23–4).[62] This test can be applied to both serum and urine, although the urine test is more sensitive and equally specific. In a retrospective study by Wheat et al, the *H. capsulatum* polysaccharide antigen (HPA) was detected in blood, urine, or CSF in 70 of 72 HIV-associated cases (97.3%).[56,59] Negative results in urine occurred in two patients who had asymptomatic pulmonary histoplasmosis.

An important application of the HPA test is its usefulness in following the response to therapy.[56,57,59] In one study, 19 of 19 successfully treated patients demonstrated a 2-unit or more fall in serum HPA levels, and 85% of patients had at least a 2-unit fall in urine HPA levels.[57] In another study of relapsing disease, 17 of 18 urine samples demonstrated a 2-unit increase in HPA levels at the time of relapse.[58] A 2-unit increase in HPA serum levels was noted in 12 of 14 relapsing patients. The magnitude of the HPA level may be predictive of long-term outcome. Three of five patients with baseline serum HPA levels of greater than 15 units died within 1 week of initiation of therapy.[56] However, more data are required before this association can be firmly established. Although the HPA test is performed only in Wheat's laboratory, a mechanism is available for practicing clinicians to send specimens to his laboratory for testing on individual patients [for more information, call 1(800) 447-8634].

Treatment

AMB has been the gold standard therapy for disseminated histoplasmosis in HIV-infected

TABLE 23–4. SENSITIVITY (%) OF DIAGNOSTIC TESTS FOR HISTOPLASMOSIS

| Test | Type of *H. capsulatum* Disease | | |
	Disseminated	Chronic Pulmonary	Acute
Histoplasma antigen	92	21	39
Culture	85	85	15
Histopathology	43	17	9
Serology	71	100	98

Data from Joseph Wheat (personal communication).

patients. Several reports in the literature document 90% success rates in control or resolution of symptoms associated with disseminated histoplasmosis.[20,54,56] Treatment with AMB often results in rapid defervescence within a period of days. Of 29 cases reported by Wheat et al, temperature fell to less than 100°F by day 3 of therapy in 25% and by day 7 of therapy in 73%.[56] Only 7% of patients remained febrile after 2 weeks of AMB therapy. The majority of patients who die of histoplasmosis usually succumb before receiving 500 mg of AMB. Additionally, those patients who are septicemic are at higher risk of death while on therapy.

Ketoconazole, which is effective in the control of histoplasmosis in non-AIDS patients, does not work well in patients with AIDS-associated histoplasmosis.[20,54,56] As induction therapy for control of acute symptoms of disseminated histoplasmosis, ketoconazole is not effective. In one series, only 1 of 11 patients with disseminated histoplasmosis was treated successfully with initial ketoconazole therapy.[56] Even using ketoconazole as maintenance therapy, up to 50% of patients relapsed compared to a relapse rate of 50% to 80% in patients not receiving maintenance therapy. In contrast, AMB at a dose of 1 mg/kg administered 1 to 2 times per week is associated with an 80% to 90% relapse-free survival.[30,56]

As opposed to ketoconazole, itraconazole has been evaluated in controlled clinical trials as both maintenance therapy (ACTG 084) and acute induction therapy (ACTG 120). The results of the maintenance study demonstrate successful prevention of relapse in 95% of patients (40 of 42 patients) receiving itraconazole (200 mg bid), with a median follow-up time of 109 weeks.[61] Urine HPA levels converted to negative in 43% of patients, whereas serum HPA levels became negative in 75% of the patients in this study. Itraconazole was evaluated as acute primary therapy of disseminated histoplasmosis (ACTG 120). Successful outcome was observed in 50 patients (85%).[60] Among those who were judged to be nonresponders, treatment failed in six (10%) because of progressive disease, in two (4%) because of toxicity, and in one (2%) was lost to follow-up by the second week. Although this study was not designed to be a comparative trial, the overall response rate was similar to historical experience with AMB. Based on these data, most investigators favor the use of itraconazole (200 mg twice daily) as the initial therapy for nonmeningeal, nonsepticemic,

AIDS-associated disseminated histoplasmosis. It should be noted that any patient treated with itraconazole should not be receiving contraindicated concomitant medications, such as rifampin, rifabutin, phenytoin, carbamazepine, H_2 blockers, or antacid therapy, in order to assure adequate drug levels.

The use of fluconazole in the treatment of histoplasmosis remains controversial. Anecdotal experience in the literature reveals a response rate of 40% for induction therapy with fluconazole.[46] A study by the ACTG (ACTG 174) demonstrated a lower response rate among those receiving fluconazole for acute histoplasmosis (74% success) than that achieved with itraconazole (historical controls). Based on the lower response rates among the anecdotal reports in the literature, fluconazole should be reserved for patients who are unable to take itraconazole and for whom AMB is not a viable option.

COCCIDIOIDOMYCOSIS

Epidemiology and Pathogenesis

Coccidioidomycosis is caused by *Coccidioides immitis,* an organism that is endemic to the southwestern United States, northern Mexico, and portions of Central and South America. The organism lives in the soil in the mycelial phase, and, when it is disturbed, aerosolized infectious particles are inhaled into the lungs of susceptible hosts. Once in the alveolar space, the organism multiplies, resulting in a giant spherule (Color Plate II*E*). Before development of T-cell immunity, macrophages may ingest the organism but are unable to kill it. The pathogenesis is similar in many ways to that seen in histoplasmosis, with potential dissemination of the organism before development of an adequate immune system response. Once T-cell immunity develops, the organism can be killed by the cells of the immune system, and the manifestations of disease are arrested. Among patients with impaired cellular immunity, however, progressive coccidioidal disease often develops, manifesting as disseminated disease in the lung, bone, skin, or CNS.

AIDS-associated coccidioidal disease is generally confined to the endemic regions. Reports of cases outside endemic areas probably represent expression of disease after exposure within an endemic area or, potentially, reactivated disease.[1,18,19] The majority of patients who develop AIDS-associated coccidioidomycosis have CD4 counts of less than 250/mm³ and evidence of impaired T-cell function, with negative spherulin skin tests.[18] In Arizona, coccidioidomycosis is the third most frequently reported opportunistic infection after *P. carinii* pneumonia and esophageal candidiasis.[19] The issue of whether disease expression is reactivation of old, arrested disease or acquisition of new infection is not resolved. A recent study by Ampel et al estimated a cumulative incidence of coccidioidal disease of 24.6% among a cohort of HIV-infected patients followed in Arizona.[1] Importantly, the presence of a positive skin test did not predict the development of active coccidioidomycosis in this cohort. Rather, a baseline positive skin test was most associated with the presence of a higher CD4 count at study entry. Nearly 20% of the subjects developed a positive skin test while on study. However, the development of dermal hypersensitivity was not associated with the development of active coccidioidomycosis.

Clinical Manifestations

Coccidioidal infection may occur in a wide variety of forms, ranging from positive serologic tests to life-threatening pneumonitis or meningitis (reviewed in ref. 18). Focal pulmonary disease may have focal radiologic abnormalities, which may be multiple and include focal alveolar infiltrates, discrete nodules, hilar adenopathy, or cavitary disease. Rarely, pleural effusions are noted. Diffuse pulmonary disease is more common and may be indistinguishable from other opportunistic infectious processes, such as *P. carinii* pneumonia (Chapters 20 and 29). Occasionally, patients with pulmonary disease may have evidence of cutaneous coccidioidomycosis. Rarely, the skin lesions are noted in the absence of pulmonary manifestations. Unlike cryptococcal meningitis, coccidioidal meningitis is characterized by high CSF cell counts, with white blood cell counts ranging from 2/mm³ to more than 1500/mm³. CSF glucose is usually suppressed and CSF protein is elevated, but not invariably so. Interestingly, about 50% of patients will have negative CSF cultures at the time of the initial visit. Complement fixation antibody is usually detected in the CSF in the majority of meningitis patients. Localized extrapulmonary disease has been reported in thoracic as well as in extrathoracic lymph nodes. Occasionally, hepatic coccidioidal disease is identified.

The majority of patients will have positive serologic titers for *C. immitis* at the time of diagnosis with either the tube precipitin (TP) or complement fixation test.[18] In general, the complement fixation test is more sensitive than the TP test. The likelihood of seropositivity is higher in patients with extrapulmonary disease than in those with focal or diffuse pulmonary manifestations. Complement fixation titers are generally highest in patients with meningitis, with values up to 1:4096. Less than 20% of patients have reactive spherulin skin tests. The CD4 count for patients with coccidioidal disease is generally less than 200/mm³. Among HIV-infected patients, long-term outcome is clearly associated with the type of disease manifestation. Patients with cutaneous or lymph node involvement experience longer median survival times than those with diffuse pulmonary disease or low initial CD4 counts. Survival among meningitis patients is variable but generally better than among those with diffuse pulmonary disease.

Diagnosis

Diagnosis of coccidioidomycosis is made by culturing the organism from clinical specimens or by demonstration of the organism via histopathologic stains. Spherules are best identified with methenamine silver or Papanicolaou stain (Color Plate II*E*). Blood cultures are positive in less than 30% of patients. Laboratories that attempt culture of *C. immitis* should bear in mind that the organism is extremely infectious and may be easily spread in a laboratory setting. Therefore, laboratory personnel should be notified when *C. immitis* disease is suspected so that appropriate precautions can be taken.

Serologic tests for *C. immitis* are positive in up to 80% of patients with coccidioidomycosis despite evidence of profound immunodeficiency in some patients.

Treatment

AMB remains the principal initial therapy for patients with coccidioidal disease, especially in individuals with diffuse pulmonary disease or meningitis. Several studies evaluating the role of oral azoles, including fluconazole and itraconazole, have demonstrated effectiveness of these agents, especially as maintenance therapy after control of disease has been achieved with AMB.[18,19] As with other systemic mycoses in AIDS patients, chronic suppressive therapy appears warranted. The precise dosage of amphotericin that should be administered before switching to an azole remains unclear. Most investigators suggest a minimum dose of at least 500 to 700 mg of AMB as initial therapy. Itraconazole and fluconazole appear to be effective as maintenance therapy of coccidioidal disease, although the number of patients treated is small.[5,22] Ketoconazole does not work well in AIDS-associated coccidioidomycoses.[65] Some investigators have had success using fluconazole as initial therapy for coccidioidal meningitis, but further data are needed before formal recommendation of this therapy, especially in the acutely ill patient. Intrathecal AMB is reserved for those patients with refractory meningitis.

FUNGAL PROPHYLAXIS

One of the most controversial areas in AIDS therapy is the use of primary prophylaxis for systemic fungal infections.[33] Systemic mycoses occur as late manifestations of HIV disease, usually with CD4 counts of less than $100/mm^3$.[32] The overall incidence of cryptococcal disease is 8% to 10% of AIDS patients, and the incidence of histoplasmosis and coccidioidomycosis varies with exposure to endemic areas. Many clinicians argue that patients living in endemic areas and patients who have CD4 counts of less than $50/mm^3$ would benefit from chronic fluconazole prophylaxis, usually at doses of 200 mg/day.[32] Indeed, in surveys of patients with advanced HIV infection who are participating in clinical trials, up to 40% of those with CD4 counts of less than $100/mm^3$ are on primary antifungal prophylaxis (J. Feinberg, personal communication).

In addition to economic concerns, a major issue in the argument against routine antifungal prophylaxis is that indiscriminate use of these agents may lead to a higher prevalence of resistant organisms in the community.[15,33,52,64] Reports of fluconazole-resistant *C. albicans* have increased substantially over the last 3 years.

However, the actual incidence of this problem is unknown and is probably quite low. Nonetheless, appropriate concern exists over azole-resistant fungi becoming a more significant problem in the next 5 to 10 years.

Fortunately, an ACTG study (ACTG 981) was initiated in 1988–1989 to evaluate this question.[36] This study enrolled over 400 patients with CD4 counts of less than $100/mm^3$ who were participating in an ongoing study of *P. carinii* pneumonia prophylaxis. Half of the patients were assigned to receive fluconazole (200 mg/day), and the other half received clotrimazole troches 5 times per day. Median follow-up was more than 35 months. Significantly more serious systemic fungal infections occurred in the clotrimazole group than in the fluconazole group. Most notably, the incidence of cryptococcal meningitis and esophageal candidiasis was substantially higher among the clotrimazole recipients. Interestingly, there were three cases of aspergillosis in the fluconazole-treated patients compared to one in the clotrimazole group. Despite the significant benefit in preventing systemic fungal infections with fluconazole, overall mortality between the two groups was no different; in fact, fewer deaths were noted overall in the clotrimazole-treated patients, although this difference did not reach statistical significance.

These data clearly support several important observations. First, serious systemic mycoses can be prevented with fluconazole when it is used in patients with advanced (CD4 counts <100 cells/mm^3) HIV disease. Second, prevention of systemic mycoses does not necessarily translate into a survival advantage, although morbidity may be reduced. Third, a cost–benefit analysis is needed to assess the overall advantage of preventing systemic fungal infections with no resultant survival advantage vs the monetary costs and potential toxicity costs (including drug interactions and potential development of resistant organisms) in this patient population. These analyses are currently underway. Until then, routine prophylaxis with fluconazole or itraconazole is not recommended.

ACKNOWLEDGMENTS

I would like to thank Jane Garrison for her outstanding help in the preparation of this manuscript.

REFERENCES

1. Ampel NM, Dols CS, Galgiani JN: Coccidioidomycosis during human immunodeficiency virus infection: Results of a prospective study in a coccidioidal endemic area. Am J Med 94:235–240, 1993
2. Anaissie E, Fainstein V, Samo T, et al: Central nervous system histoplasmosis: An unappreciated complication of the acquired immune deficiency syndrome. Am J Med 84:215–219, 1988
3. Armstrong D: Treatment of opportunistic infections. Clin Infect Dis 16:1, 1993
4. Bozzette SA, Larsen R, Chiu J, et al: A controlled trial of maintenance therapy with fluconazole after treatment of cryptococcal meningitis in the acquired immunodeficiency syndrome. N Engl J Med 324:580–584, 1991
5. Catanzaro A, Fierer J, Friedman PJ: Fluconazole in the treatment of persistent coccidioidomycosis. Chest 97:666–669, 1990
6. Centers for Disease Control: HIV/AIDS Surveillance Report. Atlanta, Centers for Disease Control, 1991
7. Chuck SL, Sande MA: Infections with *Cryptococcus neoformans* in the acquired immunodeficiency syndrome. N Engl J Med 321:794–799, 1989
8. Clark RA, Greer D, Atkinson W, et al: Spectrum of *Cryptococcus neoformans* infection in 68 patients infected with human immunodeficiency virus. Rev Infect Dis 12:768–777, 1990
9. Coker R, Tomlinson D, Harris J: Successful treatment of cryptococcal meningitis with liposomal amphotericin B after failure of treatment with fluconazole and conventional amphotericin B. AIDS 5:231–232, 1991
10. Denning DW, Armstrong RW, Lewis BH, et al: Elevated cerebrospinal fluid pressure in patients with cryptococcal meningitis and acquired immunodeficiency syndrome. Am J Med 91:267–272, 1991
11. Denning DW, Tucker RM, Hanson LH: Itraconazole therapy for cryptococcal meningitis and cryptococcosis. Arch Intern Med 149:2301–2308, 1989
12. Diamond RD, Bennett JE: Prognostic factors in cryptococcal meningitis: A study in 111 cases. Ann Intern Med 80:176–181, 1974
13. Dismukes WE: Cryptococcal meningitis in patients with AIDS. J Infect Dis 157:624–628, 1988
14. Dismukes WE, Cloud G, Gallis H, et al: Treatment of cryptococcal meningitis with combination of amphotericin B and flucytosine for four as compared with six weeks. N Engl J Med 317:334–341, 1987
15. Dupont B, Improvisi L, Eliaszewicz M, et al: Resistance of *Candida albicans* to fluconazole in AIDS patients (Abstract 1203). Program of the 32nd Interscience Conference on Antimicrobial Agents and Chemotherapy, Anaheim, CA, 1992, p 340
16. Eng RH, Bishburg E, Smith S, et al: Cryptococcal infections in the acquired immune deficiency syndrome. Am J Med 81:19–23, 1986
17. Ennis DM, Saag MS: Cryptococcal meningitis in AIDS. Hosp Pract 28:99–112, 1993
18. Fish DG, Ampel NM, Galgiani JN, et al: Coccidioidomycosis during human immunodeficiency virus infection: A review of 77 patients. Medicine (Balt.) 69:384–391, 1990
19. Galgiani JN, Ampel NM: Coccidioidomycosis in human immunodeficiency virus-infected patients. J Infect Dis 162:1165–1169, 1990
20. Graybill JR: Histoplasmosis and AIDS. J Infect Dis 158:623–625, 1988
21. Graybill JR, Sharkey PK, Vincent D, et al: Amphotericin B lipid complex (ABLC) in treatment of cryptococcal meningitis in patients with AIDS (Abstract 289). Program of 31st the Interscience Conference on Antimicrobial Agents and Chemotherapy, American Society for Microbiology, Chicago, 1991, p 147
22. Graybill JR, Stevens DA, Galgiani JN, et al: Itraconazole treatment of coccidioidomycosis. Am J Med 89:282–290, 1990
23. Hamilton JR, Noble A, Denning DW, et al: Performance of *Cryptococcus* antigen latex agglutination kits on serum and cerebrospinal fluid specimens of AIDS patients before and after pronase treatment. J Clin Microbiol 29:333–339, 1991
24. Larsen RA, Bozzette SA, Jones BE, et al: Fluconazole combined with flucytosine for treatment of cryptococcal meningitis in patients with AIDS. Clin Infect Dis 19:741–745, 1994
25. Johnston SRD, Corbett EL, Foster O, et al: Raised intracranial pressure and visual complication in AIDS patients with cryptococcal meningitis. J Infect 24:185–189, 1992
26. Keath EJ, Kobayashi GS, Medoff G: Typing of *Histoplasma capsulatum* by restriction fragment length polymorphisms in a nuclear gene. J Clin Microbiol 30:2104–2107, 1992
27. Kovacs JA, Kovacs AA, Polis M, et al: Cryptococcosis in the acquired immunodeficiency syndrome. Ann Intern Med 103:533–538, 1985
28. Larsen RA, Bozzette S, McCutchan JA, et al: Persistent *Cryptococcus neoformans* of the prostate after successful treatment of meningitis. Ann Intern Med 111:125–128, 1989
29. Larsen RA, Leal M, Chan L: Fluconazole compared with amphotericin B plus flucytosine for cryptococcal meningitis in AIDS. Ann Intern Med 113:183–187, 1990
30. McKinsey DS, Gupta MR, Riddker SA, et al: Long-term amphotericin B therapy for disseminated histoplasmosis in patients with the acquired immunodeficiency syndrome (AIDS). Ann Intern Med 111:655–659, 1989
31. McManus EJ, Jones JM: Detection of a *Trichosporon beigelii* antigen crossreactive with *Cryptococcus neoformans* capsular polysaccharide in serum from a patient with disseminated *Trichosporon* infection. J Clin Microbiol 21:681–685, 1985
32. Nightingale SD, Cal SX, Peterson DM, et al: Primary prophylaxis with fluconazole against systemic fungal infections in HIV-positive patients. AIDS 6:191–194, 1991
33. Perfect JR: Antifungal prophylaxis: To prevent or not? Am J Med 94:233–234, 1993
34. Popovich MJ, Arthur R, Helmer E: CT of intracranial cryptococcosis. Am J Radiol 154:603–606, 1990
35. Powderly WG, Cloud GA, Dismukes WE, et al: Value of serum and cerebrospinal fluid cryptococcal antigen measurement in the management of AIDS-associated cryptococcal meningitis. Clin Infect Dis 18:789–792, 1994
36. Powderly WG, Finkelstein D, Feinberg J, et al: A randomized trial comparing fluconazole with clotrimazole troches for the prevention of fungal infections

in patients with advanced human immunodeficiency virus infection: NIAID AIDS Clinical Trial Group. N Engl J Med 332:700–705, 1995

37. Powderly WG, Saag MS, Cloud GA, et al: A randomized controlled trial of fluconazole versus amphotericin B as maintenance therapy for prevention of relapse of cryptococcal meningitis in patients with AIDS. N Engl J Med 326:793–798, 1992

38. Rinaldi MG, Drutz DJ, Howell A, et al: Serotypes of *Cryptococcus neoformans* in patients with AIDS. J Infect Dis 153:642, 1986

39. Saag MS: Clinical and host differences between infections with the two varieties of *Cryptococcus neoformans*. (Editorial response). Clin Infect Dis 21:35–36, 1995

40. Saag MS, Cloud GC, Graybill JR, et al: Comparison of fluconazole versus itraconazole as maintenance therapy AIDS associated cryptococcal meningitis. (Abstract 953). Program of the 35th Interscience Conference on Antimicrobial Agents and Chemotherapy, conference, San Francisco, 1995

41. Saag MS, Dismukes WE: Azole antifungal agents: Emphasis on new triazoles. Antimicrob Agents Chemother 32:1–8, 1988

42. Saag MS, Powderly WG, Cloud GA, et al: Comparison of amphotericin B with fluconazole in the treatment of acute AIDS-associated cryptococcal meningitis. N Engl J Med 326:83–89, 1992

43. Sabetta JR, Andriole VT: Cryptococcal infection of the central nervous system. Med Clin North Am 69:333–344, 1985

44. Sarosi GA, Johnson PC: Disseminated histoplasmosis in patients with human immunodeficiency virus. Clin Infect Dis 14:S60–S67, 1992

45. Schurmann D, De Matos MB, Grunewald T, et al: Safety and efficacy of liposomal amphotericin B in treating AIDS-associated disseminated cryptococcosis. J Infect Dis 164:620–622, 1991

46. Sharkey-Mathis PK, Velez J, Fetchick R, et al: Histoplasmosis in the acquired immunodeficiency syndrome (AIDS): Treatment with itraconazole and fluconazole. J Acquir Immune Defic Syndr 6:809–819, 1993

47. Shimizu RY, Howard DH, Clancy MN: The variety of *Cryptococcus neoformans* in patients with AIDS. J Infect Dis 154:1042, 1986

48. Speed B, Dunt D: Clinical and host differences between infections with the two varieties of *Cryptococcus neoformans*. Clin Infect Dis 21:28–34, 1995

49. Stern JJ, Hartmen BJ, Sharkey P, et al: Oral fluconazole therapy for patients with acquired immunodeficiency syndrome and cryptococcal meningitis: Experience with 22 patients. Am J Med 85:477–480, 1988

50. Sugar AM, Saunders C: Oral fluconazole as suppressive therapy of disseminated cryptococcosis in patients with acquired immunodeficiency syndrome. Am J Med 85:481–489, 1988

51. Swinne D, Nkurikiyinfura JB, Muyembe TL: Clinical isolates of *Cryptococcus neoformans* from Zaire. Eur J Clin Microbiol 5:50–51, 1986

52. Troillet N, Durussel C, Billie J, et al: Fluconazole-resistant oral candidiasis in human immunodeficiency

virus-infected patients: In vitro–in vivo correlation (Abstract 1202). Program of the 32nd Interscience Conference on Antimicrobial Agents and Chemotherapy, Anaheim, CA, 1992

53. Vander Horst C, Saag MS, Cloud G, et al: Randomized double blind comparison of amphotericin B plus fluconazole to AMB alone followed by a comparison of fluconazole to itraconazole in the treatment of acute cryptococcal meningitis in AIDS (Abstract 1198). Program of the 35th Interscience Conference on Antimicrobial Agents and Chemotherapy, conference, San Francisco, 1995

54. Wheat LJ: Histoplasmosis—diagnosis and management. Infect Dis Clin Pract 1:287–290, 1992

55. Wheat LJ, Batteiger BE, Sathapatayavongs B: *Histoplasma capsulatum* infection of the central nervous system. Medicine (Balt) 69:244, 1990

56. Wheat LJ, Connolly-Stringfield P, Baker RL, et al: Disseminated histoplasmosis in the acquired immune deficiency syndrome: Clinical findings, diagnosis and treatment, and review of the literature. Medicine (Balt) 69:361–374, 1990

57. Wheat LJ, Connolly-Stringfield P, Blair R, et al: Effect of successful treatment with amphotericin B on *Histoplasma capsulatum* variety *capsulatum* polysaccharide antigen levels in patients with AIDS and histoplasmosis. Am J Med 92:153–160, 1992

58. Wheat LJ, Connolly-Stringfield P, Blair R, et al: Histoplasmosis relapse in patients with AIDS: Detection using *Histoplasma capsulatum* variety *capsulatum* antigen levels. Ann Intern Med 115:936–941, 1991

59. Wheat LJ, Connolly-Stringfield P, Kohler RB, et al: *Histoplasma capsulatum* polysaccharide antigen detection in the diagnosis and management of disseminated histoplasmosis in patients with acquired immunodeficiency syndrome. Am J Med 897:396, 1989

60. Wheat LJ, Hafner RE, Korzun AM, et al: Itraconazole treatment of disseminated histoplasmosis in patients with AIDS. Am J Med 98:336–342, 1995

61. Wheat LJ, Hafner RE, Wulfsohn M, et al: Prevention of relapse of histoplasmosis with itraconazole in patients with the acquired immunodeficiency syndrome. Ann Intern Med 118:610–616, 1993

62. Wheat LJ, Kohler RB, Tewari RP: Diagnosis of disseminated histoplasmosis by detection of *Histoplasma capsulatum* antigen in serum and urine specimens. N Engl J Med 314:83–88, 1986

63. Wilson DE, Bennett J, Bailey JW: Serologic grouping of *Cryptococcus neoformans*. Proc Soc Exp Biol Med 127:820–823, 1968

64. Wingard JR, Merz WG, Rinaldi MG, et al: Increase in *Candida krusei* infection among patients with bone marrow transplantation and neutropenia treated prophylactically with fluconazole. N Engl J Med 325:1274–1277, 1991

65. Zar FA, Fernandez M: Failure of ketoconazole maintenance therapy for disseminated coccidioidomycosis in AIDS (Letter). J Infect Dis 164:824–825, 1991

66. Zuger A, Louie E, Holzman RS: Cryptococcal disease in patients with the acquired immunodeficiency syndrome: Diagnostic features and outcome of treatment. Ann Intern Med 104:234–240, 1986

Chapter 24

AIDS-Associated Toxoplasmosis

CARLOS S. SUBAUSTE, SIN YEW WONG,
and JACK S. REMINGTON

Toxoplasma gondii is among the most prevalent causes of latent infection of the central nervous system (CNS) throughout the world. After an acute infection, cysts of *T. gondii* persist in the CNS and in multiple extraneural tissues. Although normal human hosts maintain infection in a quiescent state, immunocompromised individuals may be at risk for reactivation and dissemination of chronic (latent) infection.[70] Defective cellular immunity in patients with AIDS results in loss of the primary arm of host defense against this parasite. Reactivation of latent infection in patients with AIDS may lead to clinically apparent disease (toxoplasmosis), which most frequently manifests as life-threatening encephalitis. Thus, patients with AIDS who have been infected previously with *T. gondii* are at considerable risk for development of CNS toxoplasmosis.

Because AIDS patients in the United States who develop toxoplasmic encephalitis are almost always chronically infected with the protozoan,[134] patients with AIDS (or even individuals without AIDS who have antibody to HIV and who are known also to have antibodies to *T. gondii*) should be considered at significant risk for development of toxoplasmic encephalitis from the outset. Published data have demonstrated that 20% to 47% of AIDS patients who are seropositive for *T. gondii* will ultimately develop toxoplasmic encephalitis.[13,80,100,143,222] Seroprevalence varies between geographic locales and even within subpopulations of the same locale.[68,82,130,135,188,223] Studies performed in our laboratory have found a prevalence of *T. gondii* antibodies among HIV-positive adults of 8% to 16% in major urban areas of the United States. The prevalence is higher ($\geq$25%) among certain ethnic groups.

Because of the increasing incidence of HIV infection in women of child-bearing years, we predict that the incidence of infants congenitally infected with HIV and *T. gondii* will increase.[145,148,158] Prospective studies are underway in Miami, Florida, and Los Angeles, California, to determine the risk of congenital toxoplasmosis in infants born to women who are dually infected with HIV and *T. gondii* (see Congenital Toxoplasmosis and the HIV-Infected Woman).

CLINICAL PRESENTATION

In the United States, AIDS patients who develop toxoplasmic encephalitis generally do so after the diagnosis of AIDS has been made.[136,154,196,219] In areas where seroprevalence of *T. gondii* infection is high, toxoplasmic encephalitis frequently is the initial manifestation of AIDS.[38,40,122,170,187,222]

Ingestion of undercooked or raw meat containing tissue cysts and of vegetables or other food products contaminated with oocysts is a major means of transmission of the parasite,[221] as is more direct contact with cat feces.[221] Independent of category of risk for acquisition of HIV infection, AIDS-associated toxoplasmosis in the United States occurs significantly more often in Hispanic than in white patients.[25] In addition, a study found the frequency of toxoplasmosis to be significantly higher in poor Mexican patients with AIDS compared to counterparts with a higher socioeconomic status.[105]

Because there frequently is multifocal involvement of the CNS, there may be a wide spec-

The work discussed in this chapter was supported in part from grants A104717 and A130230 from the National Institutes of Health, Bethesda, Maryland.

trum of clinical findings, including alteration of mental status, seizures, motor weakness, sensory abnormalities, cerebellar dysfunction, meningismus, movement disorders, and neuropsychiatric manifestations.[45,87,122,126,154,179,190] The characteristic presentation is usually one of subacute onset with focal neurologic abnormalities in 58% to 89% of patients. Altered mental status, manifested by confusion, lethargy, delusional behavior, frank psychosis, global cognitive impairment, anomia, or coma, may be present initially in as many as 60% of patients.[45,87,122,154,170] Seizures are the cause of their seeking medical attention in approximately one third of AIDS patients with toxoplasmic encephalitis.[45,87,122,126,154,170] Focal neurologic deficits are evident on neurologic examination in approximately 60%.[45,122,154,170] Although hemiparesis is the most common focal neurologic finding, patients may have evidence of aphasia, ataxia, visual field loss, cranial nerve palsies, dysmetria, hemichorea-hemiballismus, tremor, parkinsonism, akathisia, or focal dystonia.[23,24,110,154,209] In addition, infection of the spinal cord with *T. gondii* has been described in cases of transverse myelitis and conus medullaris syndrome.[90,144] A rapidly fatal panencephalitis form of diffuse cerebral toxoplasmosis also has been described.[81] Unfortunately, computed tomography (CT) of the head was unrevealing in these cases.[81,82,109]

Extracerebral sites with or without concomitant toxoplasmic encephalitis may be involved in HIV-infected individuals.[132,160,184,210] Extracerebral toxoplasmosis usually occurs in patients with CD4 counts of less than 100/mm^3.[132,184] In patients with extracerebral toxoplasmosis, ocular and pulmonary sites are most commonly involved (50% and 26% of patients, respectively).[184] However, isolated parasitemia[184] and involvement of the heart,[21,79,142,151,184,191] bone marrow,[184] lymph nodes,[184] peritoneum,[102] stomach,[200] liver,[18,184] pancreas,[142] colon,[169] pituitary and adrenal glands,[83,146] bladder,[184] testes,[43,156] skeletal muscle,[74] skin,[91,184] rhinopharynx,[184] and spinal cord[184] have also been reported.

In recent years, pulmonary disease caused by toxoplasmosis has been increasingly reported and recognized.[54,160,195] The most common clinical syndrome is a prolonged febrile illness with cough and dyspnea that is clinically indistinguishable from *Pneumocystis carinii* pneumonia. Associated extrapulmonary disease caused by *T. gondii* has been reported in approximately 50% of the patients at the time of clinical presentation. Toxoplasmic encephalitis may pre-

cede or follow pulmonary toxoplasmosis if maintenance therapy is not instituted. A highly lethal syndrome of disseminated toxoplasmosis has been described in AIDS patients that consists of fever and a sepsis-like syndrome with hypotension, disseminated intravascular coagulation, elevated lactate dehydrogenase, and pulmonary infiltrates.[132,160,184] This syndrome is usually not associated with clinical or radiologic evidence of toxoplasmic encephalitis.[132,160].

Ocular disease caused by toxoplasmosis occurs relatively infrequently in AIDS patients (when compared with the incidence of cytomegalovirus retinitis).[41,71,72,94] Ocular pain and loss of visual acuity are common complaints, and funduscopic examination typically reveals findings consistent with necrotizing retinochoroiditis. The lesions are yellow-white areas of retinitis with fluffy borders. In reported series, the lesions were multifocal in 17% to 50%,[41,94] bilateral in 18% to 40%,[41,71,94] and accompanied by optic neuritis in approximately 10%. Vitreal inflammation may vary from mild localized vitreal haze to extensive vitreous inflammation.[41,71] Vasculitis and hemorrhage are uncommon. In most patients, the ocular lesions are located away from areas of preexisting scars. This suggests that the pathogenesis of these lesions may be secondary to hematogenous seeding rather than local reactivation of infection. The presence of concurrent toxoplasmic encephalitis in AIDS patients with ocular toxoplasmosis has varied from 29% to 63%.[41,71,94] On occasion, ocular toxoplasmosis may precede toxoplasmic encephalitis.[72,94,167,216]

In contrast to the immunocompetent host with toxoplasmic retinochoroiditis, in whom gross and histopathologic examination usually will reveal marked inflammation, in patients with AIDS-associated toxoplasmic chorioretinitis there frequently is only scant retinal inflammation.[94] Thus, the features of toxoplasmic retinochoroiditis commonly observed in the immunocompetent host may be absent in patients with AIDS. Toxoplasmic optic neuritis also has been described.[71]

Endocrinopathies secondary to the syndrome of inappropriate antidiuretic hormone secretion or panhypopituitarism may be the primary manifestation or a later complication of CNS toxoplasmosis.[63,83,146]

Abnormalities in routine clinical laboratory tests are too nonspecific to be of diagnostic use. Most AIDS patients with toxoplasmic encephalitis (80% to 95%) have CD4 T-lymphocyte counts of less than 100/mm^3.[2,60,143,147,161] Furthermore, the risk of developing toxoplasmic encephalitis appears to be associated with CD4 T-lymphocyte counts.[119,161] The incidence of toxoplasmic encephalitis at 18 months was 12% for patients who had CD4 T-lymphocyte counts above 100/mm^3 at baseline.[119] This increased to 25% and 45% for patients with CD4 T-lymphocyte counts of 50 to 99/mm^3 and less than 50/mm^3, respectively.[119] Approximately 90% of patients who developed this disease had CD4 T-lymphocyte counts of less than 100/mm^3 within 4 months prior to the diagnosis.[119] A case of toxoplasmic encephalitis with laboratory abnormalities of the hypothalamic–anterior pituitary–adrenal axis has been described.[146] Cerebrospinal fluid (CSF) may be normal or reveal mild pleocytosis (predominantly lymphocytes and monocytes) and an elevated protein level, whereas the glucose content usually is normal.[63,154,214,219]

CONGENITAL TOXOPLASMOSIS AND THE HIV-INFECTED WOMAN

Women infected with HIV are at risk for transmission of *T. gondii* infection to the fetus if they are seronegative for *T. gondii* antibodies and acquire *T. gondii* infection during pregnancy or if they are seropositive for *T. gondii* antibodies and suffer reactivation of their latent *T. gondii* infection because of immune deficiency from HIV infection (Chapter 30). At present, there are insufficient data to quantify the risk of congenital transmission by HIV-infected mothers who have chronic *T. gondii* infection. Preliminary data from Mitchell et al revealed a congenital transmission rate for women who are dually infected with HIV and *T. gondii* that was more than 400-fold higher when compared to non–HIV-infected, *T. gondii*–seropositive pregnant women. Approximately 5% of infants born of dually infected mothers had congenital toxoplasmosis.[149] Furthermore, when dually infected women developed toxoplasmosis during pregnancy, 75% of their infants were born with congenital toxoplasmosis and HIV infection.[149] All infants with congenital toxoplasmosis born to mothers who were HIV infected also were infected with HIV. The initial clinical presentation of congenital toxoplasmosis in the HIV-infected infant is similar to that in the non–HIV-infected infant but appears to run a more rapid and progressive course. The infants often appear normal at birth. In the ensuing months, they fail to gain

weight or develop appropriately. The majority develop multisystem organ involvement, including the CNS, heart, and lungs.[148]

DIAGNOSIS

At present, the definitive diagnosis of toxoplasmosis in AIDS patients can be made only by demonstration of the organism in tissues (Table 24–1). Although the morbidity associated with obtaining a brain biopsy for the diagnosis of toxoplasmic encephalitis is less than that which would accrue from an erroneous diagnosis,[34] neurosurgery is often deferred because many AIDS patients with neurologic syndromes frequently have inaccessible intracerebral lesions. The desire to avoid brain biopsy has resulted in the almost universal practice of initiating empiric anti–*T. gondii* therapy in AIDS patients who have characteristic findings on neuroradiologic imaging studies. In this setting alternative causes should be sought when the patient fails to respond clinically or radiographically. Brain biopsy frequently is the only alternative in this situation.

Serology

Because toxoplasmic encephalitis in patients with AIDS in the United States almost always represents reactivation of chronic (latent) infection, the presence of IgG *T. gondii* antibodies in an AIDS patient must be regarded as a marker for the potential development of toxoplasmosis. If the serologic status of an AIDS patient with suspected toxoplasmic encephalitis is

TABLE 24–1. METHODS FOR DEFINITIVE OR PRESUMPTIVE DIAGNOSIS OF TOXOPLASMOSIS IN PATIENTS WITH AIDS

- Histologic evaluation, including immunoperoxidase staining of tissue biopsies
- Demonstration of *T. gondii* in body fluids (CSF, BAL) (Wright-Giemsa stain)
- Isolation of *T. gondii* from tissue biopsies or body fluids (CSF, blood, BAL)
- Detection of *T. gondii* DNA by PCR in body fluids (CSF, blood, BAL) or tissue biopsies
- CT scans and/or MR images of the head
- Serology (including titer in agglutination assay, IgG, IgM*)
- Intrathecal production of *T. gondii*–specific antibodies

* Useful mainly in areas of high seroprevalence.

unknown, determination of immunoglobulin (Ig)G antibody status should be performed.

Although almost all AIDS patients with toxoplasmic encephalitis have detectable IgG *T. gondii* antibodies in their serum, published series have reported a 0% to 3% seronegativity rate.[55,170,205] Although the prevalence of *T. gondii* infection has not been shown to be higher in HIV-infected individuals than in uninfected individuals,[100] recent data demonstrate that, among *T. gondii*–infected individuals, those with HIV infection have significantly higher titers of *T. gondii* antibodies than do individuals without HIV infection.[55] In some studies, significantly more elevated antibody titers have been observed in AIDS patients with toxoplasmosis compared to those with latent *T. gondii* infection.[55,80,170] Although a single determination of IgG antibody titer cannot be used to distinguish latent from active infection, we observed that the magnitude of antibody titer to formalin-fixed *T. gondii* antigen had a high predictive value for the diagnosis of toxoplasmic encephalitis.[205]

When CSF is available, measurement of intrathecal production of antibody to *T. gondii* may serve as a useful ancillary test.[162,183] A similar investigation has demonstrated little use for antibody load in the diagnosis of ocular toxoplasmosis in AIDS.[29]

IgM *T. gondii* antibodies, routinely measured to diagnose acute toxoplasmosis in non-AIDS patients, are rarely demonstrable in AIDS patients with toxoplasmic encephalitis and, when present, suggest recently acquired infection.[55,80] The specificity of the IgM immunosorbent agglutination assay (ISAGA) in AIDS patients is unclear.[17,95] IgA *T. gondii* antibodies are rarely elevated in AIDS patients with acute toxoplasmic encephalitis.[202] *T. gondii* IgE antibodies measured by enzyme-linked immunosorbent assay and ISAGA have been detected in serum in a limited number of patients with toxoplasmic encephalitis.[173,220]

Isolation Studies

Isolation of *T. gondii* from body fluids or, in the appropriate clinical setting, from tissue obtained from a patient with AIDS should be considered diagnostic of active infection. Because isolation of the organism may not be evident for 6 days to 6 weeks after mice or tissue cultures are inoculated, the results often are not helpful in initial management of the patient. Neverthe-

less, isolation of the organism may obviate future need for brain biopsy.

T. gondii readily forms plaques in tissue cultures of human foreskin fibroblasts and most other cultured cells.[51,93] The plaques, when stained with Wright-Giemsa and examined microscopically, are seen to consist of necrotic and heavily infected cells and numerous extracellular tachyzoites. *T. gondii* has been isolated from the blood in 14% to 38% of AIDS patients with toxoplasmosis.[45,50,208] Parasitemia appears to occur more frequently when toxoplasmosis involves extraneural sites.[50] *T. gondii* also may be isolated from bronchoalveolar lavage (BAL) fluid in patients with toxoplasmic pneumonitis as early as 48 hours after tissue culture inoculation.[53]

Any diagnostic microbiology or virology laboratory that can inoculate the buffy coat of blood or bronchoalveolar fluid into tissue culture has the capacity to isolate *T. gondii* from patients with active infection.[53,198]

DNA Detection

The use of the polymerase chain reaction (PCR) has enabled detection of *T. gondii* DNA in brain tissue,[18,96,97,211] CSF (approximately 50% to 70%),[58,117,165,168] BAL fluid,[16,17,116] blood (as high as 69%),[58,59,66] and aqueous humor[58] of AIDS patients with toxoplasmosis. Because *T. gondii* cysts persist in the brain for years after infection, a positive PCR in the brain does not necessarily reflect active infection. Although detection of *T. gondii* DNA by PCR can be useful for the diagnosis of toxoplasmosis, studies indicate that positive PCR can occur in blood samples from patients unlikely to have toxoplasmic encephalitis.[185]

Neuroradiologic Studies

Toxoplasmic encephalitis is the most common cause of focal intracerebral lesions in patients with AIDS.[62,181,204] Imaging studies of the brain have become indispensable for diagnosis and management of these patients.[127] Typically, multiple, bilateral, hypodense, enhancing mass lesions are found on CT scan.[61,63,154,180] Lesions have a predilection for, but are not limited to, the basal ganglia and hemispheric corticomedullary junction.[19,61,63,180] A significant degree of enhancement of intracerebral lesions generally is present on CT scan.[19,61,63,78,122,154,180,181]

T. gondii abscesses may, however, fail to enhance or be solitary and located anywhere in the brain.[35,36,47,114]

Masses demonstrated by magnetic resonance (MR) images may be absent on CT scan,[114,128] whereas the converse apparently is not true. In a review of AIDS patients with focal neurologic symptoms, a CT scan was as good as an MRI image in detecting focal brain lesions (70% vs 74%). However, in AIDS patients with nonfocal neurologic symptoms, only 22% had CT scans that revealed focal lesions, compared to 42% found by MR studies. As in CT scans, lesions found on MR images of AIDS patients with toxoplasmic encephalitis frequently are bilateral and located in the basal ganglia or cerebral corticomedullary junction.[114,182] Deep lesions, which generally range from 1 to 3 cm in diameter, may show central patterns of both low and high signal intensity, suggestive of necrosis.[47] Unlike CT scans, MR images usually reveal multiple lesions.[35,36,114,182] In fact, a single lesion seen on an MR image should alert the clinician to other possible causes of the focal neuroradiologic findings (e.g., lymphoma, fungal abscesses, tuberculoma, or Kaposi's sarcoma).[35] In the presence of a single lesion on MR image, the probability of CNS lymphoma is at least equal to or higher than the probability of toxoplasmic encephalitis.[35]

As with results of CT scans, MR findings cannot be considered pathognomonic for toxoplasmic encephalitis. Although primary CNS lymphoma cannot be distinguished from toxoplasmosis solely on the basis of neuroradiologic criteria, the most reliable feature distinguishing lymphoma from toxoplasmosis in AIDS patients was the presence of hyperattenuation on non-enhanced CT scans and subependymal location on either CT or MR.[57] The neuroradiologic response of toxoplasmic encephalitis to specific treatment is seen on CT as a reduction in mass effect, number and extent of lesions, and enhancement.[47] Although the time to resolution of lesions may vary from 20 days to 6 months, the vast majority of patients who respond clinically will show radiologic improvement (>50%) by the third week of treatment.[137] The response of abnormalities on MR image to specific therapy also varies with the location and complexity of the mass lesion. Peripheral lesions of uniform signal intensity on MRI scan frequently resolve after 3 to 5 weeks of therapy, whereas deeper lesions with complex central signal patterns, consistent with necrosis, take longer to resolve and leave residual lesion(s) at the site

of necrosis.[47] Persistent enhancement on CT scans or MR images after treatment for toxoplasmic encephalitis has been associated with a higher incidence of subsequent relapse of the encephalitis.[115] Positron emission tomography has been reported to be useful in the diagnosis of toxoplasmic encephalitis.[171] Whereas areas of decreased glucose metabolism were seen in brains of all patients with toxoplasmic encephalitis, areas with increased glucose metabolism were observed in all patients with CNS lymphoma.[171]

Histopathology

Definitive diagnosis of toxoplasmic encephalitis often requires demonstration of the organism on histopathologic sections of brain tissue obtained at biopsy. Needle brain biopsy or aspiration is limited by lack of sensitivity of the procedure to make a definitive diagnosis, because the size of the specimen may be too small or there may be sampling error.[216] Some evidence suggests the superiority of open excisional biopsy compared to needle biopsy in making the histopathologic diagnosis of toxoplasmic encephalitis.[214] Moreover, the observation of abnormal lymphocytes in areas of involvement demonstrated by needle biopsy or aspiration has led to the erroneous diagnosis of cerebral lymphoma.

The response of the brain to *T. gondii* infection can vary from a granulomatous reaction with gliosis and microglial nodule formation to a severe focal or generalized necrotizing encephalitis.[63,138,154,180,204] Granulomatous lesions with a cellular infiltrate of abnormal lymphocytes, plasma cells, neutrophils, and monocytes may enlarge and develop central regions of necrosis.[63,138,154,180] Perivascular and intimal inflammatory cell infiltrates can lead to fibrosis or necrosis, which can result in hemorrhage[218] or thrombosis, accounting for neurologic signs and symptoms. It has been suggested that the invasion and multiplication of *T. gondii* in the cerebral vascular walls causes focal fibrotic hyperplasia, which leads to an obliterative vasculitis and discrete coagulative necrosis in the CNS.[48,98]

The presence of numerous *T. gondii* tachyzoites or cysts surrounded by an inflammatory reaction is diagnostic.[188] Tachyzoites, when observed, are usually found within the inflammatory reaction surrounding areas of necrosis. Cysts or free organisms not demonstrable on routine histopathologic examination can be identified using the peroxidase-antiperoxidase method.[42,214] This method is significantly more sensitive and no less specific in making the diagnosis of toxoplasmic encephalitis than is direct visualization of the organisms in association with cerebral inflammation and necrosis.[42,122] A rapid, sensitive, and specific method for diagnosis of toxoplasmic encephalitis by electron microscopy has been described.[28] Thus, when routine histopathologic studies fail to provide a definitive diagnosis, appropriately fixed brain tissue should be stained by the immunoperoxidase technique or analyzed by electron microscopy in an attempt to identify *T. gondii* antigens or organisms.

Wright-Giemsa–stained smears or touch preparations should be made as immediately as is feasible from tissue obtained at surgery. If organisms are demonstrated, potentially life-saving therapy can be initiated promptly. Similarly, Wright-Giemsa stain of a cytocentrifuge preparation of CSF may reveal the presence of tachyzoites.[49] Tachyzoites may be visualized in Giemsa-stained smears of bronchoalveolar lavage fluid in AIDS patients with pulmonary toxoplasmosis.[15]

Differential Diagnosis

In AIDS patients with focal abnormalities on neurologic examination, multiple enhancing lesions on CT scan and a positive *T. gondii* antibody titer strongly suggest the diagnosis of toxoplasmic encephalitis. Regardless of results of *T. gondii* serology, the differential diagnosis for individuals with nonfocal symptoms and one or two lesions on CT scan includes, in addition to CNS toxoplasmosis, lymphoma, fungal abscess, mycobacterial or cytomegaloviral disease, and Kaposi's sarcoma. Because therapy is available for each of these disorders, brain biopsy for histopathologic diagnosis may be necessary for successful management of the patient. The characteristic appearance of progressive multifocal leukoencephalopathy on neuroimaging studies often permits differentiation of this disorder from other causes of intracerebral mass lesions.

MANAGEMENT

General Principles

Because toxoplasmic encephalitis generally reflects reactivation of a latent infection, all HIV-positive individuals should be tested for *T. gondii*–specific IgG antibody. Patients with positive titers are at risk for development of toxoplasmic encephalitis, and the results of the serologic tests should be clearly available in the chart in case a patient has signs suggestive of toxoplasmosis (Fig. 24–1).

An MR image should be obtained in patients with neurologic abnormalities and a negative CT scan on presentation. Patients with only one lesion on CT scan should undergo MR imaging to attempt to determine if more than a single lesion is present. In patients with nonfocal neurologic abnormalities, MR imaging is the preferred initial evaluation. Because a single lesion on MR imaging is uncharacteristic of *T. gondii* infection and more than 50% of these lesions are lymphomas,[35,36] early biopsy of the involved area should be considered. Expedient and aggressive evaluation of AIDS patients with CNS mass lesions allows earlier use of specific therapies and averts use of erroneous and potentially toxic treatment regimens.

AIDS patients with multiple focal lesions visible on neuroimaging studies should receive therapy for presumptive toxoplasmic encephalitis. Focal intracranial lesions caused by *T. gondii* may occur in association with cerebral lymphoma[129] or *Mycobacterium tuberculosis*.[181] In patients with concurrent focal and diffuse CNS disease, toxoplasmosis also has been found in association with cytomegalovirus encephalitis and cryptococcal meningitis.[26,181]

Diffuse toxoplasmic encephalitis frequently goes underdiagnosed and should be suspected when a patient with severe CD4 cell depletion and positive *T. gondii* serology experiences unexplained fever and neurologic disease.[109] When diagnostic investigations fail to disclose a specific cause in these cases, a trial of empiric anti–*T. gondii* treatment should be considered.

In regard to what can be expected in relation to clinical and radiologic response to therapy, a prospective study demonstrated that 71% of the patients had a complete or partial response.[137] The neurologic response was rapid, with 51% of patients showing signs of improvement by day 3 and 91% by day 14.[137] The 29% who were classified as treatment failures all either experienced progression of their baseline neurologic abnormalities or developed new ones within the first 12 days of empiric therapy. Thus, brain biopsy with or without change of therapy should be considered in patients whose condition worsens early in the course of therapy or in patients who do not show clinical improvement by 10 to 14 days of therapy.[137] Re-

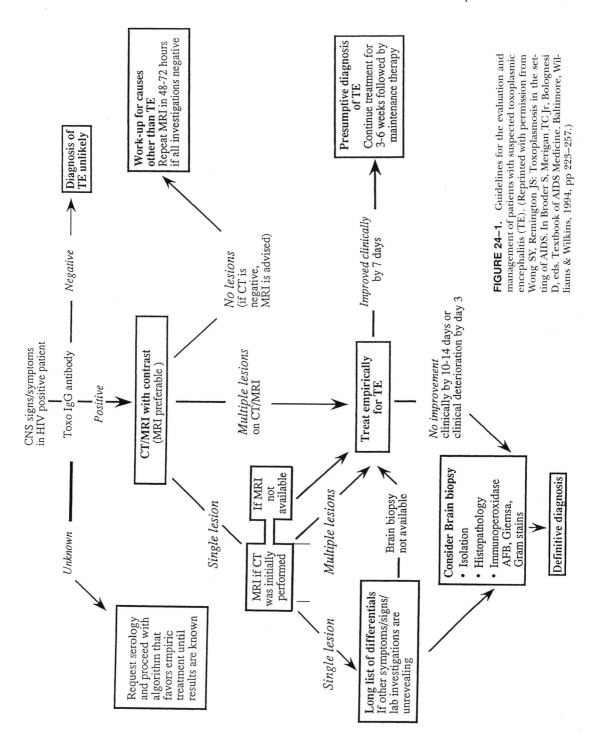

FIGURE 24–1. Guidelines for the evaluation and management of patients with suspected toxoplasmic encephalitis (TE). (Reprinted with permission from Wong SY, Remington JS: Toxoplasmosis in the setting of AIDS. In Broder S, Merigan TC Jr, Bolognesi D, eds. Textbook of AIDS Medicine. Baltimore, Williams & Wilkins, 1994, pp 223–257.)

peat neuroradiologic study by the same modality as originally selected should be performed 2 to 4 weeks after initiation of therapy in patients who demonstrate a satisfactory clinical response (or earlier if response is poor). Lesions should have diminished in size and possibly in number. Patients with extraneurologic toxoplasmosis should be evaluated for CNS disease, because most will have intracerebral involvement as well.[123,142]

Corticosteroids frequently are required for management of patients with intracranial hypertension caused by the mass effect from *T. gondii* abscesses. A recent study reported that there was no difference in the response rate and the time to response in patients who received corticosteroids when compared to those who did not.[137] At present, AIDS patients with toxoplasmic encephalitis should receive corticosteroids only when it is absolutely necessary. (If possible, no more than 2 weeks of therapy should be given.) Whether administration of anticonvulsant agents is necessary for prevention of seizures has not been determined.

It is important to distinguish between two forms of therapy for toxoplasmic encephalitis in patients with AIDS: primary therapy and maintenance therapy (Table 24–2). Primary therapy is administered during the acute disease. Maintenance therapy is administered after an adequate clinical and neuroradiologic response has been observed. Maintenance therapy should be continued for life, because the rate of relapse is prohibitively high when treatment is discontinued.

There is remarkable variability in the suscep-

tibility of different *T. gondii* strains to different antimicrobial agents,[1,5] and the potential for development of drug resistance may complicate the medical management of AIDS-associated toxoplasmosis.

Primary Therapy

It is standard practice to administer the combination of pyrimethamine plus sulfadiazine or pyrimethamine plus clindamycin. Pyrimethamine, a potent dihydrofolate reductase inhibitor, is the cornerstone of current treatment of AIDS-associated toxoplasmic encephalitis. The half-life of pyrimethamine varies from 20 to 175 hours.[217] Serum concentrations of pyrimethamine in individuals treated with the same dose of drug have great variability.[27,120,217] This variability may in part reflect erratic absorption of pyrimethamine in patients with AIDS-associated enteropathies. Although serum concentrations cannot be predicted for a given dose[120,217] or even for a given patient on a given day, serum concentrations of pyrimethamine significantly increase with increasing dose.[120] A recent study noted several patients with AIDS-associated CNS toxoplasmosis who were treated daily with 25 or 50 mg of pyrimethamine and who had peak or trough serum concentrations lower than or barely exceeding the concentration of pyrimethamine required in vitro for toxoplasmacidal activity.[103,120,139] In contrast, all patients who were treated daily with 100 mg of pyrimethamine had peak and trough serum concentrations well above the minimum con-

TABLE 24–2. GUIDELINES FOR ACUTE OR PRIMARY TREATMENT OF AIDS PATIENTS WITH TOXOPLASMIC ENCEPHALITIS

Drug	Dosage
Recommended Regimens	
Pyrimethamine	PO: 200 mg loading followed by 50–75 mg q24h
Folinic acid	PO, IV, or IM: 10–20 mg q24h
plus	
sulfadiazine	PO: 1 g q6h
or	
clindamycin	IV or PO: 600 mg q6h
Alternative Regimens	
Trimethoprim-sulfamethoxazole	PO or IV: 5 mg (trimethoprim component)/kg q6h
Pyrimethamine and folinic acid	As in recommended regimen
Plus one of the following:	
Clarithromycin	PO: 1 g q12h
Atovaquone	PO: 750 mg q6h
Azithromycin	PO: 1200–1500 mg q24h
Dapsone	PO: 100 mg q24h

centration required in vitro for toxoplasmacidal activity.[120] When CSF penetration of pyrimethamine was studied in small numbers of patients with AIDS[219] and meningeal leukemia,[73,203] the CSF concentration of drug was between 10% and 25% of the serum concentration. Data suggest that pyrimethamine may be concentrated in the brain.[121]

A prospective, randomized study of the regimens has shown clear efficacy of pyrimethamine plus clindamycin and no significant differences in clinical outcome when compared to pyrimethamine plus sulfadiazine.[45,106] A panel of experts recommended administration of 600 mg of clindamycin orally (or intravenously) every 6 hours.[190]

A few studies have revealed that trimethoprim-sulfamethoxazole (TMP-SMX) may be effective for acute therapy of toxoplasmic encephalitis,[20,89,201] achieving a 75% response rate.[20] However, TMP-SMX cannot, at present, be recommended as a first-line drug for acute therapy of toxoplasmic encephalitis because the activity of this combination against *T. gondii* is significantly inferior to that of the combination of pyrimethamine and sulfadiazine both in vitro and in animal models of toxoplasmosis.[84]

Standard therapy is limited by the high incidence of toxicity associated with both drugs in combination. The most notable toxicity of pyrimethamine is dose-related bone marrow suppression, resulting in thrombocytopenia, granulocytopenia, or megaloblastic anemia.[108,152,153] At doses of 75 to 100 mg/day, hematologic abnormalities should be anticipated but may be difficult to disassociate from those associated with HIV infection per se. Complete blood counts of patients receiving pyrimethamine should be monitored frequently for the development of drug-associated bone marrow toxicity.

Folinic acid (leucovorin calcium) may prevent marrow toxicity or be used to treat patients with marrow toxicity caused by pyrimethamine[108,188] and is not antagonistic to the activity of pyrimethamine or sulfadiazine against *T. gondii.*[69] The oral dose of folinic acid administered to these patients is usually 10 to 20 mg/day in divided doses[157] (Table 24–2). If hematologic abnormalities develop and malabsorption of the folinic acid is suspected, folinic acid may be administered parenterally. Some investigators increase folinic acid up to 50 mg/day for suspected pyrimethamine-associated hematologic toxicity.[122] Few data suggest that higher doses prevent progression of or reverse the he-

matologic toxicities. Folic acid must not be used, because it will inhibit the anti–*T. gondii* activity of pyrimethamine.[69] Although 65% to 90% of patients with toxoplasmic encephalitis will have an initial favorable response to pyrimethamine plus sulfadiazine therapy,[45,122,154] untoward reactions to this combination, most frequently rash,[45] may limit duration of therapy. Studies reveal that as many as 40% of AIDS patients who receive sulfadiazine and pyrimethamine for toxoplasmic encephalitis manifest signs of toxicity sufficiently severe to prompt discontinuation of the drug(s) during the primary phase of treatment.[85,87,122]

It is likely that sulfonamide is discontinued prematurely in many cases in which, with continuation, lessening or disappearance of the rash would occur. A number of investigators have stated that the majority of patients with AIDS who experience sulfonamide-associated cutaneous reactions can be successfully desensitized to these agents.[77,172] Crystal-induced nephrotoxicity is another well-recognized adverse reaction to sulfadiazine.[150,164,199] The most frequent adverse reactions seen in patients treated with pyrimethamine-clindamycin—skin rash and gastrointestinal and hematologic toxicity[45,106]—are similar to those seen with pyrimethamine plus sulfadiazine.[45] The substantial toxicities associated with standard anti–*T. gondii* treatment underscore the urgent need to develop safe and effective alternative drug regimens.

In the search for such regimens, most studies have evaluated the safety and efficacy of a nonsulfonamide agent in combination with pyrimethamine.[44,65,106,118] Whether toxoplasmic encephalitis can be treated effectively solely with pyrimethamine deserves further investigation.

Almost all the studies on the use of antimicrobial agents that have been described for the treatment of toxoplasmosis in AIDS patients have focused on patients with toxoplasmic encephalitis. Limited data suggest that patients with extracerebral toxoplasmosis also respond to therapy with pyrimethamine-sulfadiazine or pyrimethamine-clindamycin but that the mortality rate in patients with pulmonary or disseminated toxoplasmosis may be much higher than in patients with toxoplasmic encephalitis alone.

Investigational Drugs

A number of other agents have been tried in vitro, in animal models, and in a few case re-

TABLE 24–3. NEWER ANTIMICROBIAL/INVESTIGATIONAL AGENTS AND CYTOKINES SHOWN TO BE EFFECTIVE ALONE OR IN COMBINATION AGAINST TOXOPLASMOSIS

	References		References
Sulfa Agents		**Others**	
Dapsone (B, C)*	52,215	Rifabutin (B)	11
		Minocycline (B)	31
Macrolides/Azalides		Doxycycline (B, C)	30, 178
Azithromycin (A, B, C)	6, 64	Qinghaosu (A)	166
Clarithromycin (A, B, C)	6, 8, 65	Arpinocid (B)	133
		Pentamidine	131
Hydroxynaphthoquinones		5-Fluorouracil (A, C)	56, 86
Atovaquone (A, B, C)	39, 112	**Cytokines**	
Folic Acid Reductase Inhibitors		IFN-γ (A, B)	206
Trimetrexate (A, C)	113, 177	IFN-β (B)	163
Piritrexin (B)	2	TNF (B)	32
		IL-1 (B)	32
		IL-2 (B)	197
		IL-7 (B)	†
		IL-12 (B)	3, 99
		GM-CSF (B)	14

* A, in vitro; B, in animal models; C, in humans.
† L. Kasper, personal communication.

ports (Table 24–3) for the treatment of toxoplasmosis. It is beyond the scope of this chapter to review all of these articles, and interested readers are referred to a review on the topic.[221] Experience with the investigational agents, when they have been used as monotherapy in humans, has been that they are often associated with initial clinical improvement but subsequent relapse even when the agent is continued. *We urge that subsequent trials in humans include at least two agents in combination.*

Spiramycin, used for prevention of transplacental transmission of *T. gondii,* has been reported as ineffective for prevention, treatment, or suppression of toxoplasmic encephalitis.[125] The new macrolide-azalide antibiotics azithromycin,[1,10] roxithromycin,[31,92] and clarithromycin[33] were effective in a murine model of toxoplasmosis. A small, noncomparative clinical trial with clarithromycin plus pyrimethamine demonstrated efficacy comparable to that of the standard regimen.[65] Results of carefully controlled prospective clinical trials are needed before the new macrolide-azalide antibiotics can be recommended routinely for the treatment of acute toxoplasmic encephalitis.

Like pyrimethamine, trimetrexate inhibits *T. gondii* dihydrofolate reductase but more potently.[113] The high incidence of relapse of patients with biopsy-proven toxoplasmic encephalitis who were receiving trimetrexate suggests that this drug, when used alone, has only transient activity against this disorder.[177]

Atovaquone, a hydroxynaphthoquinone, has remarkable activity against the tachyzoite and cyst (bradyzoite) forms of *T. gondii* both in vitro and in vivo.[4,5] In a small, noncomparative salvage study completed at the National Institutes of Health, atovaquone was found safe and effective.[112] In another study of 24 patients treated presumptively with atovaquone alone for their first episode of toxoplasmic encephalitis, evaluation at 3 weeks of therapy revealed a clinical response in 66%; 13% remained stable and 17% demonstrated clinical or radiologic progression.[39] In this latter study, patients who failed to respond to atovaquone therapy responded to pyrimethamine-sulfadiazine. Relapse occurred in approximately 50% of patients in whom atovaquone was used for acute therapy and was continued alone as maintenance therapy.[39,112] Whether the combination of pyrimethamine-atovaquone will prove more efficacious is presently being examined by the AIDS Clinical Trials Groups. Atovaquone has not been approved by the Food and Drug Administration for treatment of toxoplasmosis.

Other drugs, including dapsone[215] and doxycycline,[178] have been used to treat toxoplasmic encephalitis. Studies conducted in animal models of toxoplasmosis have demonstrated anti–*T. gondii* activity of rifabutin[11] and remarkable in vivo synergy when the following combinations were used: clarithromycin plus either pyrimethamine, sulfadiazine, or minocycline[8]; azithromycin plus sulfadiazine[6]; atovaquone

TABLE 24–4. GUIDELINES FOR MAINTENANCE TREATMENT OF AIDS PATIENTS WITH TOXOPLASMIC ENCEPHALITIS

	Oral Dose	Frequency
Recommended Regimens		
Pyrimethamine* *and* sulfadiazine	25–50 mg 1 g	q24h q6h
Pyrimethamine *and* clindamycin	25–50 mg 600 mg	q24h q6h
Pyrimethamine-sulfadoxine (Fansidar)	25 mg/500 mg (1 tablet)	tiw
Alternative Regimens		
Pyrimethamine alone	50 mg	q24h
Pyrimethamine *plus one of the following:*	25–50 mg	q24h
Dapsone	100 mg	biw
Atovaquone	750 mg	q6h
Clarithromycin	1000 mg	q12h
Azithromycin	1200–1500 mg	q24h

* Folinic acid (leucovorin calcium) 10–20 mg q24h is recommended for all patients receiving pyrimethamine to help ameliorate the hematologic side effects associated with pyrimethamine. The dose of folinic acid is titrated against the patient's hematologic indices, and up to 50 mg of folinic acid has been used.

plus either pyrimethamine or sulfadiazine[7]; and rifabutin plus either pyrimethamine, sulfadiazine, clindamycin, or atovaquone.[11,12] Appropriately designed studies are needed to determine if there is a role for these compounds and combinations in the treatment or prevention of toxoplasmosis in AIDS patients.

Because of their profound defect in cellular immunity, there is the possibility that immunologic reconstitution through use of biologic response modifiers might, along with conventional antimicrobial therapy, be useful for treatment of toxoplasmosis in AIDS patients. Of particular interest is interferon (IFN)-γ, which is a known major mediator of host resistance to *T. gondii*.[206] In murine models of toxoplasmosis, significant enhancement of antimicrobial activity was observed when either roxithromycin, azithromycin, pyrimethamine, or clindamycin was combined with rIFN-γ.[9,92,101] Other biologic response modifiers, such as IFN-β,[194] interleukin (IL)-2,[197] IL-7 (L. Kasper, personal communication, 1995), IL-12,[3,99] tumor necrosis factor-α,[32] and granulocyte-macrophage colony-stimulating factor[14] also had anti-*T. gondii* activity in experimental models but have not been used to treat AIDS-associated toxoplasmosis.

Maintenance Treatment (Secondary Prophylaxis)

Whereas the combination of pyrimethamine plus sulfadiazine is highly active against the pro-liferative form, neither it nor any of the currently used drugs is effective in eradicating the cyst form of *T. gondii*. It is believed that persistence of the cyst form accounts for relapse of toxoplasmic encephalitis after therapy is discontinued. The relapse rate of toxoplasmic encephalitis in patients who do not receive maintenance therapy is 50% to 80% at 12 months.[87,170] The CT scans or MR images of patients who relapse often demonstrate mass lesions in the same location as at initial presentation.[212] Thus, it is essential that AIDS patients who complete a primary course and who have had a favorable clinical and radiologic response to therapy for toxoplasmic encephalitis be maintained on lifelong anti–*T. gondii* agents.

After successful primary therapy, drug dosages are generally decreased for lifelong maintenance therapy (Table 24–4). There is no single regimen that both is effective and has an acceptable safety profile. Although toxoplasmic encephalitis can recur during maintenance therapy,[124,170] it is important to be aware that some of these failures are due to noncompliance.[212]

The regimen of pyrimethamine plus sulfadiazine appears to have a lower rate of relapse than other regimens and is recommended.[124,140,174,190] In a prospective, randomized study, patients who received maintenance therapy with pyrimethamine-sulfadiazine (25 mg/day–500 mg four times per day) daily had a lower rate of relapse of toxoplasmic encephalitis (6% at 12 months) than patients receiving pyrimethamine-sulfadiazine twice weekly (30% at 12 months).[174] Patients on maintenance therapy with pyrimethamine-sulfadiazine most likely do not require further prophylaxis for *P. carinii*.[88,174] Although most investigators favor the daily use of pyrimethamine-sulfadiazine, many patients are unable to continue this regimen because of drug toxicity, and alternative regimens will have to be considered (Table 24–4).[46,67,124]

Maintenance therapy with pyrimethamine-clindamycin has been reported to have a relapse rate of 28%.[107] Whether the relapse rate was due to the low doses of clindamycin (1.2 g/day) used in the study remains to be determined. In addition, it is important to be aware that pyrimethamine-clindamycin does not prevent *P. carinii* pneumonia.[76,124]

Pyrimethamine-sulfadoxine (Fansidar) administered as one tablet twice weekly has been reported to be effective as maintenance therapy. Side effects were relatively common (40%), with 7% of patients discontinuing therapy because of adverse effects.[192]

Prevention (Primary Prophylaxis)

Serologic testing for *T. gondii* antibodies will distinguish those HIV-infected individuals who are at risk for reactivation of infection from those at risk for acquisition of newly acquired infection. All patients who are seronegative for *T. gondii* antibodies and who have evidence of deficient cellular immunity, especially those seronegative for *T. gondii* antibodies, should be educated about appropriate precautions to take to prevent acquisition of *T. gondii* infection (Table 24–5). Seroconversion to *T. gondii* posi-

tivity in HIV-infected individuals has been reported to occur in 2% after a mean follow-up of 2 years.[213]

Despite the availability of effective antimicrobial regimens, toxoplasmosis in AIDS patients is associated with a mortality rate of 70% by 12 months after the diagnosis of toxoplasmic encephalitis.[161] Thus, the morbidity and mortality associated with toxoplasmosis in AIDS patients strongly support the use of prophylaxis in HIV-infected patients with CD4 T-lymphocyte counts of less than 200/mm³.[141] Numerous studies have reported the efficacy of TMP-SMX,[22,155,159,175,176,193] pyrimethamine-dapsone,[37,38,175] or pyrimethamine-sulfadoxine,[111] in the prevention of toxoplasmic encephalitis in AIDS patients (Table 24–6). A prospective, randomized study that compared TMP-SMX (160 mg–800 mg orally twice daily on a thrice weekly regimen) with pyrimethamine-dapsone (50 mg–100 mg orally twice weekly) indicated that both regimens are effective as prophylaxis for toxoplasmosis.[175] However, the TMP-SMX regimen appeared to be more effective for prophylaxis of *P. carinii* pneumonia.[175] It must be emphasized that, among patients receiving primary prophylaxis with TMP-SMX,[176] pyrimethamine-dapsone,[75] or pyrimethamine-sulfadoxine, 40% to 60% will have untoward side effects, and 2% to 12% of the total number of patients will require discontinuation of therapy.

Pyrimethamine alone is currently not considered a first-line regimen for primary prophylaxis against toxoplasmic encephalitis.[119] Contrary to a previous study that reported a higher death rate among patients receiving pyrimethamine for primary prophylaxis,[104] Leport et al did not find such an association.[119] Whether the concomitant administration of folinic acid in the study by Leport et al explains the lack of increased mortality remains to be determined.[119] A trial on the use of clindamycin alone for primary prophylaxis was discontinued because of a high incidence of gastrointestinal side effects.[104] Administration of clarithromycin to AIDS patients as part of regimens for disseminated *Mycobacterium avium* complex (MAC) infections has not decreased the incidence of toxoplasmic encephalitis,[186] suggesting that clarithromycin may be ineffective for primary prophylaxis for toxoplasmic encephalitis. This failure of clarithromycin may be due to changes in its absorption and/or metabolism caused by coadministration of other drugs (didanosine, rifampin, ethambutol, ciprofloxacin).[186] Spiramycin alone has not been found

TABLE 24–5. METHODS FOR PREVENTING TOXOPLASMOSIS IN PATIENTS WITH HIV INFECTION

Individuals Should Take the Following Precautions

Cook meat to ≥66°C (well done, not pink); smoke it or cure it in brine.

Avoid touching mucous membranes of mouth and eyes while handling raw meat.

Wash hands thoroughly after handling raw meat.

Wash kitchen surfaces that come into contact with raw meat.

Wash fruits and vegetables before consumption.

Prevent access of flies, cockroaches, etc., to fruits and vegetables.

Avoid contact with materials that are potentially contaminated with cat feces (e.g., cat litter boxes) or wear gloves when handling such materials or when gardening.

Disinfect cat litter box for 5 minutes with nearly boiling water.

TABLE 24–6. REGIMENS USED FOR PRIMARY PROPHYLAXIS AGAINST TOXOPLASMOSIS IN TOXOPLASMA-SEROPOSITIVE HIV-INFECTED INDIVIDUALS WITH CD4 LYMPHOCYTE COUNT <200 mm³

Drug	Dosage Schedule
TMP-SMX	PO: 1 DS* tab qd
	PO: 2 DS tab biw
	PO: 2 DS tab tiw
Pyrimethamine-dapsone†	PO: pyrimethamine 50 mg once a week; dapsone 50 mg qd
	PO: pyrimethamine 50 mg biw; dapsone 100 mg biw
	PO: pyrimethamine 75 mg once a week; dapsone 200 mg once a week
	PO: pyrimethamine 25 mg once a week; dapsone 100 mg once a week
Pyrimethamine-sulfadoxine (Fansidar)†, ‡	PO: 3 tab every 2 weeks
	PO: 1 tab biw

* DS, double strength.

† Folinic acid (Leucovorin) 25 mg qw is recommended for all patients receiving pyrimethamine to help ameliorate the hematologic side effects associated with pyrimethamine. The dose of folinic acid is titrated against the patient's hematologic indices.

‡ Each tablet contains pyrimethamine 25 mg, sulfadoxine 500 mg.

to be useful in the primary prophylaxis of toxoplasmic encephalitis.

Because even in the absence of primary prophylaxis not all HIV-infected individuals who are seropositive for *T. gondii* antibodies develop toxoplasmic encephalitis, it would appear that other factors besides prior infection with *T. gondii* and decreased CD4 T-lymphocyte counts may be involved in determining the risk for this disease. In this regard, an association between the development of toxoplasmic encephalitis and human leukocyte antigen (HLA) molecules has been reported.[207] Compared to controls, HLA-DQ3 was significantly more frequent in white North American AIDS patients with toxoplasmic encephalitis, whereas HLA-DQ1 appeared to be less frequent in these patients.[207] Further studies may help to identify

populations at greatest risk for toxoplasmic encephalitis and thereby allow for more targeted prophylactic measures.

Although there are no data available on the use of prophylaxis against congenital toxoplasmosis in HIV-infected women who are seropositive for *T. gondii* antibodies, the high congenital transmission rate (C. Mitchell, personal communication, 1993; A. Kovacs, personal communication, 1993) strongly suggests that therapeutic intervention is warranted. Until more data are available, we recommend that these women receive spiramycin 1 g tid throughout pregnancy if their CD4 lymphocyte counts are less than 200/mm³. Whether to use TMP-SMX or pyrimethamine-sulfadiazine after the 17th week of pregnancy should be considered for those who are more severely immunosuppressed.

REFERENCES

1. Araujo FG, Guptil DR, Remington JS: Azithromycin, a macrolide antibiotic with potent activity against *Toxoplasma gondii.* Antimicrob Agents Chemother 32:755–757, 1988
2. Araujo FG, Guptil DR, Remington JS: In vivo activity of piritrexin against *Toxoplasma gondii.* J Infect Dis 156:828–830, 1987
3. Araujo FG, Hunter CA, Remington JS: Treatment with a combination of IL-12 and drugs significantly increases survival of mice with acute toxoplasmosis (Abstract G99). Program of the 35th Interscience Conference of Antimicrobial Agents and Chemotherapy, San Francisco, September 1995
4. Araujo FG, Huskinson-Mark J, Gutteridge WE, Remington JS: In vitro and in vivo activities of the hydroxynaphthoquinone 566C80 against the cyst

form of *Toxoplasma gondii.* Antimicrob Agents Chemother 36:326–330, 1992
5. Araujo FG, Huskinson J, Remington JS: Remarkable in vitro and in vivo activities of the hydroxynaphthoquinone 566C80 against tachyzoites and tissue cysts of *Toxoplasma gondii.* Antimicrob Agents Chemother 35:293–299, 1991
6. Araujo FG, Lin T, Remington JS: Synergistic combination of azithromycin and sulfadiazine for treatment of toxoplasmosis in mice. Eur J Clin Microbiol Infect Dis 11:71–72, 1992
7. Araujo FG, Lin T, Remington JS: The activity of atovaquone (566C80) in murine toxoplasmosis is markedly augmented when used in combination with pyrimethamine or sulfadiazine. J Infect Dis 167:494–497, 1993
8. Araujo FG, Prokocimer P, Lin T, Remington JS: Activ-

ity of clarithromycin alone or in combination with other drugs for treatment of murine toxoplasmosis. Antimicrob Agents Chemother 36:2454–2457, 1992

9. Araujo FG, Remington JS: Synergistic activity of azithromycin and gamma interferon in murine toxoplasmosis. Antimicrob Agents Chemother 35:1672–1673, 1991

10. Araujo FG, Shepard RM, Remington JS: In vivo activity of the macrolide antibiotics azithromycin, roxithromycin and spiramycin against *Toxoplasma gondii*. Eur J Clin Microbiol Infect Dis 10:519–524, 1991

11. Araujo FG, Slifer T, Remington JS: Rifabutin is active in the treatment of toxoplasmosis in murine models. Antimicrob Agents Chemother 38:570–575, 1994

12. Araujo FG, Suzuki Y, Remington JS: Combinations of rifabutin with atovaquone or clindamycin are effective in treatment of toxoplasmic encephalitis in a murine model (Abstract B55). Program of the 35th Interscience Conference of Antimicrobial Agents and Chemotherapy, San Francisco, September 1995

13. Aspöck H, Hassl A: Parasitic infections in HIV patients in Austria: First results of a long-term study. Zentralbl Bakteriol 272:540–546, 1990

14. Bezares R, Cueva F, Pzenni V, et al: Effects of GM-CSF (granulocyte-macrophage stimulating factor) in mice experimentally infected with *Toxoplasma gondii* (Abstract 2738). Blood 86:688a, 1990

15. Bottone EJ: Diagnosis of acute pulmonary toxoplasmosis by visualization of invasive and intracellular tachyzoites in Giemsa-stained smears of bronchoalveolar lavage fluid. J Clin Microbiol 29:2626–2627, 1991

16. Bretagne S, Costa JM, Fleury-Feith J, et al: Quantitative competitive PCR with bronchoalveolar lavage fluid for diagnosis of toxoplasmosis in AIDS patients. J Clin Microbiol 33:1662–1664, 1995

17. Bretagne S, Costa J, Vidaud M, et al: Detection of *Toxoplasma gondii* by competitive DNA amplification of bronchoalveolar lavage samples. J Infect Dis 168:1585–1588, 1993

18. Burg JL, Grover CM, Pouletty P, Boothroyd JC: Direct and sensitive detection of a pathogenic protozoan, *Toxoplasma gondii*, by polymerase chain reaction. J Clin Microbiol 27:1787–1792, 1989

19. Bursztyn EM, Lee BCP, Bauman J: CT of acquired immunodeficiency syndrome. Am J Neuroradiol 5:711–714, 1984

20. Canessa A, Del Bono V, De Leo P, et al: Cotrimoxazole therapy of *Toxoplasma gondii* encephalitis in AIDS patients. Eur J Clin Microbiol Infect Dis 11:125–130, 1992

21. Cappell MS, Mikhail N, Ortega A: *Toxoplasma* myocarditis in AIDS. Am Heart J 123:1728–1729, 1992

22. Carr A, Tindall B, Brew BJ, et al: Low-dose trimethoprim-sulfamethoxazole prophylaxis for toxoplasmic encephalitis in patients with AIDS. Ann Intern Med 117:106–111, 1992

23. Carrazana E, Rossitch E Jr, Martinez J: Unilateral "akathisia" in a patient with AIDS and a toxoplasmosis subthalamic abscess. Neurology 39:349–350, 1989

24. Carrazana E, Rossitch E Jr, Samuels MA: Parkinsonian symptoms in a patient with AIDS and cerebral toxoplasmosis. J Neurol Neurosurg Psychiatry 52:1445–1446, 1989

25. Castro KG, Selik RM, Jaffe HW, et al: Frequency of opportunistic diseases in AIDS patients by race/ethnicity and HIV transmission categories—United States (Abstract 570). Program of the 28th Interscience Conference on Antimicrobial Agents and Chemotherapy, Los Angeles, October 1988

26. Catania S, Nobili C, Trinchieri V, et al: Cryptococcal meningitis and *Toxoplasma* encephalitis in an AIDS patient. Acta Neurol (Napoli) 12:82–84, 1990

27. Cavallito JC, Nichol CA, Brenckman WD Jr, et al: Lipid-soluble inhibitors of dihydrofolate reductase. I. Kinetics, tissue distribution and extent of metabolism of pyrimethamine, metoprine, and etoprine in the rat, dog, and man. Drug Metab Dispos 6:329–337, 1978

28. Cerezo L, Alvarez M, Price G: Electron microscopic diagnosis of cerebral toxoplasmosis. J Neurosurg 630:470–472, 1985

29. Chakroun M, Meyohas MC, Pelosse B, et al: Emergence de la toxoplasme oculaire au cours du SIDA. Ann Med Interne (Paris) 141:472–474, 1990

30. Chang HR, Comte R, Pechere JC: In vitro and in vivo effects of doxycycline on *Toxoplasma gondii*. Antimicrob Agents Chemother 34:775–780, 1990

31. Chang HR, Comte R, Piguet PF, et al: Activity of minocycline against *Toxoplasma gondii* infection in mice. J Antimicrob Chemother 27:639–645, 1991

32. Chang HR, Grau GE, Pechere JC: Role of TNF and IL-1 in infections with *Toxoplasma gondii*. Immunology 69:33–37, 1990

33. Chang HR, Perchere JC: In vitro effects of four macrolides roxithromycin, spiramycin, azithromycin (CP-62,93) and A-56268 on *Toxoplasma gondii*. Antimicrob Agents Chemother 32:524–529, 1988

34. Cimino C, Lipton R, Williams A, et al: The evaluation of patients with human immunodeficiency virus-related disorders and brain mass lesions. Arch Intern Med 151:1381–1384, 1991

35. Ciricillo SF, Rosenblum ML: Imaging of solitary lesions in AIDS. J Neurosurg 74:1029, 1991

36. Ciricillo S, Rosenblum ML: Use of CT and MR imaging to distinguish intracranial lesions and to define the need for biopsy in AIDS patients. J Neurosurg 73:720–724, 1990

37. Clotet B, Sirera G, Romeu J, et al: Twice-weekly dapsone-pyrimethamine for preventing PCP and cerebral toxoplasmosis (Lett). AIDS 5:601–602, 1991

38. Clumeck N: Some aspects of the epidemiology of toxoplasmosis and *Pnemocystis* in AIDS in Europe. Eur J Clin Microbiol Infect Dis 10:177–178, 1991

39. Clumeck N, Katlama C, Ferrero T, et al: Atovaquone (14 hydroxynapthoquinone 566C80) in the treatment of acute cerebral toxoplasmosis in AIDS patients (Abstract 1217). Program of the VIIIth International Conference on AIDS, Amsterdam, The Netherlands, July 19–24, 1992

40. Clumeck N, Sonnet J, Taelman H, et al: Acquired immunodeficiency syndrome in African patients. N Engl J Med 310:492, 1984

41. Cochereau-Massin I, LeHoang P, Lautier-Frau M: Ocular toxoplasmosis in human immunodeficiency virus-infected patients. Am J Ophthalmol 114:130–135, 1992

42. Conley FK, Jenkins KA, Remington JS: *Toxoplasma gondii* infection of the central nervous system: Use

of the peroxidase-antiperoxidase method to demonstrate *Toxoplasma* in formalin-fixed, paraffin-embedded tissue sections. Hum Pathol 12: 690–698, 1981

43. Crider SR, Horstman WG, Massy GS: Toxoplasma orchitis: Report of a case and a review of the literature. Am J Med 85:421–424, 1988

44. Dannemann BR, Israelski DM, Remington JS: Treatment of toxoplasmic encephalitis and intravenous clindamycin. Arch Intern Med 148:2477–2482, 1988

45. Dannemann BR, McCutchan JA, Israelski DM, et al: Treatment of toxoplasmic encephalitis patients with AIDS: A randomized trial comparing pyrimethamine plus clindamycin to pyrimethamine plus sulfonamides. Ann Intern Med 116:33–43, 1992

46. de Gans J, Portegies P, Reiss P, et al: Pyrimethamine alone as maintenance therapy for central nervous system toxoplasmosis in 38 patients with AIDS. J Acquir Immune Defic Syndr 5:137–142, 1992

47. De La Paz RL, Enzman D: Neuroradiology of acquired immunodeficiency syndrome. In Rosenblum ML, et al, eds. AIDS and the Nervous System. New York, Raven Press, 1988, pp 121–154

48. De La Torre R, Gorraez M: *Toxoplasma*-induced occlusive hypertrophic arteritis as the cause of discrete coagulative necrosis in the central nervous system. Hum Pathol 20:604, 1989

49. Dement SH, Cox MC, Grupta PK: Diagnosis of central nervous system *Toxoplasma gondii* from the cerebrospinal fluid in a patient with AIDS. Diagn Cytopathol 3:148–151, 1987

50. Derouin F, Garin YJF: Isolement de *Toxoplasma gondii* par culture cellulaire chez les sujets infectes par le VIH. Presse Med 21:10–13, 1992

51. Derouin F, Mazeron MC, Garin YJF: Comparative study of tissue culture and mouse inoculation methods for demonstration of *Toxoplasma gondii*. J Clin Microbiol 25:1597–1600, 1987

52. Derouin F, Piketty C, Chastang C, et al: Anti-toxoplasma effects of dapsone alone and combined with pyrimethamine. Antimicrob Agents Chemother 35:252–255, 1991

53. Derouin F, Sarfati C, Beauvais B, et al: Laboratory diagnosis of pulmonary toxoplasmosis in patients with acquired immunodeficiency syndrome. J Clin Microbiol 27:1661–1663, 1989

54. Derouin F, Sarfati C, Beauvais B, et al: Prevalence of pulmonary toxoplasmosis in HIV-infected patients (Letter). AIDS 4:1036, 1990

55. Derouin F, Thulliez P, Garin YFJ: Value and limitations of toxoplasmosis serology in HIV patients. Pathol Biol (Paris) 39:255–259, 1991

56. Dhiver C, Milandre C, Poizot-Martin I, et al: 5-Fluorouracil-clindamycin for treatment of cerebral toxoplasmosis. AIDS 7:143–144, 1993

57. Dina T: Primary central nervous system lymphoma versus toxoplasmosis in AIDS. Radiology 179: 823–828, 1991

58. Dupon M, Cazenave J, Pellegrin JL, et al: Detection of *Toxoplasma gondii* by PCR and tissue culture in cerebrospinal fluid and blood of human immunodeficiency virus-seropositive patients. J Clin Microbiol 33:2421–2426, 1995

59. Dupouy-Camet J, Lavareda de Souza S, Maslo C, et al: Detection of *Toxoplasma gondii* in venous blood from AIDS patients by polymerase chain reaction. J Clin Microbiol 31:1866–1869, 1993

60. Eliaszewicz M, Lecomte I, De Sa M, et al: Relation between decreasing serial CD4 lymphocyte count and outcome of toxoplasmosis in AIDS patients: A basis for primary prophylaxis (Abstract ThB481). Program of the 6th International Conference on AIDS, San Francisco, June 1990

61. Elkin CM, Leon E, Grenell SL, et al: Intracranial lesions in the acquired immunodeficiency syndrome: Radiological (CT) features. JAMA 253: 393–396, 1985

62. Enzman DR: Imaging of Infections and Inflammations of the Central Nervous System: Computed Tomography, Ultrasound and Nuclear Magnetic Resonance. New York, Raven Press, 1984

63. Farkash AE, MacCabbee PJ, Sher JH: Central nervous system toxoplasmosis in AIDS: A clinical-pathological-radiological review of 12 cases. J Neurol Neurosurg Psychiatry 49:744–748, 1986

64. Farthing C, Rendel M, Currie B, Seidlin M: Azithromycin for cerebral toxoplasmosis. Lancet 339:437, 1992

65. Fernandez-Martin J, Leport C, Morlat P, et al: Pyrimethamine-clarithromycin combination for therapy of acute *Toxoplasma* encephalitis in patients with AIDS. Antimicrob Agents Chemother 35: 2049–2052, 1991

66. Filice G, Hitt J, Mitchell C, et al: Diagnosis of *Toxoplasma* parasitemia in patients with AIDS by gene detection after amplification with polymerase chain reaction. J Clin Microbiol 31:2327–2331, 1993

67. Foppa CU, Bini T, Gregis G, et al: A retrospective study of primary and maintenance therapy of toxoplasmic encephalitis with oral clindamycin and pyrimethamine. Eur J Clin Microbiol Infect Dis 10: 187–189, 1991

68. Frappier-Davignon L, Walker M, Adrien A, et al: Anti-HIV antibodies and other serological and immunological parameters among normal Haitians in Montreal. J Acquir Immune Defic Syndr 3: 166–172, 1990

69. Frenkel JK, Hitchings GH: Relative reversal by vitamins (*p*-aminobenzoic, folic and folinic acids) of the effects of sulfadiazine and pyrimethamine on *Toxoplasma*, mouse and man. Antibiot Chemother 7:630–638, 1957

70. Frenkel JK, Nelson BM, Arias-Stella J: Immunosuppression and toxoplasmic encephalitis. Hum Pathol 6:97–111, 1975

71. Friedman D: Neuro-ophthalmic manifestations of human immunodeficiency virus infection. Neurol Clin 9:55–72, 1991

72. Gagliuso DJ, Teich SA, Friedman AH, Orellana J: Ocular toxoplasmosis in AIDS patients. Trans Am Ophthalmol Soc 88:63–86, 1990

73. Geils GF, Scott CW Jr, Baugh CM, Butterworth CE Jr: Treatment of meningeal leukemia with pyrimethamine. Blood 38:131–137, 1971

74. Gherardi R, Baudrimont M, Lionnet F, et al: Skeletal muscle toxoplasmosis in patients with acquired immunodeficiency syndrome: A clinical and pathological study. Ann Neurol 32:535–542, 1992

75. Girard PM, Landman R, Gaudebout C, et al: Dapsone-pyrimethamine compared with aerosolized pentamidine as primary prophylaxis against *Pneu-*

mocystis carinii pneumonia and toxoplasmosis in HIV infection. N Engl J Med 328:1514–1520, 1993

76. Girard PM, Lepretre A, Detruchis P, et al: Failure of pyrimethamine-clindamycin combination for prophylaxis of *Pneumocystis carinii* pneumonia. Lancet 1:1459, 1989

77. Gluckstein D, Ruskin J: Rapid oral desensitization to trimethoprim-sulfamethoxazole (TMP-SMZ): Use in prophylaxis for *Pneumocystis carinii* pneumonia in patients with AIDS who were previously intolerant to TMP-SMZ. Clin Infect Dis 20:849–853, 1995

78. Goldstein J, Dickson D, Moser F, et al: Primary central nervous system lymphoma in acquired immunodeficiency syndrome. Cancer 67:2756–2765, 1991

79. Grange F, Kinney EL, Monsuez JJ, et al: Successful therapy for *Toxoplasma gondii* myocarditis in acquired immunodeficiency syndrome. Am Heart J 120:443–444, 1990

80. Grant IH, Gold JMW, Rosenblum M, et al: *Toxoplasma gondii* serology in HIV-infected patients: The development of central nervous system toxoplasmosis in AIDS. AIDS 4:519–521, 1990

81. Gray F, Gherard R, Wingate E, et al: Diffuse "encephalitic" cerebral toxoplasmosis in AIDS: Report of four cases. J Neurol 236:273–277, 1989

82. Greenberg AE, Thomas PA, Landesman SH, et al: The spectrum of HIV-related disease among outpatients in New York City. AIDS 6:849–859, 1992

83. Groll A, Schneider M, et al: Morphology and clinical significance of AIDS-related lesions in the adrenal and pituitary. Deutsche Med Wochenschr 115:483–488, 1990

84. Grossman PL, Remington JS: The effect of trimethoprim and sulfamethoxazole on *Toxoplasma gondii* in vitro and in vivo. Am J Trop Med Hyg 28:445–455, 1979

85. Guichard A, Zamora L, Caumes E, et al: Cutaneous side effects: A major problem in the treatment of toxoplasmosis encephalitis (Abstract MB2188). Program of the 7th International Conference on AIDS, Florence, June 1991

86. Harris C, Miklos P, Tanowitz H, Wittner M: In vitro assessment of antimicrobial agents against *Toxoplasma gondii*. J Infect Dis 157:14–22, 1988

87. Haverkos HW: Assessment of therapy for *Toxoplasma* encephalitis. Am J Med 82:907, 1987

88. Heald A, Flepp M, Chave J-P, et al: Treatment of cerebral toxoplasmosis protects against *Pneumocystis carinii* pneumonia in patients with AIDS. Ann Intern Med 115:760–763, 1991

89. Herrera G, Villalta O, Visona K, et al: Trimethoprim-sulfamethoxazole treatment of *Toxoplasma* encephalitis in AIDS patients (Abstract WB2321). Program of the 7th International Conference on AIDS, Florence, June 1991

90. Herskovitz S, Siegel SE, Schneider AT, et al: Spinal cord toxoplasmosis in AIDS. Neurology 39:1552–1553, 1989

91. Hirschmann JV, Chu AC: Skin lesions with disseminated toxoplasmosis in a patient with the acquired immunodeficiency syndrome (Letter). Arch Dermatol 124:1446–1447, 1988

92. Hofflin JM, Remington JS: In vivo synergism of roxithromycin (RU965) and interferon against *Toxoplasma gondii*. Antimicrob Agents Chemother 31:346–348, 1987

93. Hofflin JM, Remington JS: Tissue culture isolation

of *Toxoplasma* from blood of a patient with AIDS. Arch Intern Med 145:925–926, 1985

94. Holland GN, Engstrom RE Jr, Glasgow BJ, et al: Ocular toxoplasmosis in patients with the acquired immunodeficiency syndrome. Am J Ophthalmol 106:653–667, 1988

95. Holliman RE: Clinical and diagnostic findings in 20 patients with toxoplasmosis and the acquired immune deficiency syndrome. J Med Microbiol 35:1–4, 1991

96. Holliman RE, Johnson JD, Gillespie SH, et al: New methods in the diagnosis and management of cerebral toxoplasmosis associated with the acquired immune deficiency syndrome. J Infect Dis 22:281–285, 1991

97. Holliman RE, Johnson JD, Savva D: Diagnosis of cerebral toxoplasmosis in association with AIDS using polymerase chain reaction. Scand J Infect Dis 22:243–244, 1990

98. Huang TE, Chou SM: Occlusive hypertrophic arteritis as the cause of discrete necrosis in CNS toxoplasmosis in AIDS. Hum Pathol 19:1210–1214, 1988

99. Hunter CA, Candolfi E, Subauste CS, et al: Studies on the role of interleukin-12 in acute murine toxoplasmosis. Immunology 84:16–20, 1995

100. Israelski DM, Chmiel JS, Poggensee L, et al: Prevalence of *Toxoplasma* infection in a cohort of homosexual men at risk of AIDS and toxoplasmic encephalitis. J Acquir Immune Defic Syndr 6:414–418, 1993

101. Israelski DM, Remington JS: Activity of γ interferon in combination with pyrimethamine or clindamycin in treatment of murine toxoplasmosis. Eur J Clin Microbiol Infect Dis 9:358–360, 1990

102. Israelski DM, Skowren G, Leventhal JP, et al: *Toxoplasma* peritonitis in a patient with AIDS. Arch Intern Med 148:1655–1657, 1988

103. Israelski DM, Tom C, Remington JS: Zidovudine antagonizes the action of pyrimethamine in experimental infection with *Toxoplasma gondii*. Antimicrob Agents Chemother 33:30–34, 1989

104. Jacobson MA, Besch CL, Child C, et al: Primary prophylaxis with pyrimethamine for toxoplasmic encephalitis in patients with advanced human immunodeficiency virus disease: Results of a randomized trial. J Infect Dis 169:384–394, 1994

105. Jessurun J, Angeles-Angeles A, Gasman N: Comparative demographic and autopsy findings in AIDS in two Mexican populations. J Acquir Immune Defic Syndr 3:579–583, 1990

106. Katlama C: Evaluation of the efficacy and safety of clindamycin plus pyrimethamine for induction and maintenance therapy of toxoplasmic encephalitis in AIDS. Eur J Clin Microbiol Infect Dis 10:189–191, 1991

107. Katlama C, De Wit S, Clumeck N, et al: Efficacy of pyrimethamine-clindamycin for the long term suppressive therapy of toxoplasmosis encephalitis in AIDS patients (Abstract 043). Program of the 4th European Conference on Clinical Aspects and Treatment of HIV Infection, Milan, Italy, March 1994

108. Kaufman HE, Geisler PH: The hematologic toxicity of pyrimethamine (Daraprim) in man. Arch Ophthalmol 64:140–146, 1960

109. Khuong MA, Matheron S, Marche C, et al: Diffuse toxoplasmic encephalitis without abscess in AIDS

patients (Abstract 1157). Program of the 30th Interscience Conference on Antimicrobial Agents and Chemotherapy, Atlanta, October 1990

110. Koppel B, Daras M: "Rubrual" tremor due to midbrain toxoplasmosis abscess. Mov Disord 5: 254–256, 1990

111. Koppen S, Grunewald T, Jautzke G, et al: Prevention of *Pneumocystis carinii* pneumonia and toxoplasmic encephalitis in human immunodeficiency virus-infected patients: A clinical approach comparing aerosolized pentamidine and pyrimethamine/sulfadoxine. Clin Invest 70: 508–512, 1992

112. Kovacs JA: Efficacy of atovaquone in treatment of toxoplasmosis in patients with AIDS. Lancet 340: 637–638, 1992

113. Kovacs JA, Allergra CJ, Chabner BA, et al: Potent effect of trimetrexate, a lipid-soluble antifolate, on *Toxoplasma gondii.* J Infect Dis 155:1027–1032, 1987

114. Kupfer M, Zee CS, Colletti PM, et al: MRI evaluation of AIDS-related encephalopathy: Toxoplasmosis vs. lymphoma. MRI 8:51–57, 1990

115. Laissy JP, Soyer P, Parlier C, et al: Persistent enhancement after treatment for cerebral toxoplasmosis in patients with AIDS: Predictive value for subsequent recurrence. AJNR Am J Neuroradiol 15: 1773–1778, 1994

116. Lavrard I, Chouaid C, Roux P, et al: Pulmonary toxoplasmosis in HIV-infected patients: Usefulness of polymerase chain reaction and cell culture. Eur Respir J 8:697–700, 1995

117. Lebech M: Detection of *Toxoplasma gondii* DNA by polymerase chain reaction in cerebrospinal fluid from AIDS patients with cerebral toxoplasmosis (Letter). J Infect Dis 165:982–983, 1992

118. Leport C, Bastuju-Garin S, Perronne C, et al: An open study of the pyrimethamine-clindamycin combination in AIDS patients with brain toxoplasmosis. J Infect Dis 160:577–578, 1989

119. Leport C, Chene G, Morlat P, et al: Pyrimethamine for primary prophylaxis of toxoplasmic encephalitis in patients with human immunodeficiency virus infection: A double blind placebo-controlled trial. (In press).

120. Leport C, Meulemans A, Robine D, et al: Levels of pyrimethamine in serum and penetration into brain tissue in humans. AIDS 6:1040–1041, 1992

121. Leport C, Meulemans A, Robine D, et al: Penetration of pyrimethamine into human brain tissue after a single dose administration (Abstract 248). Program of the 29th Interscience Conference on Antimicrobial Agents and Chemotherapy, Houston, September 1989

122. Leport C, Raffi F, Katlama C, et al: Treatment of central nervous system toxoplasmosis with pyrimethamine/sulfadiazine combination in 35 patients with acquired immunodeficiency syndrome. Am J Med 84:94–100, 1988

123. Leport C, Remington JS: Toxoplasmose au cours du SIDA. La Presse Medicale 21:1165–1171, 1992

124. Leport C, Tournerie C, Raguin G, et al: Long-term follow-up of patients with AIDS on maintenance therapy for toxoplasmosis. Eur J Clin Microbiol Infect Dis 10:191–193, 1991

125. Leport C, Vilde JL, Katlama C, et al: Failure of spiramycin to prevent neurotoxoplasmosis in immunosuppressed patients. JAMA 255:2290, 1987

126. Levy RM, Bredesen DE: Central nervous system dysfunction in acquired immunodeficiency syndrome. J Acquir Immune Defic Syndr 1:41–64, 1988

127. Levy RM, Breit R, Russell R, Dal Canto MC: MRI-guided stereotaxic brain biopsy in neurologically symptomatic AIDS patients. J Acquire Immune Defic Syndr 4:254–260, 1991

128. Levy RM, Mills CM, Posin JP, et al: The efficacy nd clinical impact of brain imaging in neurological symptomatic AIDS patients: A prospective CT/MRI study. J Acquir Immune Defic Syndr 3:461–471, 1990

129. Levy RM, Rosenbloom S, Perrett LV: Neuroradiological findings in AIDS: A review of 200 cases. AJNR Am J Neuroradiol 7:833–839, 1986

130. Liesnard C, Van Vooren JP, Farber CM: Risk of cerebral toxoplasmosis according to toxoplasmosis seroprevalence in African and European HIV seropositive patients and recommendations for cerebral toxoplasmosis primary prevention (Abstract FB426). Program of the 6th International Conference on AIDS, San Francisco, June 1990

131. Lindsay DS, Balgburn BL, Hall JE, Tidwell RR: Activity of pentamidine and pentamidine analogs against *Toxoplasma gondii* in cell cultures. Antimicrob Agents Chemother 35:1914–1916, 1991

132. Lucet JC, Bailly MP, Bedos JP, et al: Septic shock due to toxoplasmosis in patients infected with human immunodeficiency virus. Chest 104:1054–1058, 1993

133. Luft BJ: Potent in vivo activity of arpinocid, a purine analogue, against murine toxoplasmosis. J Infect Dis 154:692–694, 1986

134. Luft BJ, Brooks RG, Conley FK, et al: Toxoplasmic encephalitis in patients with AIDS. JAMA 252:913, 1984

135. Luft BJ, Castro KG: An overview of the problem of toxoplasmosis and pneumocystosis in AIDS in the USA: Implications for future therapeutic trials. Eur J Clin Microbiol Infect Dis 10:178–181, 1991

136. Luft BJ, Conley FK, Remington JS: Outbreak of central nervous system toxoplasmosis in Western Europe and North America. Lancet 1:781–784, 1983

137. Luft BJ, Hafner R, Korzun AH, et al: Toxoplasmic encephalitis in patients with the acquired immunodeficiency syndrome. N Engl J Med 329: 995–1000, 1993

138. Luft BJ, Remington JS: Toxoplasmosis of the central nervous system. In Remington JS, Swartz MN, eds. Current Topics in Infectious Disease, vol 6. New York, McGraw-Hill, 1985, pp 315–358

139. Mack DG, McLeod R: New micromethod to study the effect of antimicrobial agents on *Toxoplasma gondii:* Comparison of sulfadoxine and sulfadiazine individually and in combination pyrimethamine and study of clindamycin, metronidazole and cyclosporin A. Antimicob Agents Chemother 26:26–30, 1984

140. Madlener J, Enzensberger W, Herdt P, et al: Neurological outcome and follow-up after successful treatment of CNS toxoplasmosis. Program of the VIIIth International Conference on AIDS, Amsterdam, The Netherlands, July 19–24, 1992, p B122

141. Mallolas J, Zamora L, Gatell JM, et al: Primary prophylaxis for *Pneumocystis carinii* pneumonia: A randomized trial comparing cotrimoxazole, aerosol-

ized pentamidine and dapsone, plus pyrimethamine. AIDS 7:59–64, 1993

142. Marche C, Mayorga R, Trophilme D, et al: Pathological study of extraneurological toxoplasmosis (ENT) in AIDS (Abstract 7074). Program of the 4th International Conference on AIDS, Stockholm, June 1988

143. Matheron S, Dournon E, Garakhanian S, et al: Prevalence of toxoplasmosis in 365 AIDS and ARC patients before and during zidovudine treatment (Abstract ThB476). Program of the 6th International Conference on AIDS, San Francisco, June 1990

144. Mehren M, Burns PJ, Mamani MD, et al: Toxoplasmic myelitis mimicking intramedullary cord tumor. Neurology 38:1648–1650, 1988

145. Miller M, Remington JS: Toxoplasmosis in infants and children with HIV infection or AIDS. In Pizzo PA, Wilfert CM, eds. Pediatric AIDS: The Challenge of HIV Infection in Infants, Children, and Adolescents, Baltimore, Williams & Wilkins, 1990, pp 299–307

146. Milligan SA, Katz MS, Craven PC: Toxoplasmosis presenting as panhypopituitarism in a patient with AIDS. Am J Med 77:760–764, 1984

147. Miro JM, Buira E, Mallolas J, et al: Relation between CD4 T lymphocyte counts, tuberculosis, other opportunistic infections or Kaposi's sarcoma in Spanish AIDS patients (Abstract MB2347). Program of the 7th International Conference on AIDS, Florence, June 1991

148. Mitchell CD, Erlich SS, Mastrucci MT, et al: Congenital toxoplasmosis occurring in infants perinatally infected with human immunodeficiency virus 1. Pediatr Infect Dis J 9:512–518, 1990

149. Mitchell CD, Lewis L, McLellan S, et al: Increased risk of congenital toxoplasmosis among infants born to mothers infected with HIV-1 and *Toxoplasma gondii* (Abstract). Program of the 3rd Conference on Retroviruses and Opportunistic Infections, Washington, DC, January-February 1996

150. Molina JM, Belenfant X, Doco-LeCompte T, et al: Sulfadiazine-induced crystalluria in AIDS patients with *Toxoplasma* encephalitis. AIDS 5:587–589, 1991

151. Moskowitz L, Hensley GT, Chan JC, Adams K: Immediate cause of death in AIDS. Arch Pathol Lab Med 109:735–738, 1985

152. Myatt AV, Coatney GR, Hernandez T, et al: A further study of the toxicity of pyrimethamine (Daraprim) in man. Am J Trop Med 2:1000–1001, 1953

153. Myatt AV, Hernandez T, Coatney GR: Studies in human malaria. Am J Trop Med 2:788–795, 1953

154. Navia BA, Petito CK, Gold JWM, et al: Cerebral toxoplasmosis complicating AIDS: Clinical and neuropathological findings in 27 patients. Ann Neurol 19:224–238, 1986

155. Nicholas P, Pierone G, Lin J, et al: Trimethoprim-sulfamethoxazole in the prevention of cerebral toxoplasmosis (Abstract ThB482). Program of the 6th International Conference on AIDS, San Francisco, June 1990

156. Nistal M, Santana A, Paniaqua R, Palacios J: Testicular toxoplasmosis in two men with AIDS. Arch Pathol Lab Med 110:746, 1986

157. Nixon PF, Bertino JR: Effective absorption and utilization of oral formyl-tetrahydrofolate in man. N Engl J Med 186:175–179, 1972

158. O'Donohoe JM, Brueton MJ, Holliman RE: Concurrent congenital human immunodeficiency virus infection and toxoplasmosis. Pediatr Infect Dis J 8:627–628, 1991

159. O'Farrell N, Bradbeer C, Fitt S, et al: Cerebral toxoplasmosis and cotrimoxazole prophylaxis. Lancet 337:986, 1991

160. Oksenhendler E, Cadranel J, Sarfati C, et al: *Toxoplasma gondii* pneumonia in patients with the acquired immunodeficiency syndrome. Am J Med 88:18N–21N, 1990

161. Oksenhendler E, Charreau I, Tournerie C, et al: *Toxoplasma gondii* infection in advanced HIV infection. AIDS 8:483–487, 1994

162. Orefice G, Carrieri PB, De Marinis T, et al: Use of the intrathecal synthesis of anti-*Toxoplasma* antibodies in the diagnostic assessment and in the follow-up of AIDS patients with cerebral toxoplasmosis. Acta Neurol (Napoli) 12:79–81, 1990

163. Orellana MA, Suzuki Y, Araujo FG, Remington JS: Role of beta interferon in resistance to *Toxoplasma gondii* infection. Infect Immun 59:3287–3290, 1991

164. Oster S, Hutchison F, McCabe R: Resolution of acute renal failure in toxoplasmic encephalitis despite continuance of sulfadiazine. Rev Infect Dis 12:618–620, 1990

165. Ostergaard L, Nielsen AK, Black FT: DNA amplification on cerebrospinal fluid for diagnosis of cerebral toxoplasmosis among HIV-positive patients with signs or symptoms of neurological disease. Scand J Infect Dis 25:227–237, 1993

166. Ou-Yang K, Krug EC, Marr JJ, Berens RL: Inhibition of growth of *Toxoplasma gondii* and derivatives. Antimicrob Agents Chemother 34:1961–1965, 1990

167. Parke DW, Font RL: Diffuse toxoplasmic retinochoroiditis in a patient with AIDS. Arch Ophthalmol 104:571–575, 1986

168. Parmley S, Goebel F, Remington JS: Detection of *Toxoplasma gondii* in cerebrospinal fluid from AIDS patients by polymerase chain reactions. J Clin Microbiol 30:3000–3002, 1992

169. Pauwels A, Meyohas MC, Eliaszewicz M, et al: Toxoplasmic colitis in the acquired immunodeficiency syndrome. Am J Gastroenterol 87:518–519, 1992

170. Pedrol E, Gonzalez-Clemente J, Gatell JM, et al: Central nervous system toxoplasmosis in AIDS patients: Efficacy of an intermittent maintenance therapy. AIDS 4:511–517, 1990

171. Pierce MA, Johnson MD, Maciunas RJ, et al: Evaluating contrast-enhancing brain lesions in patients with AIDS by using positron emission tomography. Ann Intern Med 123:594–598, 1995

172. Piketty C, Gilquin J, Kazatchkine MD: Efficacy and safety of desensitization to trimethoprim-sulfamethoxazole in human immunodeficiency virus-infected patients. J Infect Dis 172:611, 1995

173. Pinon JM, Toubas D, Marx C, et al: Detection of specific immunoglobulin E in patients with toxoplasmosis. J Clin Microbiol 28:1739–1743, 1990

174. Podzamczer D, Miro JM, Bolao F, et al: Twice-weekly maintenance therapy with sulfadiazine-pyrimethamine to prevent recurrent toxoplasmic encephalitis in patients with AIDS. Ann Intern Med 123:175–180, 1995

175. Podzamczer D, Salazar A, Jimenez J, et al: Intermittent trimethoprim-sulfamethoxazole compared

with dapsone-pyrimethamine for simultaneous primary prophylaxis of pneumocystis pneumonia and toxoplasmosis in patients infected with HIV. Ann Intern Med 122:755–761, 1995

176. Podzamczer D, Santin M, Jimenez J, et al: Thrice weekly cotrimoxazole is better than weekly dapsone-pyrimethamine for the primary prevention of *Pneumocystis carinii* pneumonia in HIV-infected patients. AIDS 7:501–506, 1993

177. Polis MA, Masur H, Tuazon C, et al: Salvage therapy of trimetrexate-leucovorin for treatment of cerebral toxoplasmosis in AIDS patients. Clin Res 37: 437A, 1989

178. Pope-Pegram L, Gathe J, Bohn B, et al: Treatment of presumed central nervous system toxoplasmosis with doxycycline. (Abstract M.B. 2027). Program of the VII International Conference on AIDS, Florence, Italy, June 1991

179. Porter SB, Sande MA: Toxoplasmosis of the central nervous system in the acquired immunodeficiency syndrome. N Engl J Med 327:1643–1648, 1992

180. Post MJD, Chan JC, Hensley GT, et al: *Toxoplasma* encephalitis in Haitian adults with AIDS: A clinical-pathologic-CT correlation. AJNR Am J Neuroradiol 140:861–868, 1983

181. Post MJD, Kursunoglu SJ, Hensley GT, et al: Cranial CT in AIDS: Spectrum of disease and optimal contrast enhancement technique. AJNR Am J Neuroradiol 6:743–754, 1984

182. Post MJD, Sheldon JJ, Hensley GT, et al: Central nervous system disease in AIDS: Prospective correlation using CT, MRI and pathologic studies. Radiology 158:141–148, 1986

183. Potasman I, Resnick L, Luft BJ, Remington JS: Intrathecal production of antibodies against *Toxoplasma gondii* in patients with toxoplasmic encephalitis and AIDS. Ann Intern Med 108:49–51, 1988

184. Rabaud C, May T, Amiel C, et al: Extracerebral toxoplasmosis in patients infected with HIV. Medicine 73:306–314, 1994

185. Raffi F, Pelloux H, Dupouy-Camet J, et al: Detection of *Toxoplasma gondii* parasitemia by culture and polymerase chain reaction (PCR) in AIDS patients with suspected toxoplasma encephalitis: A prospective study (Abstract 303). Program of the 2nd National Conference on Human Retroviruses and Related Infections, Washington, DC, January-February 1995

186. Raffi F, Struillou L, Ninin E, et al: Breakthrough cerebral toxoplasmosis in patients with AIDS who are being treated with clarithromycin. Clin Infect Dis 20:1076–1077, 1995

187. Ragnaud JM, Beylot J, Lacut JY, et al: Toxoplasmic encephalitis in 73 AIDS patients (Bordeaux, France 1985–1989) (Abstract MB2090). Program of the 7th International Conference on AIDS, Florence, June 1991

188. Remington JS, McLeod R, Desmonts G: Toxoplasmosis. In Remington JS, Klein JO, eds. Infectious Diseases of the Fetus and Newborn Infant. Philadelphia, WB Saunders Co, 1995, pp 140–267

189. Remington JWS, Vilde J: Clindamycin for *Toxoplasma* encephalitis in AIDS. Lancet 338:1142–1143, 1991

190. Renold C, Sugar A, Chave J-P, et al: Toxoplasmic encephalitis in patients with the acquired immunodeficiency syndrome. Medicine (Balt) 71: 224–239, 1992

191. Roldan EO, Moskowitz L, Hensley GT: Pathology of the heart in AIDS. Arch Pathol Lab Med 111: 943–946, 1987

192. Ruf B, Schurmann D, Bergmann F, et al: Efficacy of pyrimethamine/sulfadoxine in the prevention of toxoplasmic encephalitis relapses and *Pneumocystis carinii* pneumonia in HIV-infected patients. Eur J Clin Microbiol Infect Dis 12:325–329, 1993

193. Ruskin J, LaRiviere M: Low-dose co-trimoxazole for prevention of *Pneumocystis carinii* pneumonia in human immunodeficiency virus disease. Lancet 337:468–471, 1991

194. Schmitz JL, Carlin JM, Borden EC, et al: Beta interferon inhibits *Toxoplasma gondii* growth in human monocyte-derived macrophages. Infect Immun 57:3254–3256, 1989

195. Schanpp L, Geaghan S, Campagna A, et al: *Toxoplasma gondii* pneumonitis in patients infected with the human immunodeficiency virus. Arch Intern med 152:1073–1076, 1992

196. Selik RM, Starcher ET, Curran JW: Opportunistic disease reported in AIDS patients: Frequencies, associations, and trends. J Acquir Immune Defic Syndr 1:175–182, 1987

197. Sharma SD, Hofflin JM, Remington JS: In vivo recombinant interleukin 2 administration enhances survival against a lethal challenge with *Toxoplasma gondii*. J Immunol 135:4160–4163, 1985

198. Shepp DH, Hackman RC, Conley FK, et al: *Toxoplasma gondii* reactivation identified by detection of parasitemia in tissue culture. Ann Intern Med 103:218–221, 1985

199. Simon DI, Brosius FC, Rothstein DM: Sulfadiazine crystalluria revisited. Arch Intern Med 150: 2379–2384, 1990

200. Smart PE, Weinfeld A, Thompson NE, Defortuna SM: Toxoplasmosis of the stomach: A cause of antral narrowing. Radiology 174:369–370, 1990

201. Solbreux P, Sonnet J, Zech F: A retrospective study about the use of contrimoxazole as diagnostic support and treatment of suspected cerebral toxoplasmosis in AIDS. Acta Clin Belg 45:85–96, 1990

202. Stepick BP, Thulliez P, Araujo FG, Remington JS: IgA antibodies for diagnosis of acute congenital and acquired toxoplasmosis. J Infect Dis 162:270–273, 1990

203. Stickney DR, Simmons WS, De Angelis RL, et al: Pharmacokinetics of pyrimethamine (PRM) and 2,4-diamino-5(3′,4′-dichlorophenyl)-6-methylpyrimide (DMP) relevant to meningeal leukemia. Proc Am Assoc Cancer Res 14:52, 1973

204. Strittmatter C, Lang W, Wiestler OD, Kleihues P: The changing pattern of human immunodeficiency virus associated cerebral toxoplasmosis: A study of 46 postmortem cases. Acta Neuropathol 83: 475–481, 1992

205. Suzuki Y, Israelski DM, Dannemann BR, et al: Diagnosis of toxoplasmic encephalitis in patients with AIDS by using a new serologic method. J Clin Microbiol 26:2541–2543, 1988

206. Suzuki Y, Orellana MA, Schreiber RD, et al: Interferon-γ: The major mediator of resistance against *Toxoplasma gondii*. Science 240:516–518, 1988

207. Suzuki Y, Wong SY, Grumet FC, et al: Evidence for genetic regulation of susceptibility to toxoplasmic encephalitis in AIDS patients. J Infect Dis 173: 265–268, 1996

208. Tirard V, Niel G, Rosenheim M, et al: Diagnosis of

toxoplasmosis in patients with AIDS by isolation of the parasite from the blood (Letter). N Engl J Med 324:634, 1991

209. Tolge C, Factor S: Focal dystonia secondary to cerebral toxoplasmosis in a patient with AIDS. Mov Disord 6:69–72, 1991

210. Tschirhart D, Klatt EC: Disseminated toxoplasmosis in the acquired immunodeficiency syndrome. Arch Pathol Lab Med 112:1237–1241, 1988

211. Van de Ven E, Melchers W, Galama J, et al: Identification of *Toxoplasma gondii* infections by BI gene amplification. J Clin Microbiol 19:2120–2124, 1991

212. Walckenaer G, Leport C, Longuet P, et al: Relapses of brain toxoplasmosis in 15 AIDS patients (Abstract 251). Program of the 31st Interscience Conference on Antimicrobial Agents and Chemotherapy, Chicago, 1991

213. Wallace MR, Rossetti RJ, Olson PE: Cats and toxoplasmosis risk in HIV-infected adults. JAMA 269: 76–77, 1993

214. Wanke C, Tuazon CU, Kovacs A, et al: *Toxoplasma* encephalitis in patients with acquired immune deficiency syndrome. Am J Trop Med Hyg 36: 509–516, 1987

215. Ward DJ: Dapsone/pyrimethamine for treatment of toxoplasmic encephalitis (Abstract PoB 3277). Program of the VIII International Conference on AIDS and STD World Congress, Amsterdam, July 1992

216. Weiss A, Margo CE, Ledford DK, et al: Toxoplasmic

retinochoroiditis as an initial manifestation of AIDS. Am J Opthalmol 101:248–249, 1986

217. Weiss LM, Harris C, Berger M, et al: Pyrimethamine concentrations in serum and cerebrospinal fluid during treatment of acute *Toxoplasma* encephalitis in patients with AIDS. J Infect Dis 157:580–583, 1988

218. Wijdicks EFM, Borleffs JCC, Hoepelman AIM, Jansen GH: Fatal disseminated hemorrhagic toxoplasmic encephalitis as the initial manifestation of AIDS. Ann Neurol 29:683–686, 1991

219. Wong B, Gold JWM, Brown AE, et al: Central nervous system toxoplasmosis in homosexual men and parenteral drug abusers. Ann Intern Med 100:36–42, 1984

220. Wong SY, Hadju M-P, Ramirez R, et al: Role of specific immunoglobulin E in diagnosis of acute *Toxoplasma* infection and toxoplasmosis. J Clinb Microbiol 29:2952–2959, 1993

221. Wong SY, Remington JS: Toxoplasmosis in the setting of AIDS. In Border S, Merigan TC Jr, Bolognesi D, eds. Textbook of AIDS Medicine. Baltimore, Williams & Wilkins, 1994, pp 223–258

222. Zangerle R, Allerberger F, Pohl P, et al: High risk of developing toxoplasmic encephalitis in AIDS patients seropositive to *Toxoplasma gondii*. Med Microbiol Immunol 180:59–66, 1991

223. Zumla A, Savva D, Wheeler RB, et al: *Toxoplasma* serology in Zambian and Ugandan patients infected with the human immunodeficiency virus. Trans R Soc Trop Hyg 85:227–229, 1991

Chapter 25

Bacillary Angiomatosis and Other Unusual Infections in HIV-Infected Individuals

JANE E. KOEHLER

BARTONELLA INFECTIONS

Historical Perspective

Bacillary angiomatosis (BA) was first described by Stoler and colleagues in 1983,[71] in a human immunodeficiency virus (HIV)–infected patient with multiple subcutaneous nodules. Numerous bacilli were observed by Warthin-Starry staining of the biopsied nodules, and the subcutaneous masses resolved during erythromycin therapy. Subsequently, the BA bacilli visualized using the Warthin-Starry stain were noted to have an appearance similar to that of the cat scratch disease (CSD) bacillus.[31,38] The BA bacillus remained refractory to isolation attempts for many years, impeding identification efforts. Studies of bacterial DNA extracted from BA lesions subsequently identified the bacillus as closely related to *Rochalimaea quintana*,[57] and after isolation of the bacillus from the blood of two HIV-infected patients without BA,[66] the organism was further characterized and named *R. henselae* in 1992.[54,83] In 1993, the genus *Rochalimaea* was merged with the genus *Bartonella*.[9] More recently, the genus *Grahamella* (all of which species have been isolated only from small mammals) also was merged with *Bartonella*, resulting in a genus that includes eight extant species of *Bartonella*[7]: *B. bacilliformis, B. quintana, B. vinsonii, B. henselae, B. elizabethae, B. grahamii, B. taylorii,* and *B. doshiae.* The BA bacillus was directly cultivated from cutaneous lesions for the first time in 1992, which led to the identification of two species of the genus *Bartonella* as causative agents of BA: *B. henselae* and *B. quintana.*[32] To date, only these two species are associated with bacillary angiomatosis or peliosis. *Bartonella* species are small, gram-negative bacilli, and the relationship of this genus to other organisms is shown in Figure 25–1.

Clinical Presentation of *Bartonella* Infections

Most patients with BA are immunocompromised, usually due to infection with human immunodeficiency virus type 1 (HIV-1). BA occurs as a late manifestation of HIV infection; in a recent study of 42 patients with BA, the median CD4 lymphocyte count was 21 cells/mm^3.[45] In patients with severe immunosuppression, infection with *B. henselae* and *B. quintana* can produce unique vascular proliferative lesions known as BA.[13,37] These lesions can form in many different organs, including skin, bone, brain parenchyma, lymph nodes, bone marrow, and gastrointestinal and respiratory tracts. A histopathologically different vascular proliferative response is seen in the liver and spleen, known as bacillary peliosis hepatis (BP).[52] One notable aspect of focal *Bartonella* infection, especially cutaneous BA, is the chronic, indolent nature of the disease: lesions may be present for as long as 1 year before a diagnosis is made.[32,45]

HIV-infected individuals also can develop manifestations of *Bartonella* infection that lack vascular proliferation. Bacteremia with[68] or without[53,54,66] endocarditis has been reported in HIV-infected individuals, in the absence of focal BA or BP involvement. Patients with higher CD4 cell counts can develop focal necrotizing infections due to *B. henselae* in lymph nodes, liver, or spleen that have an appearance

Alpha-Proteobacteria

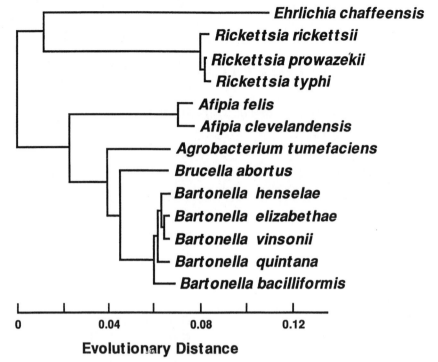

FIGURE 25–1. Species in the *Bartonella* genus and their relationship to other members of the alpha subdivision of Proteobacteria, based on 16S ribosomal RNA gene sequences. Evolutionary distance between bacteria is proportional to the summed lengths of the horizontal segments from a branch point. (From Slater LN, Welch DF: *Rochalimaea* species [recently renamed *Bartonella*]. In Principles and Practice of Infectious Diseases, ed 4. New York, Churchill Livingstone, 1994, with permission.)

similar to that of cat scratch disease in immunocompetent individuals. Rarely, HIV-infected individuals with CD4 cell counts <50 have been reported to manifest this necrotizing lymphadenitis without vascular proliferation.[85]

A case-control study identifying clinical characteristics of 42 patients with BA and BP compared with 84 control patients found that case patients were significantly more likely than controls to have fever, abdominal pain, lymphadenopathy, hepatomegaly, splenomegaly, a low CD4 cell count, anemia, or an elevated serum alkaline phosphatase concentration.[45] With the exception of cutaneous lesions, many of the clinical findings are not specific, and the major obstacle to diagnosis of *Bartonella* infection in the presence of concomitant HIV infection is recognition of the disease by the physician. Bacillary peliosis and all forms of BA can be indistinguishable from a number of other infectious or malignant conditions, and the diagnosis can usually be made only after biopsy and careful histopathologic evaluation of tissue, or by direct culture of *Bartonella* species from blood or the affected organ.[33]

Cutaneous Bacillary Angiomatosis

The most frequently diagnosed BA lesions are those affecting the skin.[33] The cutaneous BA lesions can have myriad presentations, including vascular proliferative lesions with a smooth red or eroded surface (Fig. 25–2) or papules that enlarge to form friable, exophytic lesions (Fig. 25–2). These vascular lesions of cutaneous BA are particularly difficult to distinguish clinically from Kaposi's sarcoma (KS); histopathologic examination of biopsied tissue is therefore essential. Bacillary angiomatosis may appear as a cellulitic plaque, usually overlying an osteolytic lesion (Fig. 25–3A). Less vascular-appearing lesions may be dry and scaly (Fig. 25–4) and some lesions are subcutaneous, with or without overlying erythema (Fig. 25–5). Very deep soft tissue masses (Fig. 25–6) have also been demonstrated to be a manifestation of BA.[32]

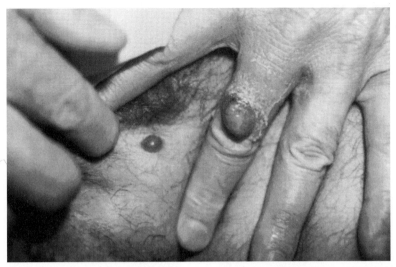

FIGURE 25–2. A friable, exophytic angiomatous BA nodule of the finger and an evolving dome-shaped vascular papule in the same patient. (From Koehler JE, LeBoit PE, Egbert BM, et al: Cutaneous vascular lesions and disseminated cat-scratch disease in patients with the acquired immunodeficiency syndrome [AIDS] and AIDS-related complex. Ann Intern Med 109:449–455, 1988, with permission.)

Osseous Bacillary Angiomatosis

Bartonella infection of the bone results in osteolytic lesions that are extremely painful. The long bones including tibia, fibula, and radius are most commonly involved,[4,33] although osseous BA involvement of a rib[4] and vertebra[24,60] have also been reported. A roentgenogram usually demonstrates well-circumscribed osteolysis (Fig. 25–3B), and these lytic lesions are always detected by technetium-99m methylene diphosphonate bone scans.[4] Osseous BA should be a primary consideration in the differential diagnosis of a lytic bone lesion in HIV-infected patients.

Splenic and Hepatic Bacillary Peliosis

Bacillary peliosis hepatis, a vascular lesion of the liver, was first described in association with bacilli in eight HIV-infected individuals by Perkocha et al.[52] *Bartonella henselae* was cultured from the blood of a patient subsequently found to have BP hepatis.[67] The symptoms of patients with BP hepatis usually include abdominal pain and fever. All eight patients reported by Perkocha et al[52] had hepatomegaly, and six also had splenomegaly. Two of the patients had a splenectomy, and histopathologic examination revealed BP of the spleen. One fourth of the patients also had cutaneous BA lesions. The alkaline phosphatase was more prominently elevated than the hepatic transaminases in these eight patients with BP. Abdominal computed tomography (CT) of the peliotic liver

usually reveals numerous hypodense lesions,[33,86] as shown in Figure 25–7, but this appearance is not specific for BP hepatis; consequently, the diagnosis of *Bartonella* infection must be confirmed by histopathologic or microbiologic evaluation. Additionally, some HIV-infected patients with hepatic *Bartonella* infection do not develop peliosis hepatis: three patients described by Slater et al[65] developed inflammatory nodules in the liver. Patients with splenic BP may have thrombocytopenia or pancytopenia, and abdominal ascites may be present.[44,61,67]

Gastrointestinal and Respiratory Tract Bacillary Angiomatosis

Histopathologically proven BA of the gastrointestinal tract has been described by several groups.[14,29,80] The lesions can involve oral, anal, peritoneal, and gastrointestinal tissue appearing as raised, nodular, ulcerated intraluminal mucosal abnormalities of the stomach and large and small intestines during endoscopy.[80] Extraluminal, intraabdominal BA presenting with massive upper gastrointestinal hemorrhage has also been described.[29] Hemorrhage occurred when the highly vascular mass eroded through small intestine; *B. quintana* was cultured from tissue obtained by transabdominal needle biopsy of the mass.

Bacillary angiomatosis lesions of the respiratory tract have been observed in the larynx,[14,81] and, in one patient, enlarged to cause

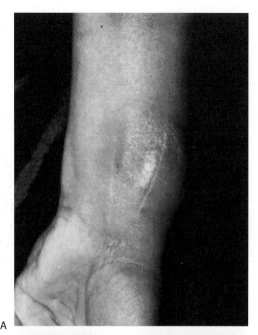

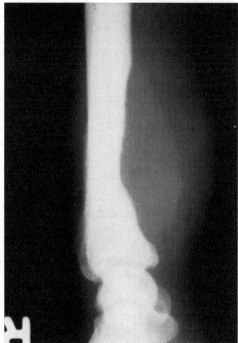

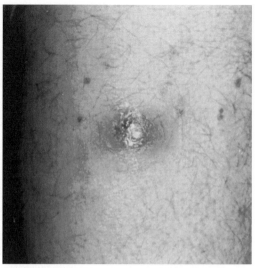

FIGURE 25–4. Unusual appearing erythematous, dry, scaling plaque of cutaneous BA mimicking staphylococcal pyoderma. *Bartonella quintana* was cultured from this lesion. (From Koehler JE, Tappero JW: AIDS Commentary: Bacillary angiomatosis and bacillary peliosis in patients infected with human immunodeficiency virus. Clin Infect Dis 17: 612–624, 1993, with permission.)

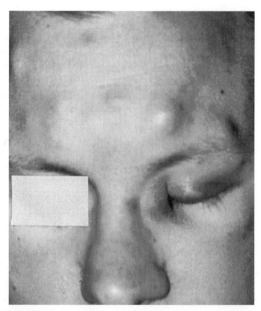

FIGURE 25–3. *A,* A tense, firm, erythematous wrist mass due to BA. *B,* A roentgenogram of the wrist of the same patient, demonstrating cortical bone erosion of the radius, with active periostitis, adjacent to the vascular soft tissue mass. (From Koehler JE, LeBoit PE, Egbert BM, et al: Cutaneous vascular lesions and disseminated cat-scratch disease in patients with the acquired immunodeficiency syndrome [AIDS] and AIDS-related complex. Ann Intern Med 109: 449–455, 1988, with permission.)

FIGURE 25–5. Multiple subcutaneous BA nodules in a patient with concomitant KS of the medial left eye canthus. (From Koehler JE, Tappero JW: AIDS Commentary: Bacillary angiomatosis and bacillary peliosis in patients infected with human immunodeficiency virus. Clin Infect Dis 17: 612–624, 1993, with permission.)

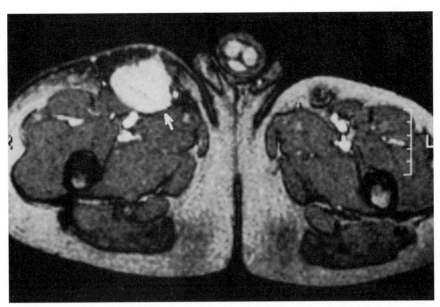

FIGURE 25–6. Magnetic resonance imaging showing a deep, highly vascular subcutaneous soft-tissue mass of BA in the anterior right thigh. (From Koehler JE, Tappero JW: AIDS Commentary: Bacillary angiomatosis and bacillary peliosis in patients infected with human immunodeficiency virus. Clin Infect Dis 17:612–624, 1993, with permission.)

an asphyxiative death.[14] Endobronchial BA lesions have been visualized during bronchoscopy, and described as polypoid lesions located in the segmental bronchi in addition to the trachea.[18,64] Several of these patients also had cutaneous BA lesions. *Bartonella* infection also can cause pulmonary nodules in the immunocompromised patient: a renal transplant patient with chemotherapy-induced immunosuppression developed high fever (41°C) and bilateral pulmonary nodules.[11] *Bartonella henselae* DNA was demonstrated in the parenchymal lung nodule specimens obtained at open lung biopsy.

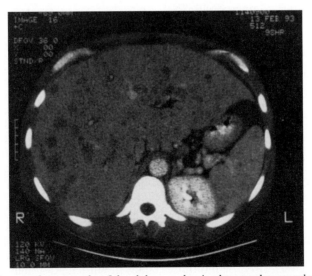

FIGURE 25–7. Computed tomography of the abdomen, showing hepatosplenomegaly with numerous low-density hepatic parenchymal lesions, in addition to pelvic ascites and pulmonary effusions. Percutaneous biopsy of the liver demonstrated peliosis hepatis by histopathology. (From Koehler JE, Tappero JW: AIDS Commentary: Bacillary angiomatosis and bacillary peliosis in patients infected with human immunodeficiency virus. Clin Infect Dis 17:612–624, 1993, with permission.)

Lymph Node Bacillary Angiomatosis

Lymph node involvement has been frequently described in association with cutaneous lesions or peliosis of the liver or spleen.[33] In these cases, the lymph nodes most commonly affected are those draining the BA lesion, and histopathologic examination may reveal angiomatous changes within the lymph node. In other cases, however, BA may involve only a single or several lymph nodes, in the absence of cutaneous or other organ involvement.

Neuropsychiatric Manifestations Associated with Bartonella Infection

Bartonella infection has been associated with aseptic meningitis,[85] parenchymal brain masses,[69] chronic central nervous system (CNS) dysfunction,[62] and acute psychiatric decompensation[3] in HIV-infected individuals. A left temporal lobe mass due to BA was reported by Spach et al[69] in an HIV-infected patient with new onset of seizures and facial nerve deficit. The cause of the mass remained undetermined for 8 months until the patient developed a cutaneous BA lesion. Treatment with erythromycin led to resolution of the cutaneous lesion and neurologic deficit; the parenchymal mass decreased in size during antibiotic treatment. In a study of HIV-infected patients with CNS dysfunction, evaluation for antibodies to *B. henselae* in serum and cerebrospinal fluid (CSF) of 50 HIV-infected patients revealed that 32% (16 of 50) of serum samples and 26% (13 of 50) of CSF samples had IgG antibodies, compared with 4% to 6% of control samples.[62] Another report detailed acute psychiatric symptoms that developed in two patients with biopsy-confirmed cutaneous BA, and resolved after the patients were treated with antibiotics appropriate for their BA infection.[3]

Unusual Bacillary Angiomatosis Presentations

Several cases of BA involving the bone marrow have been reported.[27,44,57] Hepatosplenomegaly and thrombocytopenia were noted in both of these patients, and all resolved after antibiotic treatment. Venous thrombosis of the left upper extremity occurred in an acquired immunodeficiency syndrome (AIDS) patient with *B. quintana* bacteremia during relapse.[32] The thrombosis was characterized by multiple noncontiguous, erythematous, tender, superficial thromboses in the absence of trauma or intravenous drug use, and all rapidly resolved after institution of antibiotic therapy.

Cutaneous BA complicating pregnancy in an HIV-infected woman was reported by Riley et al.[58] The cutaneous lesions resolved after antibiotic treatment, and the subsequent pregnancy and delivery were uneventful. Only one pediatric case of BA has been reported,[47] and this patient was immunocompromised due to chemotherapy, not HIV infection. However, pediatricians should be alert for the signs and symptoms of *Bartonella* infection in HIV-infected pediatric patients.

Bacteremia with Bartonella Species

Some patients with BA and BP also have bacteremia. One third of our patients with culture-positive cutaneous BA also had the corresponding *Bartonella* species simultaneously cultured from the blood (J.E. Koehler et al, unpublished data). *Bartonella* bacteremia in the absence of focal BA disease has been reported by a number of groups,[53,54,66] and may be more common than focal *Bartonella* disease. Individuals with HIV-infection and concomitant *Bartonella* bacteremia usually had systemic symptoms including fever, chills, and weight loss that resolved after antibiotic therapy. One patient with HIV infection and culture-proven *B. quintana* bacteremia was noted to have endocarditis.[68] A second case of *Bartonella* endocarditis in a patient without apparent immunocompromise was attributed to *B. elizabethae*, a new species.[16]

Diagnosis of Bartonella Infections

Histopathologic Diagnosis

OBTAINING TISSUE FOR DIAGNOSIS. Biopsy is the principal intervention available for the diagnosis of cutaneous BA. Because KS lesions can be clinically indistinguishable from those of BA, any new vascular lesion should be biopsied. In patients with previously diagnosed KS, any vascular lesion that has a different appearance or rate of growth should also be biopsied, because KS and cutaneous BA can occur simultaneously in the same patient.[6,70] Pedunculated lesions can be biopsied by shave excision, and smaller, papular, or subcutaneous lesions should be examined by punch biopsy. Biopsy of the cellulitic plaque that frequently overlies osteolytic lesions may be sufficient to yield a diagnosis of BA, but in some patients, open excisional bone biopsy is necessary.[32] Fine-needle aspiration of BA lymph nodes has not been useful in diagnosis of BA in our center, thus open excisional or incisional biopsy remains the optimal technique for diagnosis. For BP of the liver or spleen, the diagnostic procedure with greatest yield appears to be excisional wedge biopsy of the liver or splenectomy; however, peliosis hepatis has been diagnosed by either transvenous liver biopsy[43] or percutaneous liver biopsy.[67] As with cutaneous lesions, several opportunistic infections and malignancies can have a similar appearance on CT of the abdomen, and thus biopsy is extremely important to direct specific treatment. No case of hemorrhage following percutaneous biopsy of a peliotic liver has been reported; however, this remains a theoretical concern.

HISTOPATHOLOGIC CHARACTERISTICS. A characteristic vascular proliferation is seen on routine hematoxylin and eosin (H&E) staining of BA or peliotic tissue (Fig. 25–8A and Color Plate II*H*). Numerous bacilli also can be demonstrated in these lesions by modified silver staining (e.g., Warthin-Starry, Steiner, Dieterle's) or electron microscopy (Fig. 25–8*B*).[37,52,79] Other stains, such as those for tissue Gram's staining, fungi, or acid-fast mycobacteria do not stain *Bartonella* bacilli.

Cutaneous BA lesions may be misdiagnosed histopathologically, most often as KS,[1,31,38,64] angiosarcoma,[1,14,24,60] and pyogenic granuloma.[42,46,81] The histopathologic appearance of cutaneous BA lesions may be indistinguishable from pyogenic granuloma (lobular capillary hemangioma) and verruga peruana, the late, chronic phase of infection with *B. bacilliformis*.[38]

A histopathologic diagnosis of pyogenic granuloma, angiosarcoma, or peliosis of the liver or spleen in an HIV-infected patient should

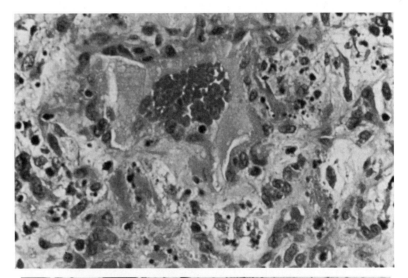

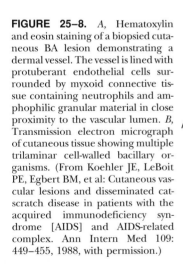

FIGURE 25–8. *A,* Hematoxylin and eosin staining of a biopsied cutaneous BA lesion demonstrating a dermal vessel. The vessel is lined with protuberant endothelial cells surrounded by myxoid connective tissue containing neutrophils and amphophilic granular material in close proximity to the vascular lumen. *B,* Transmission electron micrograph of cutaneous tissue showing multiple trilaminar cell-walled bacillary organisms. (From Koehler JE, LeBoit PE, Egbert BM, et al: Cutaneous vascular lesions and disseminated cat-scratch disease in patients with the acquired immunodeficiency syndrome [AIDS] and AIDS-related complex. Ann Intern Med 109: 449–455, 1988, with permission.)

A

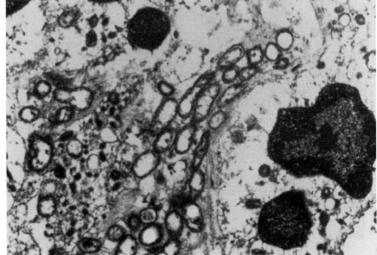

B

prompt further evaluation of the tissue for bacilli, to determine whether the lesion may actually be due to *Bartonella* infection. The presence of bacillary organisms is the diagnostic feature that distinguishes cutaneous BA, extracutaneous BA, and parenchymal BP from these other diagnoses (with the exception of the cutaneous lesions of verruga peruana, which are associated with *B. bacilliformis* bacilli).

Serologic Diagnosis

Bartonella antibodies can be detected by an indirect fluorescence antibody (IFA) test developed at the Centers for Disease Control and Prevention (CDC).[56] This test detects *Bartonella* antibodies in the serum from patients with BA.[76] Antibodies to *Bartonella* were detected in seven HIV-infected patients with biopsy-confirmed cutaneous BA, and no antibodies were detected in seven HIV-infected patients without BA. For three of the patients with *Bartonella* antibodies, examination of banked serum revealed the presence of *Bartonella* antibodies as many as 7 years prior to the development of BA disease, suggesting infection with this bacterium years before the diagnosis of BA. Prior to the diagnosis of BA in these three patients, a fourfold rise in titer occurred, raising the possibility of either relapse or reinfection. Culture-proven relapse in another BA patient[32] also was predicted by a rising serum antibody titer.[76] This IFA thus appears to be promising for the diagnosis of BA and other *Bartonella*-associated infections in HIV-infected patients, as well as in following the response to antibiotic treatment.

Culture of Bartonella Species From Blood and Tissue of Patients with BA

Slater et al[66] first reported isolation of *Bartonella* species from blood using lysis-centrifugation tubes (Isostat Tubes; Wampole, Cranbury, NJ) and plating onto fresh chocolate or heart infusion agar with 5% rabbit blood, without antibiotics. Standard blood collection tubes containing ethylenediaminetetraacetic acid (EDTA) also have been used to isolate *B. henselae* from the blood of an HIV-infected patient.[54] Detection of *B. quintana* bacteremia also has been reported using acridine orange staining of aliquots removed from Bactec blood culture bottles.[35] The use of quantitative cultures (e.g., lysis-centrifugation tubes) demonstrates that immunocompromised patients may have a high-grade bacteremia with *Bartonella,* with blood cultures yielding >1000 colony-forming-units (CFUs) per milliliter of blood.[32]

Isolation of *Bartonella* species directly from cutaneous BA lesions is difficult due to the fastidious growth characteristics of this genus. Either *B. quintana* or *B. henselae* can be isolated by mincing a sterilly obtained cutaneous,[32] lymph node,[17] splenic,[67] or hepatic biopsy specimen in inoculation media[32] and spreading onto fresh chocolate or heart infusion agar with 5% rabbit blood and incubating for at least 3 to 4 weeks in 5% CO_2. The highest recovery rate of *Bartonella* species from cutaneous BA lesions has been accomplished using an endothelial cell monolayer cocultivation system,[32] but this technique is not readily available to most microbiology labs.

Because culture of *Bartonella* species from biopsied cutaneous or hepatic tissue remains difficult, culture from blood represents the most accessible method of isolating *Bartonella* species; however, bacteremia is not always present in patients with cutaneous BA or peliosis hepatis.

Treatment of *Bartonella* Infections

Choice of Antibiotics

There have been no controlled trials for antibiotic treatment of BA. The first patient diagnosed with BA was treated empirically with erythromycin, with complete resolution of subcutaneous nodules.[71] From subsequent reports, and our experience at San Francisco General Hospital, it is evident that erythromycin is the drug of first choice for patients with BA and BP (Fig. 25–9). Oral erythromycin therapy of 500 mg four times a day is standard, but intravenous therapy should be given to patients with severe disease or those unable to tolerate oral medication. Oral doxycycline therapy with 100 mg twice a day also has been used successfully in a number of patients, and resolution of BA due to *B. henselae* also has been reported in one HIV-infected patient following oral tetracycline treatment[32] and two immunocompetent patients with *B. henselae* bacteremia.[66] Cutaneous BA in an immunocompetent patient also has been successfully treated with minocycline.[77] In several retrospective descriptions of patients with cutaneous BA, resolution of lesions was noted to be temporally related to institution of antimycobacterial therapy,[23,28,31,38,40] presumably due to the rifampin component. A summary of the apparent clinical efficacy of antibiotics for *Bartonella* infections in HIV-infected

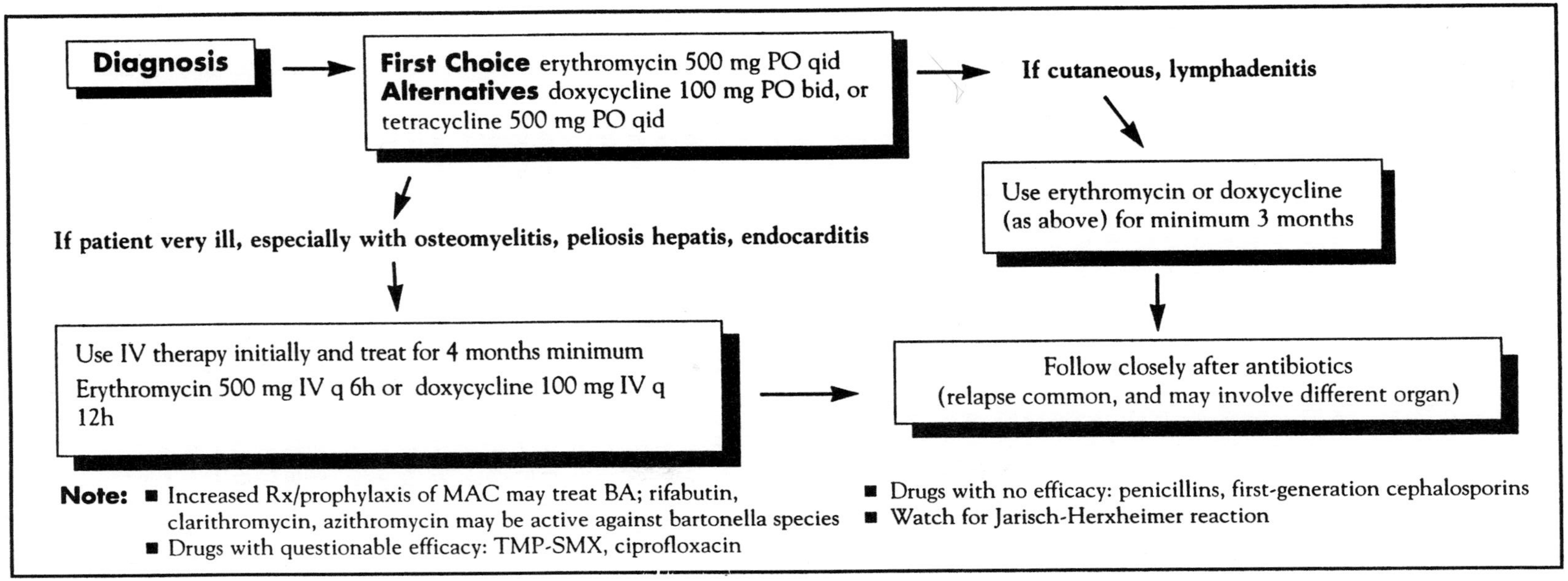
Diagnosis
First Choice erythromycin 500 mg PO qid
Alternatives doxycycline 100 mg PO bid, or tetracycline 500 mg PO qid
If cutaneous, lymphadenitis
Use erythromycin or doxycycline (as above) for minimum 3 months
If patient very ill, especially with osteomyelitis, peliosis hepatis, endocarditis
Use IV therapy initially and treat for 4 months minimum
Erythromycin 500 mg IV q 6h or doxycycline 100 mg IV q 12h
Follow closely after antibiotics
(relapse common, and may involve different organ)
Note:
■ Increased Rx/prophylaxis of MAC may treat BA; rifabutin, clarithromycin, azithromycin may be active against bartonella species
■ Drugs with questionable efficacy: TMP-SMX, ciprofloxacin
■ Drugs with no efficacy: penicillins, first-generation cephalosporins
■ Watch for Jarisch-Herxheimer reaction

FIGURE 25–9. Algorithm for treatment of *Bartonella* infections. (From Koehler J: Recurrent bacterial infections: *Bartonella*. Clin Care Options HIV 1:17–18, 1995, with permission of the publisher, Healthcare Communications Group, LLC.)

individuals is presented in Table 25–1. It is important to note that some patients develop a Jarisch-Herxheimer reaction after the first several doses of antibiotic, with exacerbation of systemic symptoms and fever.[32] This response may be attenuated by pretreatment with an antipyretic.

The clinical response of patients with BA to treatment with erythromycin, doxycycline, and tetracycline usually corresponds to the in vitro susceptibilities of *B. quintana* and *B. henselae*.[16,48,66] However, there is little correlation between the in vivo and in vitro antibiotic susceptibilities for other antibiotics, especially those that target steps in cell wall synthesis (e.g., penicillins). It is obvious from numerous reports that penicillin, penicillinase-resistant penicillins, aminopenicillins, and first-generation cephalosporins have no activity against the *B. quintana* and *B. henselae* bacilli in BA lesions.[6,31, 32,38,42,74,81] Apparent response to some antibiotics (e.g., vancomycin[81]) or a first-generation cephalosporin[42] likely represents the treatment of superinfecting skin flora. We pretreated one patient who had superinfected cutaneous BA lesions with cephradine to improve recovery of *Bartonella* organisms from the lesions.[32] The differences between in vitro and in vivo sensitivities may result because the bacilli present in BA lesions have different cell wall characteristics from those grown on agar, which changes the susceptibility to cell wall–active antibiotics. Additionally, the fastidious nature of *Bartonella* species makes accurate susceptibility testing difficult to perform.

Antibiotics included in the group with possible clinical efficacy (Table 25–1) include gentamicin and rifampin, but use of either of these drugs alone is not recommended. For severely ill patients, we administer gentamicin or rifampin in addition to a first-line drug (erythromycin or doxycycline) during the initial several weeks of therapy. For some other antibiotics listed in Table 25–1 with possible clinical efficacy, single case reports have been associated with improvement in lesions or symptoms, but the response to these antibiotics is not consistent enough to warrant their recommendation at present. It is also difficult to directly attribute improvement of symptoms to treatment with a specific antibiotic when many patients have concomitant infection with other pathogens. The clinical efficacy of ciprofloxacin, trimethoprim-sulfamethoxazole (TMP/SMX) and third-generation cephalosporins remains inconclusive. One pregnant patient received 2 weeks of ceftizoxime treatment for cutaneous BA and had complete resolution of lesions.[58] In our study of patients with BA, we have observed progression of BA lesions in patients treated with ciprofloxacin.[78] Although one patient improved when treated with TMP/SMX,[64] most patients demonstrated no improvement or had progression of lesions.[45,58,68,74]

Relapse

Both *B. quintana*[72] and *B. henselae*[41] produce recurring illness in immunocompetent hosts; it is thus not surprising that immunocompromised patients with BA or BP frequently experience relapse despite prolonged antibiotic therapy.[6,32,34,42,54,66,74,81] It should be noted that reinfection remains a possibility in these patients, but the majority of these cases probably represent relapse. The frequency of relapse appears to be increased when patients are treated with antibiotics for a shorter duration; as the result of our increased experience over the past 7 years, we have increased the duration of treatment for all presentations of BA.

Treatment of Cutaneous Bacillary Angiomatosis Lesions

Immunocompromised patients with cutaneous BA should be evaluated for parenchymal and osseous disease before beginning treatment, because presence of either of these requires treatment for a longer duration. For cutaneous disease alone, antibiotic therapy can be given orally. Response of cutaneous lesions is usually rapid, with improvement in 1 week and complete resolution by 1 month,[5] although hyperpigmentation may persist at the site of the lesion. As a result of our experience, we treat patients with cutaneous lesions alone for 12 weeks, and if relapse occurs, we extend treatment for an additional 16 weeks and occasionally, treat indefinitely.

TABLE 25–1. CLINICAL EFFICACY OF ANTIBIOTICS IN THE TREATMENT OF BACILLARY ANGIOMATOSIS AND BACILLARY PELIOSIS

Definite	Possible	Inconclusive	None
Erythromycin	Gentamicin	Ciprofloxacin	Penicillin
Doxycycline	Rifampin	Ceftriaxone	Ceph[1]
Tetracycline		Ceftizoxime	PCN-D
Minocycline		TMP/SMX	

TMP/SMX, trimethoprim-sulfamethoxazole; Ceph,[1] first-generation cephalosporins; PCN-D, penicillin derivatives (PCNase-resistant penicillins and aminopenicillins).

Treatment of Osseous Bacillary Angiomatosis Lesions

Duration of antibiotic therapy for patients with *Bartonella* osteomyelitis also is not well established. We treated one patient (see Fig. 25–3) with erythromycin, which the patient self-administered at a dose of 500 mg orally six times a day for 2 months, followed by 500 mg four times a day for an additional 2 months.[31] This patient had complete resolution of the osteolytic lesion and no relapse of BA during the subsequent 24 months, when he died of another opportunistic infection. Relapse occurred in another patient with osseous BA[32] despite 4 months of oral treatment with 500 to 1000 mg erythromycin 4 times a day; the osseous BA healed, but relapse with *B. quintana* bacteremia occurred 1 month after stopping erythromycin. For patients with osseous BA, it may be most appropriate to treat initially with several weeks of intravenous antibiotics (erythromycin or doxycycline), followed by prolonged, and perhaps indefinite, oral antimicrobial therapy. Serial technetium-99m methylene diphosphonate bone scans or roentgenograms can be used to monitor treatment efficacy, although resolution of osseous lesions is delayed, as seen with other causes of osteomyelitis.

Treatment of Hepatic and Splenic Bacillary Peliosis

Most patients with BP have severe systemic symptoms, including nausea and vomiting, which may substantially decrease absorption of oral antibiotics. Additionally, oral erythromycin or doxycycline may not be tolerated by these patients; therefore, initial treatment should be with intravenous antibiotics for several weeks, followed by oral therapy for at least 4 months, and possibly, indefinitely. Treatment progress can be monitored by liver function tests and serial CT scans, if peliotic lesions are visualized at the time of diagnosis (Fig. 25–7).

Treatment of Bartonella *Bacteremia*

If possible, *Bartonella* blood cultures should be performed for patients with all forms of BA, prior to antibiotic treatment. Because of two recent reports of endocarditis with *B. quintana* and *B. elizabethae*,[16,68] all patients with *Bartonella* bacteremia and a cardiac murmur should be evaluated further with echocardiography. Within 1 week after institution of antibiotic treatment, immunocompromised patients with isolated *Bartonella* bacteremia usually note resolution of fever and most other constitutional symptoms, although one patient did not have permanent remission of fever until he had received 8 weeks of treatment.[66] An initial period of intravenous antibiotic therapy is probably appropriate, followed by at least 3 months of oral antibiotic therapy. If endocarditis is documented, prolonged intravenous antibiotic therapy should be administered.

In summary, the drug of first choice for BA or BP is erythromycin, and for those patients unable to tolerate this antibiotic, doxycycline has demonstrated excellent clinical efficacy. If neither erythromycin nor doxycycline can be used, alternative antibiotics include tetracycline and minocycline. Patients very ill with systemic symptoms, with osteomyelitis, or with endocarditis should initially receive intravenous therapy with erythromycin or doxycycline, probably with the addition of either gentamicin or rifampin.

Epidemiology and Prevention of Bartonella Infections

Arthropods may serve as vectors of *Bartonella* species; *B. quintana* is known to be transmitted from the human reservoir via the body louse to other humans.[72] Ticks also are possible vectors: two patients reported tick bites preceding the diagnosis of *B. henselae* bacteremia.[41,83] However, at present the vector most strongly implicated in transmission of at least one *Bartonella* species, *B. henselae,* is the domestic cat.

Bartonella henselae has been identified as the principal bacterial agent causing CSD in immunocompetent individuals by serologic studies,[56] by direct culture from lymph nodes with histopathologic characteristics suggestive of CSD,[17] and by demonstration of presence of *Bartonella* DNA (but not *A. felis* DNA) in the CSD skin test antigen.[51] Similarly, an association between cat exposure and the development of BA has been noted anecdotally in many case reports.[33] The first systematic evaluation of the relationship between cat contact, numerous other environmental exposures, and development of BA was conducted by Tappero et al.[79] This case-control study found a significant epidemiologic association between development of BA and traumatic cat exposure (cat bite or cat scratch). Both CSD and BA due to *B. henselae* have been statistically associated with cat exposure,[79,87] with the cat as potential vector, reservoir, or both. The domestic cat appears to be the major reservoir for

B. henselae. The association between *B. henselae*–infected cats and development of BA in the cat owners was demonstrated in 1994, when bacteremia was detected in all seven cat contacts of four patients with BA due to *B. henselae.*[30] It was further found that about 40% of the domestic cat population sampled in the greater San Francisco Bay Area was bacteremic with *B. henselae.*[12,30]

Several lines of evidence implicate the cat flea as a potential vector of *B. henselae.* An epidemiologic association between owning a kitten with fleas and development of CSD was found by Zangwill et al.[87] Additionally, a seroprevalence survey of *B. henselae* antibodies in pet cats throughout regions of North America revealed that the regions with the highest average prevalences of antibodies coincided with the geographic areas predicted to have the highest prevalence of the cat flea (e.g., Hawaii, coastal California, the Pacific Northwest, and south central plains).[26] Finally, viable *B. henselae* bacilli were isolated from several fleas combed from one of the bacteremic cats identified by Koehler et al.[30]

Because of the high prevalence of infection in the pet cat population (there are 57 million pet cats in the United States), transmission of *B. henselae* to humans is relatively rare, and thus the benefit of these companion animals far outweighs the risk of *B. henselae* infection.[55] We suggest that several practical measures be followed to reduce the risk of *B. henselae* infection in HIV-infected individuals: (1) wash hands after petting and handling pets; (2) wash bites and scratches immediately with soap and water; (3) never allow any pet to lick an open wound; and (4) minimize infestation with fleas.

Although the domestic cat has been identified as the major reservoir and vector for *B. henselae,* it is quite evident that *B. quintana,* which causes the majority of BA infections in San Francisco, is not associated with cat contact. Further work must be undertaken to define the reservoir(s), vector(s), and method of transmission for all *Bartonella* species to facilitate further recommendations for preventing disease in the immunocompromised individual.

RHODOCOCCUS EQUI INFECTIONS

Clinical Presentation

Rhodococcus equi has been known to be a veterinary pathogen since the 1920s, but was not rec-

ognized as a human pathogen until 1967, when the first case report of pulmonary abscess in a human was published.[21] In recent years, increasing numbers of patients with *R. equi* have been described, the majority of whom have concomitant HIV infection. A comprehensive review of 72 cases revealed that 86% of the patients with *R. equi* were immunocompromised, and the majority of these patients developed pulmonary infection.[82] In contrast, the majority of the immunocompetent patients in this series had extrapulmonary disease.

The clinical presentation in HIV-infected patients with *R. equi* includes chest pain, productive cough, dyspnea, hemoptysis, and fever.[22,36,63,82] In many patients, symptoms were present for several weeks to months prior to diagnosis, and included anorexia, malaise, and weight loss.[22,36] Roentgenographic findings of *R. equi* infection in HIV-infected patients include pulmonary infiltrates, pleural effusion, empyema and, most distinctively, cavitary lung disease (more frequently in the upper lobes than the lower lobes in HIV-infected patients) (Fig. 25–10).[15,22,36,75,82] Because patients with late-stage HIV infection are less likely to develop cavitary disease with *Mycobacterium tuberculosis* infection than early after HIV infection, *R. equi* should be considered to be a likely cause of cavitary pulmonary disease in patients with very low CD4 cell counts.[82] In addition to parenchymal and cavitary disease, *R. equi* also has been associated with an endobronchial mass in an HIV-infected patient.[10]

Bacteremia developed in 53% of the immunocompromised patients with *R. equi* infection.[82] Brain abscesses due to *R. equi* have been documented in several HIV-infected patients, and were presumed to have developed from hematogenous infection in patients with extensive pulmonary disease and bacteremia.[2,63,82] One HIV-infected patient developed a foot mycetoma due to *R. equi* that progressed to sequentially involve the ipsilateral inguinal lymph nodes, pulmonary parenchyma, and, probably, brain parenchyma.[2]

Diagnosis of *Rhodococcus Equi* Infections

Rhodococcus equi infection is most readily diagnosed by isolation from sputum or bronchoalveolar lavage fluid and from normally sterile sites including blood, pleural fluid, and biopsied tissue. The organism is a gram-positive, nonmotile, non–spore-forming aerobic coccobacillus that belongs to the phylogenetic group of nocardioform actinomycetes.[19] The organism grows readily on routine bacteriologic media, including Sabouraud, Löwenstein-Jensen, sheep blood, and chocolate agars and aerobic blood culture media.[63] Distinctive, moist to mucoid, buff to salmon-pink colonies form on agar after 24 to 72 hours of incubation. In broth, bacillary forms predominate and on solid agar, cocci are usually seen.[63]

Of note, *R. equi* contains mycolic acids in the cell wall, as do species of the related genera *Mycobacteria* and *Nocardia;* thus *Rhodococcus* may stain weakly positive with acid-fast stains. Two immunocompromised patients received more than 1 month of antituberculous therapy before the acid-fast–staining bacilli from sputum smears were identified correctly as *R. equi.*[75] Additionally, *R. equi* may resemble diphtheroids in respiratory smears and cultures, leading to their erroneous identification as a respiratory contaminant.[36] When *R. equi* is isolated from sterile sites, it should never be considered a contaminating diphtheroid.[63]

Histopathologic findings in resected soft tissue or pulmonary masses include a necrotizing, granulomatous reaction with abundant polymorphonuclear leukocytes and microabscesses.[63,82] Organisms are readily stained in tissue and visualized within histiocytes using tissue Gram's and periodic acid–Schiff stains. Although organisms from young colonies on culture plates may stain acid fast using the Kinyoun stain, tissue acid-fast stains such as auramine O and modified Fite do not stain *R. equi* in tissue.[63]

Treatment of *Rhodococcus equi* Infections

Rhodococcus equi isolates usually are susceptible to erythromycin, rifampin, vancomycin, ciprofloxacin, and gentamicin.[49,82] There is usually resistance to penicillins, and even if an isolate is susceptible initially, resistance to penicillin, ampicillin, or first-generation cephalosporins can develop rapidly during treatment with these antibiotics.[19] It is important to perform antimicrobial susceptibility testing on initial patient isolates to direct antimicrobial therapy. Follow-up cultures should be obtained, and because resistance can develop during therapy with first-line antibiotics, repeat susceptibility testing is warranted for *R. equi* isolates obtained during antimicrobial therapy. The patient with

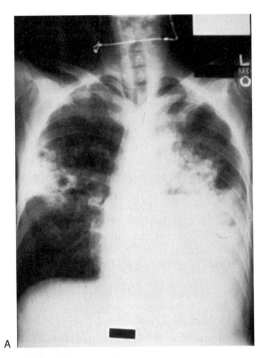

A

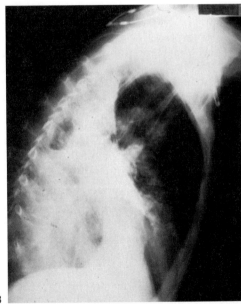

B

FIGURE 25–10. Chest roentgenograms of an HIV-infected patient with *Rhodococcus equi* pulmonary infection. Posteroantero (*A*) and lateral (*B*) views reveal bilateral pulmonary infiltrates with cavitation and air-fluid levels. An undrained empyema is also present in the left chest. (From Verville TD, Huycke MM, Greenfield RA, et al: *Rhodococcus equi* infections of humans: 12 cases and a review of the literature. Medicine 73:119–132, 1994, with permission.)

R. equi foot mycetoma, described above, was first treated with TMP/SMX and rifampin, to which the initial isolate was susceptible. However, when pulmonary disease developed, the subsequent isolate from bronchoalveolar lavage fluid was resistant to TMP/SMX.[2] The pulmonary parenchymal lesions resolved completely over the ensuing 5 months during therapy with rifampin and ciprofloxacin. Another patient was treated with rifampin and ciprofloxacin, and although the initial isolate was rifampin-sensitive, the *R. equi* isolated after recurrence of pulmonary disease was rifampin-resistant.[50] The patient was then treated with the combination of doxycycline and erythromycin and the disease stabilized for the 5 months of subsequent follow-up.

Administration of two or three drugs appears to be important for treatment of patients with concomitant HIV and *R. equi* infections. Efficacy of antibiotics for *R. equi* infection has been studied most extensively in veterinary disease: a combination of rifampin plus erythromycin is apparently superior to combinations of penicillins, aminoglycosides or TMP/SMX.[22] *Rhodococcus equi* is a facultatively intracellular organism that can infect polymorphonuclear leukocytes and macrophages, and can persist in macrophages. It is therefore recommended that the regimen include at least one and preferably two lipid-soluble drugs with good intracellular penetration.[22,36,75] Vancomycin demonstrated good activity in an animal model and has been used successfully in human regimens despite poor intracellular penetration.[82] A combination of vancomycin and imipenem was used successfully in one patient.[59] Some authors of early case reports suggest treatment may be facilitated by surgical resection of parenchymal abscesses, but in one HIV-infected patient, disease recurred after lobectomy; therefore, the benefit of this approach is unclear at present.[50]

The optimal duration for antimicrobial therapy is not known, but cumulative data from case reports indicate that prolonged, even lifelong therapy may be necessary. Treatment should be initiated with two or three antibiotics that are continued for 2 to 6 months, and subsequent therapy with one or two antibiotics is probably necessary to prevent relapse in HIV-infected individuals.[15,22,36,75] Even when patients with HIV and *R. equi* infections receive appropriate antimicrobial treatment, the infection may be fatal; one review reported that *R. equi* infection was chronic in 47% and that death occurred in 43% of patients.[82]

Epidemiology and Prevention of *Rhodococcus equi* Infections

Rhodococcus equi causes chronic suppurative bronchopneumonia in foals less than 6 months of age; pulmonary disease can be complicated by ulcerative colitis and mesenteric adenitis. *Rhodococcus equi* represents a substantial veterinary pathogen, infecting up to 10% of foals in endemic areas, and causing death in up to one third of those infected.[82] *Rhodococcus equi* is a common inhabitant of the gut of herbivores, and the presence of *R. equi* is widespread: *R. equi* has been demonstrated in the soil of all continents except Antarctica, but it is found especially frequently on horse ranches.[36,82] Both human and equine infection are presumed to result from exposure to soil contaminated with the manure from infected animals, primarily via inhalation. Ingestion also has been implicated as a route of infection, and direct soft tissue inoculation via soil contamination of superficial wounds has been well documented, especially in immunocompetent individuals.[2,63,82]

Approximately one third of patients with *R. equi* infection reported in the literature had potential exposure to contaminated soil,[82] including visiting or working on a horse farm or working as a groom.[22,36,59] Some authors have suggested that reactivation of remotely acquired *R. equi* infection may occur, although this has not been clearly demonstrated. Because the majority of HIV-infected patients do not have a defined exposure associated with developing *R. equi* infection, recommendations for prevention of infection with *R. equi* are limited to avoiding exposure to aerosolized soil contaminated with herbivore manure.[20]

PENICILLIUM MARNEFFEI INFECTIONS

Clinical Presentation

Penicillium marneffei is an unusual fungal pathogen in the United States, but is the third most common opportunistic infection in HIV-infected patients in some areas of Southeast Asia, after extrapulmonary *M. tuberculosis* infection and cryptococcosis.[73] This infection should be considered in HIV-infected patients who have traveled to or resided in Southeast Asia where *P. marneffei* is endemic, including Thailand, the Guanxi Province of China, Hong Kong, Vietnam, and Indonesia. Imported cases have been reported in the United States, France, the United Kingdom, Italy, Netherlands, and Australia.[73] The clinical presentation may be very similar to that of disseminated histoplasmosis, and this misdiagnosis has been reported in the literature.[8] In one study of 80 patients with confirmed *P. marneffei* infection, fever was the most common presenting symptom (92%) in addition to other systemic signs and symptoms including anemia (77%) and weight loss (76%).[73] Distinctive skin lesions were present in 71% of patients at the time of presentation, and the majority of these lesions (87%) had central umbilication, resembling molluscum contagiosum lesions. Larger lesions can form punched-out ulcers.[39] Reactivation after immunosuppression has been reported; disseminated *Penicillium marneffei* infection usually occurs late in HIV infection, and in two reviews, the majority of patients had a CD4 cell count <100/mm^3.[25,73]

Diagnosis of *Penicillium marneffei* Infections

Penicillium marneffei is a dimorphic fungus, first isolated from a bamboo rat in Vietnam in 1956. The fungus grows readily on routine fungal culture media in 2 to 5 days, producing an unusual, pinkish red pigment.[25] *Penicillium marneffei* is most readily isolated from blood, skin lesions, and bone marrow.[73] In endemic regions, where this infection is more frequently encountered, presumptive diagnosis is often made prior to obtaining positive culture results by examination of Wright's-stained samples of bone marrow aspirate or touch smears of skin or lymph node biopsies. In these specimens, *P.*

marneffei appears as intrahistiocytic and extracellular basophilic, spherical, oval, and elliptical yeast forms (2 to 6 μm in diameter), some of which contain a clear central septation.[73,84] In contrast, the yeast forms of *Histoplasma capsulatum* usually have narrow-based, unequal budding without septation.[84]

Treatment and Prevention of *Penicillium marneffei* Infections

The majority of patients reported in the literature were treated with amphotericin, and had a response. In the largest case series of patients from Thailand, 27 of 39 (77%) patients treated with amphotericin had clinical and microbiologic resolution of infection.[73] Seventy-five per cent (9 of 12) of patients responded to treatment with itraconazole, but only 4 of 11 (36%) responded to fluconazole. Like most other systemic fungal infections in HIV-infected patients, there is a propensity for relapse after cessation of antifungal therapy, and lifelong secondary prophylaxis with an antifungal agent (e.g., itraconazole) is recommended. Virtually nothing is known at present about transmission and, therefore, prevention, of *P. marneffei* in endemic regions, but it is important to note that the high mortality rate attributed to this infection is primarily due to failure to make a timely diagnosis and begin treatment.[73,84]

ACKNOWLEDGMENTS

This project was supported by funds from the Universitywide AIDS Research Program and the NIH grant AI36075. Dr. Koehler is a Pew Scholar in the Biomedical Sciences.

REFERENCES

1. Angritt P, Tuur SM, Macher AM, et al: Epithelioid angiomatosis in HIV infection: Neoplasm or cat-scratch disease? (Letter). Lancet 1:996, 1988
2. Antinori S, Esposito R, Cernuschi M, et al: Disseminated *Rhodococcus equi* infection initially presenting as foot mycetoma in an HIV-positive patient. AIDS 6:740–742, 1992
3. Baker J, Ruiz-Rodriguez R, Whitfeld M, et al: Bacillary angiomatosis: A treatable cause of acute psychiatric symptoms in human immunodeficiency virus infection. J Clin Psychiatry 56:161–166, 1995
4. Baron AL, Steinbach LS, LeBoit PE, et al: Osteolytic lesions and bacillary angiomatosis in HIV infection: Radiologic differentiation from AIDS-related Kaposi sarcoma. Radiology 177:77–81, 1990
5. Berger TG, Koehler JE: Bacillary angiomatosis. In Volberding P, Jacobson MA, eds. AIDS Clinical Review 1993/1994, New York, Marcel Dekker, Inc, 1993, pp 43–60
6. Berger TG, Tappero JW, Kaymen A, et al: Bacillary (epithelioid) angiomatosis and concurrent Kaposi's sarcoma in acquired immunodeficiency syndrome. Arch Dermatol 125:1543–1547, 1989
7. Birtles RJ, Harrison TG, Saunders NA, Molyneux DH: Proposals to unify the genera *Grahamella* and *Bartonella*, with descriptions of *Bartonella talpae* comb. nov., *Bartonella peromysci* comb. nov., and three new species, *Bartonella grahamii* sp. nov., *Bartonella taylorii* sp. nov., and *Bartonella doshiae* sp. nov: Int J System Bacteriol 45:1–8, 1995

8. Borradori L, Schmit JC, Stetzkowski M, et al: *Penicillium marneffei* infection in AIDS. J Am Acad Dermatol 31:843–846, 1994

9. Brenner DJ, O'Connor SP, Winkler HH, et al: Proposals to unify the genera *Bartonella* and *Rochalimaea*, with descriptions of *Bartonella quintana* comb. nov., *Bartonella vinsonii* comb. nov., *Bartonella henselae* comb. nov., and *Bartonella elizabethae* comb. nov., and to remove the family Bartonellaceae from the order Rickettsiales. Int J System Bacteriol 43:777–786, 1993

10. Canfrere I, Germaud P, Roger C: Another cause of endobronchial lesions found in HIV patients (Letter). Chest 108:587–588, 1995

11. Caniza MA, Granger DL, Wilson KH, et al: *Bartonella henselae:* Etiology of pulmonary nodules in a patient with depressed cell-mediated immunity. Clin Infect Dis 20:1505–1511, 1995

12. Chomel BB, Abbott RC, Kasten RW, et al: *Bartonella henselae* prevalence in domestic cats in California: Risk factors and association between bacteremia and antibody titers. J Clin Microbiol 33:2445–2450, 1995

13. Cockerell CJ, LeBoit PE: Bacillary angiomatosis: A newly characterized, pseudoneoplastic, infectious, cutaneous vascular disorder. J Am Acad Dermatol 22:501–512, 1990

14. Cockerell CJ, Whitlow MA, Webster GF, et al: Epithelioid angiomatosis: A distinct vascular disorder in patients with the acquired immunodeficiency syndrome or AIDS-related complex. Lancet 2:654–656, 1987

15. Cury JD, Harrington PT, Hosein IK: Successful medical therapy of *Rhodococcus equi* pneumonia in a patient with HIV infection. Chest 1619–1621, 1992

16. Daly JS, Worthington MG, Brenner DJ, et al: *Rochalimaea elizabethae* sp. nov. isolated from a patient with endocarditis. J Clin Microbiol 31:872–881, 1993

17. Dolan MJ, Wong MT, Regnery RL, et al: Syndrome of *Rochalimaea henselae* adenitis suggesting cat scratch disease. Ann Intern Med 118:331–336, 1993

18. Foltzer MA, Guiney WB Jr, Wager GC, Alpern HD: Bronchopulmonary bacillary angiomatosis. Chest 104:973–975, 1993

19. Frame BC, Petkus AF: *Rhodococcus equi* pneumonia: Case report and literature review. Ann Pharmacother 27:1340–1342, 1993

20. Glaser CA, Angulo FJ, Rooney JA: Animal-associated opportunistic infections among persons infected with the human immunodeficiency virus. Clin Infect Dis 18:14–24, 1994

21. Golub B, Falk G, Spink WW: Lung abscess due to *Corynebacterium equi.* Report of first human infection. Ann Intern Med 66:1174–1177, 1967

22. Gray BM: Case report: *Rhodococcus equi* pneumonia in a patient infected by the human immunodeficiency virus. Am J Med Sci 303:180–183, 1992

23. Hall AV, Roberts CM, Maurice PD, et al: Cat-scratch disease in patient with AIDS: Atypical skin manifestation (Letter). Lancet 2:453–454, 1988

24. Herts BR, Rafii M, Spiegel G: Soft-tissue and osseous lesions caused by bacillary angiomatosis: Unusual manifestations of cat-scratch fever in patients with AIDS. Am J Radiol 157:1249–1251, 1991

25. Hilmarsdottir I, Meynard JL, Rogeaux O, et al: Disseminated *Penicillium marneffei* infection associated with human immunodeficiency virus: A report of two cases and a review of 35 published cases. J AIDS 6:466–471, 1993

26. Jameson PH, Greene CE, Regnery RL, et al: Prevalence of *Bartonella henselae* in pet cats throughout regions of North America. J Infect Dis 172:1145–1149, 1995

27. Kemper CA, Lombard CM, Deresinski SC, et al: Visceral bacillary epithelioid angiomatosis: Possible manifestations of disseminated cat scratch disease in the immunocompromised host: A report of two cases. Am J Med 89:216–222, 1990

28. Knobler EH, Silvers DN, Fine KC, et al: Unique vascular skin lesions associated with human immunodeficiency virus. JAMA 260:524–527, 1988

29. Koehler JE, Cederberg L: Intraabdominal mass associated with gastrointestinal hemorrhage: A new manifestation of bacillary angiomatosis. Gastroenterology 109:2011–2014, 1995

30. Koehler JE, Glaser CA, Tappero JW: *Rochalimaea henselae* infection: A new zoonosis with the domestic cat as reservoir. JAMA 269:770–775, 1994

31. Koehler JE, LeBoit PE, Egbert BM, et al: Cutaneous vascular lesions and disseminated cat-scratch disease in patients with the acquired immunodeficiency syndrome (AIDS) and AIDS-related complex. Ann Intern Med 109:449–455, 1988

32. Koehler JE, Quinn FD, Berger TG, et al: Isolation of *Rochalimaea* species from cutaneous and osseous lesions of bacillary angiomatosis. N Engl J Med 327:1625–1631, 1992

33. Koehler JE, Tappero JW: AIDS Commentary: Bacillary angiomatosis and bacillary peliosis in patients infected with human immunodeficiency virus. Clin Infect Dis 17:612–624, 1993

34. Krekorian TD, Radner AB, Alcorn JM, et al: Biliary obstruction caused by epithelioid angiomatosis in a patient with AIDS. Am J Med 89:820–822, 1990

35. Larson AM, Dougherty MJ, Nowowiejski DJ, et al: Detection of *Bartonella (Rochalimaea) quintana* by routine acridine orange staining of broth blood cultures. J Clin Microbiol 32:1492–1496, 1994

36. Laskey JA, Pulkingham N, Powers MA, Dureack DT: *Rhodococcus equi* causing human pulmonary infection: Review of 29 cases. South Med J 84:1217–1220, 1991

37. LeBoit PE, Berger TG, Egbert BM, et al: Bacillary angiomatosis: The histopathology and differential diagnosis of a pseudoneoplastic infection in patients with human immunodeficiency virus disease. Am J Surg Pathol 13:909–920, 1989

38. LeBoit PE, Berger TG, Egbert BM, et al: Epithelioid haemangioma-like vascular proliferation in AIDS: Manifestation of cat-scratch disease bacillus infection? Lancet 1:960–963, 1988

39. Liu MT, Wong CK, Fung CP: Disseminated *Penicillium marneffei* infection with cutaneous lesions in an HIV-positive patient. Br J Dermatol 131:280–283, 1994

40. Lopez-Elzaurdia C, Fraga J, Sols M, et al: Bacillary angiomatosis associated with cytomegalovirus infection in a patient with AIDS. Br J Dermatol 125:175–177, 1991

41. Lucey D, Dolan MJ, Moss CW, et al: Relapsing illness due to *Rochalimaea henselae* in immunocompetent hosts: Implication for therapy and new epidemiological associations. Clin Infect Dis 14:683–688, 1992

42. Marasco WA, Lester S, Parsonnet J: Unusual presentation of cat scratch disease in a patient positive for

antibody to the human immunodeficiency virus. Rev Infect Dis 11:793–803, 1989

43. Marullo S, Jaccard A, Roulot D, et al: Identification of the *Rochalimaea henselae* 16S rRNA sequence in the liver of a French patient with bacillary peliosis hepatis (Letter). J Infect Dis 166:1462, 1992

44. Milam M, Balerdi MJ, Toney JF: Epithelioid angiomatosis secondary to disseminated cat scratch disease involving the bone marrow and skin in a patient with acquired immune deficiency syndrome: A case report. Am J Med 88:180–183, 1990

45. Mohle-Boetani JC, Koehler JE, Berger TG, et al: Bacillary angiomatosis and bacillary peliosis in patients infected with human immunodeficiency virus: Clinical characteristics in a case-control study. Clin Infect Dis 22:794–800, 1996

46. Mui BSK, Mulligan ME, George WL: Response of HIV-associated disseminated cat scratch disease to treatment with doxycycline. Am J Med 89:229–231, 1990

47. Myers SA, Prose NS, Garcia JA, et al: Bacillary angiomatosis in a child undergoing chemotherapy. J Pediatr 121:574–578, 1992

48. Myers WF, Grossman DM, Wisseman CL Jr: Antibiotic susceptibility patterns in *Rochalimaea quintana*, the agent of trench fever. Antimicrob Agents Chemother 25:690–693, 1984

49. Nordman P, Ronco E: In-vitro antimicrobial susceptibility of *Rhodococcus equi*. J Antimicrob Chemother 29:383–393, 1992

50. Nordmann P, Chavanet P, Caillon J, et al: Recurrent pneumonia due to rifampicin-resistant *Rhodococcus equi* in a patient infected with HIV (Letter). J Infect 24:104–107, 1992

51. Perkins BA, Swaminathan B, Jackson LA, et al: Case 22-1992—pathogenesis of cat scratch disease (Letter). N Engl J Med 327:1599–1601, 1992

52. Perkocha LA, Geaghan SM, Yen TSB, et al: Clinical and pathological features of bacillary peliosis hepatis in association with human immunodeficiency virus infection. N Engl J Med 323:1581–1586, 1990

53. Reed JA, Brigati DJ, Flynn SD, et al: Immunocytochemical identification of *Rochalimaea henselae* in bacillary (epithelioid) angiomatosis, parenchymal bacillary peliosis, and persistent fever with bacteremia. Am J Surg Pathol 16:650–657, 1992

54. Regnery RL, Anderson BE, Clarridge JE III, et al: Characterization of a novel *Rochalimaea* species, *R. henselae*, sp. nov., isolated from blood of a febrile, HIV-positive patient. J Clin Microbiol 30:265–274, 1992

55. Regnery RL, Childs JE, Koehler JE: Infections associated with *Bartonella* species in persons infected with human immunodeficiency virus. In USPHS/IDSA Guidelines for the Prevention of Opportunistic Infections in Persons Infected with Human Immunodeficiency Virus. Clin Infect Dis 21(Suppl 1): S94–S98, 1995

56. Regnery RL, Olson JG, Perkins BA, et al: Serological response to "*Rochalimaea henselae*" antigen in suspected cat-scratch disease. Lancet 339:1443–1445, 1992

57. Relman DA, Loutit JS, Schmidt TM, et al: The agent of bacillary angiomatosis: An approach to the identification of uncultured pathogens. N Engl J Med 323:1573–1580, 1990

58. Riley LE, Tuomala RE: Bacillary angiomatosis in a pregnant patient with acquired immunodeficiency syndrome. Obstet Gynecol 79:818–819, 1992

59. Rouquet RM, Clave D, Massip P, et al: Imipenem/vancomycin for *Rhodococcus equi* pulmonary infection in HIV-positive patient (Letter). Lancet 337:375, 1991

60. Schinella RA, Greco MA: Bacillary angiomatosis presenting as a soft-tissue tumor without skin involvement. Hum Pathol 21:567–569, 1990

61. Schwartzman WA, Marchevsky A, Meyer RD: Epithelioid angiomatosis or cat scratch disease with splenic and hepatic abnormalities in AIDS: Case report and review of the literature. Scand J Infect Dis 22: 121–133, 1990

62. Schwartzman WA, Patnaik M, Barka NE, Peter JB: *Rochalimaea* antibodies in HIV-associated neurologic disease. Neurology 44:1312–1316, 1994

63. Scott MA, Graham BS, Verrall R, et al: *Rhodococcus equi*—an increasingly recognized opportunistic pathogen. Report of 12 cases and review of 65 cases in the literature. Am J Clin Pathol 103:649–655, 1995

64. Slater LN, Min K-W: Polypoid endobronchial lesions: A manifestation of bacillary angiomatosis. Chest 102:972–974, 1992

65. Slater LN, Pitha JV, Herrera L, et al: *Rochalimaea henselae* infection in acquired immunodeficiency syndrome causing inflammatory disease without angiomatosis or peliosis: Demonstration by immunocytochemistry and corroboration by DNA amplification. Arch Pathol Lab Med 118:33–38, 1994

66. Slater LN, Welch DF, Hensel D, Coody DW: A newly recognized fastidious gram-negative pathogen as a cause of fever and bacteremia. N Engl J Med 323: 1587–1593, 1990

67. Slater LN, Welch DF, Min K-W: *Rochalimaea henselae* causes bacillary angiomatosis and peliosis hepatis. Arch Intern Med 152:602–606, 1992

68. Spach DH, Callis KP, Paauw DS, et al: Endocarditis caused by *Rochalimaea quintana* in a patient infected with human immunodeficiency virus. J Clin Microbiol 31:692–694, 1993

69. Spach DH, Panther LA, Thorning DR, et al: Intracerebral bacillary angiomatosis in a patient infected with human immunodeficiency virus. Ann Intern Med 116:740–742, 1992

70. Steeper TA, Rosenstein H, Weiser J, et al: Bacillary epithelioid angiomatosis involving the liver, spleen, and skin in an AIDS patient with concurrent Kaposi's sarcoma. Am J Clin Pathol 97:713–718, 1992

71. Stoler MH, Bonfiglio TA, Steigbigel RT, et al: An atypical subcutaneous infection associated with acquired immune deficiency syndrome. Am J Clin Pathol 80: 714–718, 1983

72. Strong RP, ed: Trench Fever: Report of Commission, Medical Research Committee, American Red Cross. Oxfords, Oxford University Press, 1918, pp 40–60

73. Supparatpinyo K, Khamwan C, Baosoung V, et al: Disseminated *Penicillium marneffei* infection in southeast Asia. Lancet 344:110–113, 1994

74. Szaniawski WK, Don PC, Bitterman SR, et al: Epithelioid angiomatosis in patients with AIDS. J Am Acad Dermatol 23:41–48, 1990

75. Takasugi JE, Godwin JD: Lung abscess caused by *Rhodococcus equi*. J Thorac Imaging 6:72–74, 1991

76. Tappero J, Regnery R, Koehler J, et al: Detection of serologic response to *Rochalimaea henselae* in patients with bacillary angiomatosis (BA) by immunofluorescent antibody (IFA) testing (Abstract

674). Program and Abstracts of the 32nd Interscience Conference on Antimicrobial Agents and Chemotherapy, Washington, DC, American Society for Microbiology, 1992, p 223

77. Tappero JW, Koehler JE, Berger TG, et al: Bacillary angiomatosis and bacillary splenitis in immunocompetent adults. Ann Intern Med 118:363–865, 1993

78. Tappero JW, Koehler JE: Cat scratch disease and bacillary angiomatosis (Letter). JAMA 266:1938–1993, 1991

79. Tappero JW, Mohle-Boetani J, Koehler JE, et al: The epidemiology of bacillary angiomatosis and bacillary peliosis. JAMA 269:770–775, 1993

80. Tuur SM, Macher AM, Angritt P, et al: AIDS case for diagnosis series, 1988. Milit Med 153:M57–M64, 1988

81. van der Wouw PA, Hadderingh RJ, Reiss P, et al: Disseminated cat-scratch disease in a patient with AIDS. AIDS 3:751–753, 1989

82. Verville TD, Huycke MM, Greenfield RA, et al: *Rhodococcus equi* infections of humans: 12 cases and a review of the literature. Medicine 73:119–132, 1994

83. Welch DF, Pickett DA, Slater LN, et al: *Rochalimaea henselae* sp. nov., a cause of septicemia, bacillary angiomatosis, and parenchymal bacillary peliosis. J Clin Microbiol 30:275–280, 1992

84. Wong KF, Tsang DNC, Chan JKC: Bone marrow diagnosis of penicilliosis (Letter). N Engl J Med 330:717–718, 1994

85. Wong MT, Dolan MJ, Lattuada CP, et al: Neuroretinitis, aseptic meningitis, and lymphadenitis associated with *Bartonella* (*Rochalimaea*) *henselae* infection in immunocompetent patients and patients infected with human immunodeficiency virus type 1. Clin Infect Dis 21:352–360, 1995

86. Wyatt SH, Fishman EK: Hepatic bacillary angiomatosis in a patient with AIDS. Abdom Imaging 18:336–338, 1993

87. Zangwill K, Hamilton DH, Perkins BA, et al: Cat scratch disease in Connecticut: Epidemiology, risk factors, and evaluation of a new diagnostic test. N Engl J Med 329:8–13, 1993

Chapter 26

Management of Herpesvirus Infections (CMV, HSV, VZV)

W. LAWRENCE DREW, MARY JEAN STEMPIEN, and KIM S. ERLICH

CYTOMEGALOVIRUS

Infection with cytomegalovirus (CMV) is extremely common in patients with AIDS and can result in several clinical illnesses, including chorioretinitis esophagitis, colitis, pneumonia and several neurologic disorders. Autopsy and clinical studies indicate that retinitis occurs in up to 40% of AIDS patients, whereas gastrointestinal disease occurs in 5% to 10%. Not all patients with blood, urine, or tissue cultures positive for CMV have clinical illness related to the infection, and diagnosis of disease caused by CMV may require tissue biopsy with histologic evidence of virus inclusions and inflammatory response. Detection of CMV antigen or nucleic acid in tissue are alternative methods for establishing that CMV is actually causing tissue disease. Viral culture is useful only if no other pathogen is identified in tissue. This section reviews the most common clinical syndromes caused by CMV and their treatment with ganciclovir (DHPG) or foscarnet.

Chorioretinitis

Ocular disease caused by CMV occurs only in patients with severe immunodeficiency and is especially common in patients with AIDS. Clinical evidence of CMV retinitis (Color Plate I*F*) occurs in as many as 40% of AIDS patients, and autopsy series have revealed that CMV retinitis is present in up to 30% of patients. With the routine use of prophylaxis against pneumocystis, retinitis is now a common presenting manifestation of AIDS, but it more often occurs months to years after the diagnosis of AIDS had been established. Decreased visual acuity, the presence of floaters, or unilateral visual field loss is often the presenting complaint. Ophthalmologic examination typically reveals large creamy to yellowish white granular areas with perivascular exudates and hemorrhages (referred to as a "cottage cheese and catsup" appearance) (Fig. 26–1). These abnormalities may be found initially at the periphery of the fundus but, if left untreated, the lesions progress within 2 to 3 weeks. Retinitis usually begins unilaterally, but progression to bilateral involvement is common because of an associated viremia. Systemic CMV infection involving other viscera is frequently present.

CMV accounts for at least 90% of HIV-related infectious retinopathies. Differentiating suspected CMV retinitis lesions from cotton wool spots is essential. Cotton wool spots appear as small, fluffy, white lesions with indistinct margins and are not associated with exudates or hemorrhages. They are common in AIDS patients, usually asymptomatic, and represent areas of focal ischemia. These lesions do not progress and often undergo spontaneous regression. Toxoplasmosis is the second most common opportunistic infection of the eye but is characterized by little if any hemorrhage. It is associated with cerebral toxoplasmosis in the majority of patients. Syphilis, herpes simplex, varicella-zoster virus (VZV), and tuberculosis are other infections that may rarely involve the retina.

Virtually all patients with CMV retinitis have CD4 lymphocyte counts of less than $50/mm^3$, and routine ophthalmologic screening of patients with pupillary dilation, as well as indirect ophthalmoscopy, may be valuable when cell counts decline to this level. It is also important to inquire about visual abnormalities, especially increased floaters, and to examine the fundus carefully when there are visual complaints. Pa-

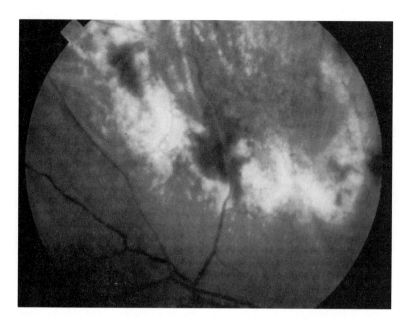

FIGURE 26–1. Funduscopic appearance of CMV retinitis, illustrating "cottage cheese and catsup" appearance resulting from perivascular exudates and hemorrhages. (Courtesy of Dr. L. Schwartz, San Francisco.)

tients with confirmed CMV chorioretinitis should be treated with ganciclovir foscarnet or cidofovir.[26,52,67] These agents are equally effective in the initial treatment of CMV chorioretinitis, although disease usually progresses despite continued treatment[34] (see Treatment).

Central Nervous System

The most characteristic neurologic syndrome caused by CMV in AIDS patients is radiculopathy, which occurs as a spinal cord syndrome with lower extremity weakness, spasticity, areflexia, urinary retention, and hypoesthesia. The cerebrospinal abnormalities are very unusual for a viral infection, namely, polymorphonuclear pleocytosis and a moderately low glucose concentration.[48] Culture of cerebrospinal fluid (CSF) may be negative, but antigen or DNA assays are usually positive. Anti-CMV therapy should be promptly administered to AIDS patients with suspected CMV encephalitis or polyradiculopathy, but limited data on efficacy are available.[40,48]

Subacute encephalitis caused by CMV probably occurs in AIDS patients. Isolation and identification of CMV in brain tissue or cerebrospinal fluid has been reported[15,16,31] (Chapter 14). CMV encephalitis in AIDS patients appears comparable to subacute encephalitis from other pathogens. Personality changes, difficulty concentrating, headaches, and somnolence frequently are present. The diagnosis can be confirmed by brain biopsy, with evidence of periventricle necrosis, giant cells, intranuclear and intracytoplasmic inclusions, and isolation or other identification of the virus—for example, by antigen or nucleic acid[31] from brain tissue or CSF.

Gastrointestinal System

Colitis

CMV colitis occurs in at least 5% to 10% of AIDS patients (Chapter 13). Diarrhea, weight loss, anorexia, and fever frequently are present. The differential diagnosis includes infection by other gastrointestinal pathogens, including *Cryptosporidium, Giardia, Entamoeba, Mycobacterium, Shigella, Campylobacter,* and *Strongyloides stercoralis,* and involvement by lymphoma or Kaposi's sarcoma. Endoscopy usually reveals diffuse submucosal hemorrhages and mucosal ulcerations, although a grossly normal-appearing mucosa may be encountered in up to 10% of those with histologic evidence of CMV colitis (Fig. 26–2). Biopsy reveals vasculitis, neutrophilic infiltration, and nonspecific inflammation, but the diagnosis is confirmed by the presence of characteristic CMV inclusions, CMV antigen, or CMV DNA, and the absence of other pathogens.

Esophagitis

Clinically evident esophagitis in AIDS patients most commonly is due to either *Candida*

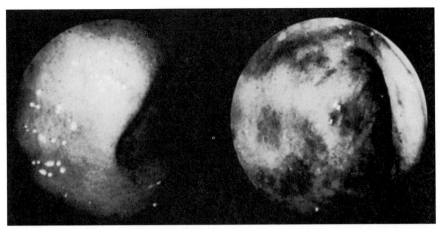

FIGURE 26–2.   Sigmoidoscopic appearance of CMV colitis (two views), demonstrating diffuse submucosal hemorrhages and mucosal ulcerations. (Courtesy of Dr. D. Dieterich, New York.)

albicans or herpes simplex virus (HSV), but may also be caused by CMV (Chapter 13). Patients with CMV esophagitis are apt to have pain on swallowing and large distal ulceration. As in colitis, diagnosis should be established through endoscopic examination and biopsy.

Treatment

Patients with symptomatic esophagitis or enterocolitis who do not have other pathogens detected by endoscopy, histology, or culture and who have CMV detected by these methods should benefit from anti-CMV treatment for 14 to 21 days and should be continued on maintenance treatment in part as a means of preventing retinitis.

The efficacy of anti-CMV treatment in patients with enterocolitis is not dramatic.[14] When compared to placebo, a significant antiviral effect was observed, but a clinical benefit was less apparent. Diarrhea and abdominal discomfort were not relieved, but in general patients seemed to improve with this therapy.[14]

Pneumonia

Isolation of CMV from pulmonary secretions or lung tissue in AIDS patients with pneumonia who undergo bronchoscopy is common, but a true pathogenic role of the virus in the disease process is not readily established. Many patients with pulmonary disease and CMV isolation from the lung have concomitant infection with other pathogens, especially *Pneumocystis carinii*. Many of the patients respond to therapy directed at *P. carinii* pneumonia alone, raising the question of whether CMV is a true pulmonary pathogen in AIDS patients. However, patients with positive CMV cultures and histologic findings from lung tissue and no other pathogens identified on diagnostic bronchoscopy may truly have invasive CMV pneumonia.

When CMV causes pulmonary disease in AIDS patients, the syndrome is that of an interstitial pneumonitis. Patients often complain of gradually worsening shortness of breath, dyspnea on exertion, and a dry, nonproductive cough. The heart and respiratory rates are elevated, but auscultation of the lungs often reveals minimal findings with no evidence of consolidation. Chest radiographs show diffuse interstitial infiltrates similar to those in patients with *P. carinii* pneumonia. Hypoxemia is invariably present.

Anti-CMV therapy should be considered when a patient has documented CMV pulmonary infection as the only pathogen identified and a progressive, deteriorating clinical course.[20,54,62]

Treatment

Ganciclovir

STRUCTURE AND MECHANISM OF ACTION. Ganciclovir (DHPG, Cytovene) is a nucleoside analog that differs from acyclovir (Zovirax) by a single carboxyl side chain. This structural change confers on the drug approximately 50 times more activity than acyclovir against CMV. Acyclovir has low activity against CMV because it is not well phosphorylated in CMV-infected cells. This is due to the absence of the gene for thymidine kinase in CMV. Ganciclovir, however, is active against CMV because it does not require thymidine kinase for phosphorylation. Instead another viral-encoded phosphorylating enzyme (UL 97) is present in CMV-infected cells.[72] It is capable of phosphorylating ganciclovir and converting it to the monophosphate. Then, cellular enzymes convert it to the active compound, ganciclovir triphosphate. Ganciclovir triphosphate acts to inhibit the viral DNA polymerase.

PHARMACOLOGY AND DOSAGE. Ganciclovir is available for clinical use in both intravenous and oral formulations. Intravenous ganciclovir is used for initial induction therapy, whereas oral ganciclovir can only be used for maintenance therapy. Oral ganciclovir is also used for prevention (see later). When administered by intravenous infusion over 1 hour in the usual dosage of 5 mg/kg, peak blood levels are approximately 8 to 9 μg/ml, and the serum half-life is 3.5 hours. The absolute bioavailability of oral ganciclovir capsules averages 9%. When administered orally as 1000 mg three times daily with food, peak serum levels are approximately 1 μg/mL, and the serum half-life is approximately 5 hours. Because ganciclovir is excreted unchanged through the kidneys, dosage must be reduced for intravenous ganciclovir in patients with renal impairment. Dosage adjustments should also be considered for oral ganciclovir. The appropriate dose reductions are presented in Table 26–1.

Initial intravenous induction treatment for CMV disease consists of 5 mg/kg twice daily for 14 to 21 days or until there is an adequate clinical response. The standard intravenous dosage for maintenance therapy is approximately one half the induction dose (i.e., 5 mg/kg/day 7 days per week or, if given orally, 1000 mg three times daily with food. Initial response in retinitis (improvement or stabilization in vision or ophthalmoscopic appearance) occurs in approximately 75% of treated patients.[67] By comparison, the disease is relentlessly progressive in 90% of patients if left untreated (Table 26–2). Visual-field defects present at the onset of therapy do not reverse, but a decrease in visual acuity caused by edema of the macula may improve with treatment. Maintenance therapy throughout the life of the patient appears critical for CMV retinitis because the virus is only suppressed by ganciclovir and is not eliminated. Oral ganciclovir maintenance therapy is associated with a risk of more rapid rate of retinitis progression compared to intravenous therapy (mean of 5 to 12 days earlier progression in three studies), but can be used where this risk is balanced by the benefit of avoiding daily intravenous infusions. Patients with stable, non–sight-threatening retinitis appear to be appropriate candidates for oral maintenance therapy. Even with continued maintenance therapy, CMV retinitis eventually progresses. This may result from viral resistance to the drug, inadequate drug delivery to the retina, or a combination of both factors. Retinal detachment may occur in later stages as the ne-

TABLE 26–1. GANCICLOVIR DOSAGE ADJUSTMENT IN PATIENTS WITH IMPAIRED RENAL FUNCTION

Creatinine Clearance* (mL/min)	IV Induction Dose (mg/kg)	Dosing Interval (hours)	Maintenance Dose (mg/kg)	Dosing Interval (hours)	Oral Dose
>70	5.0	12	5.0	24	1000 mg TID
50–69	2.5	12	2.5	24	1500 mg QD
25–49	2.5	24	1.25	24	1000 mg QD
10–24	1.25	24	0.625	24	500 mg QD
<10	1.25	3 times per week, following hemodialysis	0.625	3 times per week, following hemodialysis	500 mg 3 times per week, following hemodialysis

Creatinine clearance can be related to serum creatinine by the following formulas:

$$\text{Creatinine clearance for males} = \frac{(140 - \text{age [yrs]}) \ (\text{body wt [kg]})}{(72) \ (\text{serum creatinine [mg/dl]})}$$

$$\text{Creatinine clearance for females} = 0.85 \times \text{male value}$$

TABLE 26–2. COMPARISON OF COURSE OF CMV DISEASE IN GANCICLOVIR-TREATED VS UNTREATED CONTROL PATIENTS WITH AIDS

CMV Site	No. of Patients Improved or Stabilized/Total	
	Ganciclovir Treated (%)	Untreated Controls (%)
Retina	208/254 (82)	2/61 (3)
Gastrointestinal tract	33/39 (85)	NA
or colon	18/23 (78)	1/7 (14)
Lung		

NA, not available.

crotic retina scars and thins. Intravitreal injection of ganciclovir has been used in certain special situations, such as in patients in whom neutropenia limited the systemic use of the drug, and in one series[6] appeared effective and relatively safe. Controlled, comparative studies are underway to determine efficacy and safety. Sustained intravitreal release of ganciclovir has been accomplished using a surgically implantable device.[1,47,61] This implant, which is designed to deliver ganciclovir into the vitreous over several months, has been shown to be highly efficacious for local control of retinitis and should be available for clinical use shortly. A drawback to this approach is the lack of secondary prophylaxis afforded by systemic drug exposure; if ideal therapy is completed, it should be accomplished by systemic drug administration.

CLINICAL USE. Administration of ganciclovir is indicated for the treatment of acute CMV infection, but other herpesviruses (specifically, HSV-1, HSV-2, and VZV) are also susceptible to the drug in vitro. Because AIDS patients with severe CMV infection frequently have illnesses caused by other herpesviruses, a bonus of ganciclovir therapy may be an associated improvement of HSV and VZV infections. Ganciclovir is probably also active against Epstein-Barr virus.

VIROLOGIC RESPONSE TO GANCICLOVIR. CMV cultures of blood and urine rapidly become negative in patients treated with ganciclovir[5] (Fig. 26–3). Most of these patients had CMV retinitis, although AIDS patients with CMV infections of other organ systems are included. Of these patients, 87% had a complete virologic response (conversions of culture from positive to negative or a more than 100-fold reduction in CMV titer) in urine, and 83% had

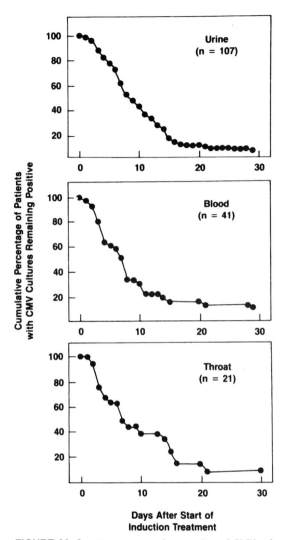

FIGURE 26–3. Time course of conversion of CMV cultures of specimens of urine, blood, or throat washings from positive (before treatment) to negative (after treatment with ganciclovir). Cultures from individual patients were performed at various times after start of treatment. Numbers in parentheses are the number of patients in whom the particular body fluid or site was sequentially cultured. (Reprinted with permission from Buhles WC Jr, Mastre BJ, Tinker AJ, et al: Ganciclovir treatment of life- or sight-threatening cytomegalovirus infection: Experience in 314 immunocompromised patients. Rev Infect Dis 10(suppl 3): S495–S504, 1988.)

a complete response in blood culture. The median time until response was 8 days for both blood and urine cultures.

RESISTANCE. Erice et al[23] reported three Minnesota patients whose clinical course suggested the emergence of resistance and whose CMV isolates exhibited increases in the concentration of ganciclovir required to inhibit the virus in tissue culture over baseline determinations. We have documented that, after 3 months of continuous ganciclovir therapy, approximately 10% of patients are excreting resistant strains of CMV (arbitrarily defined as strains that are only inhibited by four times or more the median concentration of ganciclovir required to inhibit a group of pretherapy isolates).[19] In virtually all isolates, there is a mutation in the phosphorylating gene. These strains remain sensitive to foscarnet, which may be used as an alternative therapy.[37]

TOXICITY. Toxicity may limit therapy with ganciclovir. The following adverse effects may occur.

Effects on Hematopoiesis. Leukopenia and anemia may affect up to 40% and 25%, respectively, of patients receiving intravenous ganciclovir for treatment of CMV disease. The incidence of both is lower during administration of oral ganciclovir (3000 mg daily) for either maintenance treatment of retinitis or primary prevention of CMV disease (Table 26–3). Many AIDS patients have low white blood cell counts before therapy, so the contribution of ganciclovir to leukopenia is not always clear. Neutropenia may develop at any time and is usually reversible, although at least five patients are known to have had irreversible suppression. Cytokines, such as granulocyte colony-stimulating factor (filgrastim, G-CSF), are effective in reversing ganciclovir-induced neutropenia. Severe neutropenia (absolute neutrophil count $<500/mm^3$) requires a ganciclovir dose interruption until evidence of marrow recovery is

observed and neutrophil counts have risen, preferably to greater than $1000/mm^3$. Thrombocytopenia occurs in up to 6% of ganciclovir-treated patients.

Toxicities in Other Organ Systems. Gastrointestinal adverse events, most commonly diarrhea, nausea, anorexia, and vomiting, affect a substantial number of patients treated with intravenous or oral ganciclovir. Data from a large double-blind safety comparison of oral ganciclovir (3000 mg daily) to placebo, however, suggest that the rates of these events are only modestly higher among ganciclovir patients: diarrhea (ganciclovir, 48%; placebo, 42%), anorexia (ganciclovir, 19%; placebo, 16%), and vomiting (ganciclovir, 14%; placebo, 11%). Neuropathy and paresthesia are the most frequent adverse events involving the nervous system, affecting up to 21% and 10% of patients, respectively, but only neuropathy occurred more often in ganciclovir- versus placebo-treated patients (21% versus 15%, respectively). A minority of ganciclovir-treated patients will experience modest elevations in serum creatinine (maximum levels of at least 1.5 mg/dl, or greater than 25% increases over pretreatment levels).

Therapeutic Drug Interactions

Ganciclovir Plus Zidovudine (AZT). Because both zidovudine and ganciclovir can cause neutropenia and anemia, some patients may not tolerate this combination at full dosage. The use of filgrastim (G-CSF) may counter the neutropenia caused by these drugs. Antiretroviral agents with less hematologic toxicity provide

TABLE 26–3. SELECTED LABORATORY ABNORMALITIES IN PATIENTS RECEIVING GANCICLOVIR FOR TREATMENT OF CMV RETINITIS AND PREVENTION OF CMV DISEASE

	CMV Retinitis Treatment		CMV Disease Prevention	
	Oral (3000 mg/day)	IV (5 mg/kg/day)	Oral (3000 mg/day)	Placebo
Patients	320	175	478	234
Neutropenia (ANC/μL)				
<500	18%	25%	10%	6%
500 to <749	17%	14%	16%	7%
750 to <1000	19%	26%	22%	16%
Anemia (Hgb, g/dl)				
<6.5	2%	5%	1%	<1%
6.5 to <8.0	10%	16%	5%	3%
8.0 to <9.5	25%	26%	15%	16%

Data are percentages of patients. ANC, absolute neutrophil count; Hgb, hemoglobin.

another means of maintaining antiretroviral activity during ganciclovir therapy.

Ganciclovir Plus Didanosine (ddI). Blood levels of ddI are significantly increased during concomitant ganciclovir use. The clinical significance of these increased levels is not yet known, but patients should be monitored for possible increased ddI-associated toxicity.

Gonadal Toxicity. In preclinical animal studies, ganciclovir is a potent inhibitor of spermatogenesis and may also suppress female fertility. Sperm counts in humans before and during ganciclovir therapy, however, have been performed too infrequently to provide meaningful information on spermatogenesis. Patients wishing to have children should use ganciclovir only for the strongest indications.

Teratogenesis. Because ganciclovir is a mutagen and teratogen in animals, effective contraception should be practiced by men and women with child-bearing potential during treatment. Ganciclovir should be used during pregnancy only if the potential benefit justifies the potential risk to the fetus.

Foscarnet

Foscarnet, also known as phosphonoformate or phosphonoformic acid (PFA), is a pyrophosphate that inhibits the DNA polymerase of CMV. Specifically, the drug blocks the pyrophosphate-binding site of the viral DNA polymerase, preventing cleavage of pyrophosphate from deoxyadenosine triphosphate.[8] This action is relatively selective in that CMV DNA polymerase is inhibited at concentrations less than 1% of that required to inhibit cellular DNA polymerase. Unlike such nucleosides as acyclovir and ganciclovir, foscarnet does not require phosphorylation intracellularly to be an active inhibitor of viral DNA polymerases. This biochemical fact becomes especially important in regard to viral resistance, because the principal mode of viral resistance to nucleoside analogs is a mutation that eliminates phosphorylation of the drug in virus-infected cells. Foscarnet can be used to treat patients with ganciclovir-resistant CMV, unless the virus is one of the 10% that are resistant because of a polymerase mutation and is cross-resistant to foscarnet.

PHARMACOLOGY. The recommended initial therapy with foscarnet is administered intravenously as 60 mg/kg every 8 hours or as 90 mg/kg every 12 hours. A dose of 120 mg/kg/day may be superior in efficacy to 90 mg/kg/day,[36] but this dose may also be more toxic.

CSF concentrations of foscarnet are approximately 40% of serum levels. Excretion is entirely renal without a hepatic component. Oral bioavailability is estimated at 12% to 22%, but it is poorly tolerated.

Adverse effects include renal impairment, anemia, hypocalcemia (especially ionized calcium), hypomagnesemia, and hypophosphatemia. It is important to measure renal function frequently and adjust dosage accordingly to minimize toxicity. Daily preinfusion of 1 liter of saline may reduce nephrotoxicity during maintenance therapy.

Palestine et al[52] reported a randomized control trial of foscarnet in the treatment of CMV retinitis in AIDS patients. Patients were assigned to receive either no therapy or immediate treatment with intravenous foscarnet. The justification for the design was that the lesions were peripheral and not threatening visual acuity. The mean time to progression of retinitis was 3 weeks in the control group vs 13 weeks in the treatment group, thereby proving that foscarnet is effective therapy. Also, an excellent antiviral effect was achieved in the treatment group (i.e., 9 of 13 patients had positive blood cultures for CMV at entry, and all 9 had CMV cleared from their blood by the end of the 3-week induction period). Adverse effects were seizures, hypomagnesemia, hypocalcemia, and elevated serum creatinine levels. A study comparing foscarnet with ganciclovir in the treatment of sight-threatening CMV retinitis was reported.[34] The two drugs were equivalently effective in treating retinitis. The mean time to progression of retinitis was approximately 56 days in both groups. The notable difference in the study was that patients treated with foscarnet had a 4-month longer survival time than those receiving ganciclovir. The explanation for the difference in survival time is not clear and does not seem entirely attributable to differences in the ability to take concurrent antiretroviral medications. However, this analysis was based on tabulating whether a patient had ever received any antiretroviral therapy [e.g., zidovudine, dideoxycytidine (ddC), or ddI] and did not assess the quantitative ability of patients to take these medications. Presumably, it was more difficult for the patient to be on concurrent zidovudine therapy while taking ganciclovir because of additive myelosuppression. Thus, whether the survival benefit of foscarnet was due to these other medications or was an inherent effect of foscarnet therapy itself remains unclear. Now that cytokines (e.g., granulocyte-macrophage colony stimulating factor and G-CSF) and other antiretrovirals (ddI, ddC) without extreme myelosuppressive toxicity are available, it should be possible for patients to continue receiving antiretroviral medications while taking ganciclovir.

GANCICLOVIR AND FOSCARNET. The results of a Studies of Ocular Complications of AIDS trial of combination therapy versus monotherapy for relapsed CMV retinitis were published in early 1996.[71] Combination therapy (5 mg/kg/day ganciclovir–90 mg/kg/day foscarnet) was significantly superior in delaying progression to either ganciclovir alone (10 mg/day) or foscarnet alone (120 mg/kg/day). This study also showed no advantage in switching monotherapy. That is, patients who failed monotherapy with ganciclovir and then switched to high-dose foscarnet did not do better than patients who continued ganciclovir at the higher dose. The median times to progression were: foscarnet group, 1.3 months; ganciclovir group, 2.0 months; and combination group, 4.3 months ($p < 0.001$). Side effects were not statistically significantly different in any group, but the quality of life was least in the combination group as a result of the prolonged daily infusion time of 3.1 hours.

Prevention

Ganciclovir

The oral form of ganciclovir is currently the only agent approved by the Food and Drug Administration (FDA) for prevention of CMV disease in patients with advanced HIV infection. The approval was based on a placebo-controlled study of 725 patients known to be CMV sero- or culture positive, the majority of whom had CD4 lymphocyte cell counts under $50/mm^3$. Ganciclovir taken prophylactically as 1000 mg orally three times daily decreased the cumulative risk of developing CMV disease over 12 months from 26% to 14% (an overall risk reduction of nearly 50%). Ganciclovir also effectively decreased and suppressed CMV excretion throughout the treatment period as measured by prevalence of CMV-positive urine cultures.

HERPES SIMPLEX VIRUS

Herpes simplex viruses types 1 and 2 (HSV-1, HSV-2) cause disease in both normal and immunocompromised hosts and are responsible for substantial morbidity in patients with AIDS. Most adult patients with AIDS have been infected with one or both HSV types before the development of AIDS. Although these individuals are not susceptible to primary HSV infection following new exposure, they remain at risk for disease because of reactivation of previously latent HSV infection. Viral latency occurs in nerve root ganglia that correspond to the site of initial mucocutaneous infection. Latent HSV often reactivates in the immunosuppressed population and can cause severe recurrent HSV disease, with extensive tissue destruction and prolonged viral shedding in patients with AIDS. The prevalence of HSV infection in homosexual AIDS patients exceeds that of the general population and likely reflects the common risk factor for transmission of both HSV and HIV (sexual contact). Serologic studies have revealed that up to 77% of HIV-infected patients have been previously infected with HSV, allowing for viral reactivation and clinical illness later in life.[57,65] AIDS subgroups who did not acquire HIV infection through sexual contact, such as hemophiliacs and transfusion recipients, would be expected to have lower rates of latent HSV infection.

Clinical Presentation

Because most HIV-infected patients have been infected with HSV before acquiring HIV, recurrent HSV is much more common than primary HSV infection. HSV infection in AIDS patients is often atypical compared to infection in the normal host. The severity of the illness depends on several factors, including the anatomic site of initial infection, the degree of immunosuppression, and whether the clinical episode represents initial-primary infection (no previous exposure to either HSV type), initial-nonprimary infection (previous exposure to the heterologous HSV type), or recurrent infection.

Localized mucocutaneous ulcerative lesions, without visceral or cutaneous dissemination, are the most frequent presentation of HSV infection in HIV-infected patients and may actually result in the initial diagnosis of AIDS. In an individual with no other cause of underlying immunodeficiency or who has laboratory evidence of HIV infection, ulcerative HSV infection present for longer than 1 month is diagnostic of AIDS.

Orolabial Infection

Orolabial infection in adults with AIDS is usually due to recurrent disease from previously latent infection. Primary orolabial HSV infection is more likely to occur in children with AIDS, however, because HIV infection in these patients may precede initial exposure to HSV.

The incubation period of primary HSV infection ranges between 2 and 12 days. In the normal host, primary orolabial infection may be asymptomatic or result in a gingivostomatitis.[13,49,68] Immunocompromised patients apparently are at greater risk than normal hosts of developing a severe clinical illness during primary HSV-1 infection, with a painful vesicular eruption occurring along the lip, tongue, pharynx, or buccal mucosa. The vesicles rapidly coalesce and rupture to form large ulcers covered by a whitish yellow necrotic film.[68,70] Fever, pharyngitis, and cervical lymphadenopathy frequently are present in adults, whereas infants may display poor feeding and persistent drooling.

Orolabial recurrences of HSV (fever blisters) in AIDS patients may increase in frequency and severity as immunosuppression increases. Alternatively, some AIDS patients will have only infrequent, mild, self-limiting recurrences throughout their disease.[53] Prodromal symptoms, consisting of tingling or numbness at the site of the impending recurrence, may be present from 12 to 24 hours before the onset of an HSV recurrence.

In the normal host, orolabial herpes lesions usually heal in 7 to 10 days. By comparison, AIDS patients often have a prolonged illness with markedly delayed lesion healing. If left untreated, chronic ulcerative lesions with persistent viral shedding may occur for several weeks.[70]

Genital Infection

After a 2- to 12-day incubation period, local symptoms develop in the majority of individuals with primary genital herpes.[11] Small papules appear initially and rapidly evolve into fluid-filled vesicles, which are usually painful and tender to palpation. The vesicles ulcerate rapidly and, in the normal host, heal in 3 to 4 weeks by crusting and by reepithelialization. Tender inguinal adenopathy is common, and dysuria may be present even if the urethra is not infected. Systemic symptoms, such as fever, headache, myalgias, malaise, and meningismus, also may occur during primary infection.[11]

In the normal host, recurrent genital herpes is less severe than primary infection. Compared with primary infection, recurrent herpes typically results in fewer external lesions, a shorter duration of illness, and the absence of systemic symptoms.[11,12] In AIDS patients, however, the severity and duration of recurrent genital herpes may be greater than that seen in normal hosts. Prolonged new lesion formation, with continued tissue destruction, persistent virus shedding, and severe local pain, is common. As with orolabial herpes, the frequency and severity of genital recurrences may increase with increasing immunosuppression, with symptoms lasting for several weeks.[80]

Asymptomatic genital shedding of HSV has been documented on 1% to 6% of the days on which cultures were obtained in nonimmunocompromised patients.[42] HIV-infected patients who are also infected with HSV would be expected to shed HSV at similar or even higher rates. All HSV-infected individuals (whether HIV infected or not) should be counseled about the possibility of asymptomatic HSV shedding and the possible risk of transmission of virus despite the absence of symptoms or visible lesions.

Anorectal Infection

Chronic perianal herpes was among the first reported opportunistic infections associated with AIDS. HSV is the most frequent cause of nongonococcal proctitis in sexually active homosexual men.[30,66] HSV proctitis usually results from primary HSV-2 infection but may also occur as a result of HSV-1 infection or recurrent disease caused by either viral type. Severe anorectal pain, perianal ulcerations, constipation, tenesmus, and neurologic symptoms in the distribution of the sacral plexus (sacral radiculopathy, impotence, and neurogenic bladder) are common findings of HSV proctitis and help differentiate it from proctitis resulting from other causes[30] (Fig. 26–4). Anorectal or sigmoidoscopic examination in patients with HSV proctitis typically reveals a friable mucosa, diffuse ulcerations, and occasional intact vesicular or pustular lesions.[30]

Recurrent perianal lesions caused by HSV in the absence of true proctitis are a common finding in patients with AIDS. Local pain, tenderness, itching, and pain on defecation are prominent symptoms of these lesions. Shallow ulcers in the perianal region are often visible on external examination, and ulcerative lesions frequently coalesce and extend along the gluteal crease to involve the area overlying the sacrum. These lesions often are atypical in appearance

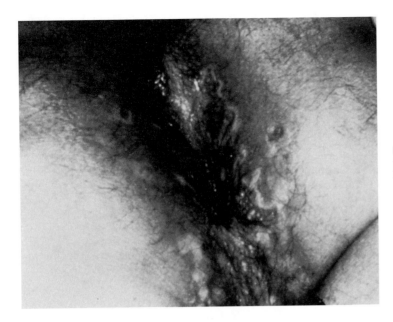

FIGURE 26-4. Perianal ulcerations typical of herpes simplex. (Courtesy of Dr. K. Erlich, Daly City, California.)

and may be confused with pressure decubiti (Color Plate II*F*). To prevent misdiagnosis, all perianal ulcerations and anal fissures in patients with AIDS should be examined for the presence of HSV by culture or direct antigen detection.

Esophagitis

Symptoms of HSV esophagitis typically include retrosternal pain and odynophagia (Chapter 13). Dysphagia may be of acute onset or chronic and may be severe enough to interfere with eating. Herpetic lesions in the oropharynx may not be present, and the clinical picture is often confused with *Candida* or CMV esophagitis. Radiographic contrast studies typically reveal a cobblestone appearance of the esophageal mucosa, although this finding is also present with esophagitis from other causes (Fig. 26-5). Definitive diagnosis of HSV esophagitis should be made by direct endoscopic visualization of the esophageal mucosa with positive viral studies and histopathologic evidence of invasive viral infection.

Encephalitis

HSV encephalitis occurs rarely in AIDS but is the most life-threatening complication of HSV infection (Chapter 14). Both HSV-1 and HSV-2 have been identified in brain tissue of AIDS patients, and simultaneous brain infections with HSV and CMV have been reported.[15,17] In adults with AIDS, HSV encephalitis usually occurs as a complication of primary or reactivated

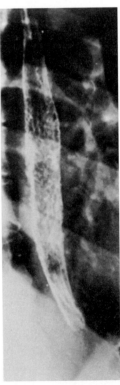

FIGURE 26-5. Barium esophagram revealing a cobblestone appearance of the esophageal mucosa. These findings are typical in both HSV esophagitis and *Candida* esophagitis. (Reprinted with permission from Farthing CF, Brown SE, Staughton RCD: A Colour Atlas of AIDS and HIV Disease Slide Set, ed 2. London, Mosby-Year Book/Wolfe, 1989.)

orolabial HSV infection. In neonates, the disease may occur as a result of primary HSV infection at the time of birth.[13]

The presentation of HSV encephalitis in adults with AIDS is often highly atypical. A subacute illness with subtle neurologic abnormalities is common in AIDS patients with HSV encephalitis, suggesting that host immune responses contribute to the clinical manifestations of the disease.[15,17] Headache, meningismus, and personality changes may develop gradually as the illness progresses. Alternatively, however, in some AIDS patients the onset of encephalitis as a result of HSV infection is acute. Abrupt onset of fever, headache, nausea, lethargy, and confusion may occur with temporal lobe abnormalities, cranial nerve defects, and focal seizures. Grand mal seizures, obtundation, coma, and death may eventually ensue.

The clinical diagnosis of HSV encephalitis may be extremely difficult because other central nervous system (CNS) infections (including HIV encephalopathy, *Cryptococcus neoformans,* and *Toxoplasma gondii*) may occur in an identical fashion. CSF usually reveals nonspecific findings, with elevated protein and a lymphocytic pleocytosis. Viral CSF cultures are usually negative.[50] Noninvasive diagnostic studies (such as computed tomography scan, radionuclide brain scan, or electroencephalography) are rarely diagnostic but may reveal localized abnormalities (often in the temporal lobes) to guide diagnostic brain biopsy. Definitive diagnosis may require brain biopsy and the recovery of virus or demonstration of viral antigens from tissue specimens.[50] The histopathologic abnormalities typically observed in normal hosts (hemorrhagic cortical necrosis and lymphocytic infiltration) may be absent in AIDS patients.[15,17] Recent studies have demonstrated the utility of detecting HSV DNA in CSF by the polymerase chain reaction technique as a method of noninvasive diagnosis of HSV encephalitis, although false-positive and false-negative results do occur.[43,44] AIDS patients with suspected HSV encephalitis should be treated with intravenous acyclovir pending results of diagnostic studies.

Acyclovir-Resistant HSV Infection

Since the initial description of acyclovir-resistant HSV infection in patients with AIDS, numerous additional reports have appeared in the literature.[22,24,25,46,59] The incidence of acyclovir-resistant HSV infections in immunocompromised hosts has been estimated as 4%

to 5%,[22] but the exact incidence of this problem in the AIDS population has not been determined. Most acyclovir-resistant HSV strains isolated from patients with AIDS have been deficient in the enzyme thymidine kinase. These mutated strains do not phosphorylate acyclovir to the active antiviral compound and are resistant to standard dosages of acyclovir. Although these thymidine kinase–deficient strains do not result in clinical disease in nonimmunocompromised hosts and have reduced virulence in animal models, they remain capable of causing severe clinical illness in patients with AIDS.[25] Most reports of acyclovir-resistant HSV have cited localized chronic mucocutaneous infection, but cases of disseminated mucocutaneous disease,[46] meningoencephalitis,[28] and esophagitis[22] caused by these strains have been described.

Treatment

Acyclovir

The prompt administration of antiviral chemotherapy to AIDS patients with acute HSV infection reduces morbidity and the risk of serious complications. Acyclovir, the antiviral agent of choice for most HSV infections in AIDS patients, can be administered orally,[18,64,69,74] intravenously,[75,79] or topically.[80] The optimum route of administration, dosage, and duration of acyclovir therapy often depend on the site and severity of the acute HSV infection.

Acyclovir has a high therapeutic ratio because it undergoes selective phosphorylation by virus-induced thymidine kinase in HSV-infected cells. Acyclovir triphosphate acts by selective inhibition of viral DNA polymerase and early termination of DNA-chain synthesis. The drug has slightly higher activity against HSV-1 than HSV-2. Acyclovir distributes into all tissues, including the brain and CSF, and is cleared by renal mechanisms. The serum half-life in patients with normal renal function is 2 to 3 hours, and the intravenous dose should be reduced in patients with impaired renal function (Table 26–4).[45]

Foscarnet

Phosphonoformic acid (PFA, foscarnet, Foscavir), a pyrophosphate, has been approved by the FDA as a treatment for CMV disease and acyclovir-resistant HSV infection. Unlike acyclovir, foscarnet does not require viral en-

TABLE 26–4. DOSAGE ADJUSTMENT OF INTRAVENOUS ACYCLOVIR IN PATIENTS WITH RENAL DYSFUNCTION

Creatinine Clearance (ml/min/1.73 m²)	Percent of Standard Dose*	Dosing Interval (hours)
>50	100	8
25–50	100	12
10–25	100	24
0–10	50	24

* Usually 5 mg/kg; 10 mg/kg is used for HSV central nervous system infections and in some instances for VZV infection.

zyme-mediated phosphorylation for activity. Hence, it remains an effective antiviral agent for treatment of acyclovir-resistant, thymidine kinase–deficient strains of HSV.[24,58,59] Foscarnet is superior to vidarabine in the treatment of acyclovir-resistant HSV infections in AIDS and is the treatment of choice for this illness.[59]

Other Antiviral Drugs

Two newer antiviral drugs, famciclovir and valacyclovir, have been approved by the FDA for treatment of recurrent HSV infection in the nonimmunocompromised host. Although these agents have more favorable bioavailability and pharmacokinetics than acyclovir, they have not been shown to be superior to acyclovir in clinical trials and are not approved for use in the immunocompromised host. Studies are currently in progress to determine whether these drugs are safe and effective in patients with AIDS.

Management of HSV Infection (Table 26–5)

The treatment of choice for most cases of HSV infections in AIDS is systemic acyclovir.

TABLE 26–5. MANAGEMENT OF HSV INFECTIONS IN AIDS

Clinical Presentation	Treatment
Mucocutaneous infection, mild	Acyclovir, 200 mg PO five times daily
Mucocutaneous infection, severe	Acyclovir, 15 mg/kg/day IV
Visceral organ infection	Acyclovir, 30 mg/kg/day IV
Recurrent mucocutaneous infection	Acyclovir, 200–400 mg tid or qid
Severe infection caused by acyclovir-resistant HSV	Foscarnet, 40 mg/kg IV tid

Modified with permission from Drew WL: The medical management of AIDS. Infect Dis Clin North Am 2:505, 1988.

Most AIDS patients with primary or recurrent mucocutaneous HSV infections are not ill enough to require hospitalization and are suitable for outpatient treatment. The usual dose of acyclovir for outpatient therapy is 200 mg five times daily, or 400 mg three times daily. Therapy can be started while awaiting results of viral culture (if the clinical suspicion is high) or when the diagnosis has been confirmed by the appropriate laboratory techniques.[64] Oral acyclovir should be continued until all external lesions are crusted.

Intravenous acyclovir should be reserved for patients with severe or extensive mucocutaneous HSV infection and for patients with viral dissemination, visceral organ infection (e.g., brain, esophagus, eye), or neurologic complications (atonic bladder, transverse myelitis). Treatment with intravenous acyclovir also may be indicated for AIDS patients who require specific antiviral chemotherapy but are unable to tolerate or absorb oral acyclovir because of nausea, dysphagia, or protracted diarrhea. The dose of intravenous acyclovir for patients with mucocutaneous HSV infection and normal renal function is 15 mg/kg/day in three divided doses.[75] Patients with life-threatening HSV infection (encephalitis, neonatal infection, disseminated infection) or visceral organ involvement (esophagitis, proctitis) should probably receive a higher dose—usually 30 mg/kg/day in three divided doses.[79] Treatment should last for a minimum of 10 days, but longer therapy in AIDS patients may be necessary. As noted, the intravenous dose should be adjusted in patients with impaired renal function (Table 26–4). If prolonged therapy is required, oral acyclovir can be substituted for intravenous therapy when the patient is ready for hospital discharge.

Topical acyclovir is less effective than either oral or intravenous therapy and has little, if any, usefulness in the clinical setting. Although topical acyclovir decreases the duration of viral shedding in compromised hosts with mucocutaneous HSV infection, it does not reduce new lesion formation or the risk of dissemination.[80] There is no apparent added benefit to the combination of topical acyclovir with either oral or intravenous acyclovir.[41]

Treatment with acyclovir should be continued until all mucocutaneous lesions have crusted or reepithelialized. Lesions may heal slowly in AIDS patients even with optimum antiviral chemotherapy. If lesions do not heal while the patient is receiving acyclovir, repeat viral cultures should be obtained, high-dose intravenous therapy (30 mg/kg/day) should be given, and acyclovir-resistant HSV infection should be considered as a possible diagnosis. If available, antiviral susceptibility testing should be performed to determine whether acyclovir-resistant HSV infection is present. If antiviral testing is not available, patients who continue to have positive cultures for HSV and no evidence of clinical response despite high-dose systemic acyclovir therapy should be treated presumptively for acyclovir-resistant infection with intravenous foscarnet.

Suppressive Acyclovir Therapy for HSV Infection

Many AIDS patients suffer from frequently recurring HSV infection or develop new HSV recurrences shortly after antiviral chemotherapy is discontinued. These patients often can be managed with suppressive acyclovir therapy.[18,69,74] AIDS patients requiring suppressive therapy should be treated initially with oral acyclovir, 200 mg tid or 400 mg bid. Increase of the daily dosage up to 400 mg qid may be necessary to control recurrences, but gastrointestinal intolerance to the drug may limit the amount that can be taken. Breakthrough recurrences that develop while the patient is receiving suppressive acyclovir therapy may be controlled by increasing the daily suppressive dose. Breakthrough recurrences may or may not represent the emergence of acyclovir-resistant strains.[51] Patients who demonstrate a good response to suppressive oral acyclovir at high doses may attempt a reduction in the daily suppressive dose. Although suppressive acyclovir therapy is approved for no longer than 12 months, patients have received daily acyclovir for up to 7 years with no evidence of adverse reactions or cumulative toxicity.[39] Studies have shown that the incidence of asymptomatic virus shedding is decreased while a patient is on acyclovir suppression.[76] Individuals maintained on long-term suppressive therapy should be cautioned, however, that recurrences likely will develop after discontinuation of therapy and that the first recurrence may be more severe than those previously experienced.[18,69,74] Many HIV-positive patients receiving acyclovir may also be taking zidovudine or other antiretroviral agents. There is no conclusive evidence that the combination of these drugs and acyclovir results in synergistic activity against HIV.

Management of Acyclovir-Resistant HSV Infection

With the increased incidence of acyclovir-resistant HSV infections observed in patients with AIDS, several studies have examined the utility of alternate antiviral agents and treatment regimens. Standard doses of intravenous or oral acyclovir have no clinical benefit if the HSV isolate is resistant to acyclovir ($ID_{50} > 3.0$ μg/ml) in vitro. Most acyclovir-resistant strains isolated from patients with AIDS have been thymidine kinase deficient and have remained susceptible in vitro to vidarabine, which is phosphorylated without thymidine kinase, and foscarnet, which does not require phosphorylation for activity. Studies have confirmed, however, that foscarnet is superior to vidarabine in the treatment of acyclovir-resistant HSV infection in AIDS and is the treatment of choice for this disease.[24,59] The dosage of foscarnet used for the treatment of acyclovir-resistant HSV infections in AIDS patients is 40 mg/kg every 8 hours (with reduction in dose for renal dysfunction).

Continuous infusion acyclovir therapy has been effective in a few AIDS patients with severe acyclovir-resistant HSV infection. Acyclovir has been administered at a dosage of 1.5 to 2.0 mg/kg/hour for 6 weeks, and complete resolution of acyclovir-resistant HSV proctitis has been observed.[21] This approach must be viewed as investigational, however, and cannot be recommended for routine use. Other investigational agents under study for treatment of mucocutaneous acyclovir-resistant HSV infections include topical trifluridine, cidofovir, and cyclobut.[46]

As with many opportunistic infections in AIDS patients, there is a high incidence of recurrent HSV disease after successful treatment for acyclovir-resistant HSV. Some (but not all) relapses in this setting have been due to acyclovir-resistant strains, suggesting that these mutant viruses are capable of causing latency in the immunocompromised host. Chronic prophylaxis with daily acyclovir, 200 to 400 mg PO tid, or foscarnet, 40 mg/kg/day intravenously can be considered in patients who are treated successfully for acyclovir-resistant HSV, although there are no data to confirm efficacy in this setting. Foscarnet-resistant strains of HSV have recently been reported.[60]

VARICELLA-ZOSTER VIRUS

Primary VZV infection is usually a childhood illness, with attack rates exceeding 90% in susceptible household contacts.[77] Most adults with AIDS have been previously infected with VZV and (as with HSV) are not susceptible to primary infection.

AIDS patients develop recurrent VZV infection (zoster) more frequently than do age-matched immunocompetent hosts. A retrospective review of 300 AIDS patients with Kaposi's sarcoma revealed that 8% of patients had at least one prior attack of zoster, an incidence seven times greater than expected by the age of the study group. Zoster also occurs with a higher-than-expected frequency in HIV-infected individuals who appear otherwise healthy. Additionally, some HIV-infected patients develop more than one episode of zoster in a relatively short period of time, an uncommon occurrence in immunocompetent hosts.[9,10,27]

Primary Infection—Varicella

Varicella in immunocompetent children is usually a benign illness. Adults, however, are more likely to develop complications during primary VZV infection. Viral dissemination to visceral organs occurs in up to one third of immunocompetent adults with primary infection.[77] Although most adults with AIDS have been previously infected with VZV and are not susceptible to primary infection,[55] for those who are, a protracted and potentially life-threatening illness could follow.

Recurrent Infection—Zoster

Unlike primary VZV infection, recurrent VZV infection (zoster) is common in patients with AIDS. The illness usually begins with radicular pain and is followed by localized or segmental erythematous rash covering one to three dermatomes. Maculopapules develop in the dermatomal area, and the patient experiences increasing pain. The maculopapules progress to fluid-filled vesicles, and contiguous vesicles may become confluent, with true bullae formation. In many HIV-infected patients, the lesions remain confined in a dermatomal distribution and heal by crusting and reepithelialization.[9,10,27] Occasionally, however, widespread cutaneous or visceral dissemination may occur.[56] Extensive cutaneous dissemination may appear identical to primary varicella. Visceral dissemination to lung, liver, or the CNS may produce a life-threatening illness.

Reactivated infection involving the ophthalmic division of the trigeminal nerve often results in infection of the cornea (zoster ophthalmicus). The presence of vesicles on the tip of the nose often is associated with involvement of the eye. Although healing without sequelae may occur, untreated patients often develop anterior uveitis, corneal scarring, and permanent visual loss.[9] Acyclovir-resistant zoster is rare but often has a peculiar dermatomal wart-like, nonhealing appearance.

Complications

Complications of VZV infection are common in immunocompromised patients and may cause prolonged morbidity and death. Dissemination of virus to the lung, liver, and CNS has been associated with a mortality rate of 6% to 17%.

Varicella pneumonia may occur during primary VZV infection or during reactivated infection with visceral dissemination in immunocompromised patients. Symptoms are variable. Many patients develop only mild respiratory symptoms, whereas others suffer from severe hypoxemia and succumb to respiratory failure. Radiographic abnormalities are usually out of proportion to the clinical findings, with diffuse nodular densities on chest radiograph and occasional pleural effusions.

Encephalitis is a rare complication of VZV infection in AIDS patients but may occur with or without visceral dissemination (Chapter 14). The illness begins 3 to 8 days after the onset of varicella or 1 to 2 weeks after the development of zoster, but occasionally AIDS patients have developed progressive neurologic disease caused by VZV up to 3 months after the onset of localized zoster.[56] Headache, vomiting, lethargy, and cerebellar symptoms (ataxia, tremors, dizziness) are prominent findings. Diagnosis based on clinical criteria alone can be difficult, because other CNS infections can present in a similar fashion. The diagnosis of VZV encephalitis is documented by finding VZV antibody in CSF. Postherpetic neuralgia, defined as prolonged pain following resolution of the cutaneous lesions from zoster, can be severe and disabling.[33,77] Although postherpetic neuralgia is a more common occurrence in elderly individuals with zoster, AIDS patients also may be at risk for this complication. Polyradiculopathy similar to that caused by CMV may rarely be due to VZV. In these cases VZV may be isolated from CSF.

TABLE 26–6. MANAGEMENT OF VZV INFECTIONS IN AIDS

Clinical Presentation	Treatment
Primary infection (varicella)	Acyclovir, 30 mg/kg/day IV, or acyclovir, 600–800 mg PO five times daily
Recurrent infection (localized zoster)	Acyclovir, 30 mg/kg/day IV, or acyclovir, 600–800 mg PO five times daily
Recurrent infection, disseminated	Acyclovir, 30 mg/kg/day IV
Severe infection caused by acyclovir-resistant VZV	Foscarnet, 40 mg/kg tid IV (not FDA approved)

Modified with permission from Drew WL: The medical management of AIDS. Infect Dis Clin North Am 2:507, 1988.

Management of VZV Infection (Table 26–6)

Oral acyclovir in the dosage used to treat herpes simplex infection (200 mg five times daily) does not result in serum drug levels adequate to inhibit VZV in tissue culture.[45] Higher doses of oral acyclovir (800 mg five times daily) have been approved by the FDA for the treatment of VZV infections.[32,33] This dose produces serum drug levels that inhibit the growth of VZV in vitro. Although somewhat effective in the treatment of VZV infections, this higher dose regimen may be poorly tolerated in some AIDS patients because of gastrointestinal side effects.

Management of primary or recurrent VZV infection in AIDS patients may require hospitalization and intravenous acyclovir therapy. Many AIDS patients with localized zoster will not be ill enough to require hospitalization, and the decision whether to hospitalize an individual patient must be based on several factors, including the severity of the infection, the immune status of the host, and whether visceral or cutaneous dissemination has occurred.

Immunocompromised hosts with primary or recurrent VZV infection treated with intravenous acyclovir have a reduction in the duration of viral shedding, new lesion formation, incidence of dissemination, and mortality rate.[2,63] All AIDS patients with disseminated VZV infec-tion, either cutaneous or visceral, should be hospitalized and treated initially with intravenous acyclovir, 30 mg/kg/day in three divided doses (with dosage adjustments for renal dysfunction; Table 26–4). Treatment should be continued for at least 7 days or until all external lesions are crusted. Oral acyclovir (800 mg five times daily) may be used for treatment of localized zoster in AIDS patients who do not require hospitalization and may prevent visceral or cutaneous dissemination. Additionally, oral acyclovir has been shown to modestly decrease the incidence and severity of postherpetic neuralgia in nonimmunocompromised hosts.[32,33] Famciclovir and valacyclovir are useful in the management of zoster in the nonimmunocompromised host because they reduce the duration of postherpetic pain.[3,73] These drugs have not been approved by the FDA for treatment of AIDS patients, however, and should not be used in this population until additional efficacy and safety data are available.

Treatment of Acyclovir-Resistant VZV Infection

Acyclovir-resistant VZV has been identified in patients with AIDS. All strains have been isolated from patients previously treated with acyclovir for recurrent VZV or HSV infection.[35] Foscarnet is clinically useful in this setting[58] but remains investigational for this purpose.

Prevention of VZV Infection

Varicella-zoster immune globulin is effective in preventing severe primary VZV infection in a susceptible (i.e., seronegative) immunocompromised host if administered within 96 hours from the time of a significant exposure. The attenuated, live vaccine has recently been licensed in the United States for nonimmunocompromised hosts.[29,78] Efficacy and safety in AIDS patients have not been reported.

SUMMARY

Herpesvirus (CMV, HSV, VZV) infections are common in AIDS patients and often exist in a chronic or progressive form. Oral ganciclovir prophylaxis can reduce the risk of developing CMV disease. CMV retinitis occurs in up to 40% of AIDS patients and can be treated effectively with ganciclovir or foscarnet. Perianal ulcers, proctitis, and other clinical syndromes caused by HSV can be treated effectively with acyclovir, which, administered daily, can prevent HSV recurrence. Herpes zoster in a young adult may be the first indication of immune deficiency resulting from HIV. Because VZV is less susceptible to acyclovir than is HSV, intravenous acyclovir or high-dose oral therapy is required to achieve inhibitory blood levels. Herpesviruses resistant to acyclovir are usually susceptible to foscarnet.

Note Added in Proof

Cidofovir (HPMPC)

In June 1996, Cidofovir, or HPMPC, was approved by the FDA for the treatment of CMV retinitis. This drug is a departure from previous nucleoside analogues since it appears to the cell as a nucleo*tide*. It has a phosphonate moiety attached to a cytosine analogue and does not require phosphorylation by virus induced enzyme. It is therefore active against the majority of ganciclovir resistant viruses which have resistance mutations in the UL97 or phosphorylating gene. The drug also has a extremely long half-life permitting it to be administered as infrequently as every 2 weeks during maintenance treatment (See Lalezari JP, Drew WL, Glutzer E, et al: (*S*)-1-[3-hydroxy-2-(phosphonylmethoxy)propyl]cytosine (Cidofovir): Results of a Phase I/II study of a novel antiviral nucleotide analogue. J Infect Dis 171:788–796, 1995, references 1–27.) Cidofovir is nephrotoxic, especially to the proximal renal tubule but this can apparently be diminished by prehydration and concomitant probenecid therapy. Renal function and toxicity must be monitored carefully and proteinuria or a rising creatinine are reasons for dosage reduction, interruption, or discontinuation. Despite its potential for toxicity, the drug is effective and convenient and it will find an important niche in anti-CMV therapy.

REFERENCES

1. Anand R, Nightingale D, Fish RH, et al: Control of cytomegalovirus retinitis using sustained release of intraocular ganciclovir. Arch Ophthalmol 111:223–227, 1993
2. Balfour HH, Bean B, Laskin OL, et al: Acyclovir halts progression of herpes zoster in immunocompromised patients. N Engl J Med 308:1448–1453, 1983
3. Beutner KR, Friedman DJ, Forszpaniak C, et al: Valaciclovir compared with acyclovir for improved therapy for herpes zoster in immunocompetent adults. Antimicrob Agents Chemother 39:1546–1553, 1995
4. Brock BV, Selke S, Benedetti J, et al: Frequency of asymptomatic shedding of herpes simplex virus in women with genital herpes. JAMA 263:418–420, 1990
5. Buhles WC Jr, Mastre BJ, Tinker AJ, et al: Ganciclovir treatment of life- or sight-threatening cytomegalovirus infection: Experience in 314 immunocompromised patients. Rev Infect Dis 10(suppl 3):S495–S504, 1988
6. Cantrill HL, Henry K, Melroe H, et al: Treatment of cytomegalovirus retinitis with intravitreal ganciclovir: Long-term results. Ophthalmology 96:367–374, 1989
7. Chatis PA, Miller CH, Schrager LE, Crumpacker CS: Successful treatment with foscarnet of an acyclovir-resistant mucocutaneous infection with herpes simplex virus in a patient with acquired immunodeficiency syndrome. N Engl J Med 320:297–300, 1989
8. Chrisp, Clissold SP: Foscarnet: A review of its antiviral activity, pharmacokinetic properties and therapeutic use in immunocompromised patients with cytomegalovirus retinitis. Drugs 41:104–109, 1991
9. Cole EL, Meisler DM, Calabrese LH, et al: Herpes zoster ophthalmicus and acquired immune deficiency syndrome. Arch Ophthalmol 102:1027–1029, 1984
10. Cone LA, Schiffman HA: Herpes zoster and the acquired immunodeficiency syndrome (Letter). Ann Intern Med 100:462, 1984
11. Corey L, Adams HG, Brown ZA, et al: Genital herpes simplex virus infections: Clinical manifestations, course, and complications. Ann Intern Med 98:958–972, 1983
12. Corey L, Homes KK: Genital herpes simplex virus infections: Current concepts in diagnosis, therapy, and prevention. Ann Intern Med 98:973–983, 1983
13. Corey L, Spear PG: Infections with herpes simplex viruses (parts 1 and 2). N Engl J Med 314:686–691, 749–757, 1986
14. Dieterich DT, Kotler DP, Busch DF: Ganciclovir treatment of cytomegalovirus colitis in AIDS: A randomized, double-blind, placebo-controlled multicenter study. J Infect Dis 167:278–282, 1993
15. Dix RD, Bredesen DE, Davis RL, Mills J: Herpesvirus neurological diseases associated with AIDS: Recovery of viruses from central nervous system (CNS) tissues, peripheral nerve, and cerebrospinal fluid (CSF) (Abstract 43). Program of the International Conference on AIDS, Atlanta, 1985
16. Dix RD, Bredesen DE, Erlich KS, et al: Recovery of herpes-viruses from cerebrospinal fluid of immunodeficient homosexual men. Ann Neurol 18:611–614, 1985
17. Dix RD, Waitzman DM, Follansbee S, et al: Herpes simplex virus type 2 encephalitis in two homosexual men with persistent adenopathy. Ann Neurol 17:203–206, 1985
18. Douglas JM, Critchlow C, Benedetti J, et al: Double

blind study of oral acyclovir for suppression of recurrences of genital herpes simplex virus infection. N Engl J Med 310:1551–1556, 1984

19. Drew WL, Miner RC, Busch DF, et al: Prevalence of resistance in patients receiving ganciclovir for serious cytomegalovirus infection. J Infect Dis 163:716–719, 1991

20. Emanuel D, Cunningham I, Jules-Elysee K, et al: Cytomegalovirus pneumonia after bone-marrow transplantation successfully treated with the combination of ganciclovir and high-dose intravenous immune globulin. Ann Intern Med 109:777–782, 1988

21. Engel JP, Englund JA, Fletcher CV, Hill EL: Treatment of resistant herpes simplex virus with continuous-infusion acyclovir. JAMA 263:1662–1664, 1990

22. Englund JA, Zimmerman ME, Swierkosz EM, et al: Herpes simplex virus resistant to acyclovir: A study in a tertiary care center. Ann Intern Med 112:416–422, 1990

23. Erice A, Chou S, Biron K, et al: Ganciclovir (GCV) resistant strains of cytomegalovirus (CMV) in GCV-treated patients with AIDS (Abstract 7190). Program of the 4th International Conference on AIDS, Stockholm, 1988

24. Erlich KS, Jacobson MA, Koehler JE, et al: Foscarnet therapy for severe acyclovir-resistant herpes simplex virus type-2 infections in patients with the acquired immunodeficiency syndrome (AIDS): An uncontrolled trial. Ann Intern Med 110:710–713, 1989

25. Erlich KS, Mills J, Chatis P, et al: Acyclovir-resistant herpes simplex virus infections in patients with the acquired immunodeficiency syndrome. N Engl J Med 320:293–296, 1989

26. Felsenstein D, D'Amico DJ, Hirsch MS, et al: Treatment of cytomegalovirus retinitis with 9-[2-hydroxy-1-(hydroxy-methyl)ethoxymethyl] guanine. Ann Intern Med 103:377–380, 1985

27. Friedman-Kien AE, Lafleur FL, Gendler E, et al: Herpes zoster: A possible early clinical sign for development of acquired immunodeficiency syndrome in high-risk individuals. J Am Acad Dermatol 14:1023–1028, 1986

28. Gateley A, Gander RM, Johnson PC, et al: Herpes simplex type 2 meningoencephalitis resistant to acyclovir in a patient with AIDS. J Infect Dis 161:711–715, 1990

29. Gershon AA, Steinberg SP, LaRussa P, et al: Immunization of healthy adults with live attenuated varicella vaccine. J Infect Dis 158:132–137, 1988

30. Goodell SE, Quinn TC, Mkrtichian F, et al: Herpes simplex proctitis in homosexual men: Clinical, sigmoidoscopic, and histopathologic features. N Engl J Med 308:868–871, 1983

31. Hawley DA, Schaefer JF, Schulz DM, Muller J: Cytomegalovirus encephalitis in acquired immunodeficiency syndrome. Am J Clin Pathol 80:874–877, 1983

32. Huff JC, Bean B, Balfour HH, et al: Therapy of herpes zoster with oral acyclovir. Am J Med 85(suppl 2A):84–89, 1988

33. Huff JC, Drucker JL, Clemmer A, et al: Effect of oral acyclovir on pain resolution in herpes zoster: A reanalysis. J Med Virol 1(suppl):93–96, 1993

34. Jabs D, and the Studies of Ocular Complications of AIDS Research Group, in collaboration with the AIDS Clinical Trial Group: Mortality in patients with the acquired immunodeficiency syndrome

treated with either foscarnet or ganciclovir for cytomegalovirus retinitis. N Engl J Med 326:213–220, 1992

35. Jacobson MA, Berger TG, Fikrig S, et al: Acyclovir (ACV)-resistant varicella zoster virus (VZV) infection following chronic oral ACV therapy in patients with AIDS. Ann Intern Med 112:187–191, 1990

36. Jacobson MA, Causey D, Polsky B: A dose-ranging study of daily maintenance intravenous foscarnet therapy for cytomegalovirus retinitis in AIDS. J Infect Dis 168:444–448, 1993

37. Jacobson MA, Drew WL, Feinberg J, et al: Foscarnet therapy for ganciclovir-resistant cytomegalovirus retinitis in patients with AIDS. J Infec Dis 163:1348–1351, 1991

38. Kahlon J, Chatterjee S, Lakeman FD, et al: Detection of antibodies to herpes simplex virus in the cerebrospinal fluid of patients with herpes simplex encephalitis. J Infect Dis 155:38–44, 1987

39. Kaplowitz LG, Baker D, Gelb L, et al: Prolonged continuous acyclovir treatment of normal adults with frequently recurring genital herpes simplex virus infection. JAMA 265:747–751, 1991

40. Kim YS, Hollander H: Polyradiculopathy due to cytomegalovirus: Report on two cases in which improvement occurred after prolonged therapy and review of the literature. Clin Infect Dis 17:32–37, 1993

41. Kinghorn GR, Abeywickreme I, Jeavons M, et al: Efficacy of combined treatment with oral and topical acyclovir in first episode genital herpes. Genitourin Med 62:186–188, 1986

42. Koelle DM, Benedetti J, Langenberg A, Corey L: Asymptomatic reactivation of herpes simplex virus in women after the first episode of genital herpes. Ann Intern Med 116:433–437, 1992

43. Lakeman FD, Whitley RJ, and the National Institute of Allergy and Infectious Diseases Collaborative Antiviral Study Group: Diagnosis of herpes simplex encephalitis: Application of polymerase chain reaction to cerebrospinal fluid from brain-biopsied patients and correlation with disease. J Infect Dis 171:857–863, 1995

44. Landry ML: False-positive polymerase chain reaction results in the diagnosis of herpes simplex encephalitis. J Infect Dis 172:1641–1643, 1995

45. Laskin O: Acyclovir: Pharmacology and clinical experience. Arch Intern Med 144:1241–1246, 1984

46. Marks GL, Nolan PE, Erlich KS, Ellis MN: Mucocutaneous dissemination of acyclovir-resistant herpes simplex virus in a patient with AIDS. Rev Infect Dis 11:474–476, 1989

47. Martin DF, Parks DJ, Mellow D, et al: Treatment of cytomegalovirus retinitis with an intraocular sustained-release ganciclovir implant. Arch Ophthalmol 112:1531–1539, 1994

48. Miller RG, Storey JR, Greco CM: Ganciclovir in the treatment of progressive AIDS-related polyradiculopathy. Neurology 40:569–574, 1990

49. Nahmias AJ, Keyserling H, Lee FK: Herpes simplex viruses 1 and 2. In Evans A, ed. Viral Infections of Humans: Epidemiology and Control, ed. 3. New York, Plenum Press, 1989

50. Nahmias AJ, Whitley RD, Visintine AN, et al: Herpes simplex virus type 2 encephalitis: Laboratory evaluations and their diagnostic significance. J Infect Dis 146:829–836, 1982

51. Nusinoff-Lehrman S, Douglas JM, Corey L, et al: Recurrent genital herpes and suppressive oral

acyclovir therapy: Relation between clinical outcome and in-vitro sensitivity. Ann Intern Med 104: 786–790, 1986

52. Palestine AG, Polis MA, De Smet MD, et al: A randomized, controlled trial of foscarnet in the treatment of cytomegalovirus retinitis in patients with AIDS. Ann Intern Med 115:665–673, 1991

53. Quinnan GV, Masur H, Rook AH, et al: Herpes simplex infections in the acquired immune deficiency syndrome. JAMA 252:72–77, 1984

54. Reed EC, Bowden RA, Dandliker PS, et al: Treatment of cytomegalovirus pneumonia with ganciclovir and intravenous cytomegalovirus immunoglobulin in patients with bone marrow transplants. Ann Intern Med 109:783–788, 1988

55. Rogers MF, Morens DM, Stewart JA, et al: National case-control study of Kaposi's sarcoma and *Pneumocystis carinii* pneumonia in homosexual men: Part 2, Laboratory results. Ann Intern Med 99:151–158, 1983

56. Ryder JW, Croen K, Kleinschmidt-DeMasters BK, et al: Progressive encephalitis three months after resolution of cutaneous zoster in a patient with AIDS. Ann Neurol 19:182–188, 1986

57. Safrin S, Arvin A, Mills J, Ashley R: Comparison of the Western immunoblot assay and a glycoprotein G enzyme immunoassay for detection of serum antibodies to herpes simplex virus type 2 in patients with AIDS. J Clin Microbiol 30:1312–1314, 1992

58. Safrin S, Berger TG, Gilson I, et al: Foscarnet therapy in five patients with AIDS and acyclovir-resistant varicella-zoster virus infection. Ann Intern Med 115: 19–21, 1991

59. Safrin S, Crumpacker C, Chatis P, et al: A controlled trial comparing foscarnet with vidarabine for acyclovir-resistant mucocutaneous herpes simplex in the acquired immunodeficiency syndrome. N Engl J Med 325:551–555, 1991

60. Safrin S, Kemmerly S, Plotkin B, et al: Foscarnet-resistant herpes simplex virus infection in patients with AIDS. J Infect Dis 169:193–196, 1994

61. Sanborn GE, Anand R, Torti RE, et al: Sustained-release ganciclovir therapy for treatment of cytomegalovirus retinitis. Arch Ophthalmol 110:188–195, 1992

62. Shepp DH, Dandliker PS, de Miranda P, et al: Activity of 9-[2-hydroxy-1-(hydroxymethyl)ethoxymethyl] guanine in the treatment of cytomegalovirus pneumonia. Ann Intern Med 103:368–373, 1985

63. Shepp DH, Dandliker PS, Meyers JD: Treatment of varicella zoster virus infection in severely immunocompromised patients. N Engl J Med 314:208–212, 1986

64. Shepp DH, Newton BA, Dandliker PS, et al: Oral acyclovir therapy for mucocutaneous herpes simplex virus infections in immunocompromised marrow transplant recipients. Ann Intern Med 102: 783–785, 1985

65. Siegel D, Golden E, Washington E, et al: Prevalence and correlates of herpes simplex infections: The population-based AIDS in Multiethnic Neighborhoods study. JAMA 268:1702–1708, 1992

66. Siegel FP, Lopez C, Hammer BS, et al: Severe acquired immunodeficiency in male homosexuals, manifested by chronic perianal ulcerative herpes simplex lesions. N Engl J Med 305:1439–1444, 1981

67. Spector SA, Weingeist T, Pollard RB, et al: A randomized, controlled study of intravenous ganciclovir therapy for cytomegalovirus peripheral retinitis in patients with AIDS. J Infect Dis 168:557–563, 1993

68. Spruance SI, Overall JC, Kern ER, et al: The natural history of recurrent herpes simplex labialis: Implications for antiviral therapy. N Engl J Med 297: 68–75, 1977

69. Straus SE, Seidlin M, Takiff H, et al: Oral acyclovir to suppress recurring herpes simplex virus infections in immunodeficient patients. Ann Intern Med 100: 522–524, 1984

70. Straus SE, Smith HA, Brickman C, et al: Acyclovir for chronic mucocutaneous herpes simplex virus infection in immunosuppressed patients. Ann Intern Med 96:270–277, 1982

71. Studies of Ocular Complications of AIDS Research Group in Collaboration with the Clinical Trials Group: Combination foscarnet and ganciclovir therapy vs monotherapy for the treatment of relapsed cytomegalovirus retinitis in patients with AIDS: The cytomegalovirus Retreatment Trial. Arch Ophthalmol 114:23–33, 1996

72. Sullivan V, Taliarico CL, Stanat SC, et al: A protein kinase homologue controls phosphorylation of ganciclovir in human cytomegalovirus-infected cells. Nature 358:162–164, 1992

73. Tyring S, Barbarash RA, Nahlik JE, et al: Famciclovir for the treatment of acute herpes zoster: Effects on acute disease and postherpetic neuralgia. A randomized, double blind, placebo controlled trial. Ann Intern Med 123:89–96, 1995

74. Wade JC, Newton B, Flournoy N, et al: Oral acyclovir for prevention of herpes simplex virus reactivation after marrow transplantation. Ann Intern Med 100: 823–828, 1984

75. Wade JC, Newton B, McLaren C, et al: Intravenous acyclovir to treat mucocutaneous herpes simplex virus infection after marrow transplantation. Ann Intern Med 96:265–269, 1982

76. Wald A, Zeh J, Barnum G, et al: Suppression of subclinical shedding of herpes simplex virus type 2 with acyclovir. Ann Intern Med 124:8–15, 1996

77. Weller TH: Varicella and herpes zoster: Changing concepts of the natural history, control, and importance of a not-so-benign virus (parts 1 and 2). N Engl J Med 309:1362–1368, 1434–1440, 1983

78. White CJ, Kuter BJ, Hidebrand CS, et al: Varicella vaccine (VARIVAX) in healthy children and adolescents: Results from clinical trials, 1987 to 1989. Pediatrics 87:604–610, 1991

79. Whitley RJ, Alford CA, Hirsch MS, et al: Vidarabine versus acyclovir therapy in herpes simplex encephalitis. N Engl J Med 314:144–149, 1986

80. Whitley RJ, Levin M, Barton N, et al: Infections caused by herpes simplex virus in the immunocompromised host: Natural history and topical acyclovir therapy. J Infect Dis 150:323–329, 1984

81. Whitley RJ, Soong SJ, Dolin R, et al: Adenine arabinoside therapy of biopsy proved herpes simplex encephalitis: National Institute of Allergy and Infectious Diseases collaborative antiviral study. N Engl J Med 297:289–294, 1977

Management of Syphilis in HIV-Infected Persons

GAIL BOLAN

The management of syphilis in persons with coexisting human immunodeficiency virus (HIV) infection is a complex problem.[35–37,60, 61,65,84,85] Epidemiologic studies have demonstrated that a history of sexually transmitted diseases (STDs), including syphilis, is associated with an increased risk for HIV infection and the acquired immunodeficiency syndrome (AIDS) and that STDs causing genital ulceration may be cofactors for acquiring HIV infection.[11,25,42] More recently, isolated case reports have suggested that coexistent HIV infection may alter the natural history of syphilis or the dosage or duration of treatment required to cure syphilis.[5,13,23,43,54] Also, reports of false-negative and false-positive serologic test results for syphilis in HIV-infected persons raise questions about the sensitivity and specificity of serologic diagnostic tests in such patients.[1,26,34,69,81] Questions about the significance of cerebrospinal fluid (CSF) abnormalities in patients with early syphilis may assume greater importance in the presence of HIV infection.[35,36,53,59–61]

Because data from prospective controlled studies are not available to answer many of these questions, definitive recommendations for managing HIV-infected patients with syphilis are limited. Management options are presented here for clinicians to consider until more definitive recommendations can be made. Options to consider in treating HIV-infected patients include (1) evaluating CSF for evidence of neurosyphilis earlier in the course of infection; (2) treating patients with penicillin regimens of longer duration, higher dose, and better CSF penetration; (3) obtaining biopsy specimens from suspicious lesions and using special stains for spirochetes in patients with serologic test results negative for syphilis; and (4) testing syphilitic patients for antibodies to HIV and testing HIV-infected patients for syphilis.

EPIDEMIOLOGY

Epidemiologic studies demonstrate that a history of an STD, including syphilis, is associated with an increased risk for HIV infection and AIDS among both homosexuals[11,42] and heterosexuals,[66] presumably because sexual behaviors that increase the risk for acquiring other STDs also increase the risk for acquiring HIV (Chapter 1). Furthermore, STDs that cause genital ulcerations have been implicated as cofactors for acquiring HIV infection.[25] Therefore, increases in the incidence of STDs in any population may presage future HIV-related disease.

Since 1982, the significant decreases seen in syphilis morbidity in the United States have occurred primarily among homosexual and bisexual men.[67] In areas reporting high rates of syphilis infection, the percentage of early syphilis cases occurring among homosexual and bisexual men decreased from 50% to 70% in the late 1970s to 5% to 15% in 1990.[67] These data presumably reflect changes in sexual practices that reduce the risk of HIV infection among homosexual and bisexual men. They suggest that education efforts encouraging safer sex practices have been effective among homosexual men. However, safer sex practices, such as oral sex without ejaculation, may reduce the risk of HIV infection but may not reduce the risk of syphilis unless a condom is used. In addition, because many patients with syphilis are not routinely tested for neurosyphilis or HIV infection and because these conditions (if diagnosed) are not reportable in many areas, the incidence of syphilis—especially neurosyphilis—in HIV-infected patients is unknown. Thus, it is not known whether patients with HIV infection are at higher risk for acquired syphilis or neurosyphilis than persons without HIV infection.

PATHOGENESIS

It is plausible that impairment of both cell-mediated and humoral immunity by HIV[6] could limit the host's defenses against *Treponema pallidum*, thereby altering the clinical manifestations or natural course of syphilis infection or both. Host immunity, especially cell-mediated immunity, plays an important role in protecting the host against syphilis.[63] In animal models, selective impairment of cell-mediated immunity alters the host response to syphilis infection. Incubation time is shorter, lesions are more numerous and widespread, and healing time is slower.[62] Furthermore, HIV-induced meningeal inflammation may facilitate penetration of spirochetes into the central nervous system (CNS) and thus contribute to the development of symptomatic neurosyphilis.

CLINICAL MANIFESTATIONS AND COURSE

Case reports have suggested that the clinical manifestations of syphilis may be unusual and the course more rapid in patients with HIV infection.[43,61] These anecdotal reports have led to the hypothesis that in patients coinfected with HIV and *T. pallidum*, symptomatic neurosyphilis may be more likely to develop, the latency period before development of meningovascular syphilis may be shorter, and the efficacy of standard therapy for syphilis may be reduced.

Neurosyphilis

Several cases of neurosyphilis have been reported in patients with HIV infection[4,27,43,47] (Chapter 14). One patient had a diffuse maculopapular rash, hepatomegaly, and unilateral facial palsy. Laboratory data were remarkable for transient elevation of serum transaminases, a rapid plasma reagin (RPR) titer of 1:512, and a positive fluorescent treponemal antibody-absorbed (FTA-abs) test result. CSF examination revealed mononuclear pleocytosis (66 cells/mm³), an elevated protein level (182 mg/dl), and a CSF–venereal disease research laboratories (VDRL) titer of 1:4. This case is consistent with secondary syphilis accompanied by acute syphilitic meningitis and cranial nerve involvement.

Another patient presented with a pure motor hemiplegia that appeared after a 2-month prodrome of fatigue, malaise, and headache. No previous history of syphilis or chancre was reported. Laboratory data were remarkable for transient elevation of serum transaminases, an RPR titer of 1:256, and a positive FTA-abs test result. CSF examination revealed lymphocytic pleocytosis (234 cells/mm³), an elevated protein level (94 mg/dl), hypoglycorrhachia (glucose, 33 mg/dl), and a CSF-VDRL titer of 1:1. This case is consistent with meningovascular syphilis. A third patient had posterior uveitis, neurosensory hearing loss, and meningovascular syphilis (pure motor hemiparesis) 4 months after the diagnosis of primary syphilis. Another patient presented with an unsteady gait, sensory deficits, generalized areflexia, and a positive Romberg sign. The RPR titer was 1:8; the FTA-abs test result was positive. CSF examination revealed lymphocytic pleocytosis (54 cells/mm³) and a CSF-VDRL titer of 1:2.

These case reports of neurosyphilis in HIV-infected persons are similar to cases reported before the AIDS epidemic.[44,57,73] Neurosyphilis may occur at any stage of syphilis. The clinical spectrum and time between primary infection and neurologic symptoms are well described.[73] Approximately 35% to 40% of persons with secondary syphilis have asymptomatic CNS involvement, with an abnormal cell count, protein level, glucose level, or reactive CSF-VDRL found on CSF examination. Acute syphilitic meningitis usually occurs within the first 2 years of infection; 10% of cases are diagnosed at the time of the secondary rash. Patients experience headache, meningeal irritation, and cranial nerve abnormalities. Typically, cranial nerves at the base of the brain (especially cranial nerves II, III, VI, VII, and VIII) are involved. Meningovascular syphilis can occur a few months to 10 years after the primary infection (average, 7 years).

Unlike the sudden onset of thrombotic or embolic stroke syndromes, meningovascular syphilis is associated with prodromal symptoms for weeks to months before focal defects of a vascular syndrome are identified. Prodromal symptoms include headache, vertigo, insomnia, and psychiatric abnormalities, such as personality changes. The focal defects initially are intermittent or progress slowly over a few days. In contrast, general paresis and tabes dorsalis are the parenchymatous forms of neurosyphilis that occur, in general, 10 to 30 years later. General paresis causes symptoms similar to those of any dementia, and syndromes similar to many psychiatric illness also have been described. Tabes dorsalis is associated with a triad of symptoms (lightning pains, dysuria, and ataxia) and a triad of signs (Argyll Robertson pupils, areflexia, and loss of proprioceptive sense).

Most symptomatic neurosyphilis cases reported among HIV-infected persons have had the early forms of neurosyphilis, namely, acute syphilitic meningitis and meningovascular neurosyphilis. Tabes dorsalis was reported in one HIV-infected man who had been treated for primary syphilis 7 years earlier[9] and in another man exposed 7 years earlier.[27] In addition, cases of syphilitic meningomyelitis with spastic paraparesis[77] and syphilitic polyradiculopathy with progressive leg pain and weakness[50] have been published.

Although it is clear that the neurosyphilis cases involving persons with concurrent HIV infection published to date do not represent unusual clinical manifestations, neurologic complications may occur more frequently and earlier in HIV-infected patients. Until better data from controlled studies are available, most experts believe that HIV-infected patients with syphilis are at increased risk of neurologic complications, but the magnitude of the risk is probably very small.[76] However, the importance of a careful neurologic evaluation in any patient with syphilis or in any patient with HIV is obvious. Of note, Lukehart et al[53] found viable *T. pallidum* in the CSF of 12 of 40 patients with primary or secondary syphilis and no neurologic symptoms. In this study, isolation of *T. pallidum* was associated with two or more abnormal CSF findings, including pleocytosis, elevated protein concentration, or a reactive CSF-VDRL test, but was not associated with coexisting HIV infection. These data suggest that asymptomatic CNS involvement at the time of early syphilis infection is common but not more common in HIV-infected individuals.

Ocular and Otologic Syphilis

A number of case reports of ocular and otologic manifestations of syphilis in HIV-infected persons have been published.[3,22,51,52,56,75,79] The most common ocular findings in patients with concurrent HIV infection are uveitis, chorioretinitis, and retrobulbar neuritis. Retinitis or neuroretinitis, papillitis, vitreitis, and optic perineuritis also have been described. The most common presenting symptoms are decreased vision, eye pain, or both. In addition

to the abnormalities of the optic cranial nerve and the ocular motor nerves III and VI that can occur with acute syphilitic meningitis, these other ocular manifestations of syphilis commonly have been associated with the secondary stage of infection and CNS involvement. One case report of a gumma of the optic nerve has been published.[74]

Otologic syphilis is one of the few forms of sensorineural hearing loss that can be reversed if diagnosed and treated appropriately. Although the incidence of otologic symptoms in patients with HIV infection apparently is low, five cases of otosyphilis in persons with coexisting HIV infection have been reported.[75] Otologic findings in these patients included progressive hearing loss, tinnitus, imbalance, and a sensation of ear fullness. Three patients had been treated for primary syphilis 2 to 5 years before the onset of symptoms. Only one patient with acute syphilis meningitis had evidence of CNS involvement coincident with the diagnosis of otosyphilis. One case report of otosyphilis from an internal auditory canal gumma has been published.[51]

These clinical manifestations of ocular and otologic syphilis among persons with concurrent HIV infection have been described among persons without HIV infection. However, as is the case for neurologic complications, it is possible that ocular and otologic findings may occur more frequently in HIV-infected persons, albeit very infrequently. Performing careful opthalmologic and otologic examinations of symptomatic HIV-infected persons and any symptomatic persons with syphilis is essential.

Mucocutaneous Syphilis

Most HIV-infected patients with *T. pallidum* have typical dermatologic clinical features of primary and secondary disease, such as chancres and diffuse maculopapular rashes.[24,35,39,41] In one study among patients seen in an STD clinic, however, patients with HIV infection were more likely to present with signs and symptoms of secondary syphilis and were more likely to have overlap between the primary and secondary stages of syphilis (i.e., chancres were still present at the time of the secondary syphilis diagnosis). In addition, atypical chancres have been reported[21] and two patients in our clinic presented with lesions that looked like a fissure and an abrasion; serous fluid from both were positive for *T. pallidum* by darkfield examination. Gummatous penile ulcerations have also been reported.[32,49]

Case reports of unusual rashes include papular or nodular eruptions,[10,26] nodular or ulcerative lesions with necrotic centers (i.e., lues maligna),[26,70,71] and keratoderma.[64] These skin lesions have been characterized as more aggressive forms of secondary syphilis in HIV-infected persons, yet the same dermatologic presentations have been described in non–HIV-infected persons. The frequency of these uncommon cutaneous findings cannot be determined by these case reports, and additional studies are needed to define the clinical spectrum of syphilis in both HIV-infected and non–HIV-infected populations.

Other Syphilis

It is important to remember that syphilis is a systemic infection that disseminates early in the course of infection and can ultimately involve any organ system. Symptomatic involvement of organs other than skin, mucous membranes, and CNS is very rare, but has been described prior to the AIDS era. Recently, case reports of one HIV-infected patient with pneumonitis and hepatitis[14] and another with osteitis[46] have been published. Gummatous syphilis, a tertiary form of syphilis, also has been described in persons with HIV infection.[12,40,48]

DIAGNOSIS

Diagnosing syphilis may be more complicated in HIV-infected patients because of false-negative and false-positive serologic test results and atypical clinical presentations in the presence of HIV infection. The diagnosis should be based on a number of factors, including the patient's history, the clinical findings, direct examination of lesion material for spirochetes, and the results of serologic tests for syphilis. The importance of a careful clinical examination of HIV-infected patients with syphilis cannot be overstated. CNS disease may occur during any stage of syphilis. Clinical evidence of neurologic involvement warrants examination of the CSF.

Darkfield examination or direct fluorescent antibody (DFA) staining of exudate from lesions suspected of being primary syphilis always should be done if feasible because in patients with suspicious lesions but negative serologies,

a positive darkfield examination or DFA stain is diagnostic. Darkfield examination or DFA staining of selected secondary lesions should be used in establishing the diagnosis of secondary syphilis. It is important to confirm by DFA that the treponema seen in darkfield-positive oral lesions are *T. pallidum,* since nonpathogenic spirochetes are found in the mouth.

Serologic tests for syphilis remain the cornerstone of diagnosing untreated syphilis infection—even in HIV-infected patients. Serum samples should be obtained from any patient in whom the diagnosis of syphilis is suspected. All patients with known HIV infection should be screened for possible untreated syphilis infection. Nontreponemal antibody test results should be reported quantitatively and titered to a final end-point.

A negative RPR or VDRL test result may not rule out syphilis in patients with HIV infection. Although the sensitivity of these serologic tests in diagnosing secondary syphilis generally is very high, case reports of seronegative secondary syphilis in patients with HIV infection have raised concerns that some patients may fail to develop a normal antibody response to *T. pallidum.*[26,34,81] Even though these patients eventually seroconverted before treatment, more data are needed on the serologic response to *T. pallidum* in HIV-infected patients. However, until better data are available, most experts believe that syphilis serologic tests appear to be accurate and reliable for diagnosis of syphilis and evaluation of treatment response in the vast majority of HIV-infected patients.[76]

When clinical syndromes compatible with primary or secondary syphilis occur and when darkfield examinations and serologic test results are negative, the prozone phenomenon (i.e., falsely reading a nontreponemal serologic test as negative because the specimen was not tested after sufficient dilution so that the high concentration of antigen did not allow detectable antigen–antibody complex formation) should be ruled out.[45] A biopsy should be performed on suspicious lesions, and such biopsy specimens should be evaluated for spirochetes, using special stains or isolation techniques or both. A silver stain, such as the Steiner stain,[78] has been used successfully. Specific DFA stains for *T. pallidum* also can be used. Because *T. pallidum* cannot be grown on artificial media, inoculation of laboratory animals (usually rabbit testicles) is the only method available to isolate the organism. This method is available only in a few research laboratories.

Clinicians should consult with infectious disease specialists or pathologists about special tests available in their areas. If spirochetes are not demonstrated on biopsy material or if special techniques are not available to identify spirochetes but clinical suspicion of syphilis remains high, the clinician may wish to treat HIV-infected patients presumptively for syphilis. Such patients should be followed closely with serial serologic testing at 1 month, 2 months, 3 months, and 6 months to detect any delayed antibody response.

The specificity of the nontreponemal serologic tests for syphilis can be compromised in HIV-infected persons.[1,16,69] Very high VDRL/RPR titers of greater than 1:64 have been reported in HIV-infected patients without syphilis (SA Larsen, personal communication). However, the majority of biologically false-positive results among HIV-infected persons are titers of less than 1:8.[54,69] The nontreponemal tests detect antibodies directed against a cardiolipin-lecithin antigen. In patients with immunoglobulin abnormalities, the RPR or VDRL test result may falsely be positive. Many persons with HIV infection have both anticardiolipin-lecithin antibodies and polyclonal gammopathy. Thus, a positive RPR or VDRL test result may not represent active syphilis infection. However, in a patient with a history of adequately treated syphilis, it is best to assume a reactive nontreponemal test indicates active disease unless a serofast state has been well documented, because reinfection is difficult to rule out and reactivation or relapse of a previously treated infection is possible in a person with HIV infection.

Treponemal tests in HIV-infected patients previously treated for syphilis may not remain reactive after treatment. Haas et al[29] demonstrated that seroreversion rates of treponemal tests were significantly associated with falling T-cell counts. Rates of seroreversion were 7% for patients with asymptomatic HIV infection and 38% for patients with AIDS. More recently, Romanowski et al[68] reported that seroreversion of treponemal tests also occurs in non–HIV-infected persons treated early in the course of their syphilis infection. In this study, 13% of microhemagglutination–*Treponema pallidum* (MHA-TP) test results and 25% of FTA-abs test results were negative at 36 months following therapy for primary syphilis. Seroreversion was not found in patients treated for secondary or early latent syphilis. With progression of HIV disease, antitreponemal antibody reactivity may be lost in patients previously treated for syphilis. However, no data about the serologic response of treponemal tests in HIV-infected persons with very low T-cell counts and active syphilis infection exist. Until additional data are available, the sensitivity of treponemal tests in HIV-infected individuals should be considered high in patients with syphilis beyond the primary stage of infection. If asymptomatic patients have a positive nontreponemal test and a negative confirmatory treponemal test result, it is unlikely that they have active syphilis.

Diagnosis of Neurosyphilis

The diagnosis of neurosyphilis is based on the CSF findings of cells, elevated protein concentration, and a positive CSF-VDRL test result. Even if the CSF-VDRL test result is negative, the finding of increased CSF leukocytes (5/mm^3) and protein (0.4 mg/ml) requires consideration of a diagnosis of neurosyphilis.[19] If the CSF-VDRL test result is negative, the diagnosis of neurosyphilis is complicated by the lack of another reliable diagnostic test and the difficulty of distinguishing between neurologic disease caused by *T. pallidum* and that caused by HIV or other CNS pathogens found in patients with AIDS.

The majority of symptomatic neurosyphilis cases among persons with coexisting HIV infection have a positive CSF-VDRL test result.[55] However, case reports of symptomatic neurosyphilis in HIV-infected patients whose initial CSF-VDRL test results were negative suggest that cases of neurosyphilis will go untreated if the CSF-VDRL is the only finding used to guide therapeutic decisions.[19] In these patients, the CSF-VDRL test result became positive after penicillin therapy. These reports underscore the need for clinical judgment in establishing the diagnosis of active neurosyphilis in HIV-infected individuals. Better diagnostic tests for neurosyphilis are needed. The CSF FTA-abs test may help rule out neurosyphilis if it is negative, but a positive result is nonspecific. Measurement of immunoglobulins or treponemal antigens and isolation of treponemes have been suggested,[82] but they have not yet been adequately studied.[30] Detection of treponemal DNA using the polymerase chain reaction (PCR) test is under development, and it may be a potentially useful test for diagnosing neurosyphilis.[8,31] Until better diagnostic tests are available, clinicians may wish to treat for neurosyphilis in patients whose CSF leukocytes and protein concentration are elevated but in whom the CSF-VDRL is negative and all other possible causes have been excluded. If this empiric approach is undertaken, then it is essential that such patients be followed closely with repeat lumbar punctures at 3, 6, and 12 months to determine if the CSF returns to normal after aqueous pencillin G therapy.

Indications for CSF Examination

It is unclear when to examine the CSF in patients with syphilis and concurrent HIV infection,[35,53,60,65] but recommendations regarding indications for CSF examination in HIV-infected patients with untreated syphilis have changed recently based on a growing body of anecdotal evidence. The Centers for Disease Control and Prevention (CDC) now recommends CSF examination in all HIV-infected patients diagnosed with latent syphilis regardless of the apparent duration of infection.[76] Previous guidelines recommended CSF examination only for HIV-infected patients who had latent syphilis for longer than 1 year. Examination of CSF for evidence of neurosyphilis also should be performed in all HIV-infected patients (or patients at risk for HIV infection) who have any unexplained behavioral abnormalities; psychologic dysfunction; or ocular, auditory, or other neurologic symptoms or signs, especially those consistent with neurosyphilis. In addition, the CSF of HIV-infected patients should be examined for evidence of neurosyphilis if treatment for primary or secondary syphilis fails (i.e., if the titer does not decrease appropriately—fourfold [two dilutions] decrease by 3 months) or if a fourfold or greater increase occurs.

Because of case reports of neurosyphilis or isolation of *T. pallidum* from the CSF of HIV-infected patients who had completed standard therapy for early syphilis, some experts believe that routine CSF examination in all HIV-infected patients with syphilis is indicated and that therapy for neurosyphilis should be offered to those patients with a positive CSF-VDRL test result or with an abnormal cell count and protein concentration.[53,60,83,84] Other clinicians believe that all HIV-infected patients should be treated empirically with neurosyphilis regimens, even if the CSF examination is entirely normal. Many experts, however, believe that these isolated case reports do not justify the need for routine CSF examinations in patients

with primary and secondary syphilis and that additional studies are needed to determine the significance of these reports. CSF abnormalities are common in HIV-infected patients with primary and secondary syphilis and are of unknown diagnostic significance. The vast majority of HIV-infected patients with primary or secondary syphilis respond appropriately to clinically recommended benzathine penicillin therapy. The CDC does not recommend routine CSF examination in patients with primary and secondary syphilis.[76] Until data are available to address the need for evaluating the CSF in patients with primary and secondary syphilis, the patients should be informed about the current dilemma, and their available treatment options should be discussed with them.

Indications for Screening for HIV Infection

Many of the diagnostic options discussed previously (e.g., lumbar punctures in patients with latent syphilis) and the therapeutic options to be discussed are recommended only for patients with coexisting HIV infection. Therefore, it is important to know the HIV antibody status of patients with syphilis when choosing diagnostic and therapeutic options. All patients with syphilis should be tested for HIV antibodies and counseled. If HIV antibody testing is not possible, the clinician provides treatment, keeping in mind that HIV coinfection may be present.

TREATMENT FAILURES

Neurosyphilis

Several cases of neurologic relapse after benzathine penicillin G and ceftriaxone therapy for syphilis have been reported in patients with HIV infection.[5,15,23,43,50,83] One patient was seen initially with eye pain, double vision, dizziness, and headache. Two weeks later, he was found in a stuporous state with hemiparesis, homonymous hemianopsia, and expressive aphasia. CSF evaluation revealed mononuclear pleocytosis (32 cells/mm^3), an elevated protein level (92 mg/dl), and a CSF-VDRL titer of 1:4. This presentation is consistent with meningovascular syphilis. The patient had been treated with benzathine penicillin G for secondary syphilis 5 months before this neurologic event, and his serum VDRL titer had decreased from 1:256 to

1:16. Although a serum VDRL titer around the time of the stroke was 1:256, careful contact tracing and close follow-up after the initial treatment suggested that reinfection did not occur.[5] Meningovascular neurosyphilis was diagnosed also in a patient within 6 months after treatment with 2 g of ceftriaxone intravenously (IV) daily for 14 days for latent syphilis.[15] Another patient developed syphilitic ophthalmitis with irreversible blindness 96 hours after starting the high-dose IV penicillin treatment for syphilitic meningitis. Twenty-four weeks after completing the 10-day course of 24 million units of crystalline penicillin G daily, she developed meningovascular neurosyphilis. Prior to her treatment for syphilitic meningitis she had recently received 7.2 million units of benzethine penicillin for early syphilis.[23]

Neurologic relapse following penicillin therapy is not unique to HIV-infected patients[2,13,73] but is uncommon in non–HIV-infected patients. Additional studies are needed to determine the response of HIV-infected patients to currently recommended therapy.

Persistence of Treponemes

Lukehart et al[53] found viable treponemes in the CSF of two of three HIV-infected patients with secondary syphilis 3 to 6 months after treatment with a single dose of 2.4 million units of benzathine pencillin G. In these two patients, no signs or symptoms of neurologic relapse were reported, CSF-VDRL titers seroreverted, and the CSF white blood cell (WBC) count decreased, and in one patient, the serum VDRL titer decreased. In another HIV-infected patient with early syphilis who was treated with a single dose of benzathine penicillin G, serum and CSF-VDRL titers were unchanged, but no treponemes were isolated 8 months after therapy. This patient also had no signs or symptoms of neurologic relapse. Long-term studies on larger numbers of patients are needed to determine whether persistence of treponemes is common and reflects inadequate therapy or whether the usual course after therapy is eventually to clear the CSF of organisms, albeit slowly.

Other Treatment Failure Issues

Clinicians have reported slow resolution of skin lesions in patients with HIV infection after penicillin therapy, although the time period from treatment to resolution of the signs and symptoms of primary or secondary syphilis has never been well defined, even in patients without HIV infection. In addition, relapse of mucocutaneous signs and symptoms of secondary syphilis has been reported[54] and was documented in a sexually inactive AIDS patient treated with penicillin for infectious syphilis 3 years earlier in our clinic. It is plausible that in addition to neurologic relapse, other signs and symptoms of syphilis recur in HIV-infected individuals after treatment. Furthermore, the question of treatment failure has been raised about HIV-infected patients whose nontreponemal serologic titers fail to decrease following therapy for early syphilis.[16] As discussed previously, a positive RPR or VDRL test result may not represent active syphilis infection but rather a high serofast state. Additional studies are needed to determine the clinical and serologic response to currently recommended therapy among HIV-infected patients. Of note, well-documented treatment failures following erythromycin therapy for primary or secondary syphilis have been reported in patients with concurrent HIV infection. In these cases, chancres and mucocutaneous signs and symptoms failed to resolve or relapsed within a few days after 2 weeks of erythromycin therapy.[17]

TREATMENT

The isolated case reports discussed previously have raised questions about the efficacy of current treatment recommendations for syphilis in the HIV-infected patient. Until further studies determine the optimum therapeutic regimen for syphilis and neurosyphilis in HIV-infected patients and the significance of abnormal CSF findings in primary and secondary syphilis, treatment in such patients will remain controversial.[20,35,37,53,60,65,87] The CDC currently recommends that pencillin regimens be used whenever possible for all stages of syphilis in HIV-infected patients (Table 27–1). Erythromycin is not recommended. Doxycycline and cephalosporins are also not recommended by the CDC because no studies establishing an effective dose and duration have been done. In addition, no proven alternative therapies to penicillin are available for treating patients with neurosyphilis, congenital syphilis, or syphilis in pregnancy. Therefore, confirmation of penicillin allergy and desensitization is recommended

TABLE 27–1. TREATMENT OF SYPHILIS IN HIV-INFECTED PATIENTS

Primary and Secondary Syphilis*
Treatment Recommended†
Benzathine penicillin G, 2.4 million units intramuscularly (IM)
Unstudied Treatment Considerations
Benzathine penicillin G, 4.8 million units IM (administered as two doses of 2.4 million units IM weekly for 2 successive weeks)
Regimens for neurosyphilis as outlined below
Latent Syphilis with Normal CSF Examination
Treatment Recommended†
Benzathine penicillin G, 7.2 million units IM (administered as three doses of 2.4 million units IM weekly for 3 successive weeks)
Unstudied Treatment Considerations
Regimens for neurosyphilis as outlined below
Neurosyphilis
Treatment Recommended†
Aqueous crystalline penicillin G, 12 to 24 million units intravenously (IV) per day for 14 days (administered as 2 to 4 million units every 4 hours each day)
 or
Aqueous procaine penicillin G, 2.4 million units IM daily for 14 days, plus probenecid, 500 mg PO four times a day for 14 days
 plus
Benzathine penicillin G, 2.4 million units IM after completion of the above aqueous penicillin G 14-day regimen

---

 * Without clinical evidence of neurosyphilis.
 † Penicillin-allergic patients should be densensitized if skin testing confirms penicillin allergy or is unavailable.

for these patients. The following treatment recommendations are based on available data and the consensus recommendations published by the CDC.[76,87] These recommendations recently were changed to include 7.2 million units of benzathine penicillin G total (administered in three doses of 2.4 million units intramuscularly [IM] weekly for 3 weeks) for treatment of nonneurologic latent syphilis regardless of the apparent duration of infection. Previous guidelines recommended only 7.2 million units of benzathine penicillin G for patients with nonneurologic latent syphilis of greater than 1 year's duration.

Treatment of Nonneurologic Primary and Secondary Syphilis

A careful clinical examination to rule out clinical evidence of neurologic involvement (e.g., optic and auditory symptoms and cranial nerve palsies) must be done before treatment of HIV-infected patients with primary and sec-

ondary syphilis. For HIV-infected patients with incubating, primary, or secondary syphilis and no clinical evidence of neurologic involvement, the same treatment regimen as for patients without HIV infection is recommended: 2.4 million units of benzathine penicillin G administered IM at a single session. In penicillin-sensitive patients, allergy should be confirmed. If compliance and close follow-up are ensured, use of doxycycline (100 mg orally two times a day for 2 weeks) may be considered if the patient refuses desensitization. However, no data are available on the efficacy of tetracyclines in treating syphilis in HIV-infected patients, and if compliance and close follow-up cannot be ensured in patients taking tetracyclines, desensitization to penicillin and management in consultation with an infectious disease expert are recommended.

Treatment of Nonneurologic Latent Syphilis

A careful clinical examination and CSF examination should precede and guide treatment of HIV-infected patients with latent syphilis. If CSF examination is not possible, patients should be treated for presumed neurosyphilis. If the CSF examination yields no evidence of neurosyphilis, administration of 7.2 million units of benzathine penicillin G total (administered as three doses of 2.4 million units by IM injection weekly for 3 successive weeks) is recommended. In penicillin-sensitive patients, allergy should be confirmed, after which desensitization to penicillin and management in consultation with an infectious disease expert are recommended. Doxycycline is not recommended.

All patients should be warned about the possibility of a Jarisch-Herxheimer reaction before any treatment is given. In addition, HIV-infected patients should be informed that currently recommended regimens may be less effective for them than for patients without HIV infection and that follow-up care is essential.

Treatment of Neurosyphilis

For HIV-infected patients with any type of symptomatic neurosyphilis (including ocular or otologic syphilis), aqueous crystalline penicillin G is the treatment of choice (12 to 24 million units IV per day [i.e., 2 to 4 million units every 4 hours for 14 days]). Penicillin-sensitive patients should be desensitized to penicillin.

If hospitalization is impossible, administration of aqueous procaine penicillin G is another option (2.4 million units IM daily plus probenecid 500 mg by mouth four times daily for 14 days). However, these injections are painful, and patient compliance may be difficult to ensure. Most experts also recommend the addition of benzathine penicillin G 2.4 million units IM after completion of aqueous crystalline or aqueous procaine penicillin G therapy to provide comparable duration of therapy for latent syphilis.

Treatment Alternatives

Other outpatient regimens have been used in the treatment of neurosyphilis patients with normal immune function. These regimens include amoxicillin (2 g with probenecid, 500 mg, by mouth three times daily for 14 days),[18,33,58] although the minimum inhibitory concentrations (MICs) of the drug for *T. pallidum* are 10 to 20 times higher than that of penicillin, doxycycline (200 mg by mouth twice a day for 21 days),[86] and ceftriaxone (1 g IM daily for 14 days).[38] However, tetracyclines and cephalosporins are less active than penicillin for syphilis therapy. The efficacy of these regimens for treating syphilis in HIV-infected patients is unknown.

Because of concerns about neurologic relapse and persistence of treponemes in the CSF in HIV-infected patients treated with benzathine penicillin G for primary and secondary syphilis, some experts believe that until better data are available, HIV-infected patients with primary and secondary syphilis and abnormal CSF (i.e., with asymptomatic neurosyphilis) should be offered treatment regimens of longer duration, higher dosage, and better CSF penetration (e.g., the antibiotic regimens for neurosyphilis outlined previously).[53] Other experts emphasize that HIV-infected patients treated for syphilis who fail to respond (as defined below) to standard benzathine penicillin G therapy should also be offered antibiotic regimens of higher dose, longer duration, and better CSF penetration. Some clinicians believe that all HIV-infected patients with syphilis should be treated with penicillin regimens effective for neurosyphilis, an approach considered by others as of unproven benefit, impractical, and costly.[35] Still other experts suggest that

HIV-infected patients with primary and secondary syphilis should receive a longer course of benzathine penicillin G therapy, such as 2.4 million units IM weekly for 2 or 3 weeks.[20,60] Others have considered adding oral amoxicillin to the benzathine penicillin G regimen to supplement levels of penicillin in the blood.[84] The justification for using any of these alternative regimens is only theoretical. No studies comparing the efficacy of 2.4 million units of benzathine penicillin G with other treatment options for the treatment of syphilis in HIV-infected patients have been completed. Eradication of *T. pallidum* from patients with HIV infection may be impossible, and such patients may require chronic penicillin therapy to control their infection.

FOLLOW-UP

Until the efficacy of treatment regimens is better defined, the importance of close follow-up of HIV-infected patients with syphilis cannot be overstated. All patients should be watched carefully for persistent or recurrent symptoms, for any signs of neurologic involvement, and for increasing serologic titers.[15]

All patients treated for syphilis should be examined and retested with a quantitative nontreponemal test at 1 to 2 weeks and at 1, 2, 3, 6, 9, and 12 months after treatment. The reasons for the follow-up intervals include verifying that the level of the nontreponemal test result falls and does not increase; documenting a Jarisch-Herxheimer reaction; monitoring resolution, persistence, or recurrence of clinical signs and symptoms and development of any new signs or symptoms, especially those involving the CNS; and ensuring compliance with treatment, effective partner notification, and safer sex practices. Although of unproven benefit, some experts recommend performing a CSF examination 6 months after therapy. Patients should be followed longer if any questions about the adequacy of their clinical or serologic response exist. Patients must be followed using the same nontreponemal test because titers from the VDRL and RPR tests are not interchangeable. In the absence of HIV infection and no previous history of *T. pallidum* infection, treatment usually produces seronegativity within 1 year in patients with primary syphilis and within 2 years in patients with secondary syphilis. The serologic response in HIV-infected patients and patients with a history of syphilis infection needs further study. One retrospective case-control study found no difference in serologic response in HIV-infected patients treated for early syphilis when compared with non–HIV-infected patients treated for a comparable stage of syphilis.[80]

Determining what constitutes a therapeutic cure for syphilis in patients with coexisting HIV infection is problematic because no simple test is available. Moreover, symptoms and signs of early syphilis may resolve even without treatment. Criteria defining treatment failure are currently based on curves of serologic response to treatment established in patients with normal immune function.[7,28,72] Treatment failure criteria include the following findings: (1) persistence or recurrence of signs or symptoms of syphilis; (2) a sustained, fourfold (two dilutions) increase in the titer of nontreponemal tests of greater than 2 weeks' duration; or (3) failure of the nontreponemal test titer in patients with primary and secondary syphilis to decrease fourfold (two dilutions) by 3 months.

Until additional follow-up data on HIV-infected patients treated for syphilis are available, it is recommended that all patients with a documented clinical or serologic relapse as evidenced by persisting or recurring signs or symptoms of syphilis or by a sustained fourfold increase in nontreponemal test titer undergo a CSF examination. If there is no evidence of neurosyphilis, retreatment with three weekly injections of benzathine penicillin G 2.4 million units IM (7.2 million units, total) is recommended.

For HIV-infected patients treated for primary and secondary syphilis whose serologic titers have not decreased fourfold at 3 months after therapy, a CSF examination is indicated. If there is no evidence of neurosyphilis, most clinicians would treat the patient with 7.2 million units of benzathine penicillin G IM (i.e., 2.4 million units IM weekly for 3 weeks) and follow the patient with repeat serologic testing every 6 months. Unless the patient has recurrent or new clinical signs or symptoms or a sustained fourfold increase in the serologic titer, no further therapy is offered.

For patients with neurosyphilis, repeat serologic testing as described previously and CSF examination at 6-month intervals are recommended until the findings have stabilized. Abnormal CSF WBC counts and protein levels should decrease by 6 months if no coexisting CNS infections are present, but CSF-VDRL tests may not return to nonreactivity. If the CSF WBC count is not normal by 2 years, retreatment using an antibiotic regimen for neurosyphilis is recommended.

For HIV-infected patients treated for latent syphilis, follow-up guidelines are less clear because limited data are available to guide the evaluation of the serologic response. Current guidelines suggest that in patients treated for latent disease in whom an initially high titer (1:32) fails to decline at least fourfold (two dilutions) within 12 months, another evaluation for neurosyphilis should be done. If the CSF examination is normal, some experts retreat with 7.2 million units of benzathine penicillin G IM (i.e., 2.4 million units IM weekly for 3 weeks), and other clinicians do not retreat but simply follow such patients for evidence of clinical or serologic relapse. Recommendations regarding management of patients treated for latent syphilis in whom the initial nontreponemal titer is low are less clear. Although of unproven benefit, some experts recommend performing a CSF examination if a low titer fails to decrease after 12 months and retreatment with 7.2 million units of benzathine penicillin G if the CSF examination is normal. Other experts follow these patients for evidence of clinical or serologic relapse.

SEXUAL CONTACTS

An effort must be made to identify and treat any possible contacts of patients with early syphilis. In patients with primary syphilis, all contacts for 3 months before the appearance of the chancre should be evaluated clinically and serologically. In patients with secondary syphilis, contacts for the prior 6 months should be evaluated clinically and serologically. In patients with early latent syphilis and no history of symptoms or signs suggestive of primary or secondary syphilis, contacts for the prior 12 months should be evaluated clinically and serologically. Efforts should be made to establish a diagnosis of syphilis by history, clinical findings, and serologic testing before treating such contacts. However, persons exposed to a patient with early syphilis within the previous 3 months may be infected and seronegative and, therefore, should be treated presumptively for early syphilis, even without an established diagnosis.

Follow-up serologic tests should also be done at 1 week and 3 months to establish the diagnosis of syphilis in these contacts if they are HIV-infected or at risk of HIV infection. All cases of infectious syphilis (primary, secondary, and early latent) must be reported to the local health department. In addition, some state and local health departments (e.g., in San Francisco) require that health care providers notify the director of STD Control about HIV-infected patients who have (1) neurosyphilis confirmed by CSF examination (i.e., positive CSF-VDRL) or histopathology (DFA or special stains of biopsy material), (2) negative serologic test results for syphilis (nontreponemal [VDRL, RPR] or treponemal [FTA-abs, MHA-TP] tests) during secondary syphilis diagnosed by darkfield microscopy or histopathology of lesion material, or (3) failed treatment for syphilis as defined previously.

EDUCATION

All patients with syphilis and their contacts must be given education and counseling to reduce their risk of future STDs. Safer sex messages should include reducing the number of sexual partners, knowing the health status of partners (if possible), avoiding unsafe sexual practices, and using condoms.

ACKNOWLEDGMENT

Our studies on the clinical management and therapy of syphilis in HIV-infected patients are supported by Public Health Service grant no. H25/CCH 904371-02.

REFERENCES

1. Augenbraun MH, Dehovitz JA, Feldman J, et al: Biological false-positive syphilis test results for women infected with human immunodeficiency virus. Clin Infect Dis 19:1040–1044, 1994
2. Bayne LL, Schmidley JW, Goodin DS: Acute syphilitic meningitis: Its occurrence after clinical and serologic cure of secondary syphilis with penicillin G. Arch Neurol 43:137–138, 1986
3. Becerra LI, Ksiazek SM, Savino PJ, et al: Syphilitic uveitis in human immunodeficiency virus infected and noninfected patients. Ophthalmology 96:1727–1730, 1989
4. Berger JR: Neurosyphilis in human immunodeficiency virus type 1-seropositive individuals. Arch Neurol 48:700–702, 1991
5. Berry CD, Hooton TM, Collier AC, Lukehart SA: Neurologic relapse after benzathine penicillin therapy for secondary syphilis in a patient with HVI infection. N Engl J Med 316:1587–1589, 1987
6. Bowen DL, Lane HC, Fauci AS: Immunopathogenesis of the acquired immunodeficiency syndrome. Ann Intern Med 103:704–709, 1985
7. Brown ST, Zaidi A, Larsen SA, Reynolds GH: Serologic response to syphilis treatment: A new analysis of old data. JAMA 253:1296–1299, 1985
8. Burstain JM, Frimprel E, Lukehart SA, et al: Sensitive detection of *Treponema pallidum* by using the polymerase chain reaction. J Clin Microbiol 29:62–69, 1991
9. Calderon W, Danville H, Nigro M, et al: Concomitant syphilitic and HIV infection: A case report. Acta Neurol 45:132–137, 1990
10. Cusini M, Zerboni R, Muratori S, et al: Atypical early syphilis in a HIV-infected homosexual male. Dermatologica 177:300–304, 1988
11. Darrow WW, Echenberg DF, Jaffe HW, et al: Risk factors for human immunodeficiency virus (HIV) infections in homosexual men. Am J Public Health 77:479–483, 1987
12. Dawson S, Evans BA, Lawrence AG: Benign tertiary syphilis and HIV infection. AIDS 2:315–316, 1988
13. DiNubile MJ, Copare FJ, Gekowski KM: Neurosyphilis developing during treatment of secondary syphilis with benzathine penicillin in a patient without serologic evidence of human immunodeficiency virus infection. Am J Med 88:5-45N–5-48N, 1990
14. Dooley DP, Tomski S: Syphilitic pneumonitis in an HIV-infected patient. Chest 105:629–631, 1994
15. Dowell ME, Ross PG, Musher DM, et al: Response of latent syphilis or neurosyphilis to ceftriaxone therapy in persons infected with human immunodeficiency virus. Am J Med 93:481–488, 1992
16. Drabick JJ, Tramont EC: Utility of the VDRL test in HIV-seropositive patients. N Engl J Med 322:271, 1990
17. Duncan WC: Failure of erythromycin to cure secondary syphilis in a patient infected with the human immunodeficiency virus. Arch Dermatol 125:82–84, 1989
18. Faber WR, Bos JD, Reitra PJ, et al: Treponemicidal levels of amoxicillin in cerebrospinal fluid after oral administration. Sex Transm Dis 10:148–150, 1983
19. Feraru ER, Aronow HA, Lipton RB: Neurosyphilis in AIDS patients: Initial CSF VDRL may be negative. Neurology 40:541–543, 1990
20. Fiumara N: Human immunodeficiency virus infection and syphilis. J Am Acad Dermatol 21:141–142, 1989
21. Garcia-Silva J, Velasco-Benito JA, Pena-Penabad C: Primary syphilis with multiple chancres and porphyria cutanea tarda in an HIV-infected patient. Dermatology 188:163–165, 1994
22. Gass JD, Braunstein RA, Chenoweth RG: Acute syphilitic posterior placoid chorioretinitis. Ophthalmology 97:1288–1297, 1990
23. Gordon SM, Eaton ME, George R, Larsen S, et al: The response of symptomatic neurosyphilis to high-dose intravenous penicillin G in patients with human immunodeficiency virus infection. N Eng J Med 331:1469–1473, 1994
24. Gourevitch MN, Selwyn PA, Davenny K, et al: Ann Intern Med 118:350–355, 1993
25. Greenblatt RM, Lukehart SA, Plummer FA, et al: Genital ulcerations as a risk factor for human immunodeficiency virus infection. AIDS 2:47–50, 1988

26. Gregory N, Sanchez M, Buchness MR: The spectrum of syphilis in patients with human immunodeficiency virus infection. J Am Acad Dermatol 22:1061–1067, 1990

27. Gue JW, Wang SJ, Lin YY, et al: Neurosyphilis presenting as tabes dorsalis in a HIV-carrier. China Med J 51:389–391, 1993

28. Guinan ME: Treatment of primary and secondary syphilis: Defining failure at three- and six-month follow-up. JAMA 257:359–360, 1987

29. Haas JS, Bolan G, Larsen SA, et al: Sensitivity of treponemal tests for detecting prior treated syphilis during human immunodeficiency virus infection. J Infect Dis 162:862–866, 1990

30. Hart G: Syphilis tests in diagnostic and therapeutic decision making. Ann Intern Med 104:368–376, 1986

31. Hay PE, Clark JR, Taylor-Robinson D, Goldmeier D: Detection of treponemal DNA in the CSF of patients with syphilis and HIV infection using the polymerase chart reaction. Genitourin Med 66:428–432, 1990

32. Hay PE, Tam FWK, Kitchen VS, et al: Gummatous lesions in men infected with human immunodeficiency virus and syphilis. Genitourin Med 66:374–379, 1990

33. Hay PE, Taylor-Robinson D, Waldron S, Goldmeier D: Amoxicillin, syphilis, and HIV infection. Lancet 335:474–475, 1990

34. Hicks CB, Benson PM, Lupton GP, Tramont EC: Seronegative secondary syphilis in a patient infected with the human immunodeficiency virus (HIV) with Kaposi's sarcoma: A diagnostic dilemma. Ann Intern Med 107:492–495, 1987

35. Hook EW III: Syphilis and HIV infection. J Infect Dis 160:530–534, 1989

36. Hook EW III: Treatment of syphilis: Current recommendations, alternatives and continuing problems. Rev Infect Dis 11:S1511–S1517, 1989

37. Hook EW III: Management of syphilis in human immunodeficiency virus-infected patients. Am J Med 93:477–479, 1992

38. Hook EW III, Baker-Zander SA, Moskovitz BL, et al: Ceftriaxone therapy for asymptomatic neurosyphilis. Case report and Western blot analysis of serum and cerebrospinal fluid IgG response to therapy. Sex Transm Dis (Suppl 3):185S–188S, 1986

39. Hook EW III, Marra CM: Acquired syphilis in adults. N Engl J Med 326:1060–1069, 1992

40. Horowitz HW, Valsamis MP, Wicher V, et al: Cerebral syphilitic gumma confirmed by the polymerase chain reaction in a man with human immunodeficiency virus infection. N Engl J Med 331:1488–1491, 1994

41. Hutchinson CM, Hood EW III, Shepherd M, et al: Altered clinical presentation of early syphilis in patients with human immunodeficiency virus infection. Ann Intern Med 121:94–99, 1994

42. Jaffe HW, Choi K, Thomas PA, et al: National case-control study of Kaposi's sarcoma and *Pneumocystis carinii* pneumonia in homosexual men. Part 1. Epidemiologic results. Ann Intern Med 99:145–151, 1983

43. Johns DR, Tierney M, Felsenstein D: Alteration in the natural history of neurosyphilis by concurrent infection with the human immunodeficiency virus. N Engl J Med 316:1569–1572, 1987

44. Jordan KG: Modern neurosyphilis—a critical analysis. West J Med 149:47–57, 1988

45. Jurado RL, Campbell J, Martin PD: Prozone phenomenon in secondary syphilis. Arch Intern Med 153:2496–2498, 1993

46. Kastner RJ, Malone JL, Decker CF: Syphilitic osteitis in a patient with secondary syphilis and concurrent human immunodeficiency virus infection. Clin Infect Dis 18:250–252, 1994

47. Katz DA, Berger JR: Neurosyphilis in acquired immunodeficiency syndrome. Arch Neurol 46:895–898, 1989

48. Kerns G, Pogrel MA, Honda G: Intraoral tertiary syphilis (gumma) in a human immunodeficiency virus-positive man. J Oral Maxillofac Surg 51:85–88, 1993

49. Kitchen VS, Cook T, Doble A, Harris JR: Gummatous penile ulceration and generalized lymphadenopathy in homosexual man: Case report. Genitourin Med 64:276–279, 1988

50. Lanska MJ, Lanska DJ, Schmidley JW: Syphilitic polyradiculopathy in an HIV-positive man. Neurology 38:1297–1301, 1988

51. Little JP, Gardner G, Acker JD, Land MA: Otosyphilis in a patient with human immunodeficiency virus: Internal auditory canal gumma. Otolaryngol Head Neck Surg 112:488–492, 1995

52. Levy JH, Liss RA, Maguire AM: Neurosyphilis and ocular syphilis in patients with concurrent human immunodeficiency virus infection. Retina 9:175–180, 1989

53. Lukehart SA, Hook EW III, Baker-Zander SA, et al: Invasion of the central nervous system by *Treponema pallidum*: Implications for diagnosis and treatment. Ann Intern Med 109:855–862, 1988

54. Malone JR, Wallace MR, Hendrick BB, et al: Syphilis and neurosyphilis in a human immunodeficiency virus type-1 seropositive population: Evidence for frequent serologic relapse after therapy. Am J Med 99:55–63, 1995

55. Matlow AG, Rachlis AR: Syphilis serology in human immunodeficiency virus-infected patients with symptomatic neurosyphilis: Case report and review. Rev Infect Dis 12:703–707, 1990

56. McLeish WM, Pulido JS, Holland S, et al: The ocular manifestations of syphilis in the human immunodeficiency virus type-1 infected host. Ophthalmology 97:196–203, 1990

57. Merritt HH, Adams RD, Soloman HC: Neurosyphilis. New York, Oxford University Press, 1946

58. Morrison RE, Harrison SM, Tramont EC: Oral amoxicillin: An alternative treatment for neurosyphilis. Genitourin Med 61:359–362, 1985

59. Musher DM: How much penicillin cures early syphilis? Ann Intern Med 109:849–851, 1988

60. Musher DM: Syphilis, neurosyphilis, penicillin and AIDS. J Infect Dis 163:1201–1206, 1991

61. Musher DM, Hamill RJ, Baughn RE: Effect of human immunodeficiency virus (HIV) infection on the course of syphilis and on the response to treatment. Ann Intern Med 113:872–881, 1990

62. Pacha N, Metzger M, Smogor W, et al: Effects of immunosuppressive agents on the course of experimental syphilis in rabbits. Arch Immunol Ther 27:45–51, 1979

63. Pavia CS, Folds JD, Baseman JB: Cell-mediated immunity during syphilis: A review. Br J Venereal Dis 54:144–150, 1978

64. Radolph JD, Kaplan RP: Unusual manifestations of

secondary syphilis and abnormal humoral immune response to *Treponema pallidum* antigens in a homosexual man with asymptomatic human immunodeficiency virus infection. J Am Acad Dermatol 18: 423–428, 1988

65. Recommendations for diagnosing and treating syphilis in HIV-infected patients. MMWR 37:600–602, 607–608, 1988

66. Risk factors for AIDS among Haitians in the United States. Evidence of heterosexual transmission. The Collaborative Study Group of AIDS in Haitian-Americans. JAMA 257:635–639, 1987

67. Rolfs RT, Nakashima AK: Epidemiology of primary and secondary syphilis in the United States: 1981–1989. JAMA 264:1432–1437, 1990

68. Romanowski B, Sutherland R, Fick GH, et al: Serologic response to treatment of infectious syphilis. Ann Intern Med 144:1005–1009, 1991

69. Rompalo AM, Cannon RO, Quinn TC, Hook EW III: Association of biologic false-positive reactions for syphilis with human immunodeficiency virus infection. J Infect Dis 165:1124–1126, 1992

70. Sands M, Markus A: Lues maligna, or ulceronodular syphilis, in a man infected with human immunodeficiency virus: Case report and review. Clin Infect Dis 20:387–390, 1995

71. Schlossbert D, Morley J, Montero M, Krouse T: Rupia syphilitica. Arch Dermatol 129:514–515, 1993

72. Schroeter AL, Lucas JB, Price EV, Falcone VH: Treatment for early syphilis and reactivity of serologic tests. JAMA 221:471–476, 1972

73. Simon RP: Neurosyphilis. Arch Neurol 42:606–613, 1985

74. Smith JL, Byrne SF, Cambron GR: Syphiloma/gumma of the optic nerve and human immunodeficiency virus seropositivity. J Clin Neurol Ophthalmol 10: 175–184, 1990

75. Smith ME, Canalis RF: Otologic manifestations of AIDS: The otosyphilis connection. Laryngoscope 99:365–372, 1989

76. STD: 1993 sexually transmitted diseases treatment guideline. MMWR 42:RR-14, 1993

77. Strom T, Schneck SA: Syphilis meningomyelitis. Neurology 41:325–326, 1991

78. Swisher BL: Modified Steiner procedure for microwave staining of spirochetes and non-filamentous bacteria. J Histotechnol 10:241–243, 1987

79. Tamesis RR, Foster CS: Ocular syphilis. Ophthalmology 97:1281–1287, 1990

80. Telzak EE, Greenberg MSZ, Harrison J, et al: Syphilis treatment response in HIV-infected individuals. AIDS 5:591–595, 1991

81. Tikjob G, Russel M, Petersen CS, et al: Seronegative secondary syphilis in a patient with AIDS: Identification of *Treponema pallidum* in biopsy specimen. J Am Acad Dermatol 24:506–508, 1991

82. Tomberlin MG, Holtom PD, Owens JL, Larsen RA: Evaluation of neurosyphilis in human immunodeficiency virus-infected individuals. Clin Infect Dis 18: 288–294, 1994

83. Tramont EC: Persistence of *Treponema pallidum* following penicillin G therapy: Report of 2 cases. JAMA 236:2206–2207, 1976

84. Tramont EC: Syphilis in the AIDS era. N Engl J Med 316:1600–1601, 1987

85. Tramont EC: Syphilis in adults: From Christopher Columbus to Sir Alexander Fleming to AIDS. Clin Infect Dis 21:1361–1371, 1995

86. Yim CW, Flynn NM, Fitzgerald FT: Penetration of oral doxycycline into the cerebrospinal fluid of patients with latent or neurosyphilis. Antimicrob Agents Chemother 28:347–348, 1985

87. Zenker PN, Rolfs RT: Treatment of syphilis, 1989. Rev Infect Dis 12:S590–S609, 1990

Chapter 28

Malignancies Associated with AIDS

LAWRENCE D. KAPLAN and DONALD W. NORTHFELT

Malignancies as a complication of immuno-deficiency have been well described in the literature, being recognized long before the advent of the HIV epidemic.[37,63,70] The incidence of both Kaposi's sarcoma and non-Hodgkin's lymphoma are markedly increased in immunosuppressed allograft recipients. It is therefore not surprising that patients with HIV infection, who also have profound defects in cell-mediated immunity, develop these two malignancies. The marked rise in the incidence of both Kaposi's sarcoma and B-cell lymphoma in populations at risk for HIV infection in the years since 1982 strongly suggests a causal relationship between immunodeficiency and the development of these malignancies.[60] As a result of this relationship, these neoplasms are included in the AIDS case definition established by the Centers for Disease Control and Prevention (CDC).[12] Recently, it has been recognized that women with HIV infection develop human papillomavirus (HPV)–associated cervical intraepithelial neoplasia and invasive cervical carcinoma with high frequency. Thus, invasive cervical cancer has been added to the revised CDC AIDS case definition. Thus, these three neoplasms are referred to as "AIDS-defining" malignancies. They are listed in Table 28–1 with a variety of other malignancies that have been reported in HIV-infected individuals for which a causal relationship is uncertain. Data reported from the Pittsburg component of the Multicenter AIDS Cohort Study (MACS) indicated that, among 430 seropositive homosexual men, a combined frequency of all cancers other than Kaposi's sarcoma, non-Hodgkin's lymphoma, central nervous system lymphoma, and non-melanoma skin cancers were statistically significantly increased in comparison to both 769 seronegative patients as well as the general population. This increase appeared to be secondary to an unusually increased frequency of both seminoma and Hodgkin's disease.[100] The data reported from the San Francisco City Clinic Cohort study[65] also suggest a possible increased risk of Hodgkin's disease in this patient population. In the case of cervical and anal carcinomas and interepithelial neoplasias, accumulating evidence suggests a relationship between immune function and the risk of invasive disease.[11,103]

Regardless of the causal relationship between various malignancies and the underlying immunodeficiency state, reports in the literature suggest that the natural history of cancer may be altered in the setting of HIV infection.[32,135,167] Patients tend to present with more advanced disease that is more rapidly progressive and responds less well to therapy than in the non–HIV-infected population. However, for neoplastic disease that is normally highly responsive to therapeutic intervention, such as testicular germ cell tumors, treatment of these neoplasms when they occur in the setting of HIV infection can be highly successful.[5,164]

Management of the HIV-infected patient with a malignancy imposes obstacles rarely encountered in the non–HIV-infected population. Poor bone marrow reserve and the risk of intercurrent opportunistic infections, problems frequently observed in this patient population, can compromise the delivery of adequate dose intensity. In addition, administration of chemotherapy may lead to further immunosuppression, resulting in a greater likelihood of opportunistic infection. Finally, toxicity to chemotherapeutic agents, antibiotics, and radiation therapy are excessive and often severe, further impairing the physician's ability to administer adequate therapy.

This chapter focuses on the AIDS-defining neoplasms from primarily a clinical perspective. Kaposi's sarcoma, non-Hodgkin's lymphoma,

TABLE 28–1. MALIGNANCIES IN HIV INFECTION

AIDS-Defining Malignancies	Non–AIDS-Defining Malignancies	References
Kaposi's sarcoma	Hodgkin's disease	71,73,146
B-cell lymphoma	Squamous carcinoma	19,32,54,103,167
Cervical carcinoma	Head and neck	
	Anus	
	Melanoma	165
	Plasmacytoma	167
	Adenocarcinoma colon	10
	Small-cell lung carcinoma	54,167
	Germ cell (testicular) tumor	163
	Basal cell tumor	66

and the HPV-associated anogenital neoplasms are discussed. The natural history of these malignancies is presented along with various therapeutic options.

KAPOSI'S SARCOMA

Kaposi's sarcoma (KS), once a rarely reported malignancy, is the most common neoplasm affecting HIV-infected individuals. It is seen primarily in homosexual men and has only rarely been reported in IV drug users or other risk groups.[109,142] The proportion of AIDS patients with KS as the initial AIDS diagnosis has changed since the first cases were reported in 1981.[22] In New York City, KS was the initial AIDS diagnosis in 50% of non–IV-drug-using homosexual men diagnosed between 1981 and 1983. Between 1984 and 1987, however, this proportion had fallen to 30%. Similar trends have been reported from San Francisco.[141] However, in a study of infectious diseases and cancers among persons dying of HIV infection, national multiple-cause mortality data showed no significant trend in the prevalence of KS between 1987 (10.4%) and 1992 (12.1%).[148]

The pathogenesis of KS in HIV-infected patients remains uncertain. The decline in the incidence of KS in the homosexual male population during a period of time when sexual practices were changing and the nearly exclusive confinement of this neoplasm to the homosexual male population support the concept of another sexually transmitted agent's being involved in the pathogenesis of KS.[25] When KS occurs in women, it is seen almost exclusively in women whose sexual partners are bisexual males.[3] Laboratory studies have implicated a variety of endothelial growth factors, including basic fibroblast growth factor, interleukin (IL)-1, and tumor necrosis factor, in the etiology of KS.[27,115,143] The roles of IL-6 and oncostatin M have received particular attention. It has been demonstrated that HIV-associated KS tissue produces large amounts of immunoreactive IL-6 and that HIV-associated KS-derived cell lines produce and respond to IL-6 in an autocrine growth loop.[107] Oncostatin M, produced by activated T cells, may be the most potent stimulus to KS spindle cell proliferation and appears to be capable of producing phenotypic changes in vascular smooth muscle cells that resemble the KS spindle cell.[106] It has also been observed that male mice transgenic for the HIV *tat* gene develop KS-like tumors.[169] Additional laboratory studies have demonstrated that the proliferation of KS spindle cells in vitro observed in response to HIV *tat* is accompanied by an increase in IL-6 production by these same cells.[138] What the precise roles of these various factors may be in the pathogenesis and growth of KS in the clinical setting are the subject of investigation. A better understanding of the pathogenesis of this disease may have significant implications for future therapeutic strategies.

Figure 28–1 illustrates how viral infections, including HIV, might activate a cytokine cascade, resulting in stimulation of spindle cell proliferation and neoangiogenesis. The reason for the male predominance in Kaposi's sarcoma is not clear. IL-6 production in cultured KS-derived spindle cells was enhanced by glucocorticoids and testosterone,[47] whereas marked inhibition of IL-6 production was noted with the addition of 17-beta-estradiol.[47,175] Other in vitro studies have suggested inhibitory activity of beta-human chorionic gonadotropin against cultured spindle cells.[99] These observations may also be significant for the development of future therapeutic clinical trials.

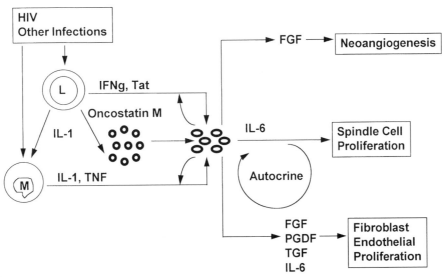

FIGURE 28–1. KS pathogenesis. Proposed cytokine cascade that may give rise to KS. Lymphocytes and monocytes activated by HIV or other infections produce a variety of cytokines. Oncostatin M may be responsible for maintaining the spindle cell phenotype, whereas other cytokines activate spindle cells to produce large quantities of IL-6 that, in an autocrine growth loop, stimulate their own growth. Other growth factors in turn produced by this spindle cell population may result in the neoangiogenesis and proliferation of fibroblasts and endothelial cells characteristic of the KS lesion. (Modified with permission from Ensoli B, Barillari G, Gallo RC: Pathogenesis of AIDS-associated Kaposi's sarcoma. Hematol Oncol Clin North Am 5: 281–295, 1991.)

Clinical Presentation and Diagnosis

Unlike the more indolent, endemic form of KS, KS in the HIV-infected individual usually is an aggressive and unpredictable disease.[109,142] The skin most commonly is the first site of presentation. Palpable, firm, cutaneous nodules ranging from 0.5 to 2 cm in diameter frequently are observed. However, in early stages, smaller, nonpalpable lesions may be seen. Some early lesions can appear like small ecchymoses. In more advanced disease, cutaneous lesions can become confluent and form large tumor masses involving extensive cutaneous surfaces. In light-skinned individuals, the lesions are typically violaceous in appearance (Color Plate I*G*), whereas in dark-skinned individuals, the lesions acquire a more hyperpigmented appearance, appearing brown or even black. KS lesions may follow Langer's lines, may be symmetrical, and have a particular predilection for the tip of the nose and the penis. Rather than being limited to a single cutaneous site as in classic KS, KS in an individual with HIV infection can involve any cutaneous surface. Involvement of the head and neck is frequent, and the appearance of oral KS lesions is often the first sign of disease (Color Plate I*H*).

The natural history of KS associated with HIV infection more closely resembles that observed in immunosuppressed allograft recipients. The disease tends to progress with time and is associated with the appearance of larger and more numerous cutaneous lesions. However, the course of the disease is unpredictable. A patient may have relatively few lesions that remain stable over time. New cutaneous lesions may not appear for many months but may be followed by a sudden and rapid increase in disease activity. Visceral involvement with KS is extremely common and can involve almost any visceral site. Careful endoscopic examination will reveal gastrointestinal (GI) sites of disease in 40% of patients with asymptomatic cutaneous KS at the time of diagnosis.[35]

Although KS is usually not a direct cause of death in HIV-infected patients, the morbidity associated with more advanced disease can be significant. Bulky cutaneous lesions may become painful and, if large cutaneous surfaces are involved, can restrict movement. Lymphatic obstruction is common and can result in severe edema, most commonly involving the extremities (Color Plate I*E*) or the face. Visceral spread of KS is rarely symptomatic, particularly when it involves the GI tract. However, rare cases of obstruction, perforation, or GI bleeding have been reported.[34] Often, pulmonary KS results in cough, bronchospasm, and dyspnea, and death caused by respiratory failure is not uncommon.[75,122] Finally, the social problems associated with this disfiguring neoplasm in the setting of an already socially stigmatizing disease cannot be over-emphasized.

Pulmonary involvement with KS deserves special attention because this is becoming an increasingly common complication of KS. In contrast to other visceral sites of involvement, pulmonary KS is generally symptomatic. This complication tends to occur in the setting of poor immune function, and most individuals will have a CD4 lymphocyte count of less than 100/mm³.[42] Pulmonary involvement also tends to occur more frequently in individuals who have more than 50 cutaneous lesions, although the disease has been seen in individuals with minimal or even absent cutaneous KS.[75] The disease may be rapidly progressive when it involves the lungs and clinically may be difficult to distinguish from a rapidly progressive pneumonitis. Survival is relatively short in these patients, with median survival times of between 2 and 6 months reported.[42,75] The typical chest radiographic appearance is variable, with the characteristic reticular-nodular pattern being seen in approximately one third of patients[75] (Chapter 29). More commonly, diffuse interstitial infiltrates are observed that may be difficult to distinguish from *Pneumocystis carinii* pneumonitis.[20,42,75,122] Pleural effusions are seen frequently,[20,42,75,122] and hilar adenopathy is observed in approximately 50% of cases.[42] Death caused by respiratory failure is not uncommon in the patient with pulmonary KS.

Careful examination of the skin and oral cavity at each clinic visit is the key to early diagnosis. Once lesions are identified, histologic confirmation should be obtained. This is particularly important because other cutaneous diseases, some of which can mimic KS, are common in the HIV-infected patient (Chapter 11). For cutaneous lesions, a small punch biopsy specimen generally is obtained. Conventional biopsy techniques can be used at other sites. In patients with suspected pulmonary KS, violaceous endobronchial lesions are typically observed on bronchoscopic examination. Unfortunately, attempts at endobronchial biopsy frequently are unsuccessful because of the submucosal nature of the lesions. However, bronchoscopic visualization of typical lesions is generally accepted for the purpose of diagnosis of pulmonary disease in patients who have had KS

at other sites.[75] In the patient for whom treatment with chemotherapy is anticipated for KS at other sites and who has respiratory symptoms or an abnormal chest radiograph, gallium scanning can be sufficient to rule out a pulmonary opportunistic infection, making chemotherapy administration more acceptable. KS is not gallium avid.[75]

Although historically the most common cause of death in individuals with HIV and KS is opportunistic infection, there is evidence that, as survival is prolonged in individuals with HIV infection as a result of improvements in medical care, pulmonary involvement with KS is becoming an increasingly common cause of death.

Staging

Currently used staging systems are based primarily on tumor bulk. A modification of this staging system to include the presence or absence of constitutional symptoms is shown in Table 28–2. Unfortunately, these systems have not proved useful because a majority of patients fall into the most advanced stages. In addition, tumor bulk may not be the most important predictor of survival in this group of patients.

Analysis of data from 190 individuals with HIV-associated KS at the University of California at Los Angeles Medical Center demonstrated that the most important predictor of survival is the absolute CD4⁺ lymphocyte count[162]

TABLE 28–2. STAGING OF KAPOSI'S SARCOMA

Stage	Characterics
I	Limited cutaneous lesions (<10 or in one anatomic area)
II	Disseminated cutaneous lesions (>10 or in more than one anatomic area)
III	Visceral lesions only (gastrointestinal, lymph node)
IV	Cutaneous and visceral lesions
Subtypes	
A	No systemic signs or symptoms
B	Fevers >37.8°C unrelated to identifiable infection for >2 weeks or weight loss >10% of body weight

Reprinted with permission from Mitsuyasu RT, Groopman JE: Biology and therapy of Kaposi's sarcoma. Semin Oncol 11:53–59, 1984.

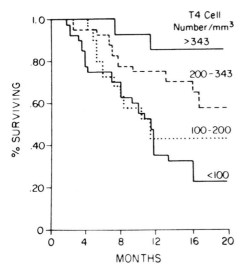

FIGURE 28–2. Relationship of various levels of T4 (CD4) cell numbers to survival in AIDS Kaposi's sarcoma patients (Kaplan-Meier graph). (Reprinted with permission from Taylor J, Afrasiabi R, Fahey JL, et al: Prognostically significant classification of immune changes in AIDS with Kaposi's sarcoma. Blood 67:666–671, 1986.)

(Fig. 28–2). Only 30% of patients with fewer than 100 CD4 lymphocytes survived for 1 year. Other features associated with a negative impact on survival in various studies have included prior history of opportunistic infection,[110] bulky tumor,[110,113] the presence of constitutional symptoms,[110,113] and initial presentation that involves a mucosal surface or cutaneous site other than the lower extremities or the lymph nodes.[113]

Based on these known predictors of survival in patients with AIDS-associated KS, the Oncology Subcommittee of the National Institute of Health–sponsored AIDS Clinical Trials Group (ACTG) has proposed and is using a new staging classification, illustrated in Table 28–3.[88] This system takes into account tumor bulk, immune function, and the presence of other systemic illness, including history of opportunistic infection by the presence of constitutional symptoms. This staging system has recently been validated by comparing survival times among patients staged using this classification who participated in ACTG KS clinical trials between 1986 and 1994.[7]

Treatment

Because most patients do not die as a direct result of KS, it would seem unlikely that therapy directed toward this neoplasm would have a significant impact on survival. Although the data are retrospective, a review of 194 cases of KS by Volberding et al[171] suggests that this is, in fact, the case. There was no significant difference in survival time between the group of patients treated with chemotherapy (or alpha-interferon) and those who received no treatment.

Some patients with KS do require treatment.

TABLE 28–3. PROPOSED STAGING CLASSIFICATION FOR KAPOSI'S SARCOMA

Good Risk (0): All of the Following	Poor Risk (1): Any of the Following
Tumor (I)	
Confined to skin and/or lymph nodes and/or minimum oral disease*	Tumor-associated edema or ulceration
	Extensive oral Kaposi's sarcoma (KS) lesions
	Gastrointestinal KS lesions
	KS lesions in other nonnodal viscera
Immune System (I)	
CD4 cells ≥200/μl	CD4 cells <200/μl
Systemic Illness (S)	
No history of opportunistic infection (OI) or thrush	History of OI or thrush or both
No "B" symptoms†	B symptoms present
Karnofsky performance status ≥70	Karnofsky performance status <70
	Other HIV-related illness (e.g., neurologic disease, lymphoma)

Modified with permission from Krown SE, Metroka C, Wernz J: Kaposi's sarcoma in the acquired immune deficiency syndrome: A proposal for uniform evaluation, response, and staging criteria. J Clin Oncol 7:1201–1207, 1989.

* Minimum oral disease in nonnodular KS confined to the palate.

† B symptoms are unexplained fever, night sweats, >10% involuntary weight loss, or diarrhea persisting for more than 2 weeks.

Subgroups of patients must be defined in terms of whom treatment will benefit most. The primary goals of therapy for patients with KS are palliation of symptoms and cosmesis. Achievement of good cosmetic results may not only improve appearance but also significantly improve the patient's overall outlook.

Palliative therapy may be indicated in the following situations:

1. Painful or uncomfortable intraoral or pharyngeal lesions can interfere with eating or swallowing. Bulky KS can even result in airway compromise.

2. Lymphedema is a common complication of advanced KS. Because of its propensity for infiltrating lymphatic tissue, obstruction and edema formation can occur relatively early. The face and the lower extremities are the sites most commonly affected. Lower extremity edema can form as a result of bulky lymphadenopathy in the femoral, inguinal, or iliac regions, in the setting of confluent bulky cutaneous lesions, or even in the absence of bulky visible KS.

3. Painful or bulky lesions can occur at any site. Lesions involving the plantar surfaces of the feet may be particularly uncomfortable during ambulation.

4. Pulmonary KS is frequently symptomatic and can result in a variety of respiratory symptoms. This is becoming a more frequent complication of KS as patients survive for longer periods of time with the disease. Disease progression can be rapid, resulting in severe respiratory compromise and death.[42,75]

Another indication for therapy is rapidly progressive disease. Although it is impossible to prove benefit without a randomized trial, it is likely that, without treatment, such patients will rapidly develop either symptomatic disease requiring palliative therapy or cosmetically problematic disease.

Treatment options include a variety of local therapies, such as radiation, cryotherapy, and intralesional chemotherapy, as well as systemic therapy (e.g., chemotherapy, alpha-interferon). Systemic chemotherapy can result in subjective toxicities, myelosuppression, and immunosuppression, leaving the patient more susceptible to a variety of opportunistic infections. Thus, the use of systemic chemotherapy should be approached cautiously. Local forms of therapy should be selected whenever possible.

Local Therapy

RADIATION THERAPY. Radiation therapy has been the most frequently used local therapeutic modality. A single dose of 800 cGy or the equivalent fractionated dose can be highly effective in achieving local palliation.[14,67]

Radiation therapy is not appropriate for the patient with widespread symptomatic disease but is best suited for the patient with a single or a few locally symptomatic areas. It is highly effective in relieving facial edema and can be applied to a field encompassing the whole face. Generally, electron-beam therapy is used in treating the face. Radiation therapy has been frequently used, although less effectively, in the treatment of lower extremity edema.[67] In addition, larger facial lesions, painful lesions, or other unsightly cutaneous lesions can be treated with this modality as are intraoral and pharyngeal lesions. However, a high frequency of severe mucositis has been observed in the latter two groups of patients.[67]

INTRALESIONAL CHEMOTHERAPY. Small cutaneous lesions can be treated with intralesional chemotherapy for cosmetic purposes.[119] This is generally accomplished by intralesional injection of 0.01 mg of vinblastine in 0.1 ml sterile water using a tuberculin syringe. Repeated treatments may be necessary. A hyperpigmented area frequently remains after treatment.

CRYOTHERAPY. Cryotherapy using liquid nitrogen has been used successfully for the treatment of isolated small KS lesions.[161] This treatment modality is particularly useful for the treatment of cosmetically unsightly lesions.

PHOTODYNAMIC THERAPY. Phase I results of the use of photodynamic therapy using intravenously administered Photofrin 48 hours prior to exposure to 100 to 300 J/cm^2 of 630-nm light demonstrated that up to 68% of lesions exposed to 300 J/cm^2 showed evidence of partial response.[7] This therapeutic approach remains investigational at the present time but may be useful for small, cosmetically unsightly lesions.

Systemic Therapy

For the patient with more rapidly progressive disease or with advanced widespread symptomatic disease, systemic therapy may be most appropriate. Several antineoplastic agents used alone or in combination are active against KS (Table 28–4).

VINCRISTINE AND VINBLASTINE. Vincristine[108] and vinblastine[170] have been used commonly for systemic therapy in patients with HIV-associated KS because each is subjectively well tolerated and the incidence of serious toxicity is low. However, when administered on a weekly

TABLE 28–4. CHEMOTHERAPY IN AIDS—KAPOSI'S SARCOMA

Agents	Dose	Reported Response (%)	Reference
Vincristine	2 mg/week	20–59	108
Vinblastine	0.05–0.1 mg/kg/week	25–30	170
Etoposide	150 mg/m^2 IV qd for 3 days every 3–4 weeks, or 50 mg PO qd	75	92
Doxorubicin (Adriamycin)	20 mg/m^2 every other week	53	44
Bleomycin	10–15 U/m^2 every 2 weeks		
Liposomal doxorubicin	20 mg/m^2 every 2–3 weeks	30–95	61,64F
Liposomal daunorubicin	40 mg/m^2 every 2–3 weeks	30–95	134,150E
Taxol	135 mg/m^2 every 2–3 weeks or 100 mg/m^2 every 2 weeks	53	43,68
Combination Chemotherapy			
Vincristine	2 mg	45	74
plus vinblastine	0.1 mg/kg (alternate weeks)		
Vincristine	2 mg	100	42
plus bleomycin	10 mg/m^2 (every 14 days)		
Doxorubicin	10–20 mg/m^2	87	44
plus bleomycin	10 mg/m^2		
plus vincristine	2 mg (every 14 days)		

basis, vinblastine can cause significant myelosuppression, necessitating dose reduction, and vincristine can cause significant peripheral neuropathy. The cumulative toxicities of each of these drugs can be reduced by administering each drug on an alternate-week basis.[74]

ETOPOSIDE (VP16). Etoposide also is an active agent in treating KS.[92] The frequent occurrence of alopecia in patients treated with etoposide makes it a poor choice for patients being treated primarily for cosmetic purposes. However, the more recent availability of an oral formulation of etoposide makes this an attractive agent for systemic therapy in other situations. When administered orally, etoposide is 50% bioavailable. Therefore, an appropriate oral dose is generally twice the standard IV dose. The use of daily administration of low-dose oral etoposide is under study.

DOXORUBICIN (ADRIAMYCIN). Doxorubicin may be the most active single agent against HIV-associated KS[44] and may be useful in the management of patients with more advanced disease or in those in whom prior therapy has failed to produce a response. A randomized trial has suggested that the combination regimen of doxorubicin (Adriamycin), bleomycin, and vincristine (ABV) is more efficacious against KS than doxorubicin used as a single agent.[44] This regimen has been used successfully in patients with widespread, advanced KS, including those with peripheral edema and pulmonary involvement.[42,171] It is not unusual to see rapid improvement in peripheral edema or in respiratory symptoms after administration of this combination. In one study, the overall response rate to ABV in pulmonary KS was 60%.[42] The major short-term toxicity associated with doxorubicin is myelosuppression, which may require periodic dose reductions or the use of a myeloid growth factor.

The combination of vincristine and bleomycin has significant antitumor activity and may be especially useful for those patients with granulocytopenia, who are likely to be intolerant of more myelosuppressive regimens.[42,48,50,108]

Phase I and II studies have shown the liposome-encapsulated anthracyclines, doxorubicin and daunorubicin, to be a promising new approach to the administration of chemotherapy to individuals with KS. In one trial, intralesional concentrations of doxorubicin after administration of the liposome-encapsulated doxorubicin were shown to be 5 to 11 times the levels achieved after administration of the non-liposome-encapsulated agent.[121] Subsequent phase II trials with both liposome-encapsulated daunorubicin and doxorubicin have demonstrated response rates of 30% to 100% in patients treated with the single agents.[51,134] Most of the treated individuals had advanced KS with visceral involvement and were refractory to previous chemotherapy. Significant responses have also been observed in patients previously unresponsive to doxorubicin-containing combination chemotherapy regimens.[61,134] The results of a phase III clinical trial in which liposomal doxorubicin was compared to the standard ABV regimen have been reported.[120] This trial demonstrated that liposome-encapsulated doxorubicin is associated with a lower incidence of toxicities such as nausea, fatigue, and alopecia. Mild mucositis appears to occur more commonly with liposomal doxorubicin than with the non-liposome-encapsulated product, and neutropenia occurs as frequently with the liposomal drugs as with the standard combination regimen. In this study, liposomal doxorubicin was associated with a significantly higher response rate than ABV when used as initial therapy.[120] Both liposomal agents have received recent Food and Drug administration approval and are currently available for use in patients with KS.

Clinical trials of the drug paclitaxel (taxol) have demonstrated significant antitumor activity in patients with both previously untreated[43] and refractory KS.[43,144] Response rates are over 50% regardless of prior therapy. Outstanding clinical responses have been seen in patients with advanced refractory symptomatic disease. The drug has been well tolerated, with generally only mild toxicities reported. Paclitaxel is significantly myelosuppressive, and most patients in these trials have required adjunctive therapy with a myeloid colony-stimulating factor (CSF).

The recent availability of the myeloid growth factors granulocyte colony-stimulating factor (G-CSF) and granulocyte-macrophage colony-stimulating factor (GM-CSF) may make it possible to administer myelosuppressive chemotherapy to individuals in whom this may not have been possible in the past. Because many individuals with advanced KS have poor myeloid reserve, these agents can be valuable adjuncts to chemotherapy. For most individuals with KS, the use of a CSF is unnecessary. The use of a relatively nonmyelosuppressive regimen, such as vincristine with bleomycin, will be adequate therapy for many patients. At San Francisco General Hospital, we usually reserve the use of myeloid growth factors for those patients who are severely symptomatic from their KS and who, in our opinion, require the use of an anthracycline as a part of their chemotherapeutic regimen and who have a neutrophil count of less than 1500/mm³ before initiating therapy. Although no specific guidelines exist for administrations of CSFs in this setting, we generally

begin administration 1 to 3 days following the chemotherapy. In our experience, a dose of 300 μg (5 μg/kg) administered on alternate days for a total of five doses often is adequate. However, therapy must be individualized, and frequent neutrophil counts should be made during the first cycle of therapy to establish the optimal dosage regimen.

INTERFERON. Alpha-interferon is an attractive agent for use in the treatment of AIDS-associated KS because it possesses both antiproliferative[86] and apparent anti-HIV activity.[84,91] Alpha-interferon used as a single agent in the treatment of HIV-associated KS has significant antitumor activity, as demonstrated in a large number of clinical trials.[24,53,86,136,139,172,173] The importance of dose intensity in the administration of alpha-interferon is demonstrated in Table 28–5. These data, compiled from several institutions,[53,136,139,173] demonstrate that high doses (>20 million units/m²) of alpha-interferon are more effective in inducing antitumor responses than are lower doses. Several studies have demonstrated that patients with better immune function (higher CD4 cell counts), without a prior history of opportunistic infection and without B symptoms, are more likely to respond to alpha-interferon than those whose cellular immune function is more compromised and who have had a prior opportunistic infection and are symptomatic.[86,168]

Despite the frequency of objective responses and reports of long disease-free remissions, the use of alpha-interferon in high doses as a single agent has been limited by its toxicity. With chronic administration, many patients experience a flu-like syndrome, with low-grade fever, anorexia, malaise, myalgias, and weight loss. Al-

TABLE 28–5. ALPHA-INTERFERON IN AIDS-RELATED KAPOSI'S SARCOMA: EFFICACY OF LOW-DOSE VS HIGH-DOSE THERAPY

Response	Low Dose (<20 Million U/m²), n = 65	High Dose (≥20 Million U/m²), n = 105
Complete	1 (2%)	18 (17%)
Partial	3 (5%)	27 (26%)
Minor or stable	13 (20%)	17 (16%)
Progression	48 (74%)	43 (41%)

Data compiled from published studies at San Francisco General Hospital, the University of California at Los Angeles, Memorial Sloan-Kettering Cancer Center, the M.D. Anderson Hospital and Tumor Institute, and the National Cancer Institute.

though many patients develop tachyphylaxis to these symptoms during the first several weeks of treatment, these symptoms may persist and become sufficiently disabling to warrant either dosage reduction or discontinuation of the agent.

Most patients who go on to have significant antitumor response usually show evidence of tumor regression after 4 to 8 weeks of high-dose treatment. Often 6 or more months of therapy are required to achieve maximum tumor regression. Because tumor recurrence is usual after discontinuation of treatment, it is suggested that alpha-interferon therapy be maintained for as long as the antitumor response persists.

Alpha-Interferon and Nucleoside Analogs

The use of combinations of interferon and nucleoside analogs investigated in several phase I and II trials is underway, as is continuing investigation in large clinical trials. From the standpoint of antiretroviral therapy the combination of alpha-interferon with a nucleoside analog is an attractive one, because each of these agents appears to inhibit HIV-1 replication at a different stage of the viral life cycle, and the combination has shown synergistic in vitro inhibition of HIV-1 replication.[62] Although the nucleoside analogs have failed to show any significant antitumor activity in patients with KS when used as single agents,[90] the use of these agents is associated with improvement in immune function, a factor clearly associated with responsiveness of KS to interferon. Furthermore, the use of alpha-interferon is not associated with the decline in immune function normally associated with the use of standard cytotoxic chemotherapeutic agents.

The results of three clinical trials investigating the use of combination alpha-interferon with zidovudine are shown in Table 28–6. It appears that daily 600-mg doses of zidovudine can be combined safely with alpha-interferon doses of 4 to 18 million units daily. The most common dose-limiting toxicity has been neu-

tropenia. Response rates of over 40% have been observed in all these trials and apparently are better at all levels of immune function when the results of treatment with these two agents are compared with historical data for the use of single-agent alpha-interferon. These response rates are particularly striking in view of the fact that alpha-interferon doses used in these trials were significantly lower than those known to have single-agent antitumor activity. The ability to use these lower doses of alpha-interferon may significantly reduce the incidence of subjective toxicities that frequently are dose limiting in patients treated with high-dose single-agent alpha-interferon.

Because the most common dose-limiting toxicity of the combination of alpha-interferon and zidovudine is neutropenia, two clinical trials have explored the addition of GM-CSF to this regimen.[89,145] Scadden et al[145] found that GM-CSF administered at a dosage of 125 $\mu g/m^2$ reversed neutropenia in patients whose neutrophil counts fell to less than 1000/mm^3 while on the drug combination. Krown et al[89] titrated the dose of GM-CSF to maintain neutrophil counts between 1000 and 5000/mm^3 in patients receiving 1200 mg zidovudine and 5, 10, or 20 million units of alpha-interferon daily. On average, a dose of only 1.25 $\mu g/kg/day$ was sufficient to maintain the neutrophil count within this range.

Because the addition of a CSF to the combination of alpha-interferon and zidovudine adds an additional expense of a potentially toxic agent, it would seem more appropriate to combine alpha-interferon with other relatively nonmyelosuppressive antiretroviral agents. An ongoing ACTG clinical trial is investigating combinations of alpha-interferon with didanosine without a CSF. Therapy appears to be well tolerated, and antitumor responses have been seen in both arms of the study, including those patients receiving alpha-interferon doses as low as 1 million units/day (ACTG 206). Other investigators have also documented responses with

TABLE 28–6. TRIALS OF ALPHA-INTERFERON WITH ZIDOVUDINE FOR KAPOSI'S SARCOMA

Alpha-Interferon	Alpha-Interferon Doses or Range	Zidovudine Doses (mg q4h)	Complete or Partial Response Total (%)	Reference
α-2A or α-nl	4, 5, 9, 18 million	100 or 200	17/37 (46)	87
α-2 or α-nl	9, 18, 27 million	100 or 200	20/43 (47)	30
α-nl	<5 to >25	50, 100, or 250	11/26 (42)	83
TOTAL			48/108 (45)	

combinations of antiretroviral therapy and a 1-million-unit dose of alpha-interferon.[152] It is unclear whether response rates with this very low dose are comparable to those seen with somewhat higher interferon dosages.

Appropriate candidates for therapy with alpha-interferon and antiretrovirals include those patients with relatively intact immune function (CD4 count not much below $200/mm^3$) whose KS is not significantly symptomatic, given that tumor regression may not be observed for up to 8 weeks after initiation of therapy. At San Francisco General Hospital, we generally begin patients on an alpha-interferon dose of 5 million units/day administered by subcutaneous injection 5 days/week. Patients are instructed in self-administration of their medication. Any antiretroviral agent or combination of agents is acceptable to use concurrently with interferon; however, nonmyelosuppressive agents are preferable (excluding zidovudine) so as to avoid overlapping myelosuppression with alpha-interferon.

Antiretroviral Agents

A variety of antiretroviral agents are currently available for the management of HIV disease. These may include the nucleoside analogs (zidovudine, didanosine, zalcitabine, stavudine, and lamivudine); nonnucleoside reverse transcriptase inhibitors (nevarapine, delavridine); and protease inhibitors (ritonavir, saquinavir and indinavir). The effect of concurrent administration of antiviral therapy with chemotherapy on HIV replication and disease activity is not known. However, because viral replication undoubtedly continues in the presence of chemotherapeutic agents and because these agents are immunosuppressive, it is suggested that antiviral therapy be continued or instituted while chemotherapy is being administered. Any agent or combination of antiviral agents are acceptable; however, it is recommended that zidovudine not be administered because of the potential for overlapping myelosuppression in the presence of myelosuppressive chemotherapeutic agents.

Therapeutic Recommendations

Table 28–7 summarizes the recommendations for treatment of patients with AIDS-associated KS. Patients with minimal disease (<25 cutaneous lesions), unless cosmetically unsightly or in pain, are generally not candidates for KS-directed therapy. They may benefit from antiretroviral therapy or from participation in

TABLE 28–7. KAPOSI'S SARCOMA: RECOMMENDATIONS FOR TREATMENT

Minimal disease	
Stable or slowly progressive	1. Observation only 2. Investigational agents 3. Antivirals with or without alpha-interferon
Rapidly progressive	1. Vincristine and vinblastine 2. Alpha-interferon with or without antivirals
Widespread symptomatic	1. Liposomal doxorubicin, daunorubicin 2. Adriamycin, bleomycin, vincristine (ABV)
Locally symptomatic	1. Radiotherapy 2. Laser (oral lesions)
Local cosmesis	1. Intralesional chemotherapy 2. Radiotherapy 3. Cryotherapy 4. Photodynamic therapy
Cytopenic patients	1. Vincristine *and/or* 2. Bleomycin

clinical trials of investigational agents. Systemic therapy is recommended for patients with asymptomatic but rapidly progressive disease or for patients with widespread symptomatic disease.

The doxorubicin-containing regimens or single-agent liposomal anthracylenes generally should be reserved for patients with more advanced disease or patients with previously unsuccessful therapy. Vincristine with or without bleomycin may benefit those patients with cytopenias. Alternatively, myeloid growth factors may be used to reduce myelotoxicity. Localized therapy, generally radiation, can palliate locally symptomatic disease. Local cosmetic problems can be treated successfully with radiation therapy, intralesional chemotherapy, or cryotherapy. Alpha-interferon as a single agent is best reserved for those individuals with CD4 lymphocyte counts of less than $200/mm^3$, but for most patients, the high doses required will prove too toxic. The use of low doses of alpha-interferon with a nucleoside analog or combination of nonmyelosuppressive antiretroviral agents makes this a much more tolerable treatment approach to the patient with systemic KS.

NON-HODGKIN'S LYMPHOMA

The non-Hodgkin's lymphomas (NHLs) are a heterogeneous group of malignancies. Their biologic behavior ranges from indolent, requiring no therapy, to aggressive with few long-term survivors. Approximately 70% of NHLs originate in B cells, and another 20% derive from T cells.

In the most commonly used classification system for the NHLs,[118] these malignancies are divided into three major categories, low grade, intermediate grade, and high grade, according to pathologic characteristics of involved lymph nodes and morphologic criteria of the lymphoma cells.

The first cases of NHL in homosexual men were reported in 1982,[176] and increasing numbers of cases have been reported since that time. The finding of an intermediate or high-grade B-cell NHL in an HIV-infected individual constitutes an AIDS diagnosis as defined by the CDC.[12] Advanced extranodal disease is commonly found at presentation, and median survival times have been short.

Epidemiology

The incidence of NHL is increased markedly in individuals with impaired cell-mediated immunity.[37,70] The best described of these groups is immunosuppressed allograft recipients, a group in which the incidence of NHL is 30 to 50 times that of the general population.[70,126,127] Similarly, Harnly et al[60] have demonstrated a statistically significant increase in the incidence of NHL among never-married men ages 25 to 44 years in San Francisco in the years 1980 to 1985. The increase in census tracts with a high incidence of AIDS was greater than the increase in other San Francisco census tracts. In 1985, the incidence of NHL was five times greater than the rate in 1980. However, increases in incidence rates were not observed for other malignancies. Similar trends have been observed for New York City.[85]

Despite suggestions that the incidence of NHL in HIV-infected individuals receiving long-term antiretroviral therapy may be as high as 29% at 36 months, in a small group of patients with HIV disease, data do not indicate a rise in incidence out of proportion to the rising incidence of new AIDS diagnoses.[131] In the study by Pluda et al,[131] a high incidence of NHL was seen in patients receiving either zidovudine or dideoxyinosine. Most had CD4 lymphocyte counts of less than 50/mm^3, and most developed primary central nervous system (CNS) lymphoma. There are indications, however, that as treatment for the underlying HIV disease becomes more successful and as patients survive for longer periods of time without opportunistic infections, more cases of lymphoma will appear in this patient population. It was estimated that for 1992 HIV-associated NHL would account for 8% to 27% of all NHL diagnosed in the United States.[38] A large prospective observational study indicates an incidence of approximately 1.6% per year that is constant over time in a population with advanced HIV infection treated with zidovudine.[112] Recent data indicate a continuing rise in the prevalence of NHL among patients dying with HIV disease.[148]

Pathogenesis/Etiology

The etiology of NHL in patients with HIV infection is not known. In immunosuppressed allograft recipients, molecular data have implicated Epstein-Barr virus (EBV) as a potential causative agent in the development of NHL. Several studies have documented the presence of EBV DNA sequences in the vast majority of B-cell lymphomas from transplant recipients.[58,126,151] The majority of lymphomas described in this population have been classified as immunoblastic lymphomas. However, in this patient population, aggressive lymphoproliferative processes also have been described that apparently are polyclonal by both immunologic and morphologic criteria.[36,58,59] In some of these cases, a typical monoclonal lymphoma has subsequently developed.[57]

Although the finding of chromosome 8;14 translocations, like those seen with Burkitt's lymphoma, and the finding of EBV nuclear antigen in some tumors[6,13,55,129] suggested that EBV might also be implicated in the etiology of HIV-associated lymphomas, more recent observations indicate that EBV DNA sequences are present in a minority of patients with HIV-associated lymphoma.[72,104,154,159] However, there is also information suggesting that EBV DNA sequences may be present in a majority of primary CNS lymphomas in patients with HIV infection.[101,104] Other viruses have been implicated in the pathogenesis of specific subcategories of HIV-associated NHL. The observation of clonally integrated HIV genome in either the malignant cells themselves or tumor-associated macrophages within certain HIV-associated T-cell lymphomas has raised the possibility of a more direct role for HIV in lymphomagenesis in a small number of cases.[64,153] In addition, recent laboratory studies have identified HHV8 sequences associated with HIV-associated body cavity lymphomas.[114] In fact, viruses such as HIV or HHV8, by infecting macrophages, may act in a nonspecific way to enhance cytokine expression. Cytokine overexpression may then drive polyclonal B-cell proliferation.

Evaluation of immunoglobulin gene rearrangements using Southern blot hybridization techniques demonstrates that, although many of the B-cell tumors observed in this patient population have clonal immunoglobulin gene rearrangements, clonal rearrangements are not observed in other lymphomas.[21,104,154,158] These tumors may represent polyclonal processes not unlike those observed in allograft recipients.[59]

Emilie et al[26] recently demonstrated high levels of the cytokine IL-6 associated with immunoblastic lymphoma. Others have identified overexpression of both IL-6 and IL-10 in some HIV-NHLs (M. G. McGrath, et al, unpublished data, 1992), suggesting the possibility that a cytokine-driven process may be involved in pathogenesis.

This heterogeneity of molecular characteristics, including clonality and the presence or absence of EBV, suggests that lymphomagenesis may occur through several different mechanisms. Although EBV may be involved in the pathogenesis of some HIV-associated lymphomas, other viruses, spontaneous genetic changes, cytokines, or even the underlying immune disregulation itself may give rise to NHL.

Clinical Characteristics

Like the molecular features of the lymphomas themselves, the individuals with HIV-associated NHL are also a heterogeneous group. Individuals with HIV-associated NHL are not all severely immunocompromised. Patients seen at San Francisco General Hospital with peripheral (as opposed to primary CNS) NHL have exhibited a wide range of CD4 lymphocyte counts, with a mean value of $200/mm^3$ ($n = 95$). Over one third of these individuals had CD4 lymphocyte counts above $200/mm^3$. NHL was the initial AIDS-defining diagnosis in 70%. Patients with primary CNS lymphoma represent a very different patient population. These individuals are almost universally severely immunocompromised, with CD4 lymphocyte counts below $50/mm^3$.[95]

The vast majority of the NHLs observed in patients with HIV infection are classified as B-cell malignancies.[94,174] A small number of NHLs of other histologic and immunologic subtypes have been observed, including T-cell lymphoma[72,116,133] and others of uncertain lineage.[82] Of 327 cases reported in the literature from five centers, 73% of the lymphomas were classified as high grade, 24% as intermediate grade, and 3% as low grade.[4,45,72,81,98,174] Most B-cell lymphomas in these individuals are classified as diffuse large-cell tumors of either intermediate-grade type or the high-grade immunoblastic type (Color Plate II*G*). In addition, approximately one third of patients have tumors of the high-grade, small, noncleaved cell variety.

Widespread disease involving extranodal sites is the hallmark of AIDS-associated lymphoma at the time of diagnosis. Ziegler et al[174] reported that 95% of patients had evidence of extranodal disease, 42% of patients had CNS disease, and 33% had bone marrow involvement. In a series of 89 patients diagnosed at New York University, 87% had extranodal disease at presentation.[81] The most common sites of disease included the GI tract, CNS, bone marrow, and liver. At San Francisco General Hospital, two thirds of the patients had stage IV disease, and 31% had extranodal disease alone, with no identifiable site of nodal disease.

As observed in other immunosuppressed patients with NHL, unusual extralymphatic presentations are common. Sites of disease have included the rectum,[9] heart and pericardium,[1,56] and common bile ducts.[77] GI involvement has been reported in up to 27% of individuals with lymphoma,[34] and virtually any site in the GI tract or hepatobiliary tree can be involved. In the San Francisco General Hospital series, other unusual sites of disease included subcutaneous and soft tissue, epidural space, appendix, gingiva, parotid gland, and paranasal sinus.[72]

NHL confined to the CNS frequently has been reported in association with HIV infection.[2,31,46,156] The most common presenting symptoms have been confusion, lethargy, and memory loss. Other symptoms have included hemiparesis, aphasia, seizures, cranial nerve palsies, and headache. Single or multiple discrete contrast-enhancing lesions are the most common findings on computed tomographic (CT) or magnetic resonance imaging (MRI) scans of the brain. The radiographic appearance of primary CNS lymphoma is generally not easily distinguished from that of toxoplasmosis.

Solitary lesions are observed in approximately 21% of MRI scans from individuals with toxoplasmosis, and therefore solitary lesions are somewhat more likely to be associated with lymphoma. However, 50% of CNS lymphomas present as multiple lesions, creating an even more difficult diagnostic dilemma.[15]

Patients with neurologic symptoms should be evaluated promptly with CT or MRI scans of the brain. Lumbar puncture should be performed if not contraindicated by the CT findings. A serum specimen from patients with focal lesions should be sent for cryptococcal antigen and toxoplasma titers. Because toxoplasmosis is infrequent in individuals with negative *Toxoplasma* serologies,[52,132] brain biopsy should be performed in a timely fashion in this group of patients. Individuals with focal intracerebral lesions and positive serologic studies for *Toxoplasma* typically are started on antitoxoplasma therapy and observed closely for signs of improvement or deterioration.

Treatment and Prognosis

The use of multiagent chemotherapeutic regimens for the treatment of intermediate and high-grade NHL in the non–HIV-infected individual has resulted in a dramatic improvement in prognosis for this group.[23] A complete response rate as high as 86% and long-term survival rates as high as 65% have been reported in patients treated for aggressive, large-cell lymphomas.[16]

In HIV-infected individuals, however, the use of similar chemotherapeutic regimens has not resulted in as favorable an outcome (Table 28–8). Complete response rates are lower than the corresponding rates in the non–HIV-infected population, and these responses are usually of short duration. In a retrospective review by Ziegler et al[174] of patients treated at multiple institutions, 53% of 66 patients who could be evaluated achieved complete response to combination chemotherapy. However, 54% of the complete responders subsequently relapsed. In a series of patients from San Francisco General Hospital, 54% of 59 patients who could be evaluated and who were treated with a variety of combinations of chemotherapeutic regimens had complete responses.[72] Twenty-three percent of these complete responders subsequently relapsed (Fig. 28–3).

Morphologic subtype appeared to predict response to chemotherapy in one series of patients reported from New York University.[81] The best complete response rate was reported for those patients classified as having a large, noncleaved cell lymphoma (52%), whereas those having a small, noncleaved cell and immunoblastic lymphoma had response rates of 26% and 21%, respectively. One group has reported a 64% complete response rate in a series of 11 patients treated with the methotrexate, doxorubicin, cyclophosphamide, vincristine, prednisone, and bleomycin (MACOP-B) regimen.[4] However, it cannot be determined from this small number of patients whether this represents significant improvement in the complete response rate over that observed in other series of patients.

TABLE 28–8. RESPONSE TO CHEMOTHERAPY AND SURVIVAL TIMES IN HIV-ASSOCIATED NON-HODGKIN'S LYMPHOMA

Institution	No of Patients	Treatment Regimen	Complete Response (%)	Median Survival Time (mo)	Reference
USC	22	m-BACOD and others	45	NA	45
NYU	83	Various	33	5.0	81
UCSF	65	Various	54	5.5	72
MSKCC	30	Various	56	6.0	98
Pacific Medical Center	31	CHOP and MACOP-B	39	7.0	4
MultiCenter	66	Various	53	NA	174
ACTG	36	m-BACOD	42	NA	96
Italian Cooperative Group	72	Various	35	4.0	71

NA, not applicable; USC, University of Southern California; NYU, New York University; UCSF, University of California, San Francisco; MSKCC, Memorial Sloan-Kettering Cancer Institute; ACTG, AIDS Clinical Trial Group, National Institutes of Health; Multicenter: UCSF, USC, NY Hospital/Cornell, University of Texas/M.D. Anderson, NYU/Kaplan Cancer Center, and MSKCC; m-BACOD, methotrexate, bleomycin, doxorubicin, cyclophosphamide, vincristine, and dexamethasone; CHOP, cyclophosphamide, doxorubicin, vincristine, and prednisone; MACOP-B, methotrexate, doxorubicin, cyclophosphamide, vincristine, prednisone, and bleomycin.

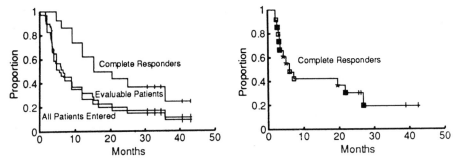

FIGURE 28–3. *Left,* Overall survival in patients with AIDS-related lymphoma. Tick marks indicate patients who are alive at the given time interval. *Right,* Event-free survival in 16 complete responders. Tick marks indicate patients who are still alive in continuous complete remission; dark boxes, development of intercurrent HIV-related illness; open boxes, development of relapse of lymphoma; asterisks, death from unknown cause. Event-free survival is taken from the time of achievement of complete remission to the time of relapse, HIV-related illness, or death. (Reprinted with permission from Levine AM, Wernz JC, Kaplan L, et al: Low-dose chemotherapy with central nervous system prophylaxis and zidovudine maintenance in AIDS-related lymphoma. JAMA 266:84–88, 1991. Copyright 1991 American Medical Association.)

Survival times from a number of large series of patients reported in the literature are shown in Table 28–8. Median survival times in these groups range from 4 to 7 months. In the series of 23 patients who received chemotherapy at the Pacific Medical Center, the median survival time was 20 months in those patients achieving complete response to therapy.[4]

Although overall survival times in patients with AIDS-associated NHL are disappointing, subgroups of patients can be identified in which the therapeutic outcome is significantly better than for other groups of patients. Morphologic subtypes predictive of response to therapy in patients treated at New York University were also predictive of survival in this same series.[81] Patients with intermediate-grade large-cell lym-

phoma had the longest median survival time (7.5 months), those with small, noncleaved cell lymphoma had a median survival time of 5.5 months, and those with immunoblastic lymphoma had a median survival time of only 2 months.

In the San Francisco General Hospital series, median survival time for all patients receiving chemotherapy ($n = 65$) was only 5.5 months. However, life-table analysis for subgroups within this population illustrates the importance of prognostic features (Table 28–9). Those features identified as being predictive of significantly improved survival time included an absolute CD4+ lymphocyte count greater than 100/mm^3, absence of a prior AIDS diagnosis, Karnofsky performance score of 70% or greater, and the absence of an extranodal site of disease. Multivariate analysis of pretreatment characteristics from patients enrolled in a large, multicenter, randomized trial (192 patients) demonstrated the following factors to be associated with shortened survival: absolute CD4 count less than 100, stage III/IV disease, age greater than 35, and IV drug use.[157]

Evaluation of newly diagnosed patients for these prognostic features may help determine how to approach therapy in the individual with this disease. The patient without a prior AIDS diagnosis whose immune function is relatively good is a much better candidate for therapy than is a patient whose diagnosis of lymphoma comes after a history of multiple opportunistic infections. Because many patients will fall between these extremes, these prognostic characteristics can serve only as rough guidelines in determining which patients to treat.

TABLE 28–9. PREDICTORS OF SURVIVAL IN CHEMOTHERAPY-TREATED HIV-ASSOCIATED NON-HODGKIN'S LYMPHOMA ($n = 65$)

Characteristics	Median Survival Time	p Value
CD4 count		0.01
<100/mm^3	4.1	
>100/mm^3	24	
Prior AIDS		0.0001
Yes	2.2	
No	8.3	
Karnofsky performance scale		0.03
<70%	3.8	
≥70%	6.8	
Extranodal disease		0.01
Yes	4.2	
No	12.2	

What the most appropriate therapeutic regimen will be for a given patient also must be individualized, because there is no known best regimen. Poor bone marrow reserve and the occurrence of opportunistic infections often result in dose reductions and delays in therapy. In addition, the risk of further immunosuppression when treating HIV-infected patients with aggressive combination chemotherapy must be considered.

Contrary to the belief that more intensive chemotherapy is associated with improved clinical outcome in non–HIV-associated lymphoma, retrospective data from two centers have suggested that, in HIV-infected individuals with NHL, survival may be improved in those treated with less aggressive regimens. Survival data from the San Francisco General Hospital cohort of chemotherapy-treated patients with NHL revealed that patients receiving chemotherapy regimens containing 1 g/m^2 or more of cyclophosphamide had a median survival time of only 4.6 months compared to those treated with regimens containing less than 1 g/m^2 of cyclophosphamide, who had a median survival time of 12.2 months ($p = 0.02$).[72] Similarly, in a study of nine patients treated with a novel, more aggressive chemotherapeutic regimen consisting of high-dose cytosine arabinoside, L-asparaginase, vincristine, prednisone, cyclophosphamide (high dose), methotrexate, and leucovorin, only three patients achieved complete remission.[45] This intesive regimen was associated with a high risk of mortality caused by opportunistic infection.

Two different approaches to therapy have been studied and reported. In the first of these clinical trials, 35 patients with HIV-associated NHL and a mean CD4 lymphocyte count of 150/mm^3 were treated with a modification of the standard methotrexate, bleomycin, doxorubicin, cyclophosphamide, vincristine, and dexamethasone (m-BACOD) regimen. Instead of administering cyclophosphamide at 600 mg/m^2 and doxorubicin at 45 mg/m^2, these two agents were administered at 300 mg/m^2 and 25 mg/m^2, respectively. All patients received CNS prophylaxis and zidovudine maintenance after the completion of chemotherapy. Complete remission was observed in 16 of 35 individuals (46%), and the median survival time for the 35 patients who could be evaluated was 6.5 months. These results are not significantly different from those reported previously using a variety of more standard chemotherapeutic regimens. However, these results were achieved at the expense of

significantly less hematologic toxicity, with only 10% of chemotherapeutic cycles complicated by an absolute neutrophil count of less than 500/mm^3. Fifteen cycles (12%) were delayed because of neutropenia. The survival curves shown in Figure 28–3 demonstrate that durable, complete remissions were achieved in some individuals, with a median survival time of 15 months in the 16 complete responders. It is noteworthy, however, that when a similar regimen was used in a group of individuals with a mean CD4 count of 35/mm^3,[166] only 19% achieved complete remission and the median survival was only 3 months. These observations again point out the strong relationship between immune function and clinical outcome.

In a second approach to therapy, more standard doses of cyclophosphamide, doxorubicin, vincristine, and prednisone (CHOP) chemotherapy were used in a trial in which patients receiving chemotherapy were randomized either to receive concurrent therapy with GM-CSF or no further adjunctive treatment.[76] Table 28–10 demonstrates that individuals receiving GM-CSF had significantly higher mean nadir of absolute neutrophil counts and a significantly shorter duration of life-threatening neutropenia compared with those in the control group. As a result, those patients who received GM-CSF spent a mean time of 5.9 days in the hospital for febrile neutropenic episodes through the course of their treatment, compared with a mean of 18.6 days in the control group. This small clinical trial was not designed to evaluate response or survival, but it clearly demonstrated that one of the most significant morbidities associated with chemotherapy in this patient population can be reduced with the adjunctive use of a myeloid growth factor.

A French-Italian trial indicates that an aggressive, multiagent chemotherapy regimen can be tolerated by patients with good immune function (CD4 count >200/mm^3).[49] In this study, 140 patients received the aggressive LNH84 regimen. Treatment was associated with a complete remission rate of 63% and median survival of 9 months. It is more likely, however, that these results simply reflect the favorable outcome associated with good immune function rather than an advance in chemotherapy.

The ACTG 142 study was a large, multicenter, randomized clinical trial designed to directly address the question of the importance of chemotherapy dose intensity in determining clinical outcome of treatment for HIV-associated NHL. In this study, 198 patients were

TABLE 28–10. HEMATOLOGIC VARIABLES IN PATIENTS RECEIVING rGM-CSF VS CONTROL

	Treatment Group				
	Control ($n = 10$)		r-GM-CSF ($n = 11$)		
	No.	*(Range)*	*No.*	*(Range)*	*p*
Total number of chemotherapy cycles	42		41		
Nadir of absolute neutrophil count (ANC), mean (range)	0.360	(0–1.90)	0.886	(0–4.70)	0.009
Days ANC <0.5 × 10^9/l, mean (range)	5.0	(0–26)	1.3	(0–12)	0.02
Nadir platelet count, † mean (range)	129	(16–302)	106	(13–210)	0.1
Peak eosinophil count, † mean (range)	0.105	(0–0.60)	1.37	(0–5.70)	0.001

Reprinted with permission from Kaplan LD, Kahn JO, Crowe S, et al: Clinical and virologic effects of recombinant human granulocyte-macrophage colony-stimulating factor in patients receiving chemotherapy for human immunodeficiency virus-associated non-Hodgkin's lymphoma: Results of a randomized trial. J Clin Oncol 9:929–940, 1991.
  † Expressed as cells × 10^9/l.

randomized to receive either standard-dose m-BACOD chemotherapy with adjunctive administration of GM-CSF or the same low-dose m-BACOD regimen described earlier with GM-CSF administered only as required for management of neutropenia.[79] The results of this trial demonstrated no significant difference in response rate or survival time; the complete response rate was approximately 50% and median survival was approximately 8 months in each of the two treatment arms. However, toxicity was more severe in those patients randomized to standard-dose therapy, particularly with respect to the occurrence of grade IV neutropenia. Survival differences were not even observed for those patients with CD4 counts above 100/mm³, suggesting that most individuals with HIV-associated NHL should be treated with a low-dose chemotherapeutic regimen.

It is clear that, ultimately, variations in standard cytotoxic regimens will probably not have a major impact on survival. In the presence of the underlying immunodeficiency state, more novel approaches using nonmyelosuppressive and nonimmunosuppressive treatment modalities, either alone or as an adjunct to cytotoxic therapy, are needed. Clinical trials are currently evaluating the use of monoclonal immunotoxins directed toward cell surface determinants that are unique to HIV-associated NHLs. It is hoped that, as we continue to learn more about the biology of the HIV-associated lymphomas, we can develop more rational and effective treatment modalities that take advantage of the unique molecular characteristics of these tumors.

Treatment of Primary Central Nervous System Lymphoma

Primary CNS lymphoma has been particularly difficult to treat. Many cases have been diagnosed at autopsy,[174] and those occurring antemortem often have been in patients who had advanced immunodeficiency and had suffered multiple previous bouts of opportunistic infections.[2]

In the largest published series of treated patients reported in the literature, Baumgartner et al[2] observed that 76% of 29 patients treated with 4000 cGy of whole-brain radiation therapy showed evidence of significant clinical improvement, and 69% demonstrated complete or partial radiographic response. Similar results have been reported in smaller series from other institutions. In a series reported by Formenti et al,[31] complete responses to cranial irradiation occurred in 6 of the 10 patients. Despite this good response rate, survival times remain short, with median survival time for treated patients reported as between 2 and 5 months.[2,31] In patients with CNS lymphoma, opportunistic infection has been the most common cause of death.[2,31] In Formenti's series,[31] 50% of the patients died of opportunistic infection, and only two died of recurrent lymphoma. In Baumgartner's series,[2] of those patients undergoing postmortem examination, the only patient who died as a result of uncontrolled lymphoma developed a site of disease outside of the radiation portal in the cervical spinal cord. However, in a University of California at San Francisco series of 56 patients with HIV-associated primary CNS lymphoma, 29 of whom received radiation therapy, CNS lymphoma was the most commonly documented cause of death (63%), with only 21% dying of opportunistic infection.

Because most CNS lymphoma patients have severe immunodeficiency, they are highly susceptible to a variety of opportunistic infections. In addition, at least 20% do not respond to therapeutic intervention directed at the CNS lymphoma. Progress in the management of this disease will therefore depend on advances in the management of both the neoplastic disease and the underlying HIV infection. Protocols are currently in progress to evaluate the effect of the addition of combination chemotherapy to whole-brain irradiation in the management of this disease.

Treatment Recommendations

In selecting therapy for patients with HIV-associated NHL, emphasis should be placed on individualized therapy. Although standard-dose chemotherapy may be appropriate for the patient with good immune function and without a prior opportunistic infection, a lower dose treatment regimen might be selected for the patient with more severe immunologic compromise, marginal performance score, and a history of opportunistic infection. For some patients who are severely ill, a decision may be made to withhold therapy altogether. These decisions must take into account not only the patient's history and present condition but also the patient's own desires for a given therapeutic approach. Regardless of the chemotherapeutic approach used, it is strongly recommended that all patients treated with chemotherapy receive adjunctive antibiotic prophylaxis against *P. carinii* pneumonia. Clinical trials investigating the use of less immunosuppressive treatment approaches are in progress.

HODGKIN'S DISEASE

As discussed previously, Hodgkin's disease is not an AIDS-defining illness. The precise relationship of this malignancy to the underlying immunodeficiency state is unclear. Hodgkin's disease rarely has been reported in patients with primary immunodeficiency disorders[37] and has not been reported in immunosuppressed transplant recipients.[63] The observation that the frequency of Hodgkin's disease in the single male population ages 20 to 49 years in San Francisco has not increased in the years since 1979, when HIV seroprevalence markedly increased,[73,85] argues against a direct causal relationship between HIV-related immunodeficiency and the occurrence of Hodgkin's disease in this population. This is in striking contrast to the earlier sharp rise in the frequency of NHL observed in the same population during the same time period.[60,85] However, data from several recently reported epidemiologic studies, including the San Francisco Clinic Cohort study,[65] the MACS,[100] and a large Italian study,[81] suggest a significantly increased risk of Hodgkin's disease in HIV-seropositive individuals. The reported relative risks fall between two and fivefold, significantly lower than that observed for NHL, possibly explaining why a greater period of observation of larger populations was required to identify these differences compared with the seronegative population.

Clinical observations suggest that Hodgkin's disease in a patient with HIV infection has a different natural history and therapeutic outcome when compared to cases of Hodgkin's disease in the general population. The clinical features and therapeutic outcome in 14 homosexual men with Hodgkin's disease diagnosed at San Francisco General Hospital have been compared with those in a group of 35 single men 20 to 49 years of age diagnosed with Hodgkin's disease between the years 1973 and 1979.[73] Mixed cellularity was the most common histologic pattern among the 14 risk-group patients, whereas nodular sclerosis was significantly more common in the control population. All but one of the risk-group patients had advanced (stage III or IV) disease. Bone marrow and liver were the most common sites of extranodal disease. Similar observations were made in a series of 22 patients reported from a cooperative study of six hospitals[149] in which 68% of patients presented with either mixed cellularity or lymphocyte-depleted histology and 91% presented with stage III or IV disease.

The outcome of therapy in these patients has been disappointing. Of 12 patients treated at San Francisco General Hospital who could be evaluated, 7 were complete responders to either nitrogen mustard, vincristine, procarbazine, and prednisone (MOPP) or MOPP with doxorubicin, bleomycin, vinblastine, and dacarbazine (MOPP-ABVD).[73] Six of these seven complete responders subsequently relapsed. Eight patients (62%) developed *P. carinii* pneumonia during treatment. None of these patients is alive. One half of the patients died with advanced Hodgkin's disease, and the remaining patients died as a result of opportunistic infections. Median survival time was less than 1 year in this population, compared with 12 years in the control population. There were no differences in either response or survival time between those patients treated with MOPP alone and those treated with MOPP-ABVD.

The mean dose intensity of chemotherapy delivered to our patients was only 41% of the planned therapeutic dose. This was a result of the need for frequent dose reductions and delays in chemotherapy because of poor bone marrow reserve and intercurrent opportunistic infections. The very low dose intensity of chemotherapy may account for the high relapse rate observed in complete responders.

The Italian cooperative group for AIDS-related tumors more recently reported on 35 cases of Hodgkin's disease occurring in HIV-infected individuals.[71] Eighty-nine percent of these patients were IV drug abusers, 3% were homosexual males, and 9% were IV drug–using homosexual males. Fifty-three percent of the patients had mixed-cellularity histologic type, 31% had nodular sclerosis, and 16% had lymphocyte depletion. Seventy-eight percent of patients had either stage III or stage IV disease. Seventeen patients were treated with either MOPP, ABVD, ABV, or MOPP alternating with ABVD. Only 8 patients (30%) achieved complete remission. Of 13 patients who died, 7 (54%) died of opportunistic infections, 3 died of progression of Hodgkin's disease, and 2 died of disseminated intravascular coagulation. In one patient, the cause of death could not be determined. The median survival time of these patients with Hodgkin's disease was 15 months.

In a series of 22 patients in Spain treated with a variety of standard combination chemotherapeutic regimens,[149] the median survival for all patients was 18 months. No significant differences were found between survival and stages of Hodgkin's disease, histologic subgroup, or CD4 count; however, the sample size was quite small. Nonetheless, patients with a prior AIDS-defining diagnosis had a median survival of 13 months, which was significantly shorter than that in other patients.

As is the case for NHLs in HIV-seropositive patients, experience does not suggest that survival with Hodgkin's disease will be improved with more aggressive chemotherapeutic regimens. Poor bone marrow reserve and the occurrence of opportunistic infections have made it difficult to administer full doses of standard Hodgkin's disease chemotherapy to these pa-

tients. Preliminary results of a clinical trial using a relatively nonmyelosuppressive combination chemotherapeutic regimen for patients with Hodgkin's disease in patients with HIV infection were reported and were encouraging.[78] This treatment regimen used a combination of bleomycin, vincristine, streptozocin, and etoposide. Of the first five patients treated with this regimen, four of five had complete responses to chemotherapy alone, and a fifth had a complete response following completion of both chemotherapy and radiation therapy. Myelosuppression was not observed, and all patients remain alive and well. Future therapeutic approaches will focus on the use of more standard chemotherapeutic regimens with hematopoietic growth factors. Because a significant proportion of these patients will die as a result of opportunistic infection, prophylaxis against *P. carinii* pneumonia is strongly encouraged during chemotherapy.

HUMAN PAPILLOMAVIRUS INFECTION AND ANOGENITAL NEOPLASIA

Published reports suggest that HIV-induced immunodeficiency may promote the development of neoplasia in the cervical and anal mucosa. Cervical and anal cancers probably will become increasingly common manifestations of HIV disease as patients with profound immunodeficiency who would have succumbed to opportunistic infections earlier in the epidemic survive for extended periods of time because they receive more effective antiretroviral, prophylactic, and antimicrobial therapies. The resulting state of prolonged, severe immunodeficiency provides the necessary milieu for the emergence of diseases that develop after longer latency, such as anogenital carcinomas.

HPV Infection, Immunosuppression, and Anogenital Neoplasia

Anogenital neoplasia has a recognized association with chronic immunodeficiency. Studies of cohorts of immunosuppressed organ transplant recipients, for example, have demonstrated a 100-fold increase in incidence of vulvar and anal carcinomas and a 14-fold increase in the incidence of cervical carcinoma as compared with controls.[125,128]

Considerable evidence links the development of anogenital carcinoma to HPV infection. The so-called oncogenic HPV genotypes (HPV-16, HPV-18, and HPV-31) have been detected in 80% to 90% of cervical intraepithelial neoplasia (CIN) grade 3 lesions and invasive cervical cancers.[130] HPV infection has been presumed to play a similar causative role in the development of anal carcinoma, as suggested by the presence of HPV DNA and mRNA in tumor tissues from that site.[41] The high incidence of anogenital cancer in immunosuppressed transplant recipients is probably a consequence of the high prevalence of detectable anogenital HPV infection in that population. The prevalence of HPV infection is 5 to 17 times greater in immunosuppressed transplant recipients than in the general population.[155]

HIV Infection and Cervical Neoplasia

Over the past 5 years, a number of anecdotal reports have appeared about the possible connection between HIV-induced immunodeficiency and cervical neoplasia (Chapter 32). In one study, cytologic preparations of cervicovaginal smears from 35 HIV-infected women and 23 uninfected women were examined by one cytologist who was blinded to the individuals' HIV status.[147] Thirty-one percent of HIV-infected women had cytologic squamous atypia, compared to 4% of HIV-seronegative women ($p = 0.019$). Twenty-six percent of HIV-infected women had cytologic or histopathologic findings suggestive of genital HPV infection, compared to 4% of HIV-seronegative women ($p = 0.072$).

Feingold et al[28] extended these observations by obtaining molecular evidence of HPV infection in the cervicovaginal epithelium of women with HIV infection using Southern blot hybridization. Forty-nine percent of the HIV-infected women studied had HPV infection, compared with 25% of a group of non–HIV-infected women with similar sociodemographic and behavioral characteristics ($p < 0.05$). Forty percent of the HIV-infected women had squamous intraepithelial lesions on cervical cytology, compared with 9% of the noninfected women ($p < 0.01$). Women with concurrent HIV and HPV infection were 42 times more likely to have a cytologic abnormality than were women without evidence of either virus. In addition, 50% of women with symptomatic HIV infection (AIDS,

persistent generalized lymphadenopathy, oral candidiasis) had a cytologic abnormality, whereas only 23% with asymptomatic HIV infection did. These data suggest that more prolonged or more severe immunosuppression may allow progression of HPV-mediated cytologic abnormalities. The results of a variety of studies of this nature are summarized in Table 28–11.

An important report by Maiman et al[103] described a cohort of HIV-infected women in New York with invasive and preinvasive cervical neoplasia. In comparison to a group of non–HIV-infected women from the same institution, cervical neoplasia in HIV-infected women was more advanced at presentation, was more likely to recur, was associated more commonly with perianal involvement, and was associated more often with cytologic or histologic evidence of HPV infection (97% vs 56%; $p < 0.01$). The authors concluded that HPV-related neoplasia is having a significant impact in the HIV-infected women whom they serve. In a study expanding on their initial observations, the same authors confirmed that HIV-infected women appear to have more advanced disease at initial presentation with cervical cancer.[102] They also showed that standard treatment approaches for advanced cervical cancer in HIV-infected women resulted in significantly shorter mean time intervals until disease recurrence and death than were experienced by uninfected women.

Despite the apparent high prevalence of cervical neoplasia in HIV-infected women, only a few cases of invasive cervical cancer have been reported.[103,111,137] However, experience with immunosuppressed transplant recipients sug-

---

TABLE 28–11. SUMMARY OF FINDINGS FROM STUDIES OF ANOGENITAL INTRAEPITHELIAL NEOPLASIA IN PERSONS WITH HIV INFECTION

1. HIV-infected subjects are more likely to have cervical or anal intraepithelial neoplasia than non–HIV-infected controls.
2. HIV-infected subjects are more likely to have detectable cervical or anal HPV infection than non–HIV-infected controls.
3. Cervical or anal intraepithelial neoplasia is more common among HIV-infected subjects with lower CD4+ T-lymphocyte counts or more advanced clinical stage of HIV disease.
4. Detectable cervical or anal HPV infection is more common among HIV-infected subjects with lower CD4+ T-lymphocyte counts.

gests that a prolonged period of immunosuppression (mean of 88 months) may be necessary to permit development of anogenital cancer.[125] Most patients with HIV infection die of opportunistic infections much earlier in the course of symptomatic HIV disease and, therefore, may not survive long enough to develop cervical cancer. Improvements in survival times are being achieved through the use of effective antiretroviral, prophylactic, and antimicrobial therapies.[39,93] These successes may permit the emergence of cervical carcinoma among HIV-infected women with a high prevalence of cervical neoplasia.

HIV Infection and Anal Neoplasia

The relationship of HIV infection, HPV infection, and anal neoplasia also has been described. Although an association of anal neoplasia and HPV infection in homosexual men has been recognized for some time,[18,69] it is now apparent that HIV-infected, immunosuppressed men are particularly at risk for the development of HPV-related anal neoplasia.

Several early investigations provided preliminary evidence of the relationship of HIV infection, HPV infection, and anal neoplasia. Two small studies demonstrated HPV in neoplastic anal lesions of homosexual men by histopathologic and immunohistochemical techniques.[17,40] One individual in each study had a diagnosis of AIDS at the time that anal neoplasia was found. Frazer et al[33] examined a larger cohort of homosexual men using anorectal cytologic smears, HIV antibody testing, and T-lymphocyte phenotyping. They found that HIV seropositivity, lower CD4[+] T-lymphocyte counts, and lower CD4[+]:CD8[+] ratios were significantly associated with more pronounced cytologic atypia.

More recently, Palefsky et al[124] assessed the prevalence of anal HPV infection and precancerous abnormalities of the anal epithelium in 97 severely immunodeficient, HIV-infected homosexual men. Thirty-nine percent of the men had abnormal anal cytology, and 54% had HPV DNA in their anal cytologic specimens. Abnormalities on anal cytologic smear were significantly associated with the presence of HPV DNA (risk ratio, 4.6), and median CD4[+] T-lymphocyte counts of men with abnormal cytologic findings were significantly lower than those of men with normal findings ($p = 0.05$).

Another cohort of 105 homosexual men, including men with and without HIV infection, took part in a similar study conducted by Caussy et al.[11] HPV DNA was found in anal cytologic specimens from 53% of HIV-infected men, compared to 29% of non–HIV-infected men ($p = 0.012$). Anal neoplasia was present more frequently in HIV-infected men (24% vs 7%; $p = 0.03$). Multivariate logistic regression analysis of data from the HIV-infected men showed that low CD4[+] T-lymphocyte count was an independent risk factor for detection of HPV DNA ($p = 0.04$). Similar findings have been reported from a study of 120 Danish homosexual men[105] and from a study of 101 homosexual men attending a sexually transmitted diseases clinic in Seattle.[80] The results of a variety of studies of this nature are summarized in Table 28–11.

Lorenz et al[97] reviewed the surgical experience with anal carcinoma in HIV-infected men at the University of California at San Francisco. They noted poor treatment outcomes and short survival in their patients, similar to the experience described above with HIV-associated cervical cancer. Reports of single cases have described varying treatment outcomes with standard therapeutic approaches, with a suggestion that HIV-infected patients can benefit from standard therapies for anal cancer when immune system function is relatively intact.[117,160]

A retrospective review of the anal cancer treatment outcomes of seven HIV-seropositive patients and 55 patients whose HIV serostatus was negative or unknown found that the HIV-infected patients required more treatment delays and hospitalizations because of treatment-related toxicities.[68] Relapses were more common, and the mean time to treatment failure was shorter, in HIV-infected patients.

Clinical Implications of HIV-Related Anogenital Neoplasia

The studies cited previously demonstrate that anogenital HPV infection and neoplasia are common in persons with HIV infection. Information on the natural history of these conditions is limited, but it should be presumed that these lesions are precancerous and likely to evolve into invasive cancer over time. Early detection of preinvasive or minimally invasive cancers of the anogenital region can provide the opportunity to cure these diseases, as has been demonstrated by the successful use of Papanicolaou (Pap) smears in screening programs in the

TABLE 28–12. PROPOSED GUIDELINES FOR MANAGEMENT OF HIV-ASSOCIATED ANOGENITAL NEOPLASIA

Screening for Cervical Neoplasia

All HIV-infected women
  Annual Papanicolaou (Pap) smear of cervix
  Consider baseline colposcopy
HIV-infected women at high risk for HPV infection*
  Pap smear every 6 months
  Careful inspection of vulvar, vaginal, and anal epithelium

Treatment for Cervical Neoplasia

Refer to a gynecologist for standard treatment

Screening for Anal Neoplasia

HIV-infected men with history of anal intercourse
  Anal Pap smear†
  Anoscopy on a routine basis
  Biopsy of any abnormality identified on anoscopy
  Frequent anoscopic follow-up if abnormalities were identified previously

Treatment for Anal Neoplasia

Anal intraepithelial neoplasia: electrocautery or cryotherapy

Invasive Cancer

Surgical excision or radiation therapy or both

---

  * Those with a history of multiple sexual partners or sexual partners with HIV infection.
  † Studies evaluating the use of anal Pap smears currently are underway.

general population. It therefore seems reasonable that some patients with HIV infection, particularly those with relatively better prognosis (higher CD4+ T-lymphocyte count, no prior opportunistic infections or malignancies), would benefit from early detection and treatment of anogenital neoplasia. Palefsky, of the University of California, San Francisco,[123] has proposed guidelines (Table 28–12) for the management of cervical and anal neoplasia in HIV-infected persons.

A study is underway in which a large population of HIV-infected men will be examined with anal Pap smears and biopsies to validate the use of the Pap smear as a screening tool in this setting (J. Palefsky, personal communication). Recommendations about the widespread use of the anal Pap smear for population screening must await the results of this or similar studies.

Cervical cancer and anal cancer are likely to become more common problems in patients with HIV-induced immunodeficiency as the epidemic progresses. Observations about the development of malignancies in other states of immunosuppression suggest that these cancers will become more frequent as therapeutic interventions prolong survival. Strategies for prevention, detection, and treatment of HIV-associated anogenital malignancies will be needed.

SUMMARY

Patients with HIV infection, like immunosuppressed transplant recipients, are at high risk for the development of both Kaposi's sarcoma and B-cell non-Hodgkin's lymphoma. Although other malignancies may occur in the HIV-infected patient, epidemiologic evidence does not suggest a causal relationship between the underlying immunodeficiency state and the subsequent development of malignancy. Whether causally related or not, however, any malignancy occurring in a patient with HIV infection is likely to have a more aggressive course and to be associated with short survival time.

KS is the most common malignancy seen in HIV-infected patients. The etiology of KS is uncertain, as are the reasons for its nearly exclusive confinement to the homosexual male population with HIV infection. Prognosis is related to the extent of the disease, immune function, and the presence of systemic and local symptoms. A variety of local and systemic therapeutic modalities are available, including radiation therapy, cryotherapy, chemotherapy, and alpha-interferon. Which treatment approach is most appropriate for an individual depends on the extent of disease; the presence of local symptoms, including pain or edema; and the presence of cosmetically unsightly disease. Early studies suggest that the concurrent use of alpha-interferon and zidovudine may make the use of lower doses of alpha-interferon possible. The concurrent use of zidovudine with other chemotherapeutic regimens is being explored.

Patients with B-cell lymphoma tend to present with advanced extranodal disease, and primary lymphoma of the CNS frequently has been reported as well. Not unlike B-cell lymphoma seen in allograft recipients, lymphoma in the presence of HIV infection appears to arise out of a background of polyclonal B-cell activation. Although a viral cause has been suspected, the cause of lymphoma in these patients remains unknown. Response to therapy in these patients has been disappointing. Response rates to chemotherapy have been lower than those observed in other lymphoma patients, and treatment has been complicated by lack of adequate bone marrow reserve and by the occurrence of frequent opportunistic infections. Although overall survival times have been short, factors predictive of improved survival time include better immune function, absence of a prior AIDS diagnosis, good performance score, and absence of an extranodal site of disease. Experience suggests that, in some patients, more aggressive chemotherapy may be associated with shortened survival time. Recent clinical trials have demonstrated that either the use of reduced dosage chemotherapeutic regimens or the use of myeloid growth factors can reduce the morbidity associated with chemotherapy for this disease. Determining which of these treatment approaches will be of the greatest benefit with respect to response and survival time must await the results of ongoing clinical trials.

Cervical and anal neoplasia related to HPV infection also can occur as a consequence of HIV-induced immunodeficiency. Long-standing, profound immunodeficiency increases the risk of developing HPV-related anogenital neoplasia, as has been described in transplant recipients requiring prolonged immunosuppression. As the survival time of patients with HIV infection is extended through the use of more effective antiretroviral, prophylactic, and antimicrobial therapies, the resulting state of profound, prolonged immunodeficiency will provide the necessary milieu for the emergence of anogenital neoplasia.

Treatment of the patient with an HIV-associated malignancy imposes obstacles and challenges that are unique in medicine. For this reason, it is especially important that treatment be individualized carefully, with the patient playing an important role in determining which therapeutic alternative is most appropriate.

Note Added in Proof

Recently, novel herpes virus DNA sequences have been identified in association with the majority of cases of HIV-associated Kaposi's sarcoma (Cheng Y, et al: Identification of herpesvirus-like DNA sequences in AIDS-associated Kaposi's sarcoma. Science 266:1864–1865, 1994). This virus was termed human herpes virus 8 (HHV8) and has now been identified in association with all of the various epidemiological forms of KS in addition to AIDS (Huang YQ, Li JJ, Kaplan MH, et al: Human herpesvirus-like nucleic acid in various forms of Kaposi's sarcoma. Lancet 345:759–761, 1995; Moore PS, Chang Y: Detection of herpesvirus-like DNA sequences in Kaposi's sarcoma in patients with and those without HIV infection. N Engl J Med 332:1181–1185, 1995). This virus has recently been cultured from a body-cavity based lymphoma cell line and intact virions have been visualized (Renne R, Zhong W, Herndier B, et al: Lytic growth of Kaposi's sarcoma-associated herpesvirus (human herpesvirus 8) in culture. Nature Medicine 2:342–346, 1996). Partial sequencing of the viral genome has resulted in identification of viral genes with homology to genes encoding cyclin D (Moore PS, Gao SJ, Dominguez G, et al: Primary characterization of a herpesvirus agent associated with Kaposi's sarcoma. J Virol 70:549–558, 1996) suggesting that this virus may be capable of influencing the cell division cycle. What the precise role of this virus might be in the development of Kaposi's sarcoma is still not clearly understood and is the subject of intensive laboratory investigation.

REFERENCES

1. Balasubramanyam A, Waxman M, Kazal HL, Lee MH: Malignant lymphoma of the heart in acquired immunodeficiency syndrome. Chest 90:243–246, 1986
2. Baumgartner J, Rachlin J, Beckstead J, et al: Primary central nervous system lymphomas: Natural history and response to radiation therapy in 55 patients with acquired immunodeficiency syndrome. J Neurosurg 73:206–211, 1990
3. Beral V, Peterman TA, Berkelman RL, et al: Kaposi's sarcoma among persons with AIDS: A sexually transmitted infection? Lancet 1:123, 1990
4. Bermudez M, Grant K, Rodvien R, Mendes F: Non-Hodgkin's lymphoma in a population with or at risk for acquired immunodeficiency syndrome: Indications for intensive chemotherapy. Am J Med 86:71–76, 1989
5. Bernardi D, Salvioni R, Vaccher E, et al: Testicular germ cell tumors and HIV infection: A report of 26 cases. J Clin Oncol, 1995
6. Bernheim A, Berger R: Cytogenetic studies of Burkitt lymphoma-leukemia in patients with acquired immunodeficiency syndrome. Cancer Genet Cytogenet 32:67–74, 1988
7. Bernstein ZP, Wilson D, Summers K, et al: Pilot/phase I study—photodynamic therapy (PDT) for treatment of AIDS-associated Kaposi's sarcoma (AIDS/KS). Proc Am Soc Clin Oncol 14:289, 1995
8. Brooks JJ: Kaposi's sarcoma: A reversible hyperplasia. Lancet 2:1309–1311, 1986
9. Burkes RL, Meyer PR, Gill PS, et al: Rectal lymphoma in homosexual men. Arch Intern Med 146:913–915, 1986
10. Cappell MS, Yao F, Cho KC: Colonic adenocarci-

noma associated with the acquired immunodeficiency syndrome. Cancer 62:616–619, 1988

11. Caussy D, Goedert JJ, Palefsky J, et al: Interaction of human immunodeficiency and papilloma viruses: Association with anal intraepithelial abnormality in homosexual men. Int J Cancer 46:214–219, 1990

12. Centers for Disease Control: Revision of the case definition of acquired immunodeficiency syndrome for national reporting—United States. MMWR 4: 373–374, 1985

13. Chaganti R, Jhanwar S, Koziner B, et al: Specific translocations characterize Burkitt's-like lymphoma of homosexual men with the acquired immunodeficiency syndrome. Blood 61:1269–1272, 1983

14. Chak LY, Gill PS, Levine AM, et al: Radiation therapy for AIDS-related Kaposi's sarcoma. J Clin Oncol 6:863–867, 1988

15. Ciricillo S, Rosenblum M: Use of CT and MR imaging to distinguish intracranial lesions and to define the need for biopsy in AIDS patients. J Neurosurg 73:720–724, 1990

16. Connors JM, Klimo P: MACOP-B chemotherapy for malignant lymphomas and related conditions: 1987 update and additional observations. Semin Hematol 25(suppl 2):41–46, 1988

17. Croxson T, Chabon AB, Rorat E, Barash IM: Intraepithelial carcinoma of the anus in homosexual men. Dis Colon Rectum 27:325–330, 1984

18. Daling JR, Weiss NS, Hislop TG, et al: Sexual practices, sexually transmitted disease, and the incidence of anal cancer. N Engl J Med 317:973–977, 1987

19. Daling JR, Weiss NS, Klopfenstein LL, et al: Correlates of homosexual behavior and the incidence of anal cancer. JAMA 247:1988–1990, 1982

20. Davis SD, Henschke CI, Chamides BK, Westcott JL: Intrathoracic Kaposi sarcoma in AIDS patients: Radiographic–pathologic correlation. Radiology 163:495–500, 1987

21. Delecluse HJ, Raphael M, Magaud JP, Felman P: Variable morphology of human immunodeficiency virus-associated lymphomas with c-myc rearrangements. Blood 82:552–563, 1993

22. Des Jarlais DC, Stoneburner R, Thomas P: Declines in proportion of Kaposi's sarcoma among cases of AIDS in multiple risk groups in New York City. Lancet 2:1024–1025, 1987

23. DeVita VT, Hubbard SM, Young RC, Longo DL: The role of chemotherapy in diffuse aggressive lymphomas. Semin Hematol 25(suppl 2):2–10, 1988

24. deWit R, Schatenkerk JKME, Boucher CAB, et al: Clinical and virological effects of high-dose recombinant interferon-α in disseminated AIDS-related Kaposi's sarcoma. Lancet 2:1214–1217, 1988

25. Drew WL, Mills J, Hauer LB, et al: Declining prevalence of Kaposi's sarcoma in homosexual AIDS patients paralleled by fall in cytomegalovirus transmission. Lancet 1:66, 1988

26. Emilie D, Coumbaras J, Raphael M, et al: Interleukin 6 production in high-grade B lymphomas: Correlation with the presence of malignant immunoblasts in acquired immunodeficiency syndrome and in human immunodeficiency virus-seronegative patients. Blood 80:498–504, 1992

27. Ensoli B, Nakamura S, Salahuddin SZ, et al: AIDS-Kaposi's sarcoma-derived cells express cytokines with autocrine and paracrine growth factors. Science 243:223–226, 1989

28. Feingold AR, Vermund SH, Burk RD, et al: Cervical cytologic abnormalities and papillomavirus in women infected with human immunodeficiency virus. J Acquir Immune Defic Syndr 3:896–903, 1990

29. Fischl MA, Richman DD, Greico MH, et al: The efficacy of azidothymidine (AZT) in the treatment of patients with AIDS and AIDS-related complex: A double-blind, placebo-controlled trial. N Engl J Med 317:185–191, 1987

30. Fischl MA, Uttamchandani R, Resnick L, et al: A phase I study of recombinant human interferon alfa-2 or human lymphoblastoid interferon alfa-n1 and concomitant zidovudine in patients with AIDS-related Kaposi's sarcoma. J Acquir Immun Defic Syndr 4:4–10, 1991

31. Formenti SC, Gill PS, Rarick M, et al: Primary central nervous system lymphoma in AIDS: Results of radiation therapy. Cancer 63:1101–1107, 1989

32. Frager DH, Wolf EL, Competiello LS, et al: Squamous cell carcinoma of the esophagus in patients with acquired immunodeficiency syndrome. Gastrointest Radiol 13:358–360, 1988

33. Frazer IH, Crapper RM, Medley G, et al: Association between anorectal dysplasia, human papillomavirus, and human immunodeficiency virus infection in homosexual men. Lancet 2:657–660, 1986

34. Friedman SL: Gastrointestinal and hepatobiliary neoplasms in AIDS. Gastroenterol Clin North Am 17:465–486, 1988

35. Friedman SL, Wright TL, Altman DF: Gastrointestinal Kaposi's sarcoma in patients with acquired immunodeficiency syndrome: Endoscopic and autopsy findings. Gastroenterology 89:102–108, 1985

36. Frizzera G, Hanto DW, Gajl Peczalkska K, et al: Polymorphic diffuse B-cell hyperplasias and lymphomas in renal transplant recipients. Cancer Res 41:4262–4279, 1981

37. Frizzera G, Rosai J, Dehner LP, et al: Lymphoreticular disorders in primary immunodeficiencies: New findings based on an up-to-date histologic classification of 35 cases. Cancer 46:692–699, 1980

38. Gail MH, Pluda JM, Rabkin CS, et al: Projections of the incidence of non-Hodgkin's lymphoma related to acquired immunodeficiency syndrome. J Natl Cancer Inst 83:695–701, 1991

39. Gail MH, Rosenberg PS, Goedert JJ: Therapy may explain recent deficits in AIDS incidence. J Acquir Immun Defic Syndr 3:296–306, 1990

40. Gal AA, Meyer PR, Taylor CR: Papillomavirus antigens in anorectal condyloma and carcinoma in homosexual men. JAMA 257:337–340, 1987

41. Gal AA, Saul SH, Stoler MH: In situ hybridization analysis of human papillomavirus in anal squamous cell carcinoma. Mod Pathol 2:439–443, 1989

42. Gill PS, Akil B, Colletti P, et al: Pulmonary Kaposi's sarcoma: Clinical findings and results of therapy. Am J Med 87:57–61, 1989

43. Gill PS, Hadienberg J, Espina BM, et al: Low dose paclitaxel (taxol) every two weeks over 3 hours is safe and effective in the treatment of advanced AIDS-related Kaposi's sarcoma (Abstract 1516). ASH, 39th Annual Meeting, Seattle, WA, 1995

44. Gill PS, Krailo M, Slater L, et al: Randomized trial of ABV (Adriamycin, bleomycin and vinblastine)

vs A (Adriamycin) in advanced Kaposi's sarcoma (KS) (Abstract 11). Proc Am Soc Clin Oncol, New Orleans, LA, 1988, p 3

45. Gill P, Levine A, Krailo M, et al: AIDS-related malignant lymphoma: Results of prospective treatment trials. J Clin Oncol 5:1322–1328, 1987

46. Gill PS, Levine A, Meyer P, et al: Primary central nervous system lymphoma in homosexual men. Am J Med 78:742–748, 1985

47. Gill PS, Naidu Y, Nakamura S, et al: IL-6 regulation by steroid hormones and autocrine activity in Kaposi's sarcoma. AIDS Res Human Retroviruses 7:220, 1991

48. Gill PS, Rarick MU, Espina B, et al: Advanced acquired immune deficiency syndrome-related Kaposi's sarcoma: Results of pilot studies using combination chemotherapy. Cancer 65: 1074–1078, 1990

49. Gisselbrecht C, Oksenhendler E, Tirelli U, et al: High-dose chemotherapy (LNH84) for HIV-associated non-Hodgkin's lymphoma. Am J Med 95: 188–196, 1993

50. Glaspy J, Miles S, McCarthy S: Treatment of advanced stage Kaposi's sarcoma with vincristine and bleomycin (Abstract 10). Proc Am Soc Clin Oncol, Los Angeles, CA, 1986, p 3

51. Goebel FD, Bogner JR, Spathling S, et al: Efficacy and toxicity of liposomal doxorubicin in advanced AIDS-related Kaposi's sarcoma (KS): An open study (Abstract WSB15-6). Program of the IXth International Conference on AIDS, Berlin, Germany, 1993, p 120

52. Grant I, Gold J, Armstrong D: Risk of CNS toxoplasmosis in patients with acquired immune deficiency syndrome (Abstract 441). Program of the Interscience Conference on Antimicrobial Agents and Chemotherapy New Orleans, LA, 1986, p 177

53. Groopman JE, Gottlieb MS, Goodman J, et al: Recombinant alpha-2 interferon therapy for Kaposi's sarcoma associated with the acquired immunodeficiency syndrome. Ann Intern Med 100:671–676, 1984

54. Groopman JE, Mayer K, Zipoli T, et al: Unusual neoplasms associated with HTLV-III infection (Abstract 14). Proc Am Soc Clin Oncol, Los Angeles, CA, 1986, p 4

55. Groopman J, Sullivan J, Mulder C, et al: Pathogenesis of B-cell lymphoma in a patient with AIDS. Blood 67:612–615, 1986

56. Guarner J, Brynes RK, Chan WC, et al: Primary non-Hodgkin's lymphoma of the heart in two patients with the acquired immunodeficiency syndrome. Arch Pathol Lab Med 111:254–256, 1987

57. Hanto DW, Frizzera G, Gajl-Peczalkska K, et al: Epstein-Barr virus induced B-cell lymphoma after renal transplantation. N Engl J Med 306:913–918, 1982

58. Hanto DW, Frizzera G, Purtilo D, et al: Clinical spectrum of lymphoproliferative disorders in renal transplant recipients and evidence for the role of Epstein-Barr virus. Cancer Res 41:4253–4261, 1981

59. Hanto DW, Gajl-Peczalkska KJ, Frizzera G, et al: Epstein-Barr virus-induced polyclonal and monoclonal B-cell lymphoproliferative disease occurring after renal transplantation. Ann Surg 198: 356–369, 1983

60. Harnly ME, Swan SH, Holly EA, et al: Temporal trends in the incidence of non-Hodgkin's lymphoma and selected malignancies in a population with a high incidence of acquired immunodeficiency syndrome (AIDS). Am J Epidemiol 128: 261–267, 1988

61. Harrison M, Tomlinson D, Stewart S: Liposomal-entrapped doxorubicin: An active agent in AIDS-related Kaposi's sarcoma. J Clin Oncol 13:914–920, 1995

62. Hartshorn KL, Vogt MW, Chou TC, et al: Synergistic inhibition of human immunodeficiency virus in vitro by azidothymidine and recombinant interferon alpha-A. Antimicrob Agent Chemother 31: 168–172, 1987

63. Harwood AR, Osoba D, Hofstader SL, et al: Kaposi's sarcoma in recipients of renal transplants. Am J Med 67:759–765, 1979

64. Herndier BG, Shiramizu BT, Jewett NE, et al: Acquired immunodeficiency syndrome-associated T-cell lymphoma: Evidence for human immunodeficiency virus type 1-associated T-cell transformation. Blood 79:1768–1774, 1992

65. Hessol NA, Katz MH, Liu JY, et al: Increased incidence of Hodgkin disease in homosexual men with HIV infection. Ann Intern Med 117:309–311, 1992

66. Heyer DM, Desmond S, Volberding P, Kahn J: Changing prevalence of malignancies in men at San Francisco General Hospital during the HIV epidemic (Abstract W.B.O.19). Program of the Vth International Conference on AIDS, Montreal, Canada 1989, p 206

67. Hill DR: The role of radiotherapy for epidemic Kaposi's sarcoma. Semin Oncol 14(suppl 3):1207, 1987

68. Holland JM, Swift PS: Tolerance of patients with human immunodeficiency virus and carcinoma to treatment with combined chemotherapy and radiation therapy. Radiology 193:251–254, 1994

69. Holly EA, Whittemore AS, Aston DA, et al: Anal cancer incidence: Genital warts, anal fissure or fistula, hemorrhoids, and smoking. J Natl Cancer Inst 81: 1726–1731, 1989

70. Hoover R, Fraumeni JF: Risk of cancer in renal transplant recipients. Lancet 2:55–57, 1973

71. Italian Cooperative Group for AIDS-Related Tumors: Malignant lymphomas in patients with or at risk for AIDS in Italy: Reports. J Natl Cancer Inst 80: 855–860, 1988

72. Kapaln LD, Abrams DI, Feigal E, et al: AIDS-associated non-Hodgkin's lymphoma in San Francisco. JAMA 261:719–724, 1989

73. Kaplan LD, Abrams DA, Volberding PA: Clinical course and epidemiology of Hodgkin's disease in homosexual men in San Francisco (Abstract M.11.3). Program of the IIIrd International Conference on AIDS, Washington, DC, 1987

74. Kaplan LD, Abrams D, Volberding P: Treatment of Kaposi's sarcoma in acquired immunodeficiency syndrome with an alternating vincristine-vinblastine regimen. Cancer Treat Rep 70:1121–1122, 1986

75. Kaplan LD, Hopewell PC, Jaffe H, et al: Kaposi's sarcoma involving the lung in patients with the acquired immunodeficiency syndrome. J Acquir Immune Defic Syndr 1:23–30, 1988

76. Kaplan LD, Kahn JO, Crowe S, et al: Clinical and virologic effects of recombinant human granulo-

cyte-macrophage colony-stimulating factor in patients receiving chemotherapy for human immunodeficiency virus-associated non-Hodgkin's lymphoma: Results of a randomized trial. J Clin Oncol 9:929–940, 1991

77. Kaplan L, Kahn J, Jacobson M, et al: Primary bile duct lymphoma in the acquired immunodeficiency syndrome (AIDS). Ann Intern Med 110: 162, 1989

78. Kaplan L, Kahn J, Northfelt D, et al: Novel combination chemotherapy for Hodgkin's disease (HD) in HIV-infected individuals (Abstract 7). Proc Am Soc Clin Oncol, Houston, TX, 1991, p 33

79. Kaplan L, Straus D, Testa M, et al: Randomized trial of standard-dose mBACOD with GM-CSF vs. reduced dose mBACOD for systemic HIV-associated lymphoma: ACTG 142. Proc Am Soc Clin Oncol, Los Angeles, CA, 1995, p 288

80. Kiviat N, Rompalo A, Bowden R, et al: Anal human papillomavirus infection among human immunodeficiency virus-seropositive and seronegative men. J Infect. Dis 162:358–361, 1990

81. Knowles DM, Chamulak G, Subar M, et al: Lymphoid neoplasia associated with the acquired immunodeficiency syndrome (AIDS). Ann Intern Med 108: 744–753, 1988

82. Knowles DM, Inghirami G, Ubraico A, Dalla-Favera R: Molecular genetic analysis of three AIDS-associated neoplasms of uncertain lineage demonstrates their B-cell derivation and the possible pathogenic role of Epstein-Barr virus. Blood 73:792–799, 1989

83. Kovacs JA, Deyton L, Davey R, et al: Combined zidovudine and interferon-α therapy in patients with Kaposi's sarcoma and the acquired immunodeficiency syndrome (AIDS). Ann Intern Med 111: 280–286, 1989

84. Kovacs JA, Lance HC, Masur H, et al: A phase III, placebo-controlled trial of recombinant alpha interferon in asymptomatic individuals seropositive for the acquired immunodeficiency syndrome. Clin Res 35:479A, 1987

85. Kristal AR, Nasca PC, Burnett WS, Mikl J: Changes in the epidemiology of non-Hodgkin's lymphoma associated with epidemic human immunodeficiency virus (HIV) infection. Am J Epidemiol 128: 711–718, 1988

86. Krown SE: The role of interferon in the therapy of epidemic Kaposi's sarcoma. Semin Oncol 14(suppl 3):27–33, 1987

87. Krown SE, Gold JWM, Niedzwiecki D, et al: Interferon-α with zidovudine: Safety, tolerance, and clinical and virologic effects in patients with Kaposi sarcoma associated with the acquired immunodeficiency syndrome (AIDS). Ann Intern Med 112:812–821, 1990

88. Krown SE, Metroka C, Wernz JC: Kaposi's sarcoma in the acquired immunodeficiency syndrome: A proposal for uniform evaluation, response, and staging criteria. J Clin Oncol 7:1201–1207, 1989

89. Krown SE, Paredes J, Bundow D, et al: Interferon-α, zidovudine, and granulocyte-macrophage colony-stimulating factor: A phase I AIDS clinical trials group study in patients with Kaposi's sarcoma associated with AIDS. J Clin Oncol 10:1344–1351, 1992

90. Lane HC, Falloon J, Walker RE, et al: Zidovudine in patients with human immunodeficiency virus (HIV) infection and Kaposi's sarcoma. Ann Intern Med 111:41–50, 1989

91. Lane HC, Feinberg J, Davery V, et al: Anti-retroviral effects of interferon-alpha in AIDS-associated Kaposi's sarcoma. Lancet 2:1218–1222, 1988

92. Laubenstein LJ, Krigel RL, Odajnyk CM, et al: Treatment of epidemic Kaposi's sarcoma with etoposide or a combination of doxorubicin, bleomycin and vinblastine. J Clin Oncol 2:1115–1120, 1984

93. Lemp GF, Payne SF, Neal D, et al: Survival trends for patients with AIDS. JAMA 263:402–406, 1990

94. Levine A, Meyer P, Begandy M, et al: Development of B-cell lymphoma in homosexual men. Ann Intern Med 100:7–13, 1984

95. Levine AM, Sullivan-Halley J, Pike MC, et al: Human immunodeficiency virus-related lymphoma: Prognostic factors predictive of survival. Cancer 68: 2466–2472, 1991

96. Levine AM, Wernz JC, Kaplan L, et al: Low-dose chemotherapy with central nervous system prophylaxis and zidovudine maintenance in AIDS-related lymphoma. JAMA 266:84–88, 1991

97. Lorenz HP, Wilson W, Leigh B, et al: Squamous cell carcinoma of the anus and HIV infection. Dis Colon Rectum 34:336–338, 1991

98. Lowenthal D, Straus D, Campbell S, et al: AIDS-related lymphoid neoplasia: The Memorial Hospital Experience. Cancer 61:2325–2337, 1988

99. Lunardi-Iskandar Y, Bryant JL, Zeman RA, et al: Tumorigenesis and metastasis of neoplastic Kaposi's sarcoma cell line in immunodeficient mice blocked by a human pregnancy hormone. Nature 375:64–68, 1995

100. Lyter DW, Bryant J, Thackeray R, et al: Incidence of human immunodeficiency virus-related and non-related malignancies in a large cohort of homosexual men. J Clin Oncol 13:2540–2546, 1995

101. MacMahon EME, Glass JD, Hayward SD, et al: Epstein-Barr virus in AIDS-related primary central nervous system lymphoma. Lancet 338:969–973, 1991

102. Maiman M, Fructer RG, Guy L, et al: Human immunodeficiency virus infection and invasive cervical carcinoma. Cancer 71:402–406, 1993

103. Maiman M, Fruchter RG, Serur E, et al: Human immunodeficiency virus infection and cervical neoplasia. Gynecol Oncol 38:377–382, 1990

104. Meeker TC, Shiramizu B, Kaplan L, et al: Evidence for molecular subtypes of HIV-associated lymphoma: Division into peripheral monoclonal, polyclonal and central nervous system lymphoma. AIDS 5:669–674, 1991

105. Melbye M, Palefsky J, Gonzales J, et al: Immune status as a determinant of human papillomavirus detection and its association with anal epithelial abnormalities. Int J Cancer 46:203–206, 1990

106. Miles SA, Martinez-Maza O, Rezai A, et al: Oncostatin M as a potent mitogen for AIDS-Kaposi's sarcoma-derived cells. Science 255:1432–1434, 1992

107. Miles SA, Rezai AR, Logan D, et al: AIDS Kaposi's sarcoma-derived cells produce and respond to interleukin 6 (Abstract S.A.66). Program of the VIth International Conference on AIDS, San Francisco, CA, 3:113, 1990

108. Mintzer DM, Real FX, Jovino L, Krown SE: Treatment of Kaposi's sarcoma and thrombocytopenia with vincristine in patients with the acquired immunodeficiency syndrome. Ann Intern Med 102: 200–202, 1985

109. Mitsuyasu RT, Groopman JE: Biology and therapy of Kaposi's sarcoma. Semin Oncol 11:53–59, 1984

110. Mitsuyasu R, Taylor J, Glaspy J, et al: Heterogeneity of epidemic Kaposi's sarcoma: Implications for therapy. Cancer 57:1657–1661, 1986

111. Monfardini S, Vaccher E, Pizzocaro G, et al: Unusual malignant tumors in 49 patients with HIV infection. AIDS 3:449–452, 1989

112. Moore RD, Kessler H, Richman DD, et al: Non-Hodgkin's lymphoma in tients with advanced HIV infection treated with zidovudine. JAMA 265:2208–2211, 1991

113. Myskowski PL, Niedzweicki D, Shurgot BA, et al. AIDS-associated Kaposi's sarcoma: Variable associated with increased survival. J Am Acad Dermatol 18:1299–1306, 1988

114. Nador RG, Cesarman E, Knowles DM, Said JW: Herpes-like DNA sequences in a body-cavity-based lymphoma in an HIV-negative patient. N Engl J Med 333:943, 1995

115. Nakamura S, Salahuddin SZ, Biberfeld P, et al: Kaposi's sarcoma cells: Long-term culture with growth factor from retrovirus-infected CD4+ T cells. Science 42:426–430, 1988

116. Nasr S, Brynes R, Garrison C, Chan W: Peripheral T-cell lymphoma in a patient with acquired immunodeficiency syndrome. Cancer 61:947–951, 1988

117. Nasti G, Santarossa S, Vaccher E, et al: Anal cancer in patients with HIV infection: A report of two cases without evidence of immunological dysfunction. AIDS 8:1507–1508, 1994

118. National Cancer Institute: NCI-sponsored study of classifications of non-Hodgkin's lymphoma: Summary and description of a working formulation for clinical usage. The Non-Hodgkin's Lymphoma Pathologic Classification Project. Cancer 49:2112–2135, 1982

119. Newman SB: Treatment of epidemic Kaposi's sarcoma (KS) with intralesional vinblastine injection (IL-VLB) (Abstract 19). Proc Am Soc Clin Oncol, New Orleans, LA, 1988, p 5

120. Northfelt DW, Dezube B, Miller B, et al: Randomized comparative trial of doxil vs. Adriamycin, bleomycin, and vincristine (ABV) in the treatment of severe AIDS-related Kaposi's sarcoma (AIDS-KS) (Abstract 1515) ASH, 39th Annual Meeting, Seattle, WA, 1995

121. Northfelt DW, Martin FJ, Kaplan LD, et al: Pharmacokinetics (PK), tumor localization (TL), and safety of doxil (liposomal doxorubicin) in AIDS patients with Kaposi's sarcoma (AIDS-KS) (Abstract 8). Proc Am Soc Clin Oncol, Orlando, FL, 1993, p 51

122. Ognibene FP, Steis RG, Macher AM, et al: Kaposi's sarcoma causing pulmonary infiltrates and respiratory failure in the acquired immunodeficiency syndrome. Ann Intern Med 102:471–475, 1985

123. Palefsky J: Human papillomavirus infection among HIV-infected individuals. Hematol Oncol Clin North Am 5:357–370, 1991

124. Palefsky JM, Gonzales J, Greenblatt RM, et al: Anal intraepithelial neoplasia and anal papillomavirus infection among homosexual males with group IV HIV disease. JAMA 263:2911–2916, 1990

125. Penn I: Cancers of the anogenital region in renal transplant recipients: Analysis of 65 cases. Cancer 58:611–616, 1986

126. Penn I: Lymphomas complicating organ transplantation. Transplant Proc 15(suppl 1):2790–2797, 1983

127. Penn I: The incidence of malignancies in transplant recipients. Transplant Proc 7:323–326, 1975

128. Penn I: Tumors of the immunocompromised patient. Annu Rev Med 39:63–73, 1988

129. Petersen JM, Tubbs RR, Savage RA, et al: Small noncleaved B-cell Burkitt-like lymphoma with chromosome t(8;14) translocation and Epstein-Barr virus nuclear-associated antigen in a homosexual man with acquired immune deficiency syndrome. Am J Med 78:141–148, 1985

130. Pfister H: Relationship of papillomaviruses to anogenital cancer. Obstet Gynecol Clin North Am 14:349–361, 1987

131. Pluda JM, Venzon DJ, Tosato G, et al: Parameters affecting the development of non-Hodgkin's lymphoma in patients with severe human immunodeficiency virus infection receiving antiretroviral therapy. J Clin Oncol 11:1099–1107, 1993

132. Porter SB, Sande MA: Toxoplasmosis of the central nervous system in the acquired immunodeficiency syndrome. N Engl J Med 327:1643–1648, 1992

133. Presant CA, Gala K, Wiseman C, et al: Human immunodeficiency virus-associated T-cell lymphoblastic lymphoma in AIDS. Cancer 60:1459–1461, 1987

134. Presant CA, Scolaro M, Kennedy P, et al: Liposomal daunorubicin treatment of HIV-associated Kaposi's sarcoma. Lancet 341:1242–1243, 1993

135. Ravalli S, Chabon AB, Khan AA: Gastrointestinal neoplasia in young HIV-positive patients. Am J Clin Pathol 91:458–461, 1989

136. Real FX, Oettgen HF, Krown SE: Kaposi's sarcoma and the acquired immunodeficiency syndrome: Treatment with high and low doses of leukocyte A interferon. J Clin Oncol 4:544–551, 1986

137. Rellihan MA, Dooley DP, Burke TW, et al: Rapidly progressing cervical cancer in a patient with human immunodeficiency virus infection. Gynecol Oncol 36:435–438, 1990

138. Rezai A, Martinez-Maza O, Gaynor R, et al: HIV-tat increases production by and proliferation of AIDS-KS derived cells (Abstract 6). Proc Am Soc Clin Oncol, Houston, TX, 1991, p 33

139. Rios A, Mansell PWA, Newell GR, et al: Treatment of acquired immunodeficiency syndrome-related Kaposi's sarcoma with lymphoblastoid interferon. J Clin Oncol 3:506–512, 1985

140. Rogo KO, Kavoo-Linge: Human immunodeficiency virus seroprevalence among cervical cancer patients. Gynecol Oncol 37:87–92, 1990

141. Rutherford GW, Schwarcz SK, Lemp GF, et al: The epidemiology of AIDS-related Kaposi's sarcoma in San Francisco. J Infect Dis 159:569–572, 1989

142. Safai B: Pathophysiology and epidemiology of epidemic Kaposi's sarcoma. Semin Oncol 2(suppl 3):7–12, 1987

143. Salahuddin SZ, Nakamura S, Biberfeld P, et al: Angiogenic properties of Kaposi's sarcoma-derived cells after long-term culture in vitro. Science 242:430–433, 1988

144. Saville MW, Lietzau J, Pluda JM, et al: Activity of paclitaxel (taxol) as therapy for HIV-associated Kaposi's sarcoma (KS). Proc Am Soc Clin Oncol 14:290, 1995

145. Scadden DT, Bering HA, Levine JD, et al: Granulocyte-macrophage colony-stimulating factor mitigates the neutropenia of combined interferon

alpha and zidovudine treatment of acquired immune deficiency syndrome-associated Kaposi's sarcoma. J Clin Oncol 9:802–808, 1991

146. Schoeppel SL, Hoppe RT, Dorfman RF, et al: Hodgkin's disease in homosexual men with generalized lymphadenopathy. Ann Intern Med 102:68–70, 1985

147. Schrager LK, Friedland GH, Maude D, et al: Cervical and vaginal squamous abnormalities in women infected with human immunodeficiency virus. J Acquir Immun Defic Syndr 2:570–575, 1989

148. Selik RM, Chu SY, Ward JW: Trends in infectious disease and cancers among persons dying of HIV infection in the United States from 1987 to 1992. Ann Intern Med 123:933–936, 1995

149. Serrano M, Bellas C, Campo E, et al: Hodgkin's disease in patients with antibodies to human immunodeficiency virus: A study of 22 patients. Cancer 65:2248–2254, 1990

150. Sharma D, Muggia F, Lucci L, et al: Liposomal daunorubicin (VS103): Tolerance and clinical effects in AIDS-related Kaposi's sarcoma (KS) during a phase I study (Abstract 9). Proc Am Soc Clin Oncol, Washington, DC, 1990, p 4

151. Shearer WT, Ritz J, Finego MJ, et al: Epstein-Barr virus-associated B-cell proliferations of diverse clonal origins after bone marrow transplantation in a 12-year-old patient with severe combined immunodeficiency. N Engl J Med 312:1151–1159, 1985

152. Shepherd F, Beaulieu R, Murphy K, et al: A randomized trial of 2 doses of alpha interferon (IFN) added to AZT for the treatment of epidemic Kaposi's sarcoma (KS). Proc Am Soc Clin Oncol, Dallas, TX, 1994, p 50

153. Shiramizu B, Herndier BG, McGrath MS: Identification of a common clonal human immunodeficiency virus integration site in human immunodeficiency virus-associated lymphomas. Cancer Res 54:2069–2072, 1994

154. Shiramizu B, Herndier B, Meeker T, et al: Molecular and immunophenotypic characterization of AIDS-associated EBV-negative polyclonal lymphoma. J Clin Oncol 10:383–389, 1992

155. Sillman FH, Sedlis A: Anogenital papillomavirus infection and neoplasia in immunodeficient women. Obstet Gynecol Clin North Am 14:537–558, 1987

156. So YT, Beckstead J, Davis R: Primary central nervous system lymphoma in acquired immunodeficiency syndrome: A clinical and pathological study. Ann Neurol 20:566–572, 1986

157. Straus D, Huang J, Testa M, et al: Prognostic factors in the treatment of HIV-associated non-Hodgkin's lymphoma (HANHL): Analysis of ACTG 142 (low-dose vs. standard-dose mBACOD + GM-CSF) (Abstract 2404) ASH, 39th Annual Meeting, Seattle, WA, 1995

158. Strigle SM, Martin SE, Levine AM, Rarick MU: The use of fine needle aspiration cytology in the management of human immunodeficiency virus-related non-Hodgkin's lymphoma and Hodgkin's disease. J Acquir Immune Defic Syndr 6:1329–1334, 1993

159. Subar M, Neri A, Inghirami G, et al: Frequent c-myc oncogene activation and infrequent presence of Epstein-Barr virus genome in AIDS-associated lymphoma. Blood 72:667–671, 1988

160. Svensson C, Kaigas M, Lidbrink E, et al: Carcinoma of the anal canal in a patient with AIDS. Acta Oncol 30:8986–8987, 1991

161. Tappero JW, Berger TG, Kaplan LD, et al: Cryotherapy for cutaneous Kaposi's sarcoma (KS) associated with acquired immune deficiency syndrome (AIDS): A phase II trial. J Acquir Immune Defic Syndr 4:839–846, 1991

162. Taylor J, Afrasiabi R, Fahey JL, et al: Prognostically significant classification of immune changes in AIDS with Kaposi's sarcoma. Blood 67:666–671, 1986

163. Tessler AN, Catanese A: AIDS and germ cell tumors of testis. Urology 30:203–204, 1987

164. Timmerman JM, Northfelt DW, Small EJ: Malignant germ cell tumors in men infected with the human immunodeficiency virus: Natural history and results of therapy. J Clin Oncol 13:1391–1397, 1995

165. Tindal B, Finlayson R, Mutimer K, et al: Malignant melanoma associated with human immunodeficiency virus infection in three homosexual men. J Am Acad Dermatol 20:587–591, 1989

166. Tirelli U, Errante D, Oksenhendler E, et al for the French-Italian Cooperative Study Group: Prospective study with combined low-dose chemotherapy and zidovudine in 37 patients with poor-prognosis AIDS-related non-Hodgkin's lymphoma.

167. Tirelli U, Vaccher E, Sinicco A, et al: Forty-nine unusual HIV-related malignant tumors (Abstract W.C.P.50). Program of the Vth International Conference on AIDS, Montreal, Canada, 1989, p 600

168. Vadhan-Raj S, Wong G, Gnecco C, et al: Immunological variables as predictors of prognosis in patients with Kaposi's sarcoma and the acquired immunodeficiency syndrome. Cancer 46:417–425, 1986

169. Vogel J, Hinrichs SH, Reynolds RK, et al: The HIV tat gene induces dermal lesions resembling Kaposi's sarcoma in transgenic mice. Nature 335:606–611, 1988

170. Volberding PA, Abrams DA, Conant M, et al: Vinblastine therapy for Kaposi's sarcoma in the acquired immunodeficiency syndrome. Ann Intern Med 103:335–338, 1985

171. Volberding PA, Kusick P, Feigal D: Effects of chemotherapy for HIV-associated Kaposi's sarcoma on long-term survival (Abstract 11). Proc Am Soc Clin Oncol 8:3, 1989

172. Volberding PA, Mitsuyasu R: Recombinant interferon alpha in the treatment of acquired immune deficiency syndrome-related Kaposi's sarcoma. Semin Oncol 2(suppl 5):2–6, 1985

173. Volberding PA, Mitsuyasu RT, Golando JP, et al: Treatment of Kaposi's sarcoma with interferon alfa-2b (Intron A). Cancer 59:620–625, 1987

174. Ziegler J, Beckstead J, Volberding P, et al: Non-Hodgkin's lymphoma in 90 homosexual men: Relation to generalized lymphadenopathy and the acquired immunodeficiency syndrome. N Engl J Med 311:565–570, 1984

175. Ziegler J, Katongole-Mbidde E, Wabinga H, Dollbaum CM: Absence of sex-hormone receptors in Kaposi's sarcoma. N Engl J Med 345:925, 1995

176. Ziegler JL, Drew WL, Miner RC, et al: Outbreak of Burkitt's-like lymphoma in homosexual men. Lancet 2:631–633, 1982

Section IV

SPECIAL ASPECTS
OF AIDS

Chapter 29

The Chest Film in AIDS

PHILIP C. GOODMAN

The variety of opportunistic infections and neoplasms reported in patients with the acquired immunodeficiency syndrome (AIDS) has not changed much since 1981.[20,21] However, some diseases such as Legionnaire's pneumonia are less frequently reported, whereas others such as aspergillosis are now more common. The chest radiographic features of these entities may overlap, and this has discouraged some from using the chest film as a means of distinguishing among diseases. Nevertheless, some differences in appearance have proven fairly constant and, if recognized, permit diagnoses to be ordered into a sequence of most to least probable. This chapter addresses the chest film abnormalities observed with the more usual opportunistic infections and neoplasms seen in patients with AIDS. Less commentary is given to the infrequently observed diseases associated with the syndrome.

OPPORTUNISTIC INFECTIONS

Pneumocystis carinii Pneumonia

Pneumocystis carinii pneumonia (PCP) is the most common opportunistic pulmonary infection seen in patients with AIDS.[84,95] Chest film abnormalities are frequently present, yet in 10% to 39% of cases, the chest radiograph is normal.[52,100] The diagnosis in such situations is suggested by clinical and laboratory findings such as shortness of breath, lowered concentration of Po_2, decreased diffusing capacity, and, occasionally, an abnormal gallium lung scan. The diagnosis is confirmed by observing *P. carinii* in induced sputum, bronchoalveolar lavage, or lung biopsy samples.

In most patients with PCP, chest films are abnormal and reveal diffuse bilateral and usually fairly symmetric, fine reticular opacities[33,47,54]

(Fig. 29–1). Variations in this pattern occur frequently and include unilateral or focal lung opacities of the same quality, or, rarely, focal alveolar consolidation[49] (Fig. 29–2). Occasionally, the interstitial pattern is medium to coarse, and on rare occasions a miliary pattern is observed (Fig. 29–3). Focal nodules, measuring 1 to 2 cm in diameter, with or without cavitation, have also been attributed to *P. carinii* infection[9,38] (Fig. 29–4). The cavity walls are generally thicker than those observed with pneumatoceles.[73] The outer margins may be irregular or smooth. Cavitary nodules of PCP are usually solitary and fairly pathognomonic. Occasionally, cavitary nodules of *Cryptococcus, Aspergillus, Staphylococcus,* or bronchogenic carcinoma origin may have a similar appearance.

With appropriate therapy, improvement in the radiographic findings is expected within 7 to 10 days. Without therapy, rapid progression to a worsened, diffuse heterogeneous, and in later stages, severe bilateral homogeneous consolidation may occur. Therapy with intravenous trimethoprim-sulfamethoxazole (TMP/SMX) may lead to worsening of the chest film abnormalities within 4 days of beginning treatment. This is most likely caused by pulmonary edema due to the large amount of fluid required for intravenous therapy with this antibiotic and does not necessarily indicate worsening of pneumonia.[132] If warranted, diuretic therapy will often result in rapid improvement in the patient's radiographic and clinical state. Eventually, complete resolution of radiographic abnormalities is expected, although in some instances residual interstitial opacities are observed.[108,131] Adjunctive therapy with corticosteroids has been recommended for patients with moderate to severe PCP.[14,117] Rapid improvement in the chest film findings may be observed after this regimen.[56,109] A complication of steroid use may be an increase in secondary fungal infections.[81]

443

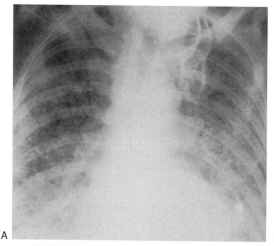
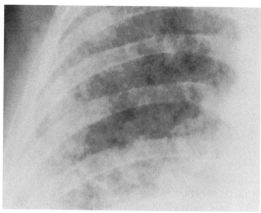

A   B

FIGURE 29–1. *Pneumocystis carinii* pneumonia (PCP). *A,* Anteroposterior (AP) chest film demonstrates moderate to severe bilateral reticular heterogeneous opacities. *B,* Close-up of the right midlung demonstrates the fine nature of the reticular opacities seen in PCP. In the peripheral areas of the lung, coalescence of these densities has produced a more homogeneous consolidation, as seen in severe episodes of infection.

A few interesting complications of PCP have been recognized with some frequency in the last several years. Spontaneous pneumothorax has been observed in approximately 5% to 10% of patients with PCP[27,53] (Fig. 29–5). The size of pneumothorax has varied from small to extremely large and may require tube thoracostomy, chemical pleurodesis, talc poudrage, or surgery.[2,64,126] Occasionally, outpatient care using a Heimlich valve has been successful.[129] Although somewhat controversial, the timing of the pneumothoraces is probably not related to treatment but apparently is due to infection with *P. carinii* itself.[113,125] Pneumothorax in AIDS patients is virtually pathognomonic of

PCP.[114] In some instances, pneumatoceles precede the appearance of pneumothorax (Fig. 29–6). In one series, 10% of patients with PCP were found to have pneumatoceles.[112] These thin-walled air-containing structures are solitary or multiple, may rapidly increase or decrease in size (Fig. 29–7), and generally resolve in 3 to 6 months. In rare instances, air-fluid levels have been noted within the pneumatoceles. These abnormalities have not been observed in AIDS patients with infections other than PCP. The mechanism for pneumatocele formation in this circumstance is unclear, and, although it may be due to a check valve mechanism, there is little pathologic proof this occurs in these pa-

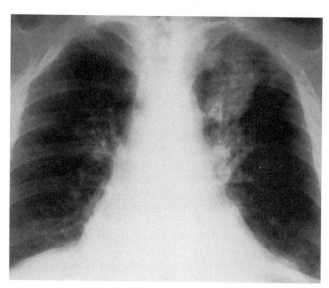

FIGURE 29–2. *Pneumocystis carinii* pneumonia (PCP). Posteroanterior (PA) chest film demonstrates a focal area of fairly homogeneous consolidation in the left upper lobe. Air bronchograms are seen in this region of alveolar opacity.

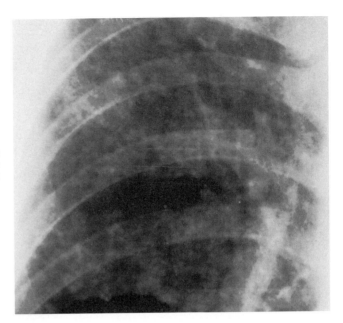

FIGURE 29–3. *Pneumocystis carinii* pneumonia (PCP). Close-up of a PA chest film demonstrates a fine to medium nodular or miliary pattern in the right upper and middle lobes.

tients.[102] Others suggest that necrosis in subpleural locations of the lung may result in pneumatoceles and subsequent pneumothorax.[39] Premature formation of bullae seen on computed tomography (CT) scans has been described in patients with AIDS.[75]

The distribution of PCP may be altered by prophylactic therapy with inhaled pentamidine. In some patients who have undergone this therapeutic regimen, new cases of PCP may be preferentially located in the upper lobes[10,16, 79,118] (Fig. 29–8). The reason for this probably is poor coverage of the upper lobes by aerosolized pentamidine. These unprotected areas are thus more likely to harbor *P. carinii* and to be selectively involved in pneumonia. Other unusual features of this therapy, including pneumothorax, pneumocystomas, pleural fluid, and lymphadenopathy, have also been reported.[2,3, 35,36,65,85] Nevertheless, the presence of pleural

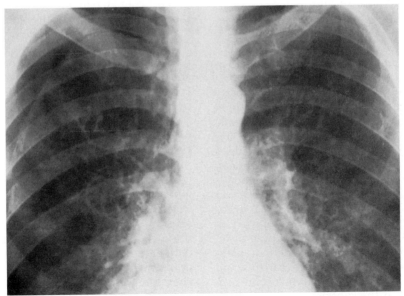

FIGURE 29–4. *Pneumocystis carinii* pneumonia (PCP). PA chest film demonstrates a solitary thick-walled cavity in the right upper lobe. PCP may appear in this fashion secondary to ischemic necrosis of affected lung.

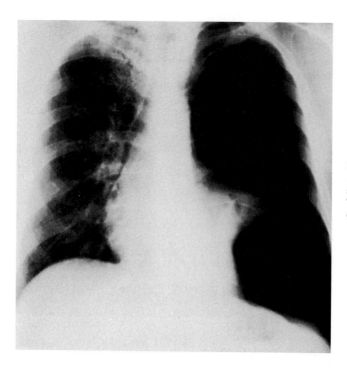

FIGURE 29–5. *Pneumocystis carinii* pneumonia (PCP) and pneumothorax. PA chest film demonstrates a large left-sided tension pneumothorax. The right lung, particularly the right upper lobe, demonstrates a medium reticulonodular pattern.

fluid or hilar or mediastinal lymphadenopathy should suggest a diagnosis other than PCP.

Mycobacterial Infections

Various mycobacterial species have been responsible for pulmonary infections in patients with AIDS.[7,18,54,63] Clearly, the majority of infections have been caused by *Mycobacterium tuberculosis* (TB) and *Mycobacterium avium* complex (MAC). The overall incidence of tuberculosis in AIDS patients has been reported to be as high as 24%.[101] More recently, in 14% of human immunodeficiency virus (HIV)–seropositive patients with known positive purified protein derivative (PPD) skin tests, TB developed within 2 years.[113a] Conversely, nearly 30% of adult non-Asian patients with tuberculosis had HIV infection.[17] The radiographic appearance of tuberculosis in this setting depends upon the stage of HIV infection.[62,104] Early in the course of infection, tuberculosis appears as it does in otherwise nonimmunosuppressed individuals; that is, patients with reactivation tuberculosis, considered the most common pathogenesis of tuberculosis in these patients, will present with heterogeneous nodular and cavitary infiltrates in the superior segments of the lower lobes and apical and posterior segments of the upper lobes (Fig. 29–9). These radio-graphic findings are not seen later in HIV infection, when diffuse and somewhat coarse interstitial opacities are observed with or without the presence of hilar or mediastinal adenopathy[50] (Fig. 29–10). Adenopathy itself may occur with different frequency within different AIDS risk groups. Thus, lymphadenopathy was found in a higher percentage (~80%) of injection drug users or Haitian patients with HIV infection and tuberculosis than in HIV-infected homosexual males with tuberculosis (~20%).[22,124] In a study from New York, 84% of patients with AIDS and tuberculosis had low-attenuation mediastinal and hilar nodes on CT scans.[103] Later in the course of HIV infection, tuberculosis may result in cavitation, but at a significantly reduced rate than in non–HIV-infected patients or those with early-stage HIV infection.[51] Pleural fluid is seen with varying incidence (9% to 22%).[50] The presence of adenopathy, pleural fluid, or a coarse bilateral heterogeneous infiltrate is much more typical of tuberculosis than of PCP.

Antituberculosis therapy should result in chest film improvement that parallels a clinical response by the patient.[119] Within weeks, the radiographic abnormalities seen with this infection should begin to resolve. Worsening of a chest film while a patient is receiving appropriate medication should prompt a workup for an alternate infection. Recently, an increase in multiple-drug-resistant TB cases has been ob-

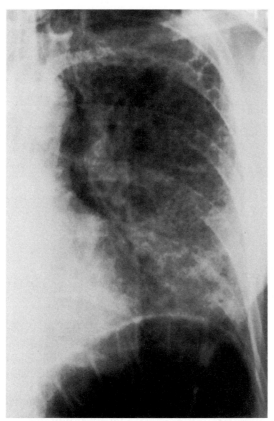

FIGURE 29–6. *Pneumocystis carinii* pneumonia (PCP) and pneumatoceles. Close-up of a PA chest film demonstrates heterogeneous medium interstitial opacities in the left lung. In the periphery of the left upper lobe, small, thin-walled, air-filled structures representing pneumatoceles are demonstrated. These usually resolve in 3 to 6 months but occasionally lead to pneumothorax.

served; consequently, appropriate individualized drug regimens have been recommended.[4,40a,77]

MAC is typically seen in the lymph nodes, liver, bone marrow, blood, and urine of patients with AIDS. Involvement of pulmonary parenchyma results in diffuse, heterogeneous, interstitial patterns with or without lymphadenopathy.[49] No definite features distinguishing this or other species of mycobacterial infection from tuberculosis have been observed on chest films. A comparison of chest films in AIDS patients with tuberculosis or MAC disease revealed that with the latter infection, approximately 50% had interstitial disease, 11% had adenopathy, and none had pleural fluid.[93] A more recent report suggests that adenopathy and pleural fluid may be noted, but that parenchymal disease due to nontuberculosis mycobacterial disease is unlikely.[6] Another article supports the

unusual occurrence of pulmonary MAC and reports chest films with consolidation, nodular infiltrates, and cavitation.[67]

Fungi

A variety of fungal infections have been observed in patients with AIDS. In regions endemic for *Histoplasma capsulatum* and *Coccidioides immitis*, these organisms have been responsible for a number of opportunistic pneumonias in HIV-infected individuals.[1,12,82,121,133,134] The radiographic appearance of these pneumonias is similar. Commonly, a diffuse, bilateral, poorly defined, nodular infiltrate is noted (Fig. 29–11). Lymphadenopathy is reported with variable incidence with both of these fungal infections. Other manifestations, including cavitation, alveolar consolidation, and pleural fluid have been reported but are less frequently observed.[83] A recent study of 50 AIDS patients with extrapulmonary histoplasmosis revealed that slightly over 50% had normal chest radiographs. The others demonstrated nodular, linear, or air-space opacities in decreasing frequency, respectively. Approximately 20% had small pleural effusions and less than 10% had adenopathy.[28]

Cryptococcal infections of AIDS patients generally affect the central nervous system (CNS), but more cases of cryptococcal pneumonia are being reported. The radiographic appearance is variable and includes single or multiple well-defined nodules with or without cavitation, diffuse reticular interstitial infiltrates, pleural fluid, and hilar or mediastinal adenopathy (Fig. 29–12).[25,26,115,124] A miliary pattern may also be seen with this and other fungal infections.[34,90]

Invasive aspergillosis in AIDS patients has been reported with increasing frequency.[72,78,92,107] Focal infiltrates of the upper lobes with or without cavitation are most commonly noted on chest films.[37,72,94,122] Occasionally, the focal opacities will remain stable for months. In one series, no air-crescent findings were noted.[91]

Cytomegalovirus

Cytomegalovirus (CMV) pneumonia was one of the initial opportunistic infections seen in patients with AIDS. However, our experience as well as others' suggests that this organism, though frequently observed in patients with AIDS, may not be responsible for pathologic lung changes.[89] Consequently, it is our

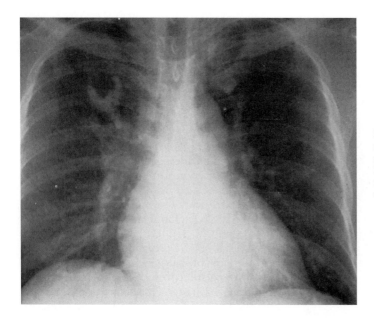

FIGURE 29–7. *Pneumocystis carinii* pneumonia (PCP). A PA chest film demonstrates multiple thin-walled pneumatoceles in both lungs. These generally will resolve over months. A pneumothorax is noted in the right hemithorax.

policy to emphasize this diagnosis less than the other opportunistic infections. In those patients reported to have CMV pneumonia, a diffuse, fine to medium reticular interstitial pattern has been observed on chest films.[123] However, it is difficult to be certain that the radiographic abnormalities have been caused by this organism because other opportunistic agents frequently coexist. It is extremely rare for CMV to be the sole pathogen responsible for pneumonia.[88,130] However, the incidence of CMV pneumonia may be increasing now

that individuals with low CD4 counts are living longer and steroids are being used more frequently.[61,97] A recent assessment of the chest film and CT abnormalities of patients with only CMV pneumonia includes focal and bilateral heterogeneous opacities, lung consolidations and ground-glass opacities, and solitary or multiple well-defined lung nodules.[87] Some reports suggest that patients shedding CMV in respiratory secretions may have a decreased inflammatory response to *P. carinii* and in fact will have a better short-term prognosis.[13]

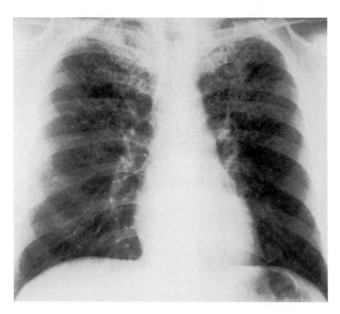

FIGURE 29–8. *Pneumocystis carinii* pneumonia (PCP). PA chest film demonstrates predominantly upper lobe medium reticular densities. This distribution of PCP may be the result of prior prophylactic aerosolized pentamidine therapy and mimics the distribution of reactivation tuberculosis.

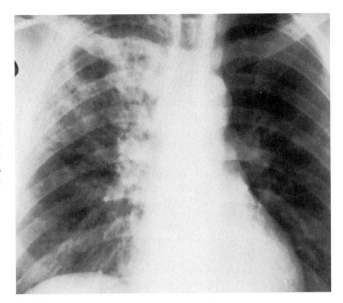

FIGURE 29–9. Tuberculosis. PA chest film demonstrates heterogeneous, medium to coarse reticular opacities in the right upper lobe. A large cavity is seen in this area. Minimal left upper lobe heterogeneous changes are seen. This pattern is typical of reactivation tuberculosis seen in the early stages of HIV infection.

Pyogenic Infection

Pneumonias caused by pyogenic organisms such as *Streptococcus pneumoniae, Haemophilus influenzae, Staphylococcus aureus,* and *Pseudomonas aeruginosa* have been reported with increasing frequency in patients with AIDS.[40,98,105,106] It has been well established that both T-cell and B-cell immune function is compromised in these patients, thus accounting for the increased frequency of pyogenic infections. The radiographic features are similar to those seen in nonimmunosuppressed individuals.[44,136] Air-space consolidation resulting in homogeneous opacity in a segment or lobe of lung is most frequently observed (Fig. 29–13). Parapneumonic effusions are also seen. Cavitation may occur in patients infected with organisms such as *Staphylococcus aureus* that can cause necrosis. A different finding has recently been

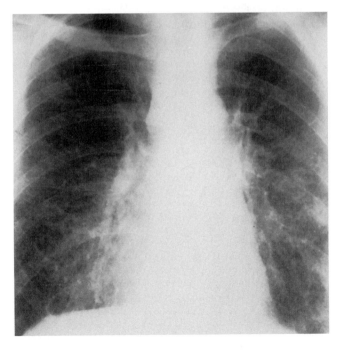

FIGURE 29–10. Tuberculosis. PA chest film demonstrates right paratracheal adenopathy and a diffuse fine to medium reticulonodular infiltrate. This is the pattern seen in patients with late-stage HIV infection and tuberculosis. Since adenopathy is not associated with PCP, it should not be considered a likely cause of disease in this patient.

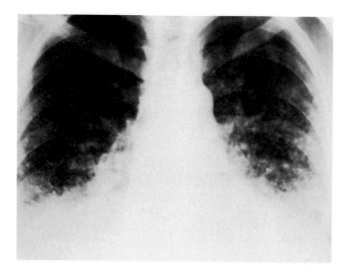

FIGURE 29–11. Histoplasmosis. Diffuse, bilateral, fairly coarse nodular opacities are seen in both lungs. This pattern is commonly reported in patients with disseminated histoplasmosis and coccidioidomycosis. Adenopathy is also associated with these diseases in patients with AIDS.

observed in a series from Switzerland in which nearly 50% of patients with bacterial pneumonias had diffuse reticulonodular opacities on chest radiographs.[80] Generally, patients with pyogenic pneumonia do not have concomitant infection with opportunistic organisms such as *P. carinii.* Response to appropriate antibiotics is similar to that of nonimmunosuppressed hosts such that radiographic improvement is seen within 1 to 2 weeks.[31] However, recurrent pneumonia and/or chronic pneumonia may require maintenance therapy.[8] It is important to consider bacterial pneumonias in differential diagnosis lists, as they may have a significant impact on patient morbidity and mortality.[98]

Rhodococcus equi is an unusual organism that has been the cause of lung disease in several HIV-infected patients. The chest films frequently reveal large moderately thick-walled cavities and empyema.[30,55,128]

Bronchitis caused by pyogenic organisms has also been seen with moderate frequency in patients with AIDS.[19] Radiographically, this is manifested by peribronchial thickening and "tram tracking" (Fig. 29–14). The latter finding is caused by bronchial mucosal edema and peribronchial inflammation and is seen as thin, parallel, linear opacities following the expected course of bronchi. This is not a feature of the pneumonia caused by *P. carinii.* Bronchiectasis in patients with AIDS has also been identified by CT.[86]

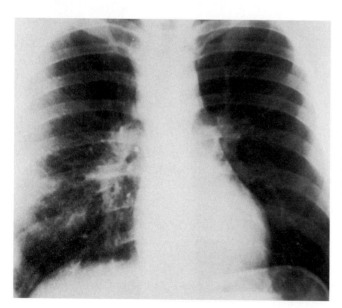

FIGURE 29–12. Cryptococcosis. PA chest film demonstrates right paratracheal and right hilar adenopathy. Occasionally, parenchymal lung nodules and reticular interstitial opacities also are seen in patients with intrathoracic cryptococcosis.

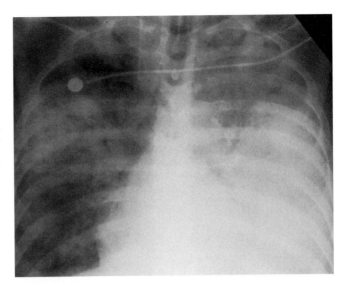

FIGURE 29–13. Pneumococcal pneumonia. AP chest film demonstrates a severe bilateral airspace consolidation, worse on the left than on the right. The findings are typical of severe pyogenic pneumonia.

NEOPLASMS

Kaposi's Sarcoma

The radiographic features of Kaposi's sarcoma are somewhat distinctive.[32,43,46,52,57,69,116] Pulmonary parenchymal involvement is manifest by coarse, poorly defined, nodular opacities scattered throughout the lungs (Fig. 29–15). Concomitant coarse, linear opacities usually distributed in a perihilar location are also frequent. Pleural fluid is reported in 35% to 50% of patients with Kaposi's sarcoma and is probably the result of pleural metastases. Kaposi's nodules generally increase slowly in size over several months. Rapid change in size of a suspected Kaposi's sarcoma pulmonary nodule with progression to lung consolidation suggests the possibility of hemorrhage in the region of these highly vascular lesions (Fig. 29–16). Hilar and mediastinal adenopathy may be observed but is uncommon (~8%). CT findings in patients with Kaposi's sarcoma reflect what is seen on chest films, with poorly marginated, nodular, and coarse perihilar opacities being most common.[96,137]

In patients with a background of intravenous drug abuse, differentiating Kaposi's sarcoma nodules from septic emboli may be impossible. However, within a few days, septic emboli will

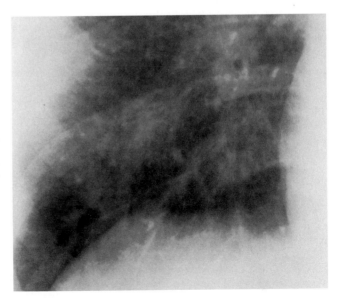

FIGURE 29–14. Bronchitis. Close-up of the right lower lobe demonstrates thin, linear opacities paralleling the course of segmental bronchi. This finding is called "tram tracking" and has been seen in AIDS patients with clinical bronchitis.

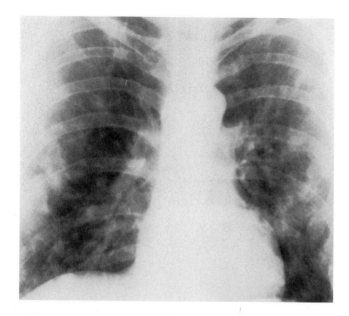

FIGURE 29–15. Kaposi's sarcoma (KS). Scattered, poorly defined nodules are seen in both lungs. This is a classic presentation of pulmonary KS. Other manifestations include pleural fluid and coarse linear interstitial opacities.

tend to cavitate, whereas Kaposi's sarcoma nodules will not. The use of sequential thallium and gallium scanning has also been proposed as a way to differentiate between pulmonary Kaposi's sarcoma and other pulmonary diseases associated with AIDS.[76] Generally, mucocutaneous Kaposi's sarcoma precedes pulmonary involvement, but occasionally lung disease is the first manifestation.[111]

Non-Hodgkin's Lymphoma

General differences in the lymphomas seen in patients with AIDS as compared to those seen in the general population include a greater stage of involvement at the time of initial discovery, greater aggressiveness of the neoplasm, an almost exclusive tendency for the lymphomas to be the non-Hodgkin's variety, and a decreased frequency of intrathoracic involvement.[60] An early study of AIDS patients with non-Hodgkin's lymphoma revealed that only 10% of patients had chest manifestations.[138] The radiographic features of non-Hodgkin's lymphoma in this setting include unilateral and bilateral pleural effusions in nearly half the patients. Hilar or mediastinal adenopathy is observed in nearly one fourth of chest films (Fig. 29–17). Pulmonary parenchymal involvement is manifest by reticulonodular interstitial infiltrates or alveolar consolidation in nearly one quarter of patients. The appearance of well-defined parenchymal nodules remarkable for their rapidity of growth has been noted (Fig. 29–18). These nodules do not tend to coalesce as do the poorly defined nodules of Kaposi's

sarcoma. Cavitation of these nodules may occur following therapy but is rare.[60]

Bronchogenic Carcinoma

There has been speculation and debate about whether HIV infection may be associated with an increased incidence of lung cancer.[23,24,110] Although a definite association has not been firmly established, there are numerous reports of bronchogenic carcinoma occurring in patients with HIV infection who are younger than the usual population with cancer. A history of intravenous drug abuse and cigarette smoking is usually elicited in these patients. Survival time in this population is significantly shortened.[42,70,120,127] The radiographic abnormalities are similar to those seen in the general population and include focal lung mass, hilar and mediastinal adenopathy, and pleural fluid.[15,41,58,135] In patients who have suspected focal PCP or fungal diseases, yet are not responding to appropriate therapy, the possibility of lung neoplasm should be raised. Diagnosis may be forthcoming with sputum cytology, bronchoscopic biopsy, or percutaneous transthoracic needle biopsy.

MISCELLANEOUS

Lymphocytic Interstitial Pneumonitis

Lymphocytic interstitial pneumonitis (LIP) is a disease of unknown cause that is characterized by an accumulation of lymphocytes and plasma cells in the pulmonary interstitial space. Al-

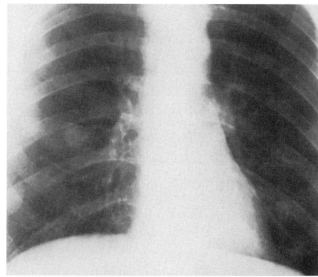

A

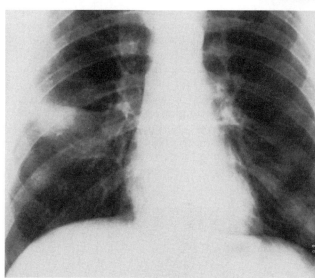

B

FIGURE 29–16. Kaposi's sarcoma (KS). *A,* PA chest film demonstrates two poorly defined nodules in the right middle lobe and one poorly defined nodule in the left retrocardiac area. These findings are typical of KS. *B,* The same patient 2 weeks later. At this time, more homogeneous consolidation is seen in the lower lobe and right middle lobe. This type of rapid change is most likely due to hemorrhage in the sites of pulmonary KS.

though even distribution is usually demonstrated, focal collections of lymphocytes may be observed.[29,48] This entity has now been recognized as an index diagnosis for AIDS in the pediatric patient. Chest films of these individuals are indistinguishable from those seen in patients with PCP. They typically demonstrate diffuse or focal, fine to medium reticular interstitial infiltrates[99] (Fig. 29–19). Some reports indicate a tendency to small nodular opacities correlating well with pathologic findings.[45] The chest radiographs remain stable initially but worsen over weeks to months. Lymphadenopathy may be seen in the late stages of disease.[59] Cystic lung disease and bronchiectasis may also develop after protracted illness.[5,11] Open lung biopsy is required for definitive diagnosis. Ste-

roid therapy may result in rapid radiographic improvement.

SUMMARY

The task of interpreting chest radiographs in patients with AIDS will be made easier, it is hoped, by applying the information contained in this chapter. Although the various infections and neoplasms seen with this syndrome occasionally have similar appearances on chest films, some patterns should allow construction of a limited differential diagnosis list. Indeed, there are findings that are nearly specific for certain processes. For example, in patients with AIDS, pneumatocele formation is seen exclusively in

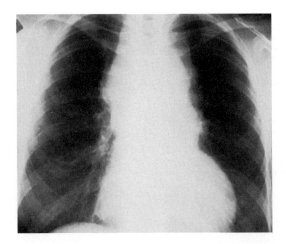

FIGURE 29–17. Non-Hodgkin's lymphoma. PA chest film demonstrates severe mediastinal adenopathy. Intrathoracic involvement in AIDS patients with non-Hodgkin's lymphoma has been observed approximately 10% of the time. Adenopathy, pleural fluid, and nodular parenchymal disease have been noted.

those with PCP. The finding of poorly defined nodular densities with associated pleural effusions is almost pathognomonic for Kaposi's sarcoma. On the other hand, some radiographic findings should dissuade one from considering certain diagnoses. For example, pleural fluid and lymphadenopathy are rarely if ever encountered in patients with PCP alone. Other entities such as non-Hodgkin's lymphoma, tuberculosis, or fungal infection should thus be considered. With experience, clinicians will develop more confidence to *interpret* the chest film, leading to better patient management.

I have emphasized the chest film abnormalities seen in patients with AIDS and have said little about the use of CT. In my experience, CT would not be a cost-beneficial modality. This has recently been confirmed in a study looking at the sensitivity and specificity of chest radiography and CT in the detection of the infections and neoplasms seen in AIDS patients. In this investigation, CT was, as expected, more sensitive to the findings of lung disease, but the authors concluded that for the majority of patients chest films were adequate and CT was not indicated.[68]

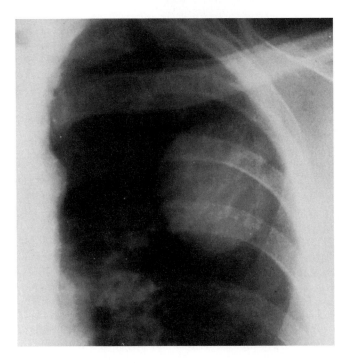

FIGURE 29–18. Non-Hodgkin's lymphoma. This large, well-defined nodule appeared over a period of 6 weeks. A needle biopsy was unrevealing, but an open lung procedure demonstrated a large non-Hodgkin's lymphoma lesion.

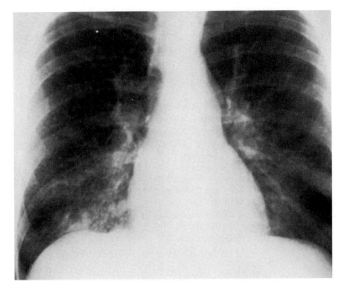

FIGURE 29–19. Lymphocytic interstitial pneumonia (LIP). PA chest film demonstrates bibasilar fine to medium reticular interstitial opacities indistinguishable from PCP. An open lung biopsy revealed LIP.

REFERENCES

1. Abrams DI, Robia M, Blumenfeld W, et al: Disseminated coccidioidomycosis in AIDS. N Engl J Med 310:986, 1984
2. Albort JV, Callejas MA, Canalis EA, et al: Surgical management of spontaneous pneumothorax in patients with AIDS. Ann Thorac Surg 55:808, 1993
3. Albrecht H, Stellbrenk HJ, Fenske S, et al: A novel variety of atypical *Pneumocystis carinii* infection after long-term prophylactic pentamidine inhalation in an AIDS patient: Large lower lobe pneumocystoma. Clin Invest 71:310, 1993
4. American Thoracic Society Centers for Disease Control: Treatment of tuberculosis and tuberculosis infection in adults and children. Am J Respir Crit Care Med 149:1359, 1994
5. Amorosa JK, Miller RW, Laraya-Cuasay L, et al: Bronchiectasis in children with lymphocytic interstitial pneumonia and acquired immune deficiency syndrome. Plain film and CT observations. Pediatr Radiol 22:603, 1992
6. Aronchick JM, Miller WT Jr: Disseminated nontuberculous mycobacterial infections in immunosuppressed patients. Semin Roentgenol 28:150, 1993
7. Bamberger DM, Driks MR, Gupta MR, et al: *Mycobacterium kansasii* among patients affected with human immunodeficiency virus in Kansas City. Clin Infect Dis 18:395, 1994
8. Baron AD, Hollander H: *Pseudomonas aeruginosa* bronchopulmonary infection in late human immunodeficiency virus disease. Am Rev Respir Dis 148:992, 1993
9. Barrio JL, Suarez M, Rodriguez JL, et al: *Pneumocystis carinii* pneumonia presenting as cavitating and non-cavitating solitary pulmonary nodules in patients with the acquired immunodeficiency syndrome. Am Rev Respir Dis 134:1094, 1986
10. Baughman RP, Dohn MN, Shipley R, et al: Increased *Pneumocystis carinii* recovery from the upper lobes in *Pneumocystis* pneumonia. The effect of aerosol pentamidine prophylaxis. Chest 103:426, 1993
11. Berdon WE, Mellins RB, Abramson SJ, et al: Pediatric HIV infection in its second decade—the changing pattern of lung involvement. Clinical, plain film, and computed tomographic findings. Radiol Clin North Am 31:453, 1993
12. Bonner JR, Alexander WJ, Dismukes WE, et al: Disseminated histoplasmosis in patients with the acquired immune deficiency syndrome. Arch Intern Med 144:2178, 1984
13. Bozzette SA, Arcia J, Bartok AE, et al: Impact of *Pneumocystis carinii* and cytomegalovirus on the course and outcome of atypical pneumonia in advanced human immunodeficiency virus disease. J Infect Dis 165:93, 1992
14. Bozzette SA, Satler FR, Chiu J, et al: A controlled trial of early adjunctive treatment with corticosteroids for *Pneumocystis carinii* pneumonia in the acquired immunodeficiency syndrome. N Engl J Med 323:1451, 1990
15. Braun MA, Killam DA, Remick SC, et al: Lung cancer in patients seropositive for human immunodeficiency virus. Radiology 175:341, 1990
16. Case Records of the Massachusetts General Hospital Case 9-1989: N Engl J Med 320:582, 1989
17. Centers for Disease Control: Advisory committee for elimination of tuberculosis and human immunodeficiency virus infection. MMWR 38:236, 1989
18. Centers for Disease Control: Diagnosis and management of mycobacterial infection and disease in persons with human immunodeficiency virus infection. Ann Intern Med 106:254, 1987
19. Chechani V, Allam AA, Smith PR, et al: Bronchitis mimicking opportunistic lung infection in patients with human immunodeficiency virus infection/AIDS. N Y State J Med 92:297, 1992
20. Centers for Disease Control: Kaposi's sarcoma and

Pneumocystis pneumonia among homosexual men: New York City and California. MMWR 30:305, 1981

21. Centers for Disease Control: *Pneumocystis* pneumonia—Los Angeles. MMWR 30:250, 1981

22. Chaisson RE, Schecter GF, Theuer CP, et al: Tuberculosis in patients with the acquired immunodeficiency syndrome: Clinical features, response to therapy, and survival. Ann Rev Respir Dis 136:570, 1987

23. Chan TK, Aranda CP, Rom WN: Bronchogenic carcinoma in young patients at risk for acquired immunodeficiency syndrome. Chest 103:862, 1993

24. Chechani V, Allam AA, Smith PR, et al: Bronchitis mimicking opportunistic lung infection in patients with human immunodeficiency virus infection/AIDS. NY State J Med 92:297, 1992

25. Chechani V, Camholz SL: Pulmonary manifestations of disseminated cryptococcosis in patients with AIDS. Chest 98:1060, 1990

26. Clark RA, Greer DL, Valaines GT, et al: *Cryptococcus neoformans* pulmonary infection in human immunodeficiency virus-1-infected patients. J Acquir Immune Defic Syndr 3:480, 1990

27. Coker RS, Moss F, Peters B, et al: Pneumothorax in patients with AIDS. Respir Med 87:43, 1993

28. Conces DJ Jr, Stockberger SM, Tarver RD, et al: Disseminated histoplasmosis in AIDS: Findings on chest radiographs. Am J Roentgenol 160:15, 1993

29. Conces DJ, Tarver RD: Noninfectious and non-malignant pulmonary disease in AIDS. J Thorac Imaging 6:53, 1991

30. Cury JD, Harrington PT, Hosein IK: Successful medical therapy of *Rhodococcus equi* pneumonia in a patient with HIV infection. Chest 102:1619, 1992

31. Dailey CL: Bacterial pneumonia in HIV-infected patients. Semin Respir Infect 8:104, 1993

32. Davis SD, Henschke CI, Chamides BK, et al: Intrathoracic Kaposi sarcoma in AIDS patients: Radiographic-pathologic correlation. Radiology 163:495, 1987

33. De Lorenzo IJ, Huang CT, Maguire GP, et al: Roentgenographic patterns of *Pneumocystis carinii* pneumonia in 104 patients with AIDS. Chest 91:323, 1987

34. Douketis JD, Kesten S: Miliary cryptococcosis in a patient with the acquired immunodeficiency syndrome. Thorax 48:402, 1993

35. Eagar GM, Friedland JA, Sagal SS: Tumefactive *Pneumocystis carinii* infection in AIDS: Report of three cases. Am J Roentgenol 160:1197, 1993

36. Edelstein H, McCabe RE: Atypical presentations of *Pneumocystis carinii* pneumonia in patients receiving inhaled pentamidine prophylaxis. Chest 98:1366, 1990

37. Fairley CK, Kent SJ, Street A, et al: Invasive aspergillosis in AIDS. Aust N Z J Med 21:747, 1991

38. Ferre C, Baguena F, Podzamczer D, et al: Lung cavitation associated with *Pneumocystis carinii* infection in the acquired immunodeficiency syndrome: A report of 6 cases and review of the literature. Eur Respir J 7:134, 1994

39. Feuerstein IM, Archer A, Pluda JM, et al: Thin-walled cavities, cysts and pneumothoraces in *Pneumocystis carinii* pneumonia: Further observations with histopathologic correlation. Radiology 174:697, 1990

40. Fimberkoff MS, El Sadr W, Schiffman G, et al: *Streptococcus pneumoniae* infections and bacteremia in patients with acquired immune deficiency syndrome with report of a pneumococcal vaccine failure. Am Rev Respir Dis 130:1174, 1984

40a. Fischl MA, Daikos GL, Uttanchandani RB, et al: Clinical presentation and outcome of patients with HIV infection and tuberculosis caused by multiple drug-resistant bacilli. Ann Intern Med 117:189, 1992

41. Fishman JR, Schwartz DS, Sais GJ, et al: Bronchogenic carcinoma in HIV-positive patients: Findings on chest radiographs and CT scans. Am J Roentgenol 164:57, 1995

42. Fraire AE, Awe RJ: Lung cancer in association with human immunodeficiency virus infection. Cancer 70:432, 1992

43. Garay SM, Belenko M, Fazzini E, et al: Pulmonary manifestations of Kaposi's sarcoma. Chest 91:39, 1987

44. Garcia-Leoni ME, Moreno S, Rodeno P, et al: Pneumococcal pneumonia in adult hospitalized patients infected with the human immunodeficiency virus. Arch Intern Med 152:1808, 1992

45. Goldman HS, Ziprowski MN, Charytan M, et al: Lymphocytic interstitial pneumonitis in children with AIDS: A perfect radiographic-pathologic correlation (Abstract). Am J Roentgenol 145:868, 1985

46. Goodman PC: Kaposi's sarcoma. J Thorac Imaging 6:43, 1991

47. Goodman PC: *Pneumocystis carinii* pneumonia. J Thorac Imaging 6:16, 1991

48. Goodman PC: Pulmonary disease in children with AIDS. J Thorac Imaging 6:60, 1991

49. Goodman PC: Pulmonary manifestations of AIDS. Curr Probl Diagn Radiol 17:81, 1988

50. Goodman PC: Pulmonary tuberculosis in patients with the acquired immunodeficiency syndrome. J Thorac Imaging 5:38–45, 1990

51. Goodman PC: Tuberculosis and AIDS. Radiol Clin North Am 33:707, 1995

52. Goodman PC, Broaddus VC, Hopewell PC: Chest radiographic patterns in the acquired immunodeficiency syndrome. Am Rev Respir Dis 129:26, 1984

53. Goodman PC, Daley C, Minagi H: Spontaneous pneumothorax in AIDS patients with *Pneumocystis carinii* pneumonia. Am J Roentgenol 147:29, 1986

54. Goodman PC, Gamsu G: Radiographic findings in the acquired immunodeficiency syndrome. Postgrad Radiol 7:3, 1987

55. Gray BM: Case report. *Rhodococcus equi* pneumonia in a patient infected by the human immunodeficiency virus. Am J Med Sci 303:180, 1992

56. Groskin SA, Stadnick ME, Dupont PG: *Pneumocystis carinii* pneumonia: Effect of corticosteroid treatment on radiographic appearance in a patient with AIDS. Radiology 180:423, 1991

57. Gruden JF, Huang L, Webb WR, et al: AIDS-related Kaposi sarcoma of the lung: Radiograph, findings and staging system with bronchoscopic correlation. Radiology 195:545, 1995

58. Gruden JF, Klein JS, Webb WR: Percutaneous transthoracic needle biopsy in AIDS: Analysis in 32 patients. Radiology 189:567, 1993

59. Haney PJ, Yale-Loehr AJ, Nussbaum AR, et al: Imaging of infants and children with AIDS. Am J Roentgenol 152:1033, 1989

60. Haskal ZJ, Lindan C, Goodman PC: Lymphoma in

the immunocompromised patient. Radiol Clin North Am 28:885, 1990

61. Hoover DR, Saah AJ, Becellar H, et al: Clinical manifestations of AIDS in the era of *Pneumocystis* prophylaxis. N Engl J Med 329:1922, 1993

62. Hopewell PC: Tuberculosis and human immunodeficiency virus infection. Semin Respir Infect 4:111, 1989

63. Hopewell PC, Luce JM: Pulmonary manifestations of the acquired immunodeficiency syndrome. Clin Immunol Allergy 6:489, 1986

64. Horowitz MD, Oliva H: Pneumothorax in AIDS patients: Operative management. Am Surg 59:200, 1993

65. Horowitz ML, Schiff M, Samuels J, et al: *Pneumocystis carinii* pleural effusion. Pathogenesis and pleural fluid analysis. Am Rev Respir Dis 148:232, 1993

66. Jayes RL, Camerow HN, Hasselquist SM, et al: Disseminated pneumocystosis presenting as a pleural effusion. Chest 103:306, 1993

67. Kalayjian RC, Toossi Z, Tomashefski JF, et al: Pulmonary disease due to infection by *Mycobacterium avium* complex in patients with AIDS. Clin Infect Dis 20:1186, 1995

68. Kang E, Staples CA, McGuinness G, et al: Detection and differential diagnosis of pulmonary infections and tumors in patients with AIDS: Value of chest radiography versus CT. Am J Roentgenol 166:15, 1996

69. Kaplan L, Hopewell PC, Jaffe H, et al: Kaposi's sarcoma involving the lung in patients with the acquired immunodeficiency syndrome. J AIDS 1:23, 1988

70. Karp J, Profeta G, Marantz PR, et al: Lung cancer in patients with immunodeficiency syndrome. Chest 103:410, 1993

71. Keiper MD, Beumont M, Elshami A, et al: CDR T lymphocyte count and the radiographic presentation of pulmonary tuberculosis. Chest 107:74, 1995

72. Klapholz A, Salomon N, Perlman DC, et al: Aspergillosis in acquired immunodeficiency syndrome. Chest 100:1614, 1991

73. Klein JS, Warnock M, Webb WR, et al: Cavitating and noncavitating granulomas in AIDS patients with *Pneumocystis* pneumonitis. Am J Roentgenol 152:753, 1989

74. Kovacs A, Forthal DN, Kovacs JA, et al: Disseminated coccidioidomycosis in a patient with acquired immune deficiency syndrome. West J Med 140:447, 1984

75. Kuhlman JE, Knowles MC, Fishman EK, et al: Premature bullous pulmonary damage in AIDS: CT diagnosis. Radiology 173:23, 1989

76. Lee VW, Fuller JD, O'Brien MJ, et al: Pulmonary Kaposi sarcoma in patients with AIDS: Scintigraphic diagnosis with sequential thallium and gallium scanning. Radiology 180:409, 1991

77. Lessnau K-D, Gorla M, Talavera W: Radiographic findings in HIV-positive patients with sensitive and resistant tuberculosis. Chest 106:687, 1994

78. Lortholary O, Meyokas MC, Dupont B, et al: Invasive aspergillosis in patients with acquired immunodeficiency syndrome: Report of 33 cases. French cooperative study group on aspergillosis in AIDS. Am J Med 95:177, 1993

79. Lowery S, Fallat R, Feigal DW, et al: Changing patterns of *Pneumocystis carinii* pneumonia on penta-

midine aerosol prophylaxis. Abstracts from Fourth International Conference on AIDS 1:419, 1988

80. Magnenat J, Nicod LP, Auckenthaler R, et al: Mode of presentation and diagnosis of bacterial pneumonia in human immunodeficiency virus-infected patients. Am Rev Respir Dis 144:917, 1991

81. Mahaffey KW, Hippenmeyer CL, Mandel R, et al: Unrecognized coccidioidomycosis complicating *Pneumocystis carinii* pneumonia in patients infected with the human immunodeficiency virus and treated with corticosteroids. A report of two cases. Arch Intern Med 153:1496, 1993

82. Mandell W, Goldberg DM, Neu HC: Histoplasmosis in patients with acquired immune deficiency syndrome. Am J Med 81:974, 1986

83. Marshall BC, Cox JK Jr, Carroll KC, et al: Case report: Histoplasmosis as a cause of pleural effusion in the acquired immunodeficiency syndrome. Am J Med Sci 300:98, 1990

84. Masur H: Prevention and treatment of *Pneumocystis* pneumonia. N Engl J Med 327:1853, 1992

85. Mayor B, Schnyder P, Giron J, et al: Mediastinal and hilar lymphadenopathy due to *Pneumocystis carinii* infection in AIDS patients. CT features. J Comput Assist Tomogr 18:408, 1994

86. McGuinness G, Naidich DP, Garay S, et al: AIDS associated bronchiectasis: CT features. J Comput Assist Tomogr 17:260, 1993

87. McGuinness G, Scholes JV, Garay SM, et al: Cytomegalovirus pneumonitis: Spectrum of parenchymal CT findings with pathologic correlation in 21 AIDS patients. Radiology 192:451, 1994

88. Miles PR, Baughman RP, Linnemann CC Jr: Cytomegalovirus in the bronchoalveolar lavage fluid of patients with AIDS. Chest 97:1072, 1990

89. Millar AB, Patou GM, Miller RF, et al: Cytomegalovirus in the lungs of patients with AIDS: Respiratory pathogen or passenger? Am Rev Respir Dis 141:1474, 1990

90. Miller WT Jr, Edelman JM, Miller WT: Cryptococcal pulmonary infection in patients with AIDS: Radiographic appearances. Radiology 175:725, 1990

91. Miller WT Jr, Sais GJ, Frank I, et al: Pulmonary aspergillosis in patients with AIDS. Chest 105:37, 1994

92. Minamoto GY, Barlam TF, Vander Els NJ: Invasive aspergillosis in patients with AIDS. Clin Infect Dis 14:66, 1992

93. Modelevsky T, Sattler FR, Barnes PF: Mycobacterial disease in patients with human immunodeficiency virus infection. Arch Intern Med 149:2201, 1989

94. Morrison DL, Granton JT, Keston S, et al: Cavitary aspergillosis as a complication of AIDS. J Can Assoc Radiol 44:35, 1993

95. Murray JF, Garay SM, Hopewell PC, et al: Pulmonary complications of the acquired immunodeficiency syndrome: An update. Am Rev Respir Dis 135:504, 1987

96. Naidich DP, Tarras M, Garay SM, et al: Kaposi's sarcoma: CT radiographic correlation. Chest 96:723, 1989

97. Nelson MR, Erskine D, Hawkins DA, Gazzard BG: Treatment with corticosteroids: A risk factor for the development of clinical cytomegalovirus disease in AIDS. AIDS 7:375, 1993

98. Nichols L, Balogh K, Silverman M: Bacterial infections in the acquired immunodeficiency syndrome. Am J Clin Pathol 92:787, 1989

99. Oldham SAA, Castillo M, Jacobson FL, et al: HIV-associated lymphocytic interstitial pneumonia: Ra-

diologic manifestations and pathologic correlation. Radiology 170:83, 1989

100. Opravil M, Marincek B, Fuchs WA, et al: Shortcomings of chest radiography in detecting *Pneumocystis carinii* pneumonia. J Acquir Immune Defic Syndr 7:39, 1994

101. Page JW, Liautaud B, Thomas F, et al: Characteristics of the acquired immunodeficiency syndrome (AIDS) in Haiti. N Engl J Med 309:945, 1983

102. Panicek DM: Cystic pulmonary lesions in patients with AIDS. Radiology 173:12, 1989

103. Pastores SM, Naidich DP, Aranda CP, et al: Intrathoracic adenopathy associated with pulmonary tuberculosis in patients with human immunodeficiency virus infection. Chest 103:1433, 1993

104. Pitchenik AE, Burr J, Suarez M, et al: Human T-cell lymphotropic virus-III (HTLV-III) seropositivity and related disease among 71 consecutive patients in whom tuberculosis was diagnosed. Am Rev Respir Dis 135:875, 1987

105. Polsky B, Gold JWN, Whimbey E, et al: Bacterial pneumonia in patients with the acquired immunodeficiency syndrome. Ann Intern Med 104:38, 1986

106. Miller RF, Foley NM, Kessel D, Jeffrey AA: Community acquired lobar pneumonia in patients with HIV infection and AIDS. Thorax 49:367, 1994

107. Pursell KJ, Telzak EE, Armstrong D: Aspergillus species colonization and invasive disease in patients with AIDS. Clin Infect Dis 14:141, 1992

108. Ramaswany G, Jagadha V, Tchnentkoff V: Diffuse alveolar damage and interstitial fibrosis in acquired immunodeficiency syndrome. Patients without concurrent pulmonary infection. Arch Pathol Lab Med 109:408, 1985

109. Rankin JA, Pella JA: Radiographic resolution of *Pneumocystis carinii* pneumonia in response to corticosteroid therapy. Am Rev Respir Dis 136:182, 1987

110. Remick SC: Lung cancer. An HIV-related neoplasm or a coincidental finding? Chest 102:1643, 1992

111. Roux FJ, Bancal C, Dombret MC, et al: Pulmonary Kaposi's sarcoma revealed by a solitary nodule in a patient with acquired immunodeficiency syndrome. Am J Respir Crit Care Med 149:1041, 1994

112. Sandhu JS, Goodman PC: Pulmonary cysts associated with *Pneumocystis carinii* pneumonia in patients with AIDS. Radiology 173:33, 1989

113. Scannell KA: Pneumothoraces and *Pneumocystis carinii* pneumonia in two AIDS patients receiving aerosolized pentamidine. Chest 97:479, 1990

113a. Selwin PA, Hartel D, Lewis BA, et al: A prospective study of the risk of tuberculosis on intravenous drug users with human immunodeficiency virus infection. N Engl J Med 320:545, 1989

114. Sepkowitz KA, Telzak EE, Gold JWM, et al: Pneumothorax in AIDS. Ann Intern Med 103:991, 1993

115. Sider L, Westcott MA: Pulmonary manifestations of cryptococcosis in patients with AIDS: CT features. J Thorac Imaging 9:78, 1994

116. Sivit CJ, Schwartz AM, Rockoff SD: Kaposi's sarcoma of the lung in AIDS. Radiologic pathologic analysis. AJR Am J Roentgenol 148:25, 1987

117. Sleasman JW, Hemenway C, Klein AS, et al: Corticosteroids improve survival of children with AIDS and *Pneumocystis carinii* pneumonia. Am J Dis Child 147:30, 1993

118. Small P, Goodman PC, Montgomery AB: Case 9-

119. Small P, Hopewell PC, Schecter GF, et al: Evolution of chest radiographs in treated patients with pulmonary tuberculosis and HIV infection. J Thorac Imaging 9:74, 1994

120. Sridhar KS, Flores MR, Raub WA Jr, et al: Lung cancer in patients with human immunodeficiency virus infection compared with historic control subjects. Chest 102:1704, 1992

121. Stansell JD: Fungal disease in HIV-infected persons: Cryptococcosis, histoplasmosis, and coccidioidomycosis. J Thorac Imaging 6:28, 1991

122. Staples CA, Kang EY, Wright JL, et al: Invasive pulmonary aspergillosis in AIDS: Radiographic, CT, and pathologic findings. Radiology 196:409, 1995

123. Stover DE, White DA, Romano PA, et al: Spectrum of pulmonary diseases associated with the acquired immune deficiency syndrome. Am J Med 78:429, 1985

124. Suster B, Akerman M, Orenstein M, et al: Pulmonary manifestations of AIDS: Review of 106 episodes. Radiology 161:87, 1986

125. Toronto Aerosolized Pentamidine Study Group: Aerosolized pentamidine and spontaneous pneumothorax in AIDS patients. Chest 97:510, 1990

126. Travaline JM, Criner GJ: Persistent bronchopleural fistula in an AIDS patient with *Pneumocystis carinii* pneumonia. Successful treatment with chemical pleurodesis. Chest 103:991, 1993

127. Vaccher E, Tirelli U, Spina M, et al: Lung cancer in 19 patients with HIV infection. The Italian Cooperative Study Group on AIDS and Tumors. Ann Oncol 4:85, 1993

128. Verville TD, Huycke MM, Greenfield RA, et al: *Rhodococcus equi* infections of humans. Twelve cases and a review of the literature. Medicine 73:119, 1994

129. Walker WA, Poate JW: AIDS-related bronchopleural fistula. Ann Thorac Surg 55:1048, 1993

130. Wallace JM, Hannah J: Cytomegalovirus pneumonitis in patients with AIDS. Chest 92:198, 1987

131. Wasserman K, Pothoff G, Kirn E, et al: Chronic *Pneumocystis carinii* pneumonia in AIDS. Chest 104:667, 1993

132. Wharton J, Coleman DL, Wofsy CB, et al: Trimethoprim-sulfamethoxazole or pentamidine for *Pneumocystis carinii* pneumonia in the acquired immunodeficiency syndrome. Ann Intern Med 105:37, 1986

133. Wheat IJ, Slama TG, Zeckel ML: Histoplasmosis in the acquired immune deficiency syndrome. Am J Med 78:203, 1985

134. Wheat J: Histoplasmosis and coccidioidomycosis in individuals with AIDS. A clinical review. Infect Dis Clin North Am 8:467, 1994

135. White CS, Haramati LB, Elder KH, et al: Carcinoma of the lung in HIV-positive patients: Findings on chest radiographs and CT scans. Am J Roentgenol 164:593, 1995

136. White S, Tsou E, Waldhorn R, et al: Life threatening bacterial pneumonia in male homosexuals with laboratory features of the acquired immunodeficiency syndrome. Chest 87:486, 1985

137. Wolff SD, Kuhlman JE, Fishman EK: Thoracic Kaposi sarcoma in AIDS: CT findings. J Comput Assist Tomogr 17:60, 1993

138. Zieler JL, Beckstead JA, Volberding PA, et al: Non-Hodgkin's lymphoma in 90 homosexual men. N Engl J Med 311:565, 1984

1989: AIDS and a cavitary pulmonary lesion (Letter). N Engl J Med 321:395, 1989

Chapter 30

Management of Pregnant Women with HIV Infection

DANIEL V. LANDERS and MAUREEN T. SHANNON

The rapid spread of HIV in women of child-bearing years has accentuated the need for clinicians to understand the effect of this infection on the pregnant woman and her unborn baby. Anonymous seroprevalence studies of antibody testing in newborns indicate that, as early as 1990, some 7130 HIV-infected women gave birth in the United States.[16] This suggests that 1.7 out of 1000 pregnant women in the United States are infected with HIV. The incidence of HIV in women is continuing to rise, and figures from 1994 through 1995 show the highest rate of increase ever.[5] It follows that infected pregnant women will continue to appear at increasingly higher rates.

Current national guidelines recommend HIV counseling and voluntary testing of all pregnant women.[6] HIV antibody testing must be accompanied by comprehensive counseling (see Chapter 15). This counseling should be provided by an experienced counselor in an informative, nonjudgmental manner, with accurate information about risks and options. Counseling for women who test positive should include the implications for both the woman and her fetus, methods of preventing transmission to others, and methods to avoid further exposure of the woman to HIV and other sexually transmitted diseases. The woman's sexual partner(s) and any other children at risk for perinatal exposure also need testing.

THE EFFECTS OF PREGNANCY ON HIV DISEASE

It has been suggested that pregnancy represents a relatively immunosuppressed state to protect the fetus from immune rejection. The evidence often cited is the susceptibility of pregnant women to more severe clinical courses with certain infections such as poliomyelitis, hepatitis A, malaria, and coccidioidomycosis. Moreover, altered numbers and ratios of CD4- and CD8-bearing T lymphocytes, decreased proliferative responses, and decreased immunoglobulin levels have all been reported in pregnancy.[3] Despite these changes, the normal pregnant woman is generally regarded as immunocompetent and capable of effectively responding to most infections. Biggar and colleagues followed CD4 counts longitudinally in HIV-infected and uninfected gravidas through the postpartum period.[2] They found that, although both groups exhibited a decrease in the number of CD4-bearing lymphocytes during pregnancy, the counts of the HIV-infected women did not recover postpartum. These findings were disconcerting considering the potential for HIV disease progression during pregnancy. In a subsequent study, Dinsmoor and Chrismas evaluated lymphocyte counts in 23 HIV-infected pregnant women, of whom 10 received zidovudine during the pregnancy. The CD4 and CD8 lymphocyte counts tended to decrease in women not taking zidovudine. They also noted a decrease in the total lymphocyte count with gestational age, which may account for the individual CD4 and CD8 decreases.[9]

Early clinical studies investigating the possible effects of pregnancy on HIV disease reported a more rapid progression to a diagnosis of AIDS or AIDS-related complex following delivery in HIV-seropositive women.[25,36] Gloeb and co-workers studied survival and disease progression after delivery. They reported findings on 103 HIV-seropositive pregnant women, and suggested that the prognosis of HIV infection may be negatively influenced by pregnancy.[13] However, the authors noted the limitations of the study and recognized the possibility of overestimation of HIV progression because of a relatively high rate of loss to follow-up. This report has also been criticized because of the absence of nonpregnant matched controls.[12] More recently, Burns et al. reported results from a prospective investigation of the effects of pregnancy on immune function in 192 HIV-infected women compared to 148 HIV-negative controls.[4] T-lymphocyte subsets were measured from the participants during the antenatal, perinatal, and postpartum periods. The HIV-infected pregnant women demonstrated a steady decline in CD4 cell count measurements throughout pregnancy and the postpartum period. Although a similar decline in CD4 cell counts in the controls was also observed during pregnancy, there was an increase in the levels noted during the third trimester and at 12 months postpartum. CD8 cell counts increased during pregnancy and returned to baseline by 6 months postpartum in both groups of women. The authors did note that other factors, such as nutritional status, may have influenced the fluctuations observed in the CD4 cell counts. Other investigators conducting prospective controlled studies of HIV-infected pregnant women have not observed any evidence that pregnancy enhances HIV disease progression in asymptomatic women.

At present, there is no clear consensus, nor are there overwhelmingly convincing data, to conclude that HIV disease progression is accelerated during or following pregnancy regardless of CD4 counts or clinical status of HIV disease. In general terms, the pregnant woman with HIV disease should be cared for in the same manner as the nonpregnant woman. The potential fetal effects and other issues regarding therapeutic interventions during pregnancy are discussed in the remainder of this chapter.

THE EFFECTS OF HIV INFECTION ON PREGNANCY

Several published studies have addressed the effects of HIV infection on pregnancy outcome. The earliest report on 50 HIV-seropositive pregnant women found that 35 (70%) had complicated prenatal courses, most commonly preterm labor or infectious complications.[14] Minkoff and co-workers reported the course of pregnancy in 91 seropositive and 126 seronegative women in Brooklyn, New York.[26] They found that seropositive women were more likely to have sexually transmitted diseases and medical complications during pregnancy than were seronegative women. However, they found no association between HIV status and birth weight, gestational age, head circumference, or Apgar score when controlling for drug and tobacco use and maternal age. These findings were in agreement with those of others who studied HIV-infected drug users during pregnancy.[17,37] All of these studies are prone to the type II statistical errors that plague studies with negative findings and insufficient power to detect real differences. This is particularly problematic in determining effects of HIV infection on infrequent complications of pregnancy such as chorioamnionitis, endometritis, and preeclampsia.

One report on 466 HIV-seropositive women in Zaire noted infants born to HIV-seropositive women were more likely to be premature, have lower birth weights, and have a higher neonatal death rate compared to infants of 606 HIV-seronegative women.[33] However, this population differed from those of the other studies in the greater (18%) number of women with AIDS included in the study population. Temmerman and co-workers studied a Nairobi cohort of 315 HIV-seropositive and 311 HIV-seronegative women prospectively through 6 weeks postpartum.[41] They found an association between HIV-1 infection and low birth weight (mean birth weight 2913 g vs 3072 g; $p = 0.003$) and prematurity (21.1% vs 9.4%; $p < 0.0001$) but no association for small for gestational age. They also found that HIV-seropositive women with CD4 counts below 30% had a higher risk of preterm delivery (26.3% vs 10.1%; $p = 0.001$). Finally, HIV-seropositive women had a higher rate of genital ulcer disease (4.7% vs 2.0%; $p = 0.06$), genital warts (4.9% vs 2.0%; $p = 0.03$), positive syphilis serology (7.9% vs 3.2%), and postpartum endometritis (10.3% vs 4.2%; $p = 0.01$). Postpartum endometritis was also inversely correlated with percentage of CD4 cells.

Langston et al. prospectively studied the outcomes of pregnancies in 124 HIV-infected women over a 4-year period of time.[21] The majority of the women were asymptomatic, with only two having been diagnosed with AIDS. There were 14 fetal losses observed (a rate of 11%) in this cohort of women. The losses occurred between 8 and 32 weeks of pregnancy, with half of these experienced by 20 weeks' gestation. HIV testing of fetal tissues revealed the presence of HIV nucleic acid in 7 of the 14 fetuses, with all of the infected fetuses demonstrating thymus gland abnormalities. In contrast, the HIV infection rate among the live-born infants in this cohort was 13%. The results of this study suggest that HIV infection of the fetus early in gestation can be toxic and result in a higher fetal loss rate.

Serious infections have been seen in HIV-seropositive pregnant women. Minkoff et al. reported an increased incidence of serious infections in 9 of 16 HIV-seropositive pregnant women with CD4 counts of less than 300 cells/mm^3. These infections included six women with *Pneumocystis carinii* pneumonia, one woman with central nervous system toxoplasmosis, one woman with bacterial pneumonia, and one woman with a postcesarean pelvic abscess.[28] Many authorities believe that the more advanced the maternal HIV disease the greater the likelihood of adverse pregnancy outcomes. Larger ongoing prospective natural history studies of HIV-infected cohorts of pregnant women, such as the National Institutes of Health (NIH)–sponsored Women and Infants Transmission Study, are hoped to provide more definitive answers regarding the relationship between HIV infection and pregnancy.

VERTICAL HIV TRANSMISSION

Another potentially devastating adverse effect of HIV disease on pregnancy outcome is the possibility of infecting the fetus or newborn with HIV. The vast majority of HIV infection in children occurs through maternal-infant transmission. Published perinatal HIV transmission rates vary widely. Most recent reviews on HIV infection in pregnancy quote rates varying from 14% to 39%.[11,29,31,43]

The three major routes of transmission are related to the timing of transmission during the course of gestation. *Intrauterine* transmission, which likely takes place well before the onset of labor and perhaps as early as the beginning of the second trimester, is thought to account for somewhere between 30% and 50% of vertical HIV transmission. *Intrapartum* transmission, occurring around the time of labor and delivery, possibly as the infant descends through the birth canal, accounts for somewhere around 50% to 60% of vertically transmitted HIV. The remainder of vertically transmitted HIV occurs *postpartum* and is thought to be associated with breast feeding.

Studies investigating risk factors for vertical transmission have reported somewhat conflicting results. Some reports have documented an increased rate of vertical transmission in women with advanced degrees of immunocompromise, a decreased CD4 lymphocyte count, an increased CD8 lymphocyte count, a decreased CD4:CD8 ratio, antigenemia, and placental membrane inflammation.[22,23,27,34,35,42] The lack of replication of these findings in larger, more heterogeneous cohorts makes it difficult to apply these findings to all populations at this time.

The European Collaborative Study group, reporting on 721 children born to 701 HIV-infected mothers, found a 14.4% vertical transmission rate.[11] Transmission was associated with maternal p24-antigenemia and a CD4 count of less than 700. They also found an association between transmission and preterm delivery (<34 weeks' gestation). Transmission rates were also higher in vaginal deliveries compared with cesarean delivery and in vaginal deliveries in which episiotomy, scalp electrodes, forceps, or vacuum extractors were used, but only in centers where these procedures were not routine. In the United States, multicenter studies of large cohorts of HIV-infected pregnant women are underway to further determine risk factors associated with an increase in perinatal transmission rates. Recent studies have demonstrated an association between perinatal transmission in women with CD4 cell levels less than 20% and duration of rupture of membranes greater than or equal to 4 hours.[24] This association was not observed in women with higher CD4 cell levels. In addition, duration of labor and mode of delivery did not correlate with perinatal transmission in this study. Previously, St. Louis and co-workers reported on a perinatal cohort in Zaire. They detected no difference in vertical transmission rates when women with duration of ruptured membranes of greater than 10 hours were compared with women with duration of 10 hours or less.[34] The data from other centers are being collected, and analyses of these data may further clarify duration of ruptured membranes as a variable associated with an increased probability of perinatal transmission.

Strategies for Preventing Vertical Transmission

Numerous approaches aimed at reducing the risk of vertical HIV transmission during pregnancy are under investigation. The focus is on intrapartum transmission because it is a relatively short interval during which infection is thought to occur. This is thought to be a major route of vertical transmission because over half of infants ultimately determined to be infected are HIV culture and polymerase chain reaction (PCR) negative in the first few days of life but positive before the second month of life. The intrapartum mode of transmission is further supported by the data on twins published by Goedert et al. showing that first-born twins are infected significantly more often than second-born twins and the effect is greatest if the first twin is delivered vaginally.[15]

The AIDS Clinical Trials Group (ACTG) protocol 076, the first interventional trial aimed at preventing mother-to-infant transmission, was closed to enrollment in February 1994, following an efficacy review by the Data and Safety Monitoring Board for ACTG protocols.[40] This study was a randomized, double-blind, placebo-controlled trial of zidovudine started in mothers between 14 and 34 weeks of gestation, with CD4 counts of 200 cells/μl or more who did not otherwise require zidovudine treatment. Zidovudine was administered orally at a dose of 100 mg five times daily and in labor as a continuous intravenous infusion of 1 mg/kg/hr following a 2 mg/kg loading dose. Infants were treated with zidovudine, 2 mg/kg orally four times daily, beginning within 8 to 12 hours after birth until 6 weeks of age. As of December 20, 1993, 477 women had been enrolled in this protocol at the 50 study sites in the United States and 9 sites in France. A total of 421 infants had been born, including six sets of twins; 363 births were included in the efficacy analysis, 180 in the zidovudine treatment, and 183 in the placebo group. HIV infection status as of 24 weeks of life was available in 233 infants. Thirteen infants in the zidovudine group and 40 in the placebo group were defined as HIV infected. This represented an 8.3% infection rate in the zidovudine-treated group, which was significantly ($p = 0.00006$) lower than the 25.5% infection rate in the placebo group. No differences were noted in the number and type of birth defects in babies whose mothers had received zidovudine or the placebo. There were no significant health hazards among the children during the first 18-month follow-up period. This represented the first major breakthrough in reducing HIV vertical transmission. These findings offer an impetus for more aggressive HIV counseling and testing programs for pregnant women because of the benefits of zidovudine treatment. The U.S. Public Health Service now recommends routine HIV counseling and vol-

untary testing for all pregnant women.[6] These recommendations are intended to provide information to reduce the risk of uninfected women acquiring HIV and to enable HIV-infected women to receive appropriate and timely medical intervention for their own health and for reducing the risk of perinatal and other modes of HIV transmission.

A number of other trials to reduce perinatal HIV transmission have begun or have been completed through the NIH-sponsored ACTG. The active immunization approach is addressed by ACTG protocols 233, 234, and 235 and 185. The first three protocols involved the administration of three similar vaccines produced by different companies using the recombinant gp120 molecule to induce increased levels of maternal antibody. Mothers were given a primary immunization at enrollment between 16 and 24 weeks' gestation followed by four monthly boosters. It was hoped that increased levels of potentially neutralizing antibodies in the mother would reduce the viral load to which the fetus is exposed. The induced antibodies are primarily of the immunoglobulin G class and would cross the placenta, potentially providing additional protection to the exposed infant. Analysis of the outcomes of these studies is ongoing.

ACTG 185 is a protocol in which mothers on zidovudine are given monthly infusions of hyperimmune HIV immunoglobulin (HIVIG) or intravenous immunoglobulin (IVIG) during the pregnancy and intravenous zidovudine during labor and delivery. Their infants receive a single infusion of either HIVIG or IVIG and 6 weeks of oral zidovudine. This approach combines passive immunization with antiretroviral infusion during labor and delivery. Lambert and co-workers recently reported preliminary data on the pharmacokinetics and safety of this study.[20] After 103 infusions, only 2 were associated with moderate adverse reactions (consisting of one episode of vomiting and another of headache). Vital testing was performed on blood samples taken from the participants prior to the IVIG or HIVIG infusion, and postinfusion at 1 hour and at 1, 7, 14, and 28 days. Analysis of the data revealed that seven women who had detectable p24 antigen levels at study entry had their p24 antigen levels decline to undetectable after receiving HIVIG. Similar analysis of p24 antigen levels in eight women with detectable levels at study entry who received IVIG did not demonstrate a decrease. Viral load testing by PCR RNA was performed as well and did not demonstrate any significant increase or decrease in viral load in either group of women.

ACTG protocol 250 is a perinatal study investigating the safety and pharmacokinetics of nevirapine. The protocol involves the oral administration of 200 mg of nevirapine to the pregnant woman when she is in active labor and an oral dose of 2 mg/kg in the infant between 48 and 72 hours after birth. The use of nevirapine in such a regimen could provide another mechanism by which perinatal HIV transmission can be reduced. In addition, the infrequent oral administration of this agent during the perinatal and early neonatal periods makes it a feasible option for use in developing countries.

There is mounting evidence that maternal HIV-1 viral load may be a determining factor in perinatal transmission. Sperling and co-workers recently reported results of maternal plasma HIV-1 RNA on samples stored from the women enrolled in ACTG 076.[39] They found that, although HIV RNA levels did correlate with transmission, transmissions did occur in both groups across all RNA levels. In another, similar report on a cohort of 151 HIV-infected pregnant women, maternal viral plasma load was higher in transmitters than nontransmitters. The difference, however, was not statistically significant and there was no threshold of viral load that predicted transmission.[18] Thus it appears that maternal viral load may be a contributing factor but certainly not the sole determinant of HIV vertical transmission.

Another approach to reducing the risk of vertical transmission particularly aimed at developing countries, where antiretrovirals and vaccines may be less feasible, is cleansing of the vaginal birth canal using microbicides effective against HIV. A variety of agents were considered, including chlorhexidine, betadine, nonoxynol-9, benzalkonium, and acidifying solutions. The virucidal properties of the solution must be weighed against the potential risk of epithelial disruption, which may occur with frequent use of certain agents. Nonoxynol-9, for example, has been associated with vaginal epithelial disruption when used frequently in concentrated doses.[32] Biggard and co-workers reported the results of the first such trial carried out in Malawi, Africa.[1] In 3637 women vaginal cleansing was performed using a 0.25% chlorhexidine solution. In another 3327 women no intervention was performed. There was no significant difference in HIV-1 transmission rates between the intervention and the nonintervention groups (26.9% vs 27.9%). It remains un-

clear whether the dosing was inadequate, the intervention did not reduce genital tract virus, or the approach simply does not work. Further studies will be necessary to determine the reason(s) for failure.

Mode of delivery has also been implicated as a risk factor in vertical HIV transmission. The data from the European Collaborative Study and from a metaanalysis indicate that significant differences exist in the vertical transmission rate depending on whether the infants were born vaginally or by cesarean section. Villari et al found in their metaanalysis a 14% transmission rate in the women delivering by cesarean compared with 20% ($p = 0.044$) in those delivering vaginally.[44] The European Collaborative Study reported a decrease in transmission from 17.6% in vaginally delivered infants to 11.7% for infants delivered by cesarean section.[10] The factors responsible for these differences are still not clear. A number of important variables must be controlled for, including duration of ruptured membranes, CD4 counts, and viral load. In the European Collaborative Study, 80% of the cesarean sections were performed with intact membranes. The obvious conclusion is that a significant number of fetuses are infected by either free or cell-associated virus in blood or in cervicovaginal secretions in the birth canal. However, first-born twins are infected more frequently even when delivered by cesarean section, indicating that time spent adjacent to or in contact with the endocervix may play a role. Infants delivered by cesarean section are also frequently covered in maternal blood to an even greater extent than those delivered vaginally.

The data regarding cesarean delivery are interesting, but the many confounding variables involved require randomized controlled trials before these findings should be used to dictate obstetrical practice in HIV-infected women. One such trial is now underway in Europe and may result in conclusive data regarding this modality. If the study shows a dramatic decrease in vertical transmission in the group randomized to cesarean delivery, we will then be challenged with determining whether the transmission prevented by cesarean delivery could have been equally prevented by zidovudine treatment. If these two modalities overlap significantly, then one might surmise that the risk of routine cesarean section may outweigh the risk of zidovudine treatment. If both modalities contribute to reduced transmission, then a close look at the risks vs the benefits would be necessary. What is even more disconcerting is that neither of these modalities is feasible on a routine basis in the developing world, where the majority of perinatal HIV transmission occurs.

PRENATAL CARE OF THE HIV-INFECTED PREGNANT WOMAN

The HIV-infected pregnant woman should receive the same routine prenatal care as all pregnant women. Moreover, attention should be afforded to potential signs of HIV disease progression and interactive sexually transmitted diseases and other opportunistic infections. A comprehensive medical and obstetric/gynecologic history should be taken, particularly in the gravida not under medical care for her HIV disease. Included in this history is an assessment of the signs and symptoms of HIV disease progression. Careful investigation of any symptom(s) suggestive of underlying pathology must be distinguished from the many and varied nonspecific symptoms of pregnancy. A review of signs and symptoms relating to potential disease progression is performed at least every trimester. The history should also include psychosocial factors to assess additional stressors that may negatively affect the woman's capacity to maintain the pregnancy and her general health. Many HIV-infected women are also at high risk for serious illness in family members (i.e., HIV disease), domestic violence, continued use or reinitiation of alcohol or other substances of abuse, and economic instability, all of which may precipitate a crisis requiring intervention.

Many women, particularly those initially screened for HIV and found to be positive during the index pregnancy, may require in-depth counseling. Sensitive, nonjudgmental, informative counseling must be provided in a supportive manner during the initial visit. This counseling should include information regarding perinatal transmission rates, the possible impact pregnancy may have on disease progression, the possible effects of HIV infection on pregnancy outcome, and therapeutic interventions and clinical trials available prenatally, in labor and delivery, and immediately postpartum. Women should also be counseled with regard to the need for specialized and ongoing primary care. Options regarding pregnancy termination should also be presented if the gestation is within the legal limits of termination. It is

frequently surprising to the clinician how often HIV-infected women will choose to continue their pregnancies, but it is necessary to respect the woman's decision and provide the best possible obstetrical care. If the clinician is unable to provide this care in a supportive manner, the woman should be referred to a qualified practitioner who can comfortably provide it.

A thorough physical exam should be performed at the initial prenatal visit, with particular attention to systems in which the patient may have reported possible HIV-related symptoms. This physical exam is repeated in each trimester or as clinically indicated. The laboratory assessment should include all of the routine prenatal laboratory testing. In addition, particular attention should be paid to ensure that the HIV-infected pregnant woman has those studies that may identify HIV-related disease processes. Papanicoulaou smears, VDRL, gonorrhea, and chlamydia testing, and any tests necessary to assess the status of HIV disease progression should be performed. A complete T-lymphocyte count (CD3, CD4, CD8, CD4:CD8 ratio) is done so that early interventions can be initiated. Other tests, such as plasma viral load, beta$_2$-microglobulin and serum neopterin, may be obtained as well if those tests are normally used by the clinician to predict HIV progression. In our institutions, tests for HIV disease progression, particularly the CD4 count, are repeated in each trimester. A baseline titer for opportunistic infections common in HIV-infected individuals that may pose additional risk to the fetus, such as toxoplasmosis, should also be performed. Tuberculosis testing should be performed as part of the usual prenatal workup (see Chapter 22). In those women with very low CD4 counts, the clinician may choose to use the chest radiograph after the first trimester to rule out active tuberculosis.

Careful antenatal clinical assessment of fetal growth and development is important in HIV-infected gravidas. Ultrasound evaluation, nonstress testing, and biophysical profiles of the fetus are performed as clinically indicated. Women in whom prenatal genetic testing is indicated should be counseled regarding the added theoretical risk of infecting an otherwise uninfected fetus by amniocentesis, chorionic villus sampling, or cordocentesis. There are very few data in HIV-infected women to determine the magnitude of this risk. Women are generally given the option to undergo genetic testing if they desire; however, given the potential added risk, few women opt for the procedure. Amniocentesis, when done, is performed under sonographic guidance with care taken to avoid puncture of the fetal skin whenever possible. The theoretical risk would be significantly higher with cordocentesis, and this procedure is avoided when amniocentesis provides sufficient genetic information.

MANAGEMENT OF HIV DISEASE IN THE PREGNANT PATIENT

Most providers of prenatal care do not have extensive experience in managing women with HIV disease. Such care should therefore be undertaken by a clinician knowledgeable in the management of HIV disease. The pregnant woman may already have such a provider or need an appropriate and immediate referral. Whenever possible, pregnant women are managed in the same manner as nonpregnant woman. There are certainly some precautions that must be taken, particularly in the first trimester, but more often than not, the indicated therapies can be continued or begun during the pregnancy.

Antiretroviral therapy is generally begun during the pregnancy using the same guidelines as in nonpregnant women. The exact regimen will be determined based on the CD4 count and the available pharmacokinetic and safety data on the various antiretroviral agents. The long-term effects of zidovudine in asymptomatic women with CD4 cell counts greater than 200 are unknown. There is concern that initiating antiretroviral therapy to reduce perinatal transmission in a woman who otherwise would not be initiating such therapy for her health may result in viral resistance. Compounding this issue is the debate surrounding the most beneficial time to initiate antiretroviral therapy in asymptomatic nonpregnant adults, and whether monotherapy or combination therapy is the best strategy.

If there is no maternal indication for antiretroviral agents, zidovudine will generally be offered to reduce the risk of perinatal transmission. The dosing for the mother is 100 mg five times per day, although many clinicians will give 200 mg three times daily to improve compliance. When in labor, 2 mg/kg intravenous load is followed by 1 mg/kg/hr continuous intravenous infusion until delivery of the infant. The infant is then treated according to the ACTG 076 protocol (see Chapter 31). The effects of this intervention on the reduction of perinatal transmission is not known for all patients. The

women enrolled in ACTG 076 were asymptomatic, with median CD4 counts over 500 and little or no prior exposure to zidovudine. Although many women may benefit from zidovudine in pregnancy to reduce transmission, the closer they resemble enrollees in ACTG 076, the more likely they can expect similar results.

Maternal side effects associated with zidovudine are similar to those reported in nonpregnant adults. Before giving zidovudine, a baseline complete blood count, differential, platelet count, liver function tests, and creatinine level should be obtained. If no significant abnormality is evident, maternal zidovudine therapy can begin, with repeat laboratory evaluations recommended 2 weeks later. If the results of these tests are within the normal range, some perinatalogists recommend monthly monitoring for hematologic and liver toxicity with a complete blood count, differential, platelet count, and liver function test. Discontinuation of zidovudine is recommended in pregnant women if there is evidence of severe anemia (e.g., hemoglobin <8 mg/dl), thrombocytopenia (platelet count <100,000/mm^3), neutropenia (granulocytes <750/mm^3), liver function abnormalities (transaminase levels more than five times the upper limit of normal), or intolerance to the drug.

Long-term follow-up of large numbers of in-utero-exposed infants is currently not available. Pharmacokinetic studies indicate that zidovudine readily crosses the placenta and equivalent levels are found in the mother and neonate. However, data from ACTG 076 revealed that the only short-term toxicity in neonates exposed to zidovudine in utero was a mild transient anemia that did not require therapeutic interventions. Continued data collection is planned in these children until they are 21 years of age (through ACTG 219) to monitor for any evidence of an adverse long-term effect. Preliminary analysis of 274 uninfected infants from this study has demonstrated no significant differences in immune characteristics, growth, or neurodevelopmental status between the zidovudine-exposed infants and the placebo controls.

Pneumocystis carinii pneumonia is the most common AIDS-defining diagnosis in pregnant women, and this opportunistic infection must be aggressively treated with prophylactic agents in women with CD4 counts below 200 cell/μl (see Chapter 20). Prophylaxis with aerosolized pentamidine has limited systemic absorption and may have little effect on the fetus. However, this approach does not provide systemic prophylaxis. The treatment of choice for *P. carinii* pneumonia prophylaxis is oral trimethoprim-sulfamethoxazole. Experience with this agent in pregnancy has been limited by the theoretical concern of newborn kernicterus. In premature newborns who received sulfonamide therapy after birth, high levels of unconjugated bilirubin have been associated with kernicterus.[38] No cases of newborn kernicterus have been reported following maternal sulfamethoxazole therapy. Cases of newborn hemolysis have been reported following maternal ingestion of long-acting sulfonamides.[3] This has not been reported following maternal sulfamethoxazole therapy. Many obstetricians use trimethoprim-sulfamethoxazole after the first trimester for prophylaxis during pregnancy in women with very low CD4 counts. There is no reported clinical experience with the use of dapsone in HIV-infected pregnancy women. Because dapsone significantly affects the glucose-6-phosphate dehydrogenase system, its use in pregnancy is of concern. No fetal abnormalities have been reported in studies using dapsone to treat leprosy and dermatitis herpetiformis.[45]

Primary prophylaxis for *Mycobacterium avium-cellulare* complex with rifabutin has been proposed for HIV-infected individuals with CD4 counts of less than 75 cells/μl.[5] Controversy exists regarding the actual efficacy of this therapy, the potential drug interactions that may occur, the cost, and the possibility of developing resistance to rifampin. No data are available regarding the use of rifabutin in HIV-infected pregnant women. Therefore, the risks versus the benefits of this prophylactic intervention during pregnancy must be carefully weighed before initiating treatment.[7]

The initiation of isoniazid therapy is recommended to prevent active tuberculosis in HIV-infected pregnant women with a positive tuberculosis skin test and a negative chest radiograph. This therapy should not be postponed until after delivery. The standard regimen of isoniazid 300 mg daily with 50 mg vitamin B_6 should be initiated and continued for 1 year. Careful monitoring for liver toxicity is indicated.

Pregnant women who do not demonstrate immunity to hepatitis B may receive recombinant hepatitis B immunizations. Usually this series is initiated after the first trimester to further reduce concerns regarding possible adverse fetal effects. Administration of pneumococcal and influenza immunizations in HIV-infected individuals have been associated with a transient increase in viral load and are of questionable efficacy in individuals with advanced immunosuppression (i.e., CD4 count <200).[19,30] The theoretical risk of giving these immunizations to pregnant women is the potential for enhancing viral transmission to the fetus during periods of increased maternal viral load. Therefore, the risks versus the benefits of administering these immunizations must be carefully considered in pregnant women. Pneumococcal and influenza immunizations can be administered to women after delivery.

INTRAPARTUM MANAGEMENT OF THE HIV-INFECTED PREGNANT WOMAN

In general terms, the care provided to the pregnant HIV-infected woman is no different than the care afforded uninfected pregnant women; however, there are some caveats that must be heeded. Routine use of scalp electrodes for fetal monitoring or routine scalp pH determinations should be avoided. The procedures have a theoretical risk of infecting an otherwise uninfected infant. When the procedure is considered necessary, it should be done only after alternative methods to assure fetal well-being have failed and alternatives such as immediate delivery have been considered. The elective use of forceps or vacuum extractors should also be avoided and used with the utmost caution when necessary. The potential risk is unknown, but abrasions and other forms of epithelial disruption to the fetal skin may increase the risk of transmission. The woman should understand the potential risks versus the benefits of any procedure that may enhance the risk of vertical transmission.

Cesarean section is performed for the usual obstetric considerations and, until definitive evidence is available, should not be offered as a method of preventing vertical transmission, especially in woman with ruptured membranes. We generally avoid the use of episiotomies unless absolutely necessary to avoid severe lacerations, with the associated risk of increased blood loss and infection.

Some clinicians use prophylactic antibiotics to prevent intrapartum and postpartum complications. Insufficient published data exist to make widespread recommendations at this time; however, studies are underway to determine exact rates of intrapartum and postpartum infectious morbidity in HIV-infected women. We currently do not use prophylactic antibiotics outside of the usual obstetric or HIV indications. However, these women must be carefully monitored for early signs of infection, and appropriate therapy instituted. Women with low CD4 counts may ultimately prove to be at greatest risk for intrapartum infections such as amnionitis and endometritis.

Health care providers must always follow universal bodily secretion precautions with all patients in labor and delivery regardless of their HIV status (see Chapter 5). This includes the use of gowns, drapes, double gloves, and eye protection. Blood, urine, vaginal fluid, amniotic fluid, saliva, and urine should all be regarded as potentially infectious. Personnel handling the infant, particularly immediately after birth, should also follow these precautions.

SUMMARY

HIV-infected women frequently choose to conceive, and those faced with an unplanned pregnancy often choose to continue their pregnancies. Although most HIV-infected women have an uneventful pregnancy, serious consideration must be given to their HIV disease. Counseling must be informative and should clearly define available options. Information about the risk of vertical transmission, management of HIV disease, and expected pregnancy outcomes will enable these women to make more informed choices. Most of all, these women need to receive care in a supportive environment that will optimize their chances for a favorable outcome.

REFERENCES

1. Biggar R, Miotti P, Taha T, et al: Perinatal HIV-1 transmission in Africa and the effect of birth canal cleansing (Abstract 27). Program of the 3rd Conference on Retroviruses and Opportunistic Infections, Washington, DC, February 1, 1996
2. Biggar RJ, Pahwa S, Minkoff H, et al: Immunosuppression in pregnant women infected with human immunodeficiency virus. Am J Obstet Gynecol 161: 1239–1244, 1989
3. Brown AK, Cevik N: Hemolysis and jaundice in the newborn following maternal treatment with sulfamethoxypyridonzine. Pediatrics 36:742–744, 1965
4. Burns D, et al: Changes in CD4 and CD8 cell levels during pregnancy and postpartum in a prospective cohort of HIV-1 seronegative and seropositive women (Abstract 14). Program of the 35th annual Interscience Conference on Antimicrobial Agents and Chemotherapy, San Francisco, September 17–20, 1995
5. Centers for Disease Control and Prevention: HIV/AIDS Surveillance Report (no. 2). Atlanta, Centers for Disease Control and Prevention, 1995, pp 29–35
6. Centers for Disease Control and Prevention: U.S. Public Health Service recommendations for human immunodeficiency virus counseling and voluntary testing for pregnant women. MMWR 44(RR-7): 1–15, 1995
7. Cotton D, Watts H: Management of HIV infection during pregnancy: New options, new questions. AIDS Clin Care 7(6):45–49, 1995
8. Coyne BA, Landers DV: Immunology of HIV disease in pregnancy. Obstet Gynecol Clin North Am 17:3, 1990
9. Dinsmoor MJ, Chrismas JT: Changes in T lymphocyte subpopulations during pregnancy complicated by human immunodeficiency virus infection. Am J Obstet Gynecol 167:1575–1579, 1992
10. European Collaborative Study: Cesarean section and the risk of vertical transmission of HIV-1 infection. Lancet 343:1464–1467, 1994
11. European Collaborative Study: Risk factors for mother-to-child transmission of HIV-1. Lancet 339: 1007–1012, 1992
12. Fuith LC, Czarnecki M, Weiss G, et al: Prognosis of human immunodeficiency virus-infected women after delivery [Letter]. Am J Obstet Gynecol 169: 752–753, 1993
13. Gloeb DJ, Lai S, Efantis J, O'Sullivan MJ: Survival and disease progression in human immunodeficiency virus-infected women after an index delivery. Am J Obstet Gynecol 167:152–157, 1992
14. Gloeb DJ, O'Sullivan MJ, Efantis J: Human immunodeficiency virus infection in women: The effect of human immunodeficiency virus on pregnancy. Am J Obstet Gynecol 159:756–761, 1988
15. Goedert JJ, Duliege A, Amos CI, et al: High risk of HIV-1 infection for first born twins. Lancet 338: 1471–1475, 1991
16. Gwinn M, Wasser S, Fleming P, et al: Increasing prevalence of HIV infection among childbearing women, United States, 1989–1991 (Abstract PO-C16-2990). Program of the 9th International Conference on AIDS, Berlin, Germany, June, 1993
17. Johnston FD, MacCallum L, Breathle R, et al: Does infection with HIV affect the outcome of pregnancy? Br Med J 196:467, 1988
18. Koup RA, Kao Y, Ho DD, et al: Lack of a maternal viral threshold for vertical transmission of HIV-1 (Abstract LB2). Program of the 3rd Conference on Retroviruses and Opportunistic Infections, Washington, DC, February 1, 1996
19. Kroon FP, vanDissel JT, de Jong JC, van Furth R: Antibody response to influenza, tetanus and pneumococcal vaccines in HIV-seropositive individuals in relation to the number of CD4 lymphocytes. AIDS 8:469–476, 1995
20. Lambert J, et al. Pharmacokinetics (PK) and safety of hyperimmune HIV immunoglobulin (HIVIG) in pregnant HIV positive women (Abstract A125). Program of the 35th annual Interscience Conference

on Antimicrobial Agents and Chemotherapy, San Francisco, September 17–20, 1995

21. Langston C, et al: Excess intrauterine fetal demise associated with maternal immunodeficiency virus infection. J Infect Dis 172:1451–1460, 1995

22. Lindgren S, Anzen B, Bohlin AB, Lidman K: HIV and childbearing: Clinical outcome and aspects of mother-to-infant transmission. AIDS 5:1111–1116, 1991

23. Mayers MM, Davenny K, Schoenbaum EE, et al: A prospective study of infants of human immunodeficiency virus seropositive and seronegative women with a history of intravenous drug-using sex partners in the Bronx, New York City. Pediatrics 88:1248–1256, 1991

24. Minkoff H, Burns D, Landesman SH, et al: The relationship of the duration of ruptured membranes to vertical transmission of HIV. Am J Obstet Gynecol 173:585–589, 1995

25. Minkoff H, de Regt RH, Landesman S, et al: *Pneumocystis carinii* pneumonia associated with acquired immunodeficiency syndrome in pregnancy: A report of three maternal deaths. Obstet Gynecol 67:284–287, 1986

26. Minkoff HL, Henderson C, Mendez H, et al: Pregnancy outcomes among mothers infected with human immunodeficiency virus and uninfected control subjects. Am J Obstet Gynecol 163:1598–1604, 1990

27. Minkoff H, Nanda D, Menez R, et al: Pregnancies resulting in infants with acquired immunodeficiency syndrome or AIDS-related complex: Follow-up of mothers, children, and subsequently born siblings. Obstet Gynecol 69:288–291, 1987

28. Minkoff HL, Willoughby A, Mendez H, et al: Serious infections during pregnancy among women with advanced human immunodeficiency virus infection. Am J Obstet Gynecol 162:30–34, 1990

29. Moreno JD, Minkoff H: Human immunodeficiency virus infection during pregnancy. Clin Obstet Gynecol 35:813–820, 1992

30. O'Brien WA, et al: Human immunodeficiency virus type 1 replication can be increased in peripheral blood of seropositive patients after influenza vaccination. Blood 86:1082–1089, 1995

31. Oxtoby M: Perinatally acquired human immunodeficiency virus infection. Pediatr Infect Dis J 9:606–609, 1990

32. Roddy RE, Cordero M, Cordero C, Fortney JA: A dosing study of nonoxynol-9 and genital irritation. Int J STD AIDS 4:165–170, 1993

33. Ryder RW, Nsa W, Hassig SE, et al: Perinatal transmission of the human immunodeficiency virus type 1 to infants of seropositive women in Zaire. N Engl J Med 320:1637–1642, 1989

34. St. Louis ME, Kamenga M, Brown C, et al: Risk factors for perinatal HIV-1 transmission according to maternal immunologic, virologic, and placental factors. JAMA 269:2853–2859, 1993

35. Scarlatti G, Lombardi V, Plebani A, et al: Polymerase chain reaction, virus isolation and antigen assay in HIV-1 antibody positive mothers and their children. AIDS 5:1173–1178, 1991

36. Scott GB, Fischl MA, Klimas N, et al: Mothers of infants with the acquired immunodeficiency syndrome: Evidence for both symptomatic and asymptomatic carriers. JAMA 253:363–366, 1985

37. Selwyn PA, Schoenbaum EE, Davenny K, et al: Prospective study of human immunodeficiency virus infection and pregnancy outcomes in intravenous drug users. JAMA 261:1289–1294, 1989

38. Silverman WA, Anderson DH, Blanc WA, Crozier DN: A difference in mortality rate and incidence of kernicterus among premature infants allotted to two prophylactic antibacterial regimens. Pediatrics 18:614–625, 1956

39. Sperling RS, Shapiro DE, Coombs R, et al: Maternal plasma HIV-1 RNA levels and the success of zidovudine in the prevention of maternal-child transmission (Abstract LB1). Program of the 3rd Conference on Retroviruses and Opportunistic Infections, Washington, DC, February 1, 1996

40. Sperling RS, Stratton P, O'Sullivan MJ, et al: A survey of zidovudine use in pregnant women with human immunodeficiency virus infection. N Engl J Med 326:857–861, 1992

41. Temmerman M, et al: Maternal HIV-1 infection and pregnancy outcome. Obstet Gynecol 83:495–501, 1994

42. Tibaldi C, Tovo PA, Ziarati N, et al: Asymptomatic women at high risk of vertical HIV-1 transmission to their fetuses. Br J Obstet Gynaecol 1090:334–337, 1993

43. Toltzis P: Rationales for treating the human immunodeficiency virus-infected woman during pregnancy. Clin Perinatol 20:47–60, 1993

44. Villari P, Spino C, Chalmers TC, et al: Cesarean section to reduce perinatal transmission of human immunodeficiency virus (Document 74). Online J Curr Clin Trials 2:July 8, 1993

45. United States Pharmacopeial Convention: Dapsone. In: United States Pharmacopeia Drug Information: Drug Information for the Health Care Professional, vol IA. Rockville, Md, United States Pharmacopeial Convention, 1990, pp 1106–1108

Chapter 31

Pediatric AIDS: Perinatal Transmission and Early Diagnosis

DIANE W. WARA and ALEJANDRO DORENBAUM

Among some groups of children and young people in the United States, acquired immunodeficiency syndrome (AIDS) has become a leading cause of death (Chapter 32). As of December 1995, over 7000 children younger than 13 years of age with AIDS had been reported to the Centers for Disease Control and Prevention (CDC). More than 3000 of these children had died. By 1990, in New York State, human immunodeficiency virus (HIV)/AIDS was the first and second leading cause of death in Hispanic and African-American children 1 through 4 years of age, accounting for 15% and 16%, respectively, of all deaths in these age/race groups.

Of all HIV-infected children who acquire their virus during 1996, over 99% will acquire it from their mothers. The risk of transmission from an HIV-infected pregnant woman to her newborn varies throughout the world from 14.1% in the European Collaborative Study,[12] to 28% in New York City, to 20% in San Francisco, to 45% in areas of Africa. The risk factors for perinatal transmission, the timing of transmission, and the early diagnosis of HIV-1 infection during infancy remain under active investigation.

To decrease the incidence of HIV-1 infection in children, it is essential to decrease HIV-1 infection in women of childbearing age. Education about risk factors for the acquisition of HIV-1 and behavior modification are powerful approaches. In addition, the incidence of HIV-1 infection in children will be modified by decreasing transmission from infected pregnant women to their infants. Two strategies are likely to prove successful during the immediate future. The first, provision of the ACTG 076 zidovudine regimen to mother and infant, decreases transmission from 25% to 8%[6]; this regimen includes the use of zidovudine orally

during pregnancy, intravenously during labor, and orally to the newborn for 6 weeks following birth.[30] The second strategy, to provide a "universal approach of offering HIV counseling and testing to all pregnant women—regardless of the prevalence of HIV infection in their community or their risk for infection—provides a uniform policy that will reach HIV-infected pregnant women in all populations and geographic areas of the United States."[36] Although this universal approach will necessitate increased resources, effective implementation of HIV counseling, and testing services for pregnant women, the ensuing medical interventions will reduce HIV-related morbidity in women and their infants and should ultimately reduce medical costs.

RISK FACTORS FOR PERINATAL TRANSMISSION

It is likely that multiple factors contribute to the risk of perinatal transmission and explain the variability of transmission rates throughout the world.[3,7,8,12,13,23] Factors that appear to influence the transmission rate from mother to infant include the severity of illness in the mother. The severity of illness is directly associated with the mother's viral burden as well as the extent of her immunodeficiency. The higher the maternal viral burden (RNA copy numbers per milliliter) the more likely a woman is to transmit HIV-1 to her newborn.[8] Dickover et al reported that all 13 pregnant women with RNA copy numbers >80,000/ml transmitted HIV to their newborns, whereas none of 63 with RNA copy numbers <20,000/ml did; other investigators have reported the absence of transmission by women with high viral load, and the presence of transmission by women with a low viral burden. Therefore, it is not possible at present to determine a direct correlation between viral burden as quantitated by RNA copy number and risk of transmission. Similarly, an association exists between CD4 count and transmission. Pregnant women with CD4 counts >600 are less likely to transmit HIV (15% transmission) than those with CD4 counts <200 (43% transmission).[23] A genetic predisposition for transmission of HIV may be important, but the precise genes responsible for increased or decreased transmission have not been identified with certainty.

Several factors occurring during delivery, including cesarean section, skin excoriation in the newborn and prematurity, appear to increase the risk of transmission. Infants born at less than 32 weeks' gestation have approximately a twofold increase in the risk of transmission when compared to those born at term.[35] Mechanisms for transmission of virus from mother to infant at the time of delivery may include the swallowing of HIV-infected maternal blood, amniotic fluid, or cervical vaginal mucus by the newborn as it passes through the birth canal and the subsequent entry of HIV-1 through the newborn gastric mucosa or skin. It is now known that prolonged ruptured membranes (>4 hours) significantly increase the risk of perinatal HIV transmission. In addition, virus may be transmitted as intracellular HIV by maternal–infant transfusion.

Postpartum, the most significant risk factor for transmission of HIV-1 from mother to infant is breastfeeding.[9,12,37,39] A review of five previously published studies estimates an incremental risk of HIV-1 transmission to infants if ever breastfed of 14%.[9] The results of these studies strongly support the recommendation that HIV-1–infected women in the United States be counseled not to breastfeed their infants.

The duration of the epidemic in an area of the world may influence the severity of illness among HIV-infected pregnant women. The more mature the epidemic is in an area of the world, the more likely it is that HIV-infected women have advanced disease. In the European Collaborative Study, the most significant predictor of transmission was the stage of maternal infection.[7] Four infants born to 13 women with clinical AIDS were infected (31%), and 14 infants born to 602 women without signs or symptoms of HIV-1 infection were infected (14%). The virologic and immunologic correlates of

progressive HIV-1 infection also predicted perinatal transmission. The presence of p24 antigen either during the third trimester or at the time of delivery increased the risk of transmission threefold, from 10% to 29%. Likewise, the transmission rate was threefold greater in those with CD4 cell counts <400/μl (19%) than in those with CD4 cell counts >700/μl (6%).

Transmission risk is increased in women with detectable virus in the peripheral blood and in those with rapidly proliferating HIV. It is likely that a quasi-species of maternal virus escapes the immune response of the mother and is transmitted to the infant, and it is possible that a specific capsular epitope within the V3 region of the virus protects against transmission.[38]

The mother's immune response to her own (autologous) virus may protect against transmission. Neutralizing antibodies in the mother directed against her own virus appear to decrease transmission of the virus.[18] It is unclear why all women do not have neutralizing antibody to autologous virus. Other immune responses, such as antibody-dependent cellular cytotoxicity,[15] do not appear to alter the risk of transmission of virus.

The newborn's gestational age as well as low birth weight, excoriation of the skin, and ever being breastfed affect the risk of transmission. Infants born at less than 32 weeks' gestational age[35] or weighing <2500 g[17] have a higher rate of transmission. The relationship between transmission and gestational age is nonlinear, with a transmission rate of approximately 30% for infants born before 32 weeks' gestation and of 14% for those born at term. Maternal IgG actively crosses the placenta at 32 weeks' gestation, and it is possible that infants born before the receipt of maternal antibody are at greater risk of infection with HIV-1. The mucosal–skin barrier of a premature infant is less intact than that of a term baby, and HIV-1 may reach the systemic circulation of a premature infant more easily after the infant swallows HIV-infected blood or amniotic fluid.

HIV-1 has been detected in breast milk and colostrum both by culture and by polymerase chain reaction (PCR). Several case reports,[39] as well as a review of experience in Rwanda,[37] strongly suggest that HIV-1 may be transmitted by breast milk from mother to infant.

TIMING OF TRANSMISSION

Infants may acquire HIV-1 in utero, intrapartum, or postpartum through breastfeeding. We hypothesize that the timing of transmission and the viral burden in the newborn are important factors in the determination of the time of onset of clinical disease as well as the rate of clinical progression. The earlier that virus is transmitted from mother to infant in utero, the more likely it is that clinical disease will begin during infancy and that disease progression will be rapid. It is likely that early intervention with antiretroviral therapy or immunomodulators or both will modify the clinical course in infants at risk for early onset and rapidly progressive disease.

The in utero model, similar to the rubella model, is supported by the identification of HIV-1 in fetal tissue as early as 8 weeks' gestation[16,33] and HIV-1 antigens in fetal thymus tissue as early as 15 weeks.[28] We hypothesize that infants infected in utero have virus detected by culture or by PCR within 48 hours of birth.[4] Approximately 30% to 50% of infants who eventually prove to be infected have virus identified shortly after birth[5,21,25,31] using virus culture or PCR.

In over 50% of infants who eventually prove to be infected, virus *cannot* be detected by culture or PCR during the first weeks of life.[11,19,20] It is likely that these infants acquired the infection intrapartum. Numerous infants studied prospectively have been reported with no evidence of HIV-1 in cord blood as assessed by PCR, or culture and with positive PCR and culture by age 1 to 2 months. The sequence of identification of virus in these patients suggests that they were infected perinatally. The finding that in twin births, the firstborn twin is more frequently infected than the secondborn twin supplies further evidence of intrapartum infection.[14] It is likely that the firstborn twin encounters higher concentrations of virus in the birth canal or is in closer proximity to the cervix for longer periods of time than the second, more quickly born twin.

The bimodal onset of HIV-related disease in infants and children further supports both in utero and intrapartum transmission. A retrospective chart review of over 200 children with AIDS whose only known route of infection was maternal revealed two populations of HIV-1–infected children.[2] Approximately 20% developed AIDS during their first year of life, with a median incubation period of 4.1 months. A second and larger group developed signs or symptoms of AIDS at a rate of 8% per year, with a median onset of disease at 4.8 years. The bimodal onset of HIV disease has been confirmed by the CDC. Recently, early-onset and rapidly progressive disease has been correlated with the following findings at birth: a positive culture or PCR, the presence of p24 antigen, the presence of hepatosplenomegaly, and a CD4 cell count of <30%.[24]

It is possible that a subset of the infants with early-onset disease were infected in utero, whereas those with a longer latency period were infected perinatally. The above observed correlation between the culture of virus, detection of genome by PCR, detection of p24 near birth, and the early onset and rapid progression of disease have implications that include potential benefit from the early initiation of antiretroviral therapy. The implications of this observation for the early initiation of antiretroviral therapy are far reaching.

EARLY DIAGNOSIS OF HIV INFECTION

The timing of HIV acquisition, the active transport of IgG across the placenta, and the relative immaturity of the newborn's immune system all influence our ability to distinguish an infected from an uninfected infant. All infants born to HIV-infected women have circulating IgG antibody to HIV. Because IgG actively crosses the placenta between 30 and 32 weeks' gestation, IgG present in the newborn may be maternal and so does not necessarily indicate that the newborn is infected. Therefore, until age 18 months, an infant's HIV status must be determined by documenting the presence of virus in the peripheral blood by culture or viral genome by PCR. After age 1 month, detection of viral antigen by immune complex–associated p24 antigen (ICD p24 ag) is adequate. In infants 18 months old or younger, positive results on two separate occasions (excluding cord blood) from one or more of the following: HIV culture, HIV PCR, and HIV antigen (ICD p24) document the presence of HIV infection. In children over 18 months of age, HIV infection during infancy may be documented by the presence of antibody determined by enzyme-linked immunosorbent assay (ELISA) and a confirmatory test. A sensitive and specific assay for IgA anti-HIV has been developed. IgA does not cross the placenta, and the presence of IgA anti-HIV may provide a serologic tool for early diagnosis.[22,29] However, the sensitivity of the IgA assay is only 77% by age 12 weeks and the assay does not reach appropriate sensitivity and specificity until infants are 6 months old. It is likely that HIV-infected infants have an incomplete early immune response to the virus because both humoral immune responses and cell-mediated cytotoxicity are frequently decreased or absent during infancy.[21]

We hypothesize that infants infected in utero have either HIV genome detected by PCR or HIV isolated from blood within 48 hours of birth. Those infected intrapartum undergo a primary viremia, and only subsequently (days 7 to 90) can virus be detected.[4] The identification of virus by culture of peripheral blood mononuclear cells (PBMC) remains the standard for diagnosis of infection in infants younger than age 18 months. Although both culture and PCR may be negative early in life, even in infants eventually proven to be infected, both approaches to diagnosis offer >90% sensitivity by age 1 month[10,27].

Current recommendations for the diagnosis of HIV during infancy include the following.

1. Offer HIV testing with counseling to all pregnant women in order to determine which infants are at risk of infection.

2. Obtain culture and PCR as close to birth as possible in those infants whose mothers are HIV infected in order to determine which infants may have had in utero infection and be most likely to have early-onset and rapidly progressive disease.

3. If there is no evidence of virus by culture and PCR close to birth, repeat at age 1 month and age 2 to 3 months.

4. If there is no evidence of virus by age 4 months, the infant is likely uninfected, and IgG anti-HIV should be obtained at age 12 and 18 months to confirm the infant's status. An infant who has had no positive culture or PCR during infancy, is seronegative at age 18 months, and has no signs or symptoms of HIV is almost certainly uninfected.

5. However, if the mother and or infant received immunomodulator or antiretroviral therapy during diagnostic testing, the infant should be tested at 12-month intervals until age 3 years.

6. An initial positive culture or PCR must be confirmed by a second culture or PCR.

SUMMARY

The ability to decrease transmission of HIV from mother to infant from 25% to 8% by the use of zidovudine orally during pregnancy, intravenously during labor, and orally to the newborn for 6 weeks provides an immediate strategy to decrease HIV-1 infection in children. Furthermore, the ability to decrease transmission utilizing this regimen strongly supports the recommended universal offering of HIV counseling and testing to all pregnant women.

Establishing the diagnosis of HIV infection with confidence prior to age 1 month is difficult. Nevertheless, the need to initiate an effective therapeutic regimen if the infant is infected or relieve the family's anxiety if the infant is uninfected support an aggressive approach to early diagnosis. It is likely that a simplified, less costly, and more sensitive and specific approach to diagnosis will be established during the next few years.

REFERENCES

1. Alimenti A, Luzuriaga K, Stechenberg B, Sullivan JL: Quantitation of human immunodeficiency virus in vertically infected infants and children. J Pediatr 119:225–229, 1991
2. Auger I, Thomas P, De Gruttola V, et al: Incubation periods for pediatric AIDS patients. Nature 336: 575–577, 1988
3. Boyer P, Dillon M, Navaie M, et al: Factors predictive of maternal-fetal transmission of HIV-1. JAMA, 271: 1925–1930, 1994
4. Bryson Y, Luzuriaga K, Sullivan J, Wara D: Establishment of a definition of the timing of vertical HIV-1 infection. N Engl J Med 327:1246–1247, 1992
5. Burgarde M, Mayayx M, Blanche S: The use of viral culture and p24 antigen testing to diagnose human immunodeficiency virus infection in neonates. N Engl J Med 327:1192–1197, 1992
6. Connor E, Sperling R, Gelber R, et al: Reduction of maternal-infant transmission of human immunodeficiency virus type 1 with zidovudine treatment. N Engl J Med 331:1173–1180, 1994
7. De Rossi A, Chieco-Bianchi L, Zacchello F, et al: The European Collaborative Study: Natural history of vertically acquired human immunodeficiency virus-1 infection. Pediatrics 94:815–819, 1994
8. Dickover R, Garratty E, Herman S, et al: Identification of levels of maternal HIV-1 RNA associated with risk of perinatal transmission. JAMA 275:599–605, 1996
9. Dunn D, Newell M, Ades A, Peckham C: Risk of human immunodeficiency virus type 1 transmission through breastfeeding. Lancet 340:585–588, 1992
10. Dunn D, Brandt C, Krivine A, et al: The sensitivity of HIV-1 DNA polymerase chain reaction in the neonatal period and the relative contributions of intra-uterine and intra-partum transmission. AIDS 9: F7–F11, 1995

11. Ehrnst A, Lindgren S, Dictor M, et al: HIV in pregnant women and their offspring: Evidence for late transmission. Lancet 338:203–207, 1991
12. European Collaborative Study: Risk factors for mother-to-child transmission of HIV-1. Lancet 339:1007–1012, 1992
13. Giaquinto C, Truscia D, De Rossi A, et al: The European Collaborative Study: Caesarian section and risk of vertical transmission of HIV. Lancet 343:1464–1467, 1994
14. Goedert J, Duliege A, Amos C, et al: High risk of HIV-1 infection for first-born twins. Lancet 338:1471–1475, 1991
15. Jenkins M, Landers D, Williams-Herman D, et al: Association between antibody-human immunodeficiency virus type 1 (HIV-1) antibody-dependent cellular cytotoxicity antibody titers at birth and vertical transmission of HIV-1 J Infect Dis 170:308–12, 1994
16. Jovaisas E, Koch MA, Schafer A: LAV/HTLV III in 20-week fetus. Lancet 2:1129, 1985
17. Kliks S, Fadem M, Wara D, Levy J: Evidence for the maternal transfer of neutralization-escape or enhancement variants into newborn infants. Eighth International Conference on AIDS, 1992
18. Kliks S, Wara D, Landers D, et al: Features of HIV-1 that could influence maternal–child transmission. JAMA 272:467–474, 1994
19. Krivine A, Firtion G, Cao L, et al: HIV replication during the first weeks of life. Lancet 339:1187–1189, 1992
20. Luzuriaga K, McQuilkin P, Alimenti A, Sullivan JL: Vertical HIV-1 infection: Intrauterine versus intrapartum transmission. Pediatr Res 31:169A, 1992
21. Luzuriaga K, McQuilken P, Alimenti A, et al: Early viremia and immune responses in vertical human immunodeficiency virus type 1 infection. J Infect Dis 167:1008–1013, 1993
22. Martin N, Levy J, Legg H: Detection of infection with human immunodeficiency virus (HIV) type 1 in infants by an anti-HIV immunoglobulin A assay using recombinant proteins. J Pediatr 118:354–358, 1991
23. Mayaux, M, Blanche S, Rouzioux C, et al: Maternal factors associated with perinatal HIV-1 transmission: The French Cohort Study & years of follow-up observation. J Acquir Immune Defic Syndr 8:188–194, 1995
24. Mayaux M, Bugard M, Telgas J, et al: Neonatal characteristics in rapidly progressive perinatally acquired HIV-1 disease. JAMA 265:606–610, 1996
25. Miles S, Balden E, Magpantay L, et al: Rapid serologic testing with immune-complex-dissociated HIV p24 antigen for early detection of HIV infection in neonates. N Engl J Med 328:297–302, 1993
26. Nair P, Alger L, Hines S, et al: Maternal and neonatal characteristics associated with HIV infection in infants of seropositive women. J Acquir Immune Defic Syndr 6:298–302, 1993
27. Owens D, Holodnly M, McDonald T, et al: A meta-analytic evaluation of the polymerase chain reaction for the diagnosis of HIV infection in infants. JAMA 275:1342–1348, 1996
28. Papiernik M, Brossard Y, Mulliez N, et al: Thymic abnormalities in fetuses aborted from human immunodeficiency virus type 1 seropositive women. Pediatrics 89:297–301, 1992
29. Quinn T, Kline R, Halsey N, et al: Early diagnosis of perinatal HIV infection by detection of viral-specific IgA antibodies. JAMA 266:3439–3442, 1991
30. Recommendations of the Public Health Service Task Force of the use of Zidovudine to reduce perinatal transmission of Human Immunodeficiency Virus: MMWR 43:1995
31. Rogers M, Ou C-Y, Rayfield M, et al: Use of the polymerase chain reaction for the early detection of the proviral sequences of human immunodeficiency virus in infants born to seropositive mothers. N Engl J Med 320:1649–1654, 1989
32. Scarlatti G, Albert J, Rossi P: Homologous and heterologous neutralization activity in sera of HIV-1-infected mothers: Correlation to transmission (Abstract WeC 1061). Eighth International Conference on AIDS, 1992
33. Sprecher S, Soumenkoff G, Pulssant F, de Gueldre M: Vertical transmission of HIV in 15 week fetus. Lancet 2:288–289, 1985
34. Thomas P, Weedon J, New York City Perinatal HIV Transmission Collaborative Study Group: Maternal predictors of perinatal HIV transmission (Abstract WeC 1059:We56). Eighth International Conference on AIDS, 1992
35. Tovo P, de Martino M, Gabiano C, et al: Mode of delivery and gestational age influence perinatal HIV-1 transmission. J Acquir Immune Defic Syndr 11:88–94, 1996
36. US Public Health Service recommendations for Human Immunodeficiency Virus counseling and voluntary testing for pregnant women: MMWR 44:1995 44, July 7, 1995
37. Van de Perre P, Simonon A, Msellati P, et al: Postnatal transmission of human immunodeficiency virus type 1 from mother to infant. N Engl J Med 325:594–598, 1991
38. Wolinsky S, Wike C, Korber B, et al: Selective transmission of human immunodeficiency virus type 1 variants from mothers to infants. Science 255:1134–1137, 1992
39. Ziegler J, Johnson R, Cooper D, et al: Postnatal transmission of AIDS-associated retrovirus from mother to infant. Lancet 1:896, 1985

Chapter 32

Gender-Specific Issues in HIV Disease

MEG D. NEWMAN and CONSTANCE B. WOFSY

EPIDEMIOLOGY

By the year 2000, 13 million women worldwide will have been infected by the human immunodeficiency virus (HIV).[104] In the United States, women constitute the fastest growing population of persons with the acquired immunodeficiency syndrome (AIDS). The proportion of cases among women increased dramatically in the period from 1993 to October 1995, with women constituting 18% of the total cases, whereas from 1981 through 1987, women accounted for only 8% of the total cases.[21,26] The incidence of HIV in male Job Corps trainees decreased from 3.6 to 2.2 per 1000 in 1992 but increased from 2.1 to 4.2 per 1000 in young women.[40] HIV has become indelibly associated with sexually transmitted diseases (STDs), and crack cocaine use.[59,99]

Nationally, 47% of women have contracted AIDS from their own personal intravenous (IV) drug use, 36% from heterosexual transmission (18% from sex with an IV drug user, 18% from other heterosexual transmission), and 5% from transfusion and other blood products; in 12%, the transmission route remains unidentified or not fully evaluated. In younger women ages 13 to 25, heterosexual contact dominates as a means of transmission, whereas it is a relatively uncommon mode of transmission in men (50% compared to 3%).[21] Injection drug use (IDU) accounts for 33% of the infections and an injecting heterosexual partner is the source in 50%. Therefore, IV drug use directly or indirectly accounts for over 60% of HIV in women, and has substantial implications for intervention and drug treatment.[3]

In the United States as of June 1995 there were 64,822 women with AIDS. Of these women, 55% were African-American and 21% were Hispanic.[21] The same population has a very high incidence of sexually transmitted diseases, including syphilis (especially congenital syphilis), and high rates of tuberculosis (TB), including multiple-drug-resistant tuberculosis now seen in metropolitan cities on the eastern seaboard of the United States and in the prison system of New York City.[23,56] Women comprise 28% of all persons with drug-resistant TB in New York City.[56] AIDS was the third leading cause of death in 1994 in women aged 25 to 44 nationally and is the leading cause of death in women of childbearing age in New York City.[29,32] By the end of 1995, maternal deaths caused by HIV/AIDS will have orphaned an estimated 24,600 children and 21,000 adolescents in the United States.[89]

Heterosexual transmission is the fastest growing risk group nationally, increasing from 3% of all AIDS cases among women in 1983 and 1984 to 36% currently.[18,20,26] The true incidence is probably even higher, but often cases are unrecognized owing to the Centers for Disease Control and Prevention (CDC) reporting hierarchy. For example, if a woman had heterosexual contact multiple times and injected intravenous drugs once, she is categorized as having IDU as the source of her infection. Of the 53,938 cases ever classified as "risk not reported or identified" through June 1995, 24,338 have been reclassified. Of these, 5305 are women and 3501 (66%) of them have been reclassified as heterosexual transmission.[21] Reports suggest that within the heterosexual transmission group, up to 50% of women did not know that they had been exposed to HIV.[18,80]

As transmission of HIV is increasingly occurring in the general population of women, prevention strategies must be generalized, because women do not constitute a focus group for whom to target outreach and intervention measures such as those used for groups with specific behaviors in common, such as IV drug use or homosexuality.

TRANSMISSION

Among HIV-discordant couples (those with only a single HIV-positive partner), heterosexual transmission is more efficient from male to female, and most infections have occurred by the vaginal route, although participation in rectal sex enhances the risk.[105,106] The cumulative incidence of transmission between discordant couples suggests an approximate 20% risk of transmission from male to female after unprotected sex over a sustained period in a fixed partnership. Other studies suggest a range of 7% to 50%. Female-to-male transmission is less efficient, at least in prospectively followed research subjects. A study showed that only 1 of 72 male partners of HIV-infected females became infected.[106] Other studies have suggested a nearly equal efficiency of transmission between men and women.[60,106] Factors associated with increased transmission include lack of condom use, anal intercourse, number of contacts, advanced disease state (measured by CD4, viral load, p24 antigen or AIDS diagnosis), genital ulcerative disease and other STDs, and intrauterine contraceptive device (IUD) use[6,60,99] (Table 32–1). Cervical ectopy is emerging as a risk for acquisition by women from HIV-infected men. It is possible that the increased levels of heterosexual transmission in adolescent women may be partially explained by the natural occurrence of cervical ectopy in this age group. Best cited in a study of African women, HIV DNA could be detected by polymerase chain reaction (PCR) in 33% of 84 cervical samples and 17% of 77 vaginal samples.[96] The yield was higher from the endocervix and was independently associated with oral contraceptive use, although numbers were small.[36] Causation between oral contraceptive use and HIV acquisition in U.S. women has not been correlated, but it is an area for future study.

HIV could be cultured from 30% of semen specimens from HIV-infected men with early disease. Sperm morphology and seminal characteristics, including those of men on zidovudine, were not affected, but direct fertility studies are not available.[77] Lack of circumcision had been associated with increased risk of transmission in Africa, and recently Kreiss et al found that uncircumcised homosexual men in the United States had a twofold increased risk of HIV infection.[74] In men, zidovudine may decrease the prevalence or titer of HIV in seminal fluid[4,61] but should not be considered as an effective means of preventing transmission in either direction.

World health leaders have universally proclaimed the need for female-controlled contraceptive antiinfectives and microbicides. Nonoxynol-9, the most promising agent because of its potent viricidal effect in vitro and effectiveness at killing other STD-causing agents,[103] is the leading candidate. However, it may produce vaginal irritation when used frequently.[102,116,135] At the Research Clinic for Prostitutes in Nairobi, Kenya, 138 seronegative prostitutes were evaluated, half routinely using a nonoxynol-9 treated sponge and half using a placebo. There were more genital ulcers and vulvitis in the nonoxynol-9 group, and the rate of HIV acquisition was similar; thus, nonoxynol-

TABLE 32–1. FACTORS ASSOCIATED WITH HETEROSEXUAL TRANSMISSION OF HIV

Factor	Male-to-Female	Female-to-Male
Lack of condom	Yes	Yes
Anal intercourse	Yes	No
Sex during menses	No	Yes
Number of sexual contacts	Yes	Yes
Advanced disease state*	Yes	Yes
Zidovudine decreases risk	Possibly	Unknown
Genital sores, infections, or inflammation	Yes	Yes
Oral contraceptives†	Yes	Unknown
Intrauterine contraceptive device (IUD) use	Possibly	Unknown
Cervical ectopy	Yes	Unknown

* As measured by CD4, p24 antigen, or AIDS diagnosis.
† Whether oral contraceptives are protective or increase the likelihood of transmission is controversial.
Modified from Padian N: Epidemiology of AIDS and heterosexually transmitted HIV in women. AIDS File 5:1–2, 1991, with permission.

9 was not protective.[75] The role of nonoxynol-9 in women with less frequent sexual contact remains to be determined. Other microbicides are under evaluation, but the lack of in vitro systems and small-animal models for testing has slowed development of these products.[111] The female condom, a latex pouch that sheaths the vagina during intercourse, is probably effective but may be too expensive and technically cumbersome for widespread use and application.

HIV IN LESBIANS

Transmission of HIV between women was documented as early as 1984.[88] A number of small studies have been conducted but are plagued by small numbers of women having sex with women (WSW) without other HIV risk factors, especially injection drug use. Through September 1989, 79 women with AIDS had reported sex with a female only, but 95% were injection drug users.[33] Sporadic cases of direct transmission have been reported, but analysis is hampered by lack of data regarding baseline serology or blood exposure during sex.[115]

When the surveillance hierarchy of risk factors is used, an infected WSW who has injected drugs or had heterosexual contact will be classified into the highest category (IDU and heterosexual transmission [HT]). Currently, WSW who are HIV-infected but have no other risk factors are classified as "no identified risk"; that is, not having reported behaviors known to efficiently transmit HIV. These regulations can shroud the true risk of HIV among WSW. Though HIV is present in the cervical and vaginal secretions of HIV-infected women, there is still a paucity of data on women's genital fluids, and risks of transmission for myriad WSW sexual practices. Of note, a recent study of 21 lesbian monogamous partners suggests strongly that bacterial vaginosis can be sexually transmitted between women.[10]

There has been no evidence of female-to-female transmission in a study of 960,000 female blood donors in the United States. Of the total, there were 96 seropositive women, of whom 3 reported sex with men and women and none with women only.[110] Lesbians have thus been considered at low risk. However, in a 1993 study of 498 women in San Francisco and Berkeley, CA, of whom 68% self-identified as lesbians and 32% as bisexuals, 81% reported having sex with men, including unprotected oral (56.3%), vaginal (39%), and anal sex (10.9%). High rates of unprotected oral, vaginal, or oral sex with gay/bisexual men (14.6%, 9.6%, and 3.2%, respectively) were also noted.[120] Other studies support these results; however, they are not ideal for deriving precise prevalence data about WSW and probably select for only parts of the WSW community. But, if providers assume that lesbians are not engaging in sex with men, especially gay men and injection-drug-using men, they may be overlooking risk behaviors that may be (or are) more common than most providers suspect. These studies reemphasize the important point that sexual identity is a poor marker for sexual behaviors. Because they have been considered "safe," lesbians have not been targeted for AIDS education and may be engaging in multiple unsafe sexual practices.

CLINICAL MANIFESTATIONS

Opportunistic Infections and HIV-Associated Infections

By the current CDC definition of AIDS, *Pneumocystis carinii* pneumonia (PCP) remains the leading AIDS-defining diagnosis in women.[20,23] Lack of access to care, minimal self-motivation, attention to the health care of their children over that of themselves, and disenfranchisement among a large proportion of women all contribute to less early detection and intervention and probably a concomitant sustained high frequency of PCP. In New York City, 544 women with first-episode PCP were compared to 2526 men. Fewer women were white, more women were admitted through emergency rooms, more women received care at hospitals that had less experience caring for PCP, and fewer women underwent bronchoscopy. In addition, more women were admitted to the intensive care unit (ICU).[6] As women themselves have said, HIV for women is an issue of access to health care, and the care system is not well suited to their needs.[21,52] AIDS-defining diagnoses seen with increasing frequency in data combined from a number of small cohorts are PCP, esophageal *Candida*, disseminated *Mycobacterium avium*, and mucocutaneous herpes simplex virus.[52] Women are not protected from any of the other AIDS-defining opportunistic infections. Bacterial infections, especially respiratory infections with such encapsulated organisms as *Streptococcus pneumoniae* and *Haemophilus influenzae*, occur more frequently in IV drug users than in homosexual men[148] and occur with equal frequency in heterosexual men and women.[60]

One of the largest prospectively followed cohorts of women with HIV comes from Rhode Island, where 200 HIV-infected women have been followed at regular intervals. The initial clinical manifestations of HIV infection in 117 symptomatic women were *Candida* vaginitis (n = 43), lymphadenopathy (n = 17), bacterial pneumonia (n = 15), acute retroviral syndrome (n = 8), and constitutional symptoms, such as unexplained weight loss of $\geq$10 pounds or diarrhea for $\geq$4 weeks (n = 8). The rest had syndromes that would suggest to most clinicians a consideration of HIV infection (i.e., thrush, tuberculosis, hairy leukoplakia, herpes zoster, PCP, AIDS encephalopathy, and cytomegalovirus [CMV] retinitis).[17] Nonspecific conditions of vaginitis, pneumonia, and constitutional symptoms associated with HIV infection were more frequent and would not suggest to other than the most alert clinician the possibility of HIV disease. In this cohort, PCP was the initial manifestation in only 20%. This cohort differs from others, particularly in having a smaller percentage of nonwhite subjects, in accord with the demographics of Rhode Island. This is in sharp contrast to national data and other cohorts in which PCP is still the leading AIDS diagnosis.[35,50,82] In a review of AIDS in women reported to the CDC by December 1990, 73% of women with AIDS were residents of large metropolitan areas of over 1 million population, mostly on the Atlantic seaboard, suggesting a target for interventions. The other 26% were from smaller cities, making it harder to target a specific population.[50]

Several factors may influence the presentation of HIV or response to therapy in women. These include altered pharmacokinetics of drugs, due either to gender or to interactions between commonly associated drugs (such as methadone or oral contraceptive pills), and possibly to differences in the immune system, since autoimmune diseases are traditionally more frequent in women than in men. Early symptoms of HIV in women, as in men, are extremely nonspecific, including night sweats, diarrhea, yeast infection, cough, and weight loss.[17,35,62] Because women frequently use emergency rooms, family planning clinics, STD clinics, youth guidance centers, jail clinic facilities, and drug treatment units, these are the sites for targeting efforts at early diagnosis and use of early intervention with antiviral and prophylactic therapies.[133]

Malignancies (Chapter 28)

Kaposi's sarcoma (KS), seen frequently in homosexual men, is found in less than 2% of HIV-infected women as an initial AIDS diagnosis. There is growing evidence that Kaposi's sarcoma in persons with or without HIV infection is associated with newly identified human herpes virus 8.[143] When KS has been seen in women, it most frequently has been associated with sex with a bisexual man, but it has been seen in women whose risk was injection drug use or transfusion.[81] In one series of 12 women, the course of KS was aggressive, even when KS was the initial manifestation of AIDS.[1,81] The case of a 22-year-old woman who went to her dentist because of a violaceous lesion on her hard palate emphasizes that all health practitioners must be alert for signs of HIV in both high-risk and seemingly low-risk populations. A recent report[47] describes a woman who presented with vulvar pain, vaginal discharge, and a vulvar mass that proved to be KS.[85] This case reemphasizes the point that unusual presentations of disease are likely to occur more often as survival is prolonged.

Limited evidence suggests an increased occurrence and aggressiveness of cervical cancer in women with HIV infection, and it now constitutes an AIDS diagnosis.[22,30] There is an increased incidence of cancer in women in Connecticut and an increase over expected cases of cervical cancer was found when the National Cancer Institute examined cancer registries nationally.[41] Non-Hodgkin's lymphoma, an AIDS-defining diagnosis, is encountered too infrequently in women to compare gender-specific incidence rates.[58,65] However, it does constitute an AIDS-defining diagnosis in both groups. To date, the occurrence of breast cancer, lung cancer, and other malignancies in HIV-infected women is not greater than in the general population.

Gynecologic Manifestations

Much attention has been given to three disorders that are more frequent, usually more severe, and less responsive to therapy in HIV-infected women, particularly those with advanced immunosuppression, than in HIV-uninfected women. They are human papillomavirus (HPV), associated cervical disorders such as cervical intraepithelial neoplasia (CIN) II and CIN III, *Candida* vaginitis, and pelvic inflammatory disease,[24,53,66,86,87] all of which are recognized as HIV-associated conditions in the expanded case definition.[22]

Cervical Disorders

An increased frequency of abnormal Papanicolaou (Pap) smear results was first noted in women attending HIV, methadone maintenance, and cervical dysplasia clinics.[24,53] In an early study, 40% of 35 HIV-positive women had squamous intraepithelial lesions on cervical cytologic examinations compared with 9% of 32 HIV-negative women.[53]

In a study of 32 HIV-infected women, 78% had a normal Pap smear result, and only 3% had cytologic findings suggesting cervical intraepithelial neoplasia. However, colposcopy associated with biopsy disclosed that 41% had cervical abnormalities.[86] This had profound implications, since colposcopy is more costly and more time consuming and requires specially trained personnel for proper interpretation. Subsequent studies have not confirmed these findings and, in fact, suggest that a correctly obtained and expertly read Pap smear (at least under research conditions) has sufficient sensitivity and specificity to detect cervical abnormalities.[51] A large, prospective, multicenter study conducted by the CDC in conjunction with investigators in Miami and New York compared 398 HIV-negative women, all of whom had Pap smears, colposcopy, and evaluation for HPV by PCR.[51,77] This controlled prospective trial confirmed numerous prior uncontrolled studies of HIV-positive cohorts in finding that cervical neoplasia is more frequent in HIV-positive women (20% in HIV-positive versus 4% in HIV-negative women) and that more advanced CIN is more likely with more advanced stage of immunosuppression. By multivariate analysis, HPV (odds ratio [OR] 9.8) and HIV infection (OR 3.5) and CD4 count (OR 2.7) were independently associated with CIN.[151,152] Because CIN is more frequent and more aggressive in women with severe immunosuppression, some practitioners routinely recommend a Pap smear every 6 months, particularly for women with more advanced immunodeficiency.[93] This large study also suggested that Pap smears were highly sensitive in HIV-positive women. Subsequent studies confirm that Pap smears also were equally sensitive for detecting cervical disorders in HIV-positive and HIV-negative women.[72] One study also demonstrated that 15% of the

dysplasia in HIV-positive women seen in a large dysplasia referral clinic was limited to vulvar, vaginal, or perianal lesions detected only by colposcopy. These lesions would have been missed if only a cervical Pap smear had been performed.[72] Although colposcopy would be the most sensitive and specific diagnostic tool, the general lack of availability and standardization require assiduous attention to appropriate Pap smear tests and follow-up. The current CDC recommendation for HIV-positive women (Table 32–2) suggests annual Pap smears if there have been two normal smears 6 months apart The CDC does not define a specific lower CD4 threshold below which Pap smears should be obtained more frequently.[101] After two normal pelvic exams and Pap smears have been obtained every 6 months, repeat exams should be performed every 12 months along with careful vulvar, vaginal, and anal inspection. Colposcopic evaluation of women should be performed with any ASCUS, AGCUS, low-grade and high-grade squamous interstitial lesion (SIL) on any Pap smear or any persistent inflammation that is unresolved after treatment for gonorrhea or *Chlamydia*. Initial colposcopy could be considered for women with poor likelihood of follow-up, or suspicion of extracervical disease.[72] Pregnancy did not affect the incidence of abnormal Pap smears in women enrolled in the Women and Infant Transmission Study.[136]

HPV prevalence, acquisition, and retention are higher in HIV-positive women than in matched controls. By DNA analysis, types 16, 18, and 33 are associated most frequently with CIN in HIV-positive women and controls.[55,84,107] In the absence of effective treatment for HPV, preventing the acquisition of the virus and early intervention in the disease process are the current goals.

Anal interstitial neoplasia (AIN) is also more prevalent and increasingly recognized in HIV-infected individuals. In a group of women IDUs

TABLE 32–2. CDC RECOMMENDED STD TREATMENT GUIDELINES FOR WOMEN WITH HIV

Initial Pap smear on diagnosis
If normal, at least one Pap test in the next 6 months
If second Pap test normal, annual screening
If inflammation/reactive atypia is present, repeat test in 3 months
If squamous interstitial lesion (SIL) or ASCUS, refer for colposcopy

Modified from 1993 Sexually transmitted disease treatment guidelines. MMWR 42:88–91, 1993, with permission.

in San Francisco, AIN was as prevalent as CIN.[147] In a small group of San Francisco men, 51% of the 37 HIV-positive men (all of whom had advanced disease) and 36% of the 28 HIV-negative men had anal HPV. Abnormal anal cytology was found in 28% of the HIV-positive men and 8% of the HIV-negative men. The risk of developing anal disease and HPV infection was highest among HIV-positive men with a CD4 count <200/mm³ who were current smokers.[109] In Seattle, 141 HIV-positive gay men were compared to 108 HIV-negative controls, and the rates of high-grade or low-grade AIN were two to three times more frequent in the HIV-positive group.[44] A review of the U.S. Anal Cancer Registry revealed a marked increase in the incidence of anal squamous cell carcinoma since the onset of the AIDS epidemic,[89] and a London study found that anal cytology was less sensitive than anal colposcopy, mimicking earlier reports of decreased sensitivity of cervical cytology in women.[46] Most clinicians, however, do not incorporate an anal Pap smear into routine clinical management of men or women and studies are ongoing in the United States.

VAGINAL CANDIDIASIS

Vaginal candidiasis, a frequent disorder in women in the general population, can be prevalent in HIV-infected women.[17,44,48,114] In the revised CDC case definition of 1993, severe vaginal candidiasis became a designated HIV-associated symptomatic disorder.[22] Vaginal candidiasis can occur early, when HIV may not be suspected. The reported rates of this as an initial HIV presentation may be falsely low, since treatment is commonly self-initiated with over-the-counter therapy. Although there have been no prospective controlled trials, in the Rhode Island cohort, *Candida* vaginitis in HIV-infected women developed when only mild immunosuppression was present.[17] Women with HIV and vaginal *Candida* had a mean CD4 count of 506/mm³, in contrast to those with esophageal *Candida* from the same population, in whom the mean CD4 count was 30/mm³. *Candida* vaginitis occurred in 44 of 200 prospectively followed HIV-infected women and, in fact, was the most frequent initial HIV-associated clinical condition. Strikingly, in no instance did new, recurrent, or more refractory *Candida* prompt the initial examining physician to evaluate or offer HIV testing.[64] A study from Rhoads found that only 24% of women with advanced HIV had recurrent severe *Candida* infections.[114] Duerr found rates of recovery of *Candida* on culture and frequency of clinical symptoms are significantly increased with progressive immune suppression.[48]

Candida can be cultured readily from the vagina in the absence of symptoms, so a diagnosis must include clinical symptoms as well as culture positivity. Recurrent or recalcitrant cases of fungal vaginitis should prompt consideration of *Torulopsis glabrata*, as it does not form hyphae or pseudohyphae, may not demonstrate a cheesy discharge, is often associated with recurrent vaginitis, and can be resistant to the imidazoles.[130,131] Culture is the mode of diagnosis. Response of vaginal *Candida* to therapy using topical antifungals, such as clotrimazole (Gyne-Lotrimin) usually is very good. Since clotrimazole preparation is available over the counter, it is important to provide the information that new and unexpected or more frequent or more refractory *Candida* in the absence of antibiotics should prompt affected women and their clinicians to consider HIV testing. The use of terconazole is usually required for non-*albicans* species. Boric acid suppositories (600 mg bid for 14 days) can also be helpful for *Torulopsis glabrata*.[130,131] Vaginal secretions maintain increased concentrations of fluconazole for 72 hours or more and 150 mg for 1 to 3 days can be extremely effective.[138] Sometimes, a higher dosage and longer duration is required for refractory cases (200 mg for 4 to 7 days). Other options include ketoconazole (200 to 400 mg/day for 14 days, followed by 5-day courses each month for 6 months, with monitoring of liver function tests).[72,93] However, both are substantially more expensive than topical therapy and require a doctor's prescription, and increasingly frequent reports of fluconazole-resistant *Candida* in men who have been exposed to oral fluconazole[12] make prescribers reluctant to routinely rely on fluconazole as a first-line therapy. Fluconazole is notable for decreased activity against non-*albicans* species like *C. krusei, glabrata,* or *lambica*.[138] Treatment needs to be individualized. The lowest effective dose should be used for a particular patient. Even topical treatment 1 time per week or a few days during the month may be quite effective for acute disease and chronic suppression.[113] Physicians who see women with recurrent or refractory vaginal candidiasis should offer HIV counseling and testing.

GENITAL ULCERATIVE DISEASE AND PELVIC INFLAMMATORY DISEASE

Severe ulcerative genital herpes was the AIDS-defining diagnosis in 18% of 44 women prospectively followed who developed AIDS.[11] Genital herpes simplex virus infections are very prevalent in the population at large and may be particularly refractory in HIV-infected men and women. Augenbraun recently demonstrated that HSV-2 shedding was nearly four times greater in HIV-positive than in HIV-negative women and that 79% of the shedding was asymptomatic.[5] As immunosuppression progresses, as measured by declining CD4 count, shedding of HSV-2 became more common.[5]

Recommended treatment is an initial course of acyclovir of 400 mg tid to qid per day for 10 days. For suppression, a course of 400 mg bid to tid for those who have more than six outbreaks a year, or significant disability with fewer outbreaks. Dose and duration of treatment may need to be individualized to avoid breakthrough. HSV unresponsive to acyclovir raises a concern for acyclovir resistance. Although these resistant infections may respond to foscarnet,[118] the therapy may be teratogenic and should be avoided in HIV-infected pregnant women. Dose and duration of treatment may need to be individualized to avoid breakthrough. New topical therapies are in early clinical trials.[79]

Giant idiopathic aphthous genital ulcers are infrequent but painful, disabling, and difficult to treat. Such ulcers should be evaluated with a full workup for HSV, CMV, syphilis, chancroid, gonorrhea, bacterial or fungal pathogens, and malignancies. The pathogenesis may be similar to giant esophageal aphthous ulcers. Anecdotal reports suggest that thalidomide may be effective for esophageal ulcers, but there is negligible experience with genital ulcers in women. A rigorous application process would be required in order to give thalidomide on a compassionate-use basis.

Genital ulcerative disease is a well-described risk factor for transmission of HIV, particularly in studies in Africa where STDs are more prevalent.[60] HIV is prevalent in women with pelvic inflammatory disease (PID), and there have been suggestions that PID may be more severe with advanced HIV disease.[63,119] Early findings of the Multicenter HIV and PID Study Group did not confirm a substantially worse presentation and found that PID responded to therapy equally in HIV-infected and HIV-uninfected groups.[66] HIV-positive patients may present with lower white blood cell counts and require more surgical intervention, especially in those with more advanced disease. Standard antibiotic regimens that include anaerobic coverage can be used. If treatment failures occur, more optimal anaerobic coverage should be instituted.[72] Most clinicians maintain a low threshold to hospitalize, especially if the HIV disease is advanced.

MENSTRUAL DISORDERS

Sporadic reports suggest that menstrual disorders are seen with greater frequency in HIV-infected women. A New York study of IV drug-using women compared 39 HIV-positive women to 39 HIV-negative women and identified more menstrual abnormalities in the HIV-positive women (41% versus 24%).[142] Amenorrhea and between-period bleeding were noted particularly. Other small studies support that approximately one third of HIV-positive women have either excessive bleeding or amenorrhea.[72] A recent small controlled trial of HIV-negative women and HIV-positive women with midstage disease found no menstrual differences between groups.[142] Larger studies are currently in progress. The fluctuations of progesterone, estradiol, and cortisol throughout the menstrual cycle of HIV-infected women with normal cycles were identical to well-established norms in the population at large.[125]

There are currently no data to suggest that diagnosis or treatment of menstrual disorders should be different from that for HIV-negative women. However, further documentation of the specific types of menstrual irregularity, the frequency, and the hormone interaction is needed. These menstrual disorders are relevant not only because of personal discomfort but because unsuspected pregnancy may masquerade as a delayed period. Menstrual irregularities make prediction of time of fertility difficult for those wishing to conceive or avoid pregnancy and may potentially increase exposure to menstrual blood for a partner.

Progression of Disease

Studies of disease progression in women are limited and, when available, are derived from three principal sources: large national databases, which usually include the diagnosis of AIDS and the date of death with little additional interval information; small to moderate sized cohort studies of 50 to 200 women, often followed for less than 3 years; and large cohort studies conducted in other regions (e.g., Africa) from which conclusions, because of great differences in economic, sociologic, and medical and public health conditions, may not be applicable to the United States or western Europe.

A recent report summarizes a dozen studies that overall reveal that the survival and course of disease in men and women is not substantially different when patients are matched for socioeconomic status, risk group, and access to care.[72] Reports from the CDC suggest that survival time of women and heterosexual men is similar. In the Bronx, NY, access to or adherence to follow-up care strongly influenced survival time, with survival substantially shortened in women who had no prior care before a severe HIV-related infection. These earlier reports are congruent with a recently published trial of 1372 patients in Baltimore, MD, that found that gender had no negative relationship with disease progression.[31] Among New York Medicaid recipients (of which 60% of men and women were IDUs), treatment with zidovudine and PCP prophylaxis was equal in IDUs. Non-IDU women were less frequently on zidovudine or PCP prophylaxis. Among drug users, women survived slightly longer than men, and among non–drug users, survival was similar for both sexes.[139] The only recent study to conflict with these findings is the Melnick-CPCRA trial in which women had an increased risk of death but not of disease progression. The risk of death was found acutely among IDUs, and the deaths were secondary to bacterial pneumonia and endocarditis, both likely related to injection drug use. The study authors concluded that these findings may represent differential access to care, treatments, or social support.[90] The most important predictors of survival or progression have been CD4 count and the specific AIDS-defining diagnosis, not gender.[8,14,43,97,117]

INFORMATION FOR WOMEN WITH AIDS AND WOMEN WITH HIV

Guidelines for Treatment of HIV and Associated Illnesses in Women

Guidelines established for licensed antiretroviral therapies, specifically zidovudine (AZT), dideoxyinosine (ddI), dideoxycitidine (ddC), lamivudine (3TC), stavudine (d4T), invirase (Saquinivir), and prophylaxis against PCP and other opportunistic infections are derived from large national studies conducted on men and women. Although men predominate in these studies, the results led to licensure and established recommendations for persons of both sexes. Data on two large early national studies from the AIDS Clinical Trials Group (ACTG 016 and 019)[54,141] comparing zidovudine versus placebo in mildly symptomatic HIV-infected patients in ACTG 016 and asymptomatic HIV-infected persons in ACTG 019 suggested no difference in benefit from zidovudine for women or nonwhite persons.[49,78] A more recent review of the impact of race on response or toxicity in antiretrovirals disclosed no significant increased risk of subjective zidovudine intolerance for blacks and Hispanics when compared with whites.[67]

In the absence of data to the contrary, the prescribing of antivirals and prophylaxis against PCP and opportunistic infections for women would follow published guidelines and clinical preference.[19,25,121,140] Potential toxicity issues affecting treatment with antiretrovirals or PCP prophylaxis include the lower mean body weight in women, lower mean hemoglobin level (with the potentially complicating effect of zidovudine or dapsone in further inducing anemia), and absence of established controls for CD4 counts in men versus women. The most frequent toxicities of ddI and ddC are rash, pancreatitis, peripheral neuropathy, and diarrhea. All of these toxicities may occur with d4T, with pancreatitis occurring only rarely. 3TC may cause insomnia, and rash, and can cause or exacerbate preexisting peripheral neuropathy. Both d4T and 3TC are well tolerated and, unlike other antiretrovirals, utilize bid dosing. Early reports of the recently licensed Saquinivir demonstrate that it is well tolerated, and side effects include abdominal discomfort, diarrhea, and nausea. None of these toxicities have a predictable or obvious female-related predilection. Some of these issues will be elucidated further in ACTG 175, which compared combination antivirals to single-drug therapy and enrolled 18% women, and in which a nested subanalysis will compare toxicity and efficacy in women patients.

Tuberculosis, bacterial endocarditis, and sepsis are seen more frequently in IV drug users. Treatment guidelines do not differ by gender, and the clinical presentation is not expected to have gender-related differences exclusive of infection of the reproductive organs.

CLINICAL MANAGEMENT DURING PREGNANCY

Antiviral Drugs

Increased rates of vertical transmission are associated with high viral load, p24 antigenemia, low CD4 levels, placental membrane inflammation, prolonged rupture of the membranes, maternal fever, and anemia.[132] Multiple recent studies in the United States and abroad document the association of high maternal viral copy number with enhanced risk of transmission, but upper and lower viral thresholds have not been firmly established.[15,16,73,123,129] The preliminary report of the results of ACTG 076 issued in February 1994 substantially altered recommendations for counseling, testing, and prescription of zidovudine and probably other antiretroviral drugs for HIV-infected pregnant women.[39] This trial demonstrated that zidovudine given during pregnancy, intrapartum, and in the first six weeks of life substantially reduces perinatal transmission of HIV. The study, conducted by the Pediatric ACTG, randomized pregnant women between 14 and 34 weeks' gestation with CD4 counts >200/mm^3 to receive either a placebo or zidovudine 100 mg five times per day throughout pregnancy, followed by intrapartum intravenous zidovudine and oral administration of zidovudine syrup for 6 weeks to the infant: 419 women were enrolled; their median age was 25 years, median CD4 count was 550/mm^3, and median gestational age was 26 weeks. The initial analysis revealed transmission in the placebo group of 25.5% versus 8.3% in the zidovudine-treated group. The ongoing analysis as of October 1995 included 419 babies (209 in the placebo group and 210 in the treatment group) with 24.9% transmission in the placebo group and 7.8% in the zidovudine group. The end-point for establishing infant infection was a positive viral culture from peripheral blood of the infant. There was no significant maternal or fetal toxicity and dropout and deaths were the same in the placebo and treated groups.[39] An interim analysis of maternal plasma HIV-1 RNA and the success of zidovudine in preventing perinatal transmission in the ACTG 076 study was recently reported.[129] Among the 210 zidovudine- and the 209 placebo-exposed mother–infant pairs, maternal RNA levels were balanced between the groups at entry but were higher overall for transmitters than nontransmitters at entry and delivery. Transmission occurred in both groups, even at the lowest RNA levels, although RNA was reduced from entry to delivery in the zidovudine group overall and the treatment effect persisted at all RNA levels. Therefore, zidovudine reduction in RNA level may only explain part of the treatment effect, raising speculation that the use of parental zidovudine during the intrapartum period or treatment of the infant may play a significant role in reduction of transmission.[129]

The U.S. Public Health Service now recommends that HIV counseling and testing be offered to all pregnant women and that zidovudine be offered to all HIV-infected pregnant women.[27,28,146] Comfort with the relative safety of zidovudine is enhanced by data gathered from a registry of women who have received zidovudine during pregnancy either by choice or inadvertently. To date, no specific adverse effects to mother or child other than a mild anemia have been reported.[39,127,128] Pharmacologic studies in humans do not suggest excessive accumulation of zidovudine in the placenta or fetal tissue, and obstetric and gynecologic specialists in HIV have routinely recommended zidovudine therapy for women with a CD4 count <200/mm^3. The new findings largely alter the recommendation for women with CD4 counts >200/mm^3. The zidovudine dose for pregnant women is the same as for nongravid women.[93,127,128]

Although the results of ACTG 076 provided an optimistic outlook for the reduction of perinatal transmission, many questions remain to be elucidated. Would other single agents be as effective? Should combination antiviral therapy, which is soon to become a frequently used standard of care for nonpregnant adults, be withheld from pregnant women, and would such combinations be even more effective at preventing perinatal transmission? Which of the three intervention times is most effective in reducing transmission? Are there any long-term effects of antiviral therapy on infants who will ultimately prove to be uninfected but are treated for 6 weeks? The feasibility of implementing the course of therapy recommended by the results of ACTG 076 is not financially possible in developing countries; therefore, trials are underway in a number of countries evaluating lower doses, fewer intervention times, or the use of other less expensive agents, including HIVIG, vaginal and cervical lavage or both, and vitamin A supplementation.[37] One such completed study conducted in Africa was designed to evaluate the role of topical cleansing of the vagina at the time of delivery. A large number of HIV-infected women who did not subsequently breast feed were randomized to receive vaginal washing with chlorhexidine or no washing at the time of delivery. There was no difference in perinatal transmission in the two groups.[11]

There has been substantially less clinical experience with ddI, ddC and 3TC, and d4T. No studies evaluating their role in prevention of transmission have been published. The World Health Organization (WHO) is currently evaluating AZT plus 3TC against placebo in Africa. The International Antiviral Pregnancy Registry is looking both prospectively and retrospectively at women on all antiretrovirals. There contact number is 1-800-722-9292 ext. 8465.

Prophylaxis for *Pneumocystis carinii* Pneumonia

No prophylactic therapies for PCP have been endorsed or approved by the U.S. Food and Drug Administration (FDA) for use in pregnancy.[70] However, based on past therapies and the growing body of community practice dictated by necessity, trimethoprim-sulfamethoxazole (TMP/SMX) has become the standard PCP prophylactic regimen used in pregnancy.[25,93,127,140] Although conventional dictum suggests that TMP/SMX therapy should be avoided in the third trimester of pregnancy because of kernicterus, this complication has not been reported, and TMP/SMX can be used through delivery in those women who can tolerate it.[93,127] Dapsone has been used without major problems in pregnant women with dermatitis herpetiformis and leprosy, conditions that necessitate daily and long-term dapsone therapy.[68] However, because of the risk of interference with dihydrofolate reductase, dapsone should be used with caution and necessitates obtaining a baseline glucose-6-phosphate dehydrogenase (G6PD) level. Aerosol pentamidine has the advantage of little systemic absorption, but evaluation of pulmonary distribution in pregnant women has not been undertaken. It is less effective than TMP/SMX in clinical trials, and aerosol pentamidine does not protect against extrapulmonary PCP.

PCP may be particularly severe during pregnancy.[93,95] For treatment of disease, TMP/SMX is the most attractive therapeutic option. Intravenous pentamidine should be avoided, and dapsone should be held in reserve until after careful risk/benefit assessment.

Virtually all of the major opportunistic infections have been reported during pregnancy, and treatment of such infections in pregnancy may be particularly problematic.[95] Of all therapies for common opportunistic disorders of HIV disease that may occur during pregnancy, no drugs are classified as category A, in which controlled clinical trials in women have demonstrated no fetal risk.[38] The clinician is left with a very difficult professional choice about treatment options, and common sense, inference from animal studies, and use of the drug for treatment of other diseases must be incorporated into making such a decision. Data from animal studies may be useful in decision-making but should be interpreted with care. Even if extensive anecdotal experience suggests that a drug is well tolerated in the pregnant woman, the decision to use the drug still must be considered on an individual basis. The patient should be informed in understandable language about the state of knowledge and the best decision tailored to the specific infection that can be made at that time. Table 32–3 shows the FDA pregnancy category and some very general guidelines for therapy, mostly from anecdotal experience of use of these therapies in serious or life-threatening disease. Although published guidelines in this emerging field are sparse, several excellent reviews address this issue and provide counseling and testing indications for pregnant women.[25,93,127,149]

Clinical Research and Access to Care

Women comprise 11% to 12% of the total AIDS population. In 1990, a group of researchers from the ACTG of the National Institutes of Health (NIH) noted that 6.7% of clinical trial subjects were women (at a time when women nationally comprised 9.8% of those with AIDS diagnoses).[42] Women most frequently were enrolled in studies of early-stage disease in large antiviral trials, which suggests that these studies are more accessible or more acceptable to women who may associate access to clinical trials with access to clinical care. Currently, 22.5% of ACTG trial subjects are women.[77] However, 26% of these are in one large trial of the role of zidovudine in interrupting perinatal

TABLE 32–3. TREATMENT OPTIONS DURING PREGNANCY

Drug	FDA Pregnancy Category*	Use in Serious Disease†
Acyclovir	C	Yes
Amikacin	D	Avoid in early pregnancy
Amphotericin B	B	Yes
Ciprofloxacin	C	Avoid
Clarithromycin	C	No experience
Clindamycin	N/A	Yes
Clofazimine	C	No experience
Clotrimazole oral troche	C	Yes
Clotrimazole vaginal suppository or cream		
Dapsone	C	Yes
Dideoxycytidine (ddC)	C	No experience
Didanosine (ddI)	B	No experience
Ethambutol	N/A	Yes
Fluconazole	C	No experience
Ganciclovir	C	No experience
Invirase (Saquinavir)	B	No experience
Isoniazid	C	Yes
Itraconazole	C	No experience
Lamividine (3TC)	C	No experience
Pentamidine IV	N/A	Avoid in preference to alternative
Pentamidine inhaled	C	Little systemic absorption; no experience
Primaquine	N/A	Avoid
Pyrazinamide (PZA)	N/A	Avoid
Pyrimethamine	C	Possibly; avoid first trimester
Rifampin		Yes
Stavudine (d4T)	B	Limited experience
Sulfadiazine	N/A	Yes
Trimethoprim	C	Seldom indicated alone
Trimethoprim-sulfamethoxazole		
	C	Yes
Zidovudine (AZT)	C	Yes

* Risk categories: N/A, classification not available; A, controlled studies in women demonstrate no risk; B, animal studies demonstrate no fetal risk, but there are no human trials, or animal studies demonstrate a risk not corroborated by human trials; C, animal studies demonstrate fetal risk but there are no human trials, or neither human nor animal studies are available; D, evidence exists for fetal risk in humans, but benefit may outweigh the risk; E, evidence exists for fetal risk in humans, and benefit is clearly outweighed by risk.

† For life-threatening condition or serious condition.

From Coleman RL: Treatment during pregnancy. AIDS File 5: 6, 1991, updated with FDA licensing data 1996, with permission.

transmission. Every effort should be undertaken to include substantial numbers of women in upcoming clinical trials and to establish guidelines for enrollment of pregnant women; standard enrollment guidelines; female-specific end-points; and guidelines about dose, body weight, and laboratory measurements standardized for women. Because women are a small percentage of the overall AIDS population, a disproportionate enrollment may be needed to allow sufficient numbers to detect a statistical difference.[45] New guidelines released by the FDA in 1993 may enhance enrollment and foster evaluation of drugs in pregnant women in clinical trials.[7,91] Specifically, the FDA is withdrawing restriction on participation of women of childbearing potential in early clinical trials, including clinical pharmacology studies and early therapeutic studies and the FDA is formalizing expectations regarding inclusion of subjects of both genders in drug development, analysis of clinical data by gender, assessment of potential pharmacokentic differences between genders and, where appropriate, assessment of pharmacodynamic differences and the conduct of specific additional studies in women.[7,91] An interesting issue to be considered is the role of the gender of the investigator in treatment design and trial enrollment.[84]

SUMMARY

The increasing frequency of HIV in women has led to a considerable body of knowledge about epidemiology, transmission, and perinatal infection. Clinical management of HIV-infected pregnant and nonpregnant women requires considerable further study about pathogenesis, infections, and malignancies of the female reproductive tract. Improvements are needed in the methods of enrolling women in epidemiologic and clinical trials to ensure adequate statistical power to find differences in end-points, mortality, and natural history. The Women's Interagency Health Study (WIHS) and HIV Epidemiologic Research Study (HERS) studies are being conducted at eight sites in the United States and will prospectively compare several thousand HIV-infected women to HIV-uninfected women. These large controlled studies should shed additional light on some of the issues obscured by low numbers.

REFERENCES

1. Aboulafia D, Mathisen G, Mitsuyasu R: Case report: Aggressive Kaposi's sarcoma and camphylobacteremia in a female with transfusion-associated AIDS. Am J Med Sci 301:256–258, 1991
2. Aboulker JP, Swart AM: Preliminary analysis of the Concorde trial. Lancet 341:889–890, 1993
3. Allen JR, Setlow VP: Heterosexual transmission of HIV—a view of the future (Editorial). JAMA 266:1695–1698, 1991
4. Anderson DJ, O'Brien TR, Politch JA, et al: Effects of disease stage and zidovudine therapy on the detection of human immunodeficiency virus 1 in semen. JAMA 267:278–2774, 1992
5. Augenbraun, M, Feldman J, Chirgwin K, et al: Increased genital shedding of herpes simplex virus type 2 in HIV-seropositive women. Ann Intern Med 123:845–847, 1995
6. Bastin L, Bennett CL, Adams J, et al: Differences between men and women with HIV-related *Pneumocystis carinii* pneumonia: Experience from 3,070 cases in New York City in 1987. J Acquir Immune Defic Syndr 6:617–623, 1993
7. Bennett JC: Inclusion of women in clinical trials—policies for population subgroups. N Engl J Med 329:288–291, 1993
8. Benson C, Sha B, Urbanski P, et al: Women with HIV disease: Clinical progression and survival in a cohort followed at a university medical center (10.15). Seventh International AIDS Conference, Amsterdam, The Netherlands, 1992
9. Beral V, Peterman TA, Berkelman RL, Jaffe HW: Kaposi's sarcoma among persons with AIDS: A sexually transmitted infection? Lancet 335:123–128, 1990
10. Berger BJ, Kolton S, Zenilman JM, et al: Bacterial vaginosis in lesbians: A sexually transmitted disease. Clin Infect Dis 21:1402–1405, 1995
11. Biggar RJ, Miotti P, Taha T, et al: Perinatal HIV-1 transmission in Africa and the effect of birth canal cleaning (Abstract 27). Third Conference on Retroviruses and Opportunistic Infections, Washington, DC, 1996, p 58
12. Boken DJ, Swindells S, Rinaldi MG: Fluconazole-resistant *Candida albicans*. Clin Infect Dis 17:1018–1021, 1993
13. Boshoff C, et al: Kaposi's sarcoma-associated herpesvirus in HIV-negative Kaposi's sarcoma. Lancet 345:1043–1044, 1995
14. Brettle RP, Leen CHS: The natural history of HIV and AIDS in women. AIDS 5:1283–1292, 1991
15. Bryson Y: Perinatal transmission: Pathogenesis and therapeutic intervention (Abstract L15). Third Conference on Retroviruses and Opportunistic Infections, Washington, DC 1996, p 169
16. Burchett SK, Kornegay J, Pitt J, et al: Assessment of maternal plasma HIV viral load as a correlate of vertical transmission (Abstract LB3). Third Conference on Retroviruses and Opportunistic Infections, Washington, DC, 1996, p 161
17. Carpenter CJ, Mayer KH, Stein MD, et al: Human immunodeficiency virus infection in North American women: Experience with 200 cases and a review of the literature. Medicine 70:307–325, 1991
18. Centers for Disease Control: AIDS in women—United States. MMWR 47:845–846, 1990
19. Centers for Disease Control: Guidelines for prophylaxis against *Pneumocystis carinii* pneumonia for persons infected with human immunodeficiency virus. MMWR 38(S5):1, 1989
20. Centers for Disease Control: HIV/AIDS Surveillance Report 5(3), 1993
21. Centers for Disease Control: HIV/AIDS Surveillance Report 7(1), 1995
22. Centers for Disease Control: 1993 Revised classification system for HIV-infection and expanded surveillance case definition for AIDS among adolescents and adults. MMWR 41(RR17):1–19, 1992
23. Centers for Disease Control: Nosocomial transmission of multidrug-resistant tuberculosis among HIV-infected persons—Florida and New York 1988–1991. MMWR 40:585–591, 1991
24. Centers for Disease Control: Risk for cervical disease in HIV-infected women, New York City. MMWR 39:826–849, 1990
25. Centers for Disease Control: USPS/IDSA Guidelines for the prevention of opportunistic infections in persons infected with the human immunodeficiency virus: A summary. MMWR 44(RR81):34, 1995
26. Centers for Disease Control: First 500,000 AIDS cases, United States, 1995. JAMA 274:1827–1828, 1995
27. Centers for Disease Control: U.S. Public Health Service recommendation for human immunodeficiency counseling and voluntary testing for pregnant women. MMWR 44(RR7): 1995
28. Centers for Disease Control: Recommendations of the U.S. Public Health Service task force on the use of zidovudine to reduce perinatal transmission of human immunodeficiency virus. MMWR 43(RR11): 1994
29. Centers for Disease Control: Update: Mortality attrib-

utable to HIV infection among persons aged 25–44 years, United States 1994. MMWR 45(6): 1996

30. Chaisson MA, Kelly KF, Williams R, et al: Invasive cervical cancer (ICC) in HIV+ women in New York City (NYC) (Abstract 412). Third Conference on Retroviruses and Opportunistic Infections, Washington, DC, 1996, p 130

31. Chaisson RE, Keruly JC, Moore RD: Race, sex, drug use, and progression of human immunodeficiency virus disease. N Engl J Med 333:751–756, 1995

32. Chu SY, Buehler JW, Berkelman RL: Impact of the human immunodeficiency virus epidemic on mortality in women of reproductive age, United States. JAMA 264:225–229, 1990

33. Chu S, Buehler JW, Fleming PL, Berkelman RL: Epidemiology of reported cases of AIDS in lesbians, United States, 1980–1989. Am J Public Health 80: 1380–1381, 1990

34. Clancy CM, Massion CT: American women's health care—a patchwork quilt with gaps (Editorial). JAMA 268:1918–1920, 1992

35. Clark RA, Brandon W, Dumestre J, et al: Clinical manifestations of infection with the human immunodeficiency virus in women in Louisiana. CIF 17: 165–172, 1993

36. Clemetson DBA, Moss GB, Willerford DM, et al: Detection of HIV DNA in cervical and vaginal secretions: Prevalence and correlates among women in Nairobi, Kenya. JAMA 269:2860–2864, 1993

37. Cohen, J: Bringing AZT to poor countries. Science 269:624–626, 1995

38. Coleman R: Treatment during pregnancy. AIDS File 5:6, 1991

39. Connor EM, Sperling RS, Gelber R, et al: Reduction of maternal-infant transmission of human immunodeficiency virus type 1 with zidovudine treatment. N Engl J Med 331:1173–1180, 1994

40. Conway GA, Epstein MR, Hayman CR, et al: Trends in HIV prevalence among disadvantaged youth. JAMA 269:2387–2391, 1993

41. Cote T, Schiffman M, Biggar R, et al: Invasive cervical cancer among women with AIDS: Results of a registry linkage (Abstract PO-B14-1637). International AIDS Conference, 1993

42. Cotton D, Feinberg J, Finkelstein D, ACTG SDAC: Participation of women in multicenter HIV clinical trials programs in the United States (Abstract TuD 114). Seventh International Conference on AIDS, Florence, Italy, 1991, p 87

43. Creagh T, Thompson M, Morris A, et al: Gender differences in the spectrum of HIV disease (Abstract 10.05). Seventh International AIDS Conference, Amsterdam, The Netherlands, 1992

44. Critchlow C, Holmes K, Daling J, et al: Risk for development of anal squamous intra-epithelial lesions among HIV (+) and HIV (−) gay men (Abstract PO-B14-1635). International AIDS Conference, Berlin, Germany, 1993

45. Currier JS, et al: Women and power: The impact of accrual rates of women on the ability to detect gender differences in toxicity rates and response to therapy in clinical trials. Seventh International AIDS Conference, Florence, Italy, June, 1991

46. de Ruiter A, Carter P, Katz D, et al: A comparison between cytology and histology to detect anal intraepithelial neoplasia (Abstract PO-B14-1638). International AIDS Conference Berlin, Germany, 1993

47. Dodd CL, Greenspan D, Greenspan JS: Oral Kaposi's sarcoma in a woman as first indication of HIV infection. J Am Dent Assoc 122:61–63, 1991

48. Duerr A, Sierra M, Clake L, et al: Vaginal candidiasis among HIV-infected women (Abstract PO-B01-0880). International AIDS Conference, 1993

49. Easterbrook PJ, Keruly JC, Creah-Kirk T, et al: Racial and ethnic differences in outcome in zidovudine-treated patients with advanced HIV disease. JAMA 266:2713–2718, 1991

50. Ellerbrock TV, Bush TJ, Chamberland ME, et al: Epidemiology of women with AIDS in the United States, 1981 through 1990. JAMA 265:2971–2975, 1991

51. Ellerbrock T, Wright TC, Chiasson MA, et al: Strong independent association between HIV infection and cervical intraepithelial neoplasia (CIN) (Abstract WS-B07-5). International AIDS Conference, Berlin, Germany, 1993

52. Farizo KM, Buehler JW, Chamberland ME, et al: Spectrum of diseases in persons with human immunodeficiency virus infection in the United States. JAMA 267:1798–1805, 1992

53. Feingold PR, Vermund SH, Burk RA, et al: Cervical cytologic abnormalities and papillomavirus in women infected with human immunodeficiency virus. J Acquir Immune Defic Syndr 3:896–903, 1990

54. Fishl MA, Richman DD, Grieco MH, et al: The efficacy of azidothymidine (AZT) in the treatment of patients with AIDS and AIDS-related complex: A double-blind, placebo controlled trial. N Engl J Med 317:185–191, 1987

55. Franco EL: Human papillomavirus and the natural history of cervical cancer. Infect Med 57–63, 1993

56. Frieden TR, Sterling T, Pablos-Mendez A, et al: The emergence of drug-resistant tuberculosis in New York City. N Engl J Med 328:521–526, 1993

57. Fullilove RE, Fullilove MT, Bowser BP, et al: Risk of sexually transmitted disease among black adolescent crack users in Oakland and San Francisco, California. JAMA 263:851–855, 1990

58. Gail MH, Pluda JM, Rabkin CS, et al: Projections of the incidence of non-Hodgkin's lymphoma related to acquired immunodeficiency syndrome. J Natl Cancer Inst 3:695–701, 1991

59. Greenberg AE, Thomas PA, Landesman SH, et al: The spectrum of HIV-1-related disease among outpatients in New York City. AIDS 6:849–859, 1992

60. Greenblatt RM, Lukehart SA, Plummer FA, et al: Genital ulceration as a risk factor for human immunodeficiency virus infection. AIDS 2:47–50, 1988

61. Hamed KA, Winters MA, Holodniy M, et al: Detection of human immunodeficiency virus type 1 in semen: Effects of disease stage and nucleoside and nucleoside therapy. J Infect Dis 167:798–802, 1993

62. Hankins CA, Handley MA: HIV disease and AIDS in women: Current knowledge and a research agenda. J Acquir Immune Defic Syndr 5:957–971, 1992

63. Hoegsberg B, Abulafia O, Sedlis A, et al: Sexually transmitted disease and human immunodeficiency virus infection among women with pelvic

inflammatory disease. Am J Obstet Gynecol 163: 1135–1139, 1990

64. Imam W, Carpenter CJ, Mayer K, et al: Hierarchical pattern of mucosal *Candida* infections in HIV-seropositive women. Am J Med 89:142–146, 1990

65. Ioachim HL, Dorsett B, Cronin W, et al: Acquired immunodeficiency syndrome-associated lymphomas. Hum Pathol 22:659–673, 1991

66. Irwin K, Rice R, O'Sullivan M, et al: The clinical presentation and course of pelvic inflammatory disease in HIV + and HIV − women: Preliminary results of a multicenter study (Abstract WS-B07-1). International AIDS Conference, 1993

67. Jacobson MA, Gundacker H, Hughes M, et al: Zidovudine side effects as reported by black, Hispanic, and white/non-Hispanic patients with early HIV disease: Combined analysis of two multicenter placebo-controlled trials. J Acquir Immune Defic Syndr 11(1):45–52, 1995

68. Jacobus Pharmaceutical: Dapsone USP. In Physician's Desk Reference. Crandall, NJ, Medical Economic Co, 1991, p 1107

69. Kamenga M, Toure CK, Nghichi JM, et al: Human immunodeficiency virus infection in women with pelvic inflammatory disease (PID) in Abidjan, Ivory Coast, Africa (Abstract WS-B07-2). International AIDS Conference, 1992

70. Kelley KF, Smith PF, Mikl J: Review of invasive cervical cancer cases for AIDS surveillance. J Acquir Immune Defic Syndr 8:102–103, 1995

71. Kennedy, MB, Scarlett, MI, Duerr AC et al: Assessing HIV risk among women who have sex with women: Scientific and communication issues. J Am Med Wom Assoc 50:103–107, 1995

72. Korn AP, Landers DV: Gynecologic disease in women infected with the immunodeficiency virus type 1. J Acquir Immune Defic Syndr 9:361–370, 1995

73. Koup RA, Yunzhen C, Ho DD, et al: Lack of maternal viral threshold for vertical transmission of HIV (Abstract LB2). Third Conference on Retroviruses and Opportunistic Infections, Washington, DC, 1996, p 161

74. Kreiss J, Hopkins S: The association between circumcision and human immunodeficiency virus infection among homosexual men. J Infect Dis 168:1404–1408, 1993

75. Kreiss J, Ngugi E, Holmes K, et al: Efficacy of nonoxynol-9 contraceptive sponge use in preventing heterosexual acquisition of HIV in Nairobi prostitutes. JAMA 268:477–482, 1992

76. Krieger JN, Coombs RW, Collier AC, et al: Fertility parameters in men infected with human immunodeficiency virus. J Infect Dis 164:464–464, 1991

77. Korvick JA, Statton P, Spino K, et al: Women's participation in AIDS Clinical Trials Group (ACTG) trials in the USA—enough or still too few? (Abstract PO-B44-2555). Ninth International Conference on AIDS, Berlin, Germany, July 1993

78. Lagakos S, Fishl MA, Stein DS, et al: Effects of zidovudine therapy in minority and other subpopulations with early HIV infection. JAMA 266:2709–2712, 1991

79. Lalezari J, Jaffe HS, Schacker T, et al: A randomized double blind placebo controlled study of Cidofovir topical gel for acyclovir resistant herpes simplex virus infections in patients with AIDS (Abstract 174). Third Conference on Retroviruses and

Opportunistic Infections, Washington, DC, 1996, p 85

80. Landesman S, Minkoff H, Holman S, et al: Serosurvey of human immunodeficiency virus infection in parturients. JAMA 258:2701–2703, 1987

81. Lassoued K, Clauvel J, Fegueux S, et al: AIDS-associated Kaposi's sarcoma in female patients. AIDS 5:877–880, 1991

82. Laurence J: Severe manifestations of common disorders in women. AIDS Reader 147–159, 1991

83. Lungu O, Sun XW, Felix J, et al: Relationship of human papillomavirus type to grade of cervical intraepithelial dysplasia. JAMA 267:2493–2496, 1992

84. Lurie N, Slater J, McGovern P, et al: Preventative care for women: Does the sex of the physician matter? N Engl J Med 329:478–482, 1993

85. Macasaet MA, Duerr A, Thelmo W, et al: Kaposi sarcoma presenting as a vulvar mass. Obstet Gynecol 86:695–697, 1995

86. Maiman M, Fruchter RG, Segur E, et al: Human immunodeficiency virus and cervical neoplasia. Obstet Gynecol 38:377–382, 1991

87. Maiman M, Tarricons N, Viera J, Suarez J: Colposcopic evaluation of human immunodeficiency virus-seropositive women. Obstet Gynecol 78:84–88, 1991

88. Marmor M, Weiss L, Lynden M, et al: Possible female-to-female transmission of human immunodeficiency virus. Ann Intern Med 105:969, 1986

89. Melbye M, Cote T, Biggar RJ, et al: High incidence of anal cancer among AIDS patients (Abstract PO-B14-1636). International AIDS Conference, Berlin, Germany, 1993

90. Melnick SL, Wertheimer WJ, Pinn VW: Survival and disease progression according to gender of patients with HIV infection. JAMA 272:1915–1921, 1994

91. Merkatz RB, Temple R, Sobel S, et al: Women in clinical trials of new drugs—a change in Food and Drug Administration policy. N Engl J Med 329:292–296, 1993

92. Michaels D, Levine C: Estimates of the number of motherless youth orphaned by AIDS in the United States. JAMA 268:3456–3461, 1992

93. Minkoff HL, DeHovitz JA: Care of women infected with the human immunodeficiency virus. JAMA 66:2253–2258, 1991

94. Minkoff HL, Moreno J: Drug prophylaxis for human immunodeficiency virus-infected pregnant women: Ethical considerations. Am J Obstet Gynecol 163:1111–1113, 1990

95. Minkoff HL, Willoughby A, Mendez H, et al: Serious infections during pregnancy among women with advanced immunodeficiency virus infection. Am J Obstet Gynecol 162:30–34, 1990

96. Moss GB, Clemetson D, D'Costa L, et al: Association of cervical ectopy with heterosexual transmission of human immunodeficiency virus: Results of a study of couples in Nairobi, Kenya. J Infect Dis 64:588–591, 1991

97. Msellati P, Leroy V, Lepage P, et al: Natural history of HIV-1 infection in African women: A prospective cohort study in Kigali (Rwanda) 1988–1991 (Abstract 10.35). Seventh International AIDS Conference, Amsterdam, The Netherlands, 1992

98. National Institute of Allergy and Infectious Disease: Clinical alert—important therapeutic information on the benefit of zidovudine for the preven-

tion of the transmission of HIV from mother to infant. Feb 22, 1994

99. Nelson KE, Vlahov D, Cohn S, et al: Sexually transmitted diseases in a population of intravenous drug users: Association with seropositivity to the human immunodeficiency virus. J Infect Dis 164:157–163, 1991

100. Ness RB, Kelly JV, Killian CD: House staff recruitment to municipal and voluntary New York City residency programs during the AIDS epidemic. JAMA 266:2843–2846, 1991

101. 1993 Sexually transmitted diseases treatment guidelines. MMWR 42:88–91, 1993

102. Niruthisard S, Roddy RE, Chutivongse S: The effects of frequent nonoxynol-9 use on the vaginal and cervical mucosa. Sex Transm Dis 18:176–179, 1991

103. Niruthisard S, Roddy RE, Chutivongse S: Use of nonoxynol-9 and reduction in rate of gonococcal and chlamydial cervical infections. Lancet 339: 1371–1374, 1992

104. Padian NS: Epidemiology of AIDS and heterosexually transmitted HIV in women. AIDS File 5:1–2, 1991

105. Padian NS, Marquis L, Francis DP, et al: Male to female transmission of human immunodeficiency virus. JAMA 258:788–790, 1987

106. Padian NS, Shiboski SC, Jewell NP: Female to male transmission of human immunodeficiency virus. JAMA 266:1664–1667, 1991

107. Palefsky J: Human papillomavirus infection among HIV-infected individuals. Hematol Oncol Clin North Am 5:357–370, 1991

108. Palefsky J, Holly EA, Ahn DK: Progression of anal cytologic changes in men with group IV HIV disease (Abstract WS-B17-6). International AIDS Conference, Berlin, Germany, 1993

109. Palefsky JM, Shiboski S, Moss A: Risk factors for anal human papillomavirus infection and cytologic abnormalities in HIV positive and HIV negative men. J Acquir Immune Defic Syndr 7:599–606, 1994

110. Petersen LR, Doll L, White C, et al: No evidence for female-to-female HIV transmission among 960,000 female blood donors. J Acquir Immune Defic Syndr 5:853–855, 1992

111. Phillips DM: Microbicide development: Progress and obstacles (Abstract S47). Third Conference on Retroviruses and Opportunistic Infections, Washington, DC, 1996, p 180

112. Plummer FA, Simones JN, Cameron DW, et al: Cofactors in male-female sexual transmission of human immunodeficiency virus type 1. J Infect Dis 163: 233–239, 1991

113. Reef SE, Levine WC, McNeil MM, et al: Treatment options for vulvovaginal candidiasis, 1993. CID 20(Suppl 1):S80–90, 1995

114. Rhoads JL, Wright C, Redfield RR, et al: Chronic vaginal candidiasis in women with human immunodeficiency virus infection. JAMA 257: 3105–3107, 1987

115. Rich JD, Buck AM, Tuomala RE, et al: Transmission of human immunodeficiency virus infection presumed to have occurred via female homosexual contact. Clin Infect Dis 17:1003–1005, 1993

116. Roddy RE, Cordero M, Cordero C, et al: A dosing study of nonoxynol-9 and genital irritation. Int J STD AIDS 4:165–170, 1993

117. Sacks H, Szabo S, Miller LH, et al: Gender differences in the natural history of HIV infection (Abstract

118. Safrin S, Assaykeen T, Follansbee S, et al: Foscarnet therapy for acyclovir-resistant mucocutaneous herpes simplex virus infection in 26 AIDS patients: Preliminary data. J Infect Dis 161:1078–1084, 1990

119. Safrin S, Dattel BJ, Haver L, et al: Seroprevalence and epidemiologic correlates of infection in women with acute pelvic inflammatory disease. Obstet Gynecol 75:666–670, 1990

120. San Francisco Department of Public Health AIDS Office Surveillance Branch, et al: Executive summary: Survey of 498 lesbians and bisexual women, 1993

121. Sande MA, Carpenter CJ, Cobbs CG, et al: Antiretroviral therapy for adult HIV-infected patients: Recommendations from a state of the art conference. JAMA 270:2583–2589, 1993

122. Schuman P, Christianen C, Sobel JD: Apthous genital ulceration in three women with AIDS (Abstract 429). Third Conference on Retroviruses and Opportunistic Infections, Washington, DC, 1996, p 133

123. Shaffer N, Chotpitayasunondh T, Roongpisuthipong A, et al: High maternal viral load predicts perinatal HIV-1 transmission and early infant progression (Abstract 38). Third Conference on Retroviruses and Opportunistic Infections, Washington, DC, 1996, p 58

124. Shah PN, Smith JR, Wells C, et al: Menstrual symptoms in women infected by the human immunodeficiency virus. Obstet Gynecol 83:397–400, 1994

125. Shelton M, Adams J, Gugino L, et al: Menstrual cycle hormone patterns in HIV-infected women (Abstract 432). Third Conference on Retroviruses and Opportunistic Infections, Washington, DC, 1996, p 134

126. Sherer R, Melnick S, Hillman D, et al: Gender, HIV-related clinical events and mortality: Preliminary observational data from the Community Programs for Clinical Research on AIDS (CPCRA) (Abstract 09.55). Seventh International AIDS Conference, Amsterdam, The Netherlands, 1992

127. Sperling RS, Stratton P, OB/GYN Working Group ACTG: Treatment options for human immunodeficiency virus-infected pregnant women. Obstet Gynecol 79:443–448, 1992

128. Sperling RS, Stratton P, O'Sullivan MJ, et al: A survey of zidovudine use in pregnant women with human immunodeficiency virus infection. N Engl J Med 326:857–861, 1992

129. Sperling RS, Shapiro DE, Coombs R, et al: Maternal plasma HIV-1 RNA in the success of zidovudine (ZDV) in the prevention of mother-child transmission (Abstract LB1). Third Conference on Retroviruses and Opportunistic Infections, Washington, DC, 1996, p 161

130. Spinillo A, Michelone G, Cvanna C, et al: Clinical and microbiological characteristics of symptomatic vulvovaginal candidiasis in HIV-seropositive women. Genitourin Med 70:268–272, 1994

131. Spinillo A, Capuzzo E, Egbe TO, et al: *Torulopsis glabrata* vaginitis. Obstet Gynecol 85:993–998, 1995

132. St. Louis ME, Munkolenkole K, Brown C, et al: Risk for perinatal transmission according to maternal immunologic, virologic and placental factors. JAMA 269:2853–2859, 1993

133. Stein MD, Liebman BD, Wachtel TJ, et al: HIV-posi-

tive women: Reasons they are tested for HIV and their clinical characteristics on entry into the health care system. J Gen Intern Med 6:286–289, 1991

134. Stephens PC, Zheng ZT, Flannery HT, et al: Incident AIDS and cervical cancer in Connecticut women: An ecological examination of time trends and age period cohort effects (Abstract WS-B17-1). International AIDS Conference, 1993

135. Stone KM, Peterson HB: Spermicides, HIV, and the vaginal sponge (Editorial). JAMA 268:521–523, 1992

136. Stratton P, Guupta P, Kalish L, et al: Immune status, STD's and cervical dysplasia on Pap smear in HIV+ pregnant and nonpregnant women in the Women and Infants Transmission Study (WITS) (Abstract 426). Third Conference on Retroviruses and Opportunistic Infections, Washington, DC, 1996, p 133

137. Sun XW, Ellerbrook TV, Lunglu O, et al: Human papillomavirus infection in human immunodeficiency virus-seropositive women. Obstet Gynecol 85:680–686, 1995

138. Tobin MJ: Vulvovaginal candidiasis: Topical vs. oral therapy. Am Fam Physician 51:1715–1720, 1995

139. Turner BJ, Markson LE, McKee LJ, et al: Health care delivery, zidovudine use, and the survival of women and men with AIDS. J Acquir Immune Defic Syndr 7:1250–1262, 1994

140. U.S. Department of Health and Human Services, Agency for Health Care Policy and Research, Evaluation and Management of Early HIV Infection, Clinical Practice Guideline number 7, January 1994

141. Volberding PA, Lagakos SW, Koch MA, et al: Zidovudine in asymptomatic human immunodeficiency virus infections: A controlled trial in persons with fewer than 500 CD-positive cells per cubic millimeter. N Engl J Med 322:941–949, 1990

142. Warne PA, Ehrhardt A, Schochter D, et al: Menstrual abnormalities in HIV + and HIV − women with a history of intravenous drug use (Abstract M.C. 3113). Seventh International AIDS Conference, Florence, Italy, 1991

143. Weiss RA: Perspectives on HHV8 and Kaposi's sarcoma. Third Conference on Retroviruses and Opportunistic Infections, Washington, DC, 1996

144. Whitby D, Howard MR, Tenant-Flowers M, et al: Detection of Kaposi's sarcoma-associated herpesvirus in peripheral blood of HIV-infected individuals and progression to Kaposi's sarcoma. Lancet 346: 799–802, 1995

145. Wilcox CM, Schwartz DA, Clark WS: Esophageal ulceration in human immunodeficiency virus infection. Ann Intern Med 122:143–149, 1995

146. Wilfert CM: Mandatory screening of pregnant women for the human immunodeficiency virus. Clin Infect Dis 19:664–666, 1994

147. Williams A, Darragh T, Osmond D, et al: Anal/cervical HPV infection and risk of anal/cervical dysplasia associated with HPV-1 (Abstract WS-B17-5). International AIDS Conference, Berlin, Germany, 1993

148. Witt DJ, Craven DE, McCable WR: Bacterial infections in adult patients with the acquired immunodeficiency syndrome (AIDS) and AIDS-related complex. Am J Med 82:900–906, 1987

149. Working Group on HIV Testing of Pregnant Women and Newborns: HIV infection, pregnant women, and newborns. JAMA 264:2416–2420, 1990

150. World Health Organization: Press release, Sept 7, 1993

151. Wright TC, Sun X, Ellerbrock T, et al: Human papillomavirus infection in HIV (+) and HIV (−) women: Prevalence, association with cervical intraepithelial neoplasia, and impact of CD4(+) count (Abstract WS-B17-2). International AIDS Conference, Berlin, Germany, 1993

152. Wright TC, Ellerbrook TV, Chiasson MA, et al: Cervical intraepithelial neoplasia in women infected with human immunodeficiency virus: Prevalence, risk factors, and validity of Papanicolaou smears. Obstet Gynecol 84:591–597, 1994

Chapter 33

HIV Nursing Care

DIANE JONES and J.B. MOLAGHAN

It would be impossible to provide a comprehensive presentation of nursing care for people with human immunodeficiency virus (HIV) disease within the confines of this chapter. There are many excellent resources with specific detailed information on specialized nursing care (see references). We have chosen to present an overview of general nursing issues that may be applicable in a variety of clinical settings.

THE RANGE AND SCOPE OF NURSING PRACTICE

Since the beginning of the acquired immunodeficiency syndrome (AIDS) epidemic, nurses have been at the forefront in the development and implementation of effective systems for delivery of care. Many of the caregiving systems and units that have evolved to meet the needs of people with AIDS were created by nurses and to this day are nurse-driven. The hospital-based nursing model has been refined and expanded to meet the unprecedented demands that the complexity of this disease has dictated. A multidisciplinary model is required to successfully integrate the efforts of AIDS care delivery to patients throughout the entire spectrum of the disease process. With the advent of health care reform and increasing prevalence of managed care health plans, the focus of care is shifting increasingly from inpatient acute care to outpatient and home-based settings. Hence, the acuity of illness is increasing in all settings, making new demands on people with HIV and their caregivers.

Acute Care

Although an HIV-dedicated inpatient unit may be ideal in large urban areas, smaller community settings may find this impractical. Clinical nurses working on a medical unit involved in the care of AIDS patients should have a solid foundation in medical nursing. It is impossible to expect nurses to become immediate experts in the knowledge of all the HIV-related opportunistic infections and malignancies, but a fundamental knowledge of the chronic progression of the HIV disease spectrum is essential. Nurse managers must plan staffing patterns to facilitate a consistent program of continuing HIV education. A clinical nurse specialist in HIV disease can enhance patient care as an on-site educator and hospitalwide consultant.

Nurse practitioners educated in either adult or family medicine can be used efficiently to provide ongoing primary care to people with HIV disease in both private office and clinical settings. Development of standardized disease process protocols by the physician and nurse practitioner is essential to ensure that patients receive quality care. In many states, nurse practitioners may prescribe medicines under these protocols.

Home care nurses have revolutionized the health care system with development of new standards of care, which include home infusion of parenteral medications. Home hospice models have been created to allow patients to die in comfort and with the support of their loved ones. With a nursing case management mode, the visiting nurse is responsible for coordinating all the services in the home, in addition to monitoring the client's status and conferring with the physician when changes are needed in the treatment plan.[33]

Ambulatory Care

Acute nursing experience in an ambulatory setting is essential, in that "health care reform" and managed care plans tend to decertify patient hospitalization days. Frequently, patients are discharged from the hospital immediately after diagnosis and it is impossible to observe them for therapeutic response to treatment as well as to reinforce patient teaching. The ambulatory care nurse should have a sound background in medical surgical and oncology nursing and should be proficient in venous access. As part of a multidisciplinary team, the nurse should be able to triage the acuity of patient problems for both scheduled primary care patients and those who drop in with urgent medical or psychosocial problems. Health care delivery systems will experience an increase in the use of ambulatory infusion centers to treat patients who need blood transfusion, intravenous (IV) antibiotics, and treatment of cytomegalovirus (CMV) retinitis.

Nurses with experience in working with substance users can greatly complement the ambulatory care team. The occupational background of health care professionals and their familiarity with drug users is likely to affect their emotional responses and attitudes.[3] Many existing models of health care will have to be modified to accommodate the unique challenges created by this frequently discriminated-against community.

Multiple treatment strategies are being explored to treat HIV disease and the associated infections and malignancies. Research nurses can mobilize their effort most efficiently by coordinating and implementing the clinical trials undertaken by principal investigators. Research nurses are invaluable not only as clinicians specializing in the gathering of data and the recruitment of clients but also as patient advocates who can guide the client through a frequently stressful experience. Research nurses should be familiar with the HIV disease process to ensure efficient monitoring of entry criteria for clinical trials.

CLINICAL MANAGEMENT AND NURSING PRACTICE

Neurologic Nursing

Neurologic complications of HIV disease are common, with pathologic changes seen in the nervous system of up to 80% of autopsied AIDS patients. Clinically, about one half to two thirds of HIV-1–seropositive patients will have significant neurologic signs or symptoms in the course of their disease.[25] Chapter 14 provides a comprehensive review of these afflictions. Nurses are likely to observe acute and chronic cognitive, behavioral, and motor changes in their patients. The insidious onset of mild behavioral changes and blunted affect may be seen in patients with HIV-related subacute encephalitis or early AIDS dementia complex (ADC). This mental deterioration may become progressive, so it is imperative that patients and family make important decisions early in the disease spectrum (e.g., durable power of attorney).

Helping patients maintain dignity and self-respect as ADC progresses is of the utmost importance. A structured environment in both acute and chronic care settings allows the patient to feel more in control. Patients may experience short-term memory loss and poor concentration. Routines should be consistent, and efforts should be made to minimize giving the patient multiple commands at any given time. Side effects of medications that can exacerbate symptoms of mental confusion should be monitored. The use of drugs with strong anticholinergic side effects, such as amitriptyline (Elavil), should be minimized.[6]

Patients with infectious or neoplastic neurologic disorders, such as central nervous system (CNS) toxoplasmosis (Chapter 24), cryptococcal meningitis (Chapter 23), and CNS lymphoma (Chapter 28), usually experience more acute neurologic changes.

Nurses should be alert to abrupt changes in mental status or motor ability. The onset of seizures, severe headaches, high fevers, vomiting, or acute visual changes should be reported to the primary care provider immediately. Appropriate monitoring of response to pharmacologic agents ordered for treatment of neurologic disorders should reflect improved neurologic function. Pharmacologic toxicities need to be monitored when such drugs as amphotericin B are used for treatment of cryptomeningitis or potentially myelosuppressive drugs are used to treat CNS lymphoma.

Many different types of peripheral neuropathies have been associated with HIV infection. The most frequent neuropathy syndrome is a distal symmetric polyneuropathy (DSPN) that causes predominantly sensory disturbances.[50] Symptoms can vary from numbness and tingling in the fingers and toes to severe burning pain. Physical mobility may be impaired. Assistive devices should be provided, with proper instruction in their use, and referrals should be made for physical therapy. Potential exacerbation of symptoms of neuropathy should be monitored. There is an increased risk of developing peripheral neuropathy when didanosine (ddI or Videx) and other neurotoxic drugs are used concurrently, or if a patient has a history of peripheral neuropathy.[40] Other potentially neurotoxic drugs frequently used in caring for patients with HIV disease include zalcitibine (ddC or HIVID), stavudine (d4T or Zerit), lamivudine (3TC or Epivir) and vincristine (Oncovin).

Since the majority of patients with HIV disease will develop neurologic complications, nurses must be supportive of the dramatic changes these patients will undergo and the effect this will have on loved ones. Nurses must be prepared to offer support when family members and partners vent their frustrations and express their grief and despair in having to witness dramatic physical and mental deterioration taking place in these patients.

Cardiovascular HIV Nursing

Clinically significant cardiac problems in AIDS patients are unusual, although cardiac abnormalities are not uncommon.[9] Specific cardiovascular disorders are covered in detail in Chapter 17. Nurses must be aware of both acute and chronic cardiovascular changes and the relationship to the underlying disease processes. Subjective complaints of acute chest pain or shortness of breath should be reported immediately. In patients with cardiomyopathy, pulmonary vascular compromise from severe or recurrent infection or interstitial lung disease gives rise to pulmonary hypertension in resulting failure of the right side of the heart.[40] Monitoring of vital signs is the single most important assessment tool. Patients who are found to have orthostatic changes in pulse and blood pressure may be exhibiting signs of hypovolemic or hemodynamic shock; patients with tachycardia, hypotension, and fever may be septic. Patients with positional orthostasis may be dehydrated. Patients with chronic orthostasis, despite intervention with fluid replacement, may be exhibiting signs of adrenal insufficiency. Prompt reporting of these changes to the primary health care provider will result in immediate corrective medical intervention and, when possible, treatment of the underlying causative disorder.

Care should be taken to monitor and report appropriate laboratory findings that may contribute to a cardiovascular abnormality. Specific changes in hemoglobin and hematocrit or abnormal serum electrolytes should be reported to the attending physician immediately. Intravenous fluid and electrolyte replacement, as well as blood transfusions, should be administered as ordered.

Respiratory Nursing

Etiology

Pulmonary manifestations frequently account for disease processes seen in people with symptomatic HIV disease in the United States.[37] Advanced nursing skills in respiratory management are among the most valuable skills needed for nurses working with people with symptomatic HIV disease.[47] There are multiple etiologies contributing to lengthy differential diagnoses of pulmonary problems, and more than one respiratory process may be occurring at any given time. Although *Pneumocystis carinii* pneumonia (PCP) is the most common respiratory infections in the latter stages of HIV infection, patients also experience a variety of other infections: fungal (cryptococcosis, histoplasmosis), bacterial, viral (especially CMV), or mycobacterial (*Mycobacterium tuberculosis* and *Mycobacterium avium* complex [MAC]) infections. Neoplasms also may cause serious respiratory disease (pulmonary Kaposi's sarcoma or non-Hodgkin's lymphoma).

Assessment

Initial symptoms may be of slow or sudden onset. Fever, fatigue, and weight loss may have been present before the onset of respiratory symptoms.[19,47] Since the advent of PCP prophylaxis, symptoms of active PCP infection also may be more subtle.[19] The most common presenting symptoms for PCP include fever, nonproductive cough, and shortness of breath. Radiologic findings may reveal diffuse interstitial infiltrates.[19] Other findings include increased respiratory rate, dyspnea on exertion, and abnormal blood gases. Diagnostic workups include sputum induction, bronchoalveolar lavage, and transbronchial lung biopsies.[19] At San Francisco General Hospital (SFGH), approximately 80% of all cases of PCP are diagnosed by sputum induction (Chapter 20).

Intervention

Nurses should maintain adequate oxygenation ($Sao_2 \geq 92\%$) in patients, titrate oxygen delivery, and be alert to sudden deterioration in respiratory status (as is seen in PCP therapy around day 4 to day 6 or in case of spontaneous pneumothorax).[47] They should administer medications (usually orally [PO] or IV) with careful monitoring of adverse reactions. Trimethoprim-sulfamethoxazole (Septra) may cause nausea, vomiting, rash, fevers, neutropenia, and thrombocytopenia. Pentamidine may cause hypoglycemia, hyperglycemia, renal toxicities, and hypertension. Low-dose morphine sulfate should be used IV for management of dyspnea and anxiety related to air hunger[34] in management of both moderate to severe PCP and pulmonary KS. Patients should limit activities to decrease their oxygen requirements. Nurses should educate patients about controlled breathing techniques, oxygen use, home safety, and smoking cessation.

Tuberculosis

Nurses must play a key role in identifying persons with risk factors for tuberculosis (TB). The incidence of TB is much higher among the homeless and people living in congregate living situations (such as community-based residential facilities for people with AIDS or in prisons). Nurses must advocate for aggressive early diagnosis and treatment (including appropriate infection-control measures), since infections can be eradicated and reactivations prevented.[1] Nondiagnosed coughing patients should be put in respiratory isolation. Sputum samples should be collected on three consecutive mornings and checked for acid-fast bacilli (AFB).[32] In San Francisco, Department of Public Health policy requires patients with active TB who live in congregate living situations with other persons with HIV disease to remain in isolation until three negative AFB sputums are obtained.

Considerable support must be given for patients to be compliant with therapy.[4] TB treatment often involves multiple drugs (usually at least isoniazid, ethambutol, and rifampin) that often have side effects. Noncompliance with therapy is contributing to increased numbers of multiple-drug-resistant cases of TB.[1] At SFGH, observed therapy is part of the intensive educational effort required to support patients through this lengthy treatment. Patients are observed while taking TB medications, rather than having the medications left at the bedside to be taken later. Health care providers must be aware of the drug–drug and drug–food interactions involving TB medications for therapy to be successful. In particular, patients receiving methadone need to have their dose increased if given rifampin, since rifampin causes increased metabolism of methadone (as well as many other drugs). Failure to address this will guarantee noncompliance with medications.[21]

Intubation and Resuscitation

The severity of infection and sudden respiratory deterioration will raise the questions of intubation and the use of mechanical ventilation. Addressing the question before facing an emergent situation will help immensely. Should the patient choose to be intubated and mechanically ventilated, nurses must advocate for timely intubation and transfer to the intensive care unit before full respiratory arrest. Prognosis is improving, especially for first-time PCP patients.[19] Mechanical ventilation can be used to keep a patient alive until the arrival of family or loved ones.

Gastrointestinal Nursing

The gastrointestinal tract is a major target for HIV disease. Patients experience a broad variety of gastrointestinal problems, ranging from minor disorders of the mouth in those with less advanced HIV disease to a profound malabsorption syndrome secondary to a variety of enteric pathogens. The entire spectrum of gastrointestinal disease is covered in Chapter 13 of this text. Clinical and pathologic changes have been found in the oral cavity, esophagus, stomach, liver, small and large intestines, and rectum.[17]

Assessments and Interventions

A variety of infections may occur in the mouth and oropharynx that can alert the health care provider to changes in the integrity of the immune system. Bacterial, fungal, viral, protozoal, and neoplastic disorders can affect the entire alimentary canal. Nurses should observe for changes in the appearance of the oral mucosa. Observation of any white coating on the buccal mucosa, ulcers or vesicles on the tongue or mucous membrane, or the appearance of any dark purple discolorations on the hard palate should be reported to the physician immediately to ensure appropriate medical intervention. Prompt treatment of oral infection will reduce discomfort and ensure adequate nutritional intake by the patient. Nurses working in a general medical setting should become familiar with these oral manifestations of HIV so that they can alert the health care team to the possibility of underlying immune dysfunction in those who may be at risk but have not yet been diagnosed with HIV infection.

Painful swallowing or dysphagia may be indicative of a fungal or viral esophagitis and should be reported immediately. Patients should be encouraged to avoid acidic or irritating foods while suffering from odynophagia. However, when treating patients for *Candida* esophagitis with ketoconazole, an acidic pH is required for optimal absorption of the medication. Since many patients experiencing gastrointestinal symptoms will have to undergo diagnostic endoscopy, teaching and explanation of procedures is of vital importance.

Cramping paraumbilical abdominal pain, weight loss, and large-volume diarrhea are common in patients with HIV disease.[6] Multiple bacterial or protozoal infections may be the sources of this diarrhea, and prompt reporting of symptoms will result in a more rapid diagnosis. Patient education about infection control is of paramount importance, as many of the enteric pathogens are very contagious. *Cryptosporidium*, for which there is no effective treatment, can be transmitted through sexual contact (oral–anal) and can also be found in the drinking water of some communities. Since the 1993 outbreak of cryptospordiosis in Milwaukee sickened 403,000 people and killed more than 100, the water-borne transmission of *Cryptosporidium* has gained increasing attention.[23] Management of symptoms of diarrhea can be a major nursing challenge. Eliminating the source of infection with medical treatment (i.e., antibiotics for shigellosis) may arrest the cause, but there is no effective treatment for such infections as cryptosporidiosis. Imodium or Lomotil may be used for treatment of diarrhea, but sometimes the condition may not improve unless tincture of opium is administered. Antidiarrheal medications are more effective when given around the clock rather than on an as-needed basis.

Constant assessment of hydration status and orthostatic blood pressure is imperative. Severe wasting may accompany the profound malabsorption syndrome. HIV-related weight loss is one of the most common manifestations of advanced HIV infection, ultimately affecting the majority of patients. The degree of involuntary weight loss in patients with AIDS has been shown to correlate with the likelihood of hospitalization and survival.[46] The use of total parenteral nutrition (TPN) as supportive treatment is controversial, since there have been no controlled studies and few anecdotal reports showing sustained weight gain.[15] Nutritional consultation referral is indicated so that dietary habits may be assessed and supplemental nutrition may be initiated. Patients need tremendous emotional support because of the dramatic physical deterioration and loss of dignity inherent in lifestyle changes, such as having to wear diapers. Loss of control of bodily functions increases the burden of adjustment to this disease.

Acute gastrointestinal bleeding is an uncommon but important manifestation of HIV disease. Symptoms of acute abdominal pain, coffee-ground emesis, and black tarry stools are signs of gastrointestinal hemorrhage and should be reported immediately.

CMV Retinitis

Ophthalmologic consultations are an important part of providing health care to people with AIDS. CMV retinitis is a late-stage manifestation that occurs in about 25% of persons with AIDS (generally with CD4 counts <50/mm^3).[13] Untreated, the patient may become blind (Chapter 26).

CMV retinitis can be asymptomatic. Patients becoming symptomatic will report painless visual loss (from loss of a portion of the visual field to blurred vision), flashes of light, floaters (either unilateral or bilateral), redness, or pain.[42]

Treatment is undergoing profound changes. The standard therapies of 2 weeks' induction followed by lifelong maintenance therapy of IV ganciclovir and/or foscarnet are in some cases being substituted with retinal implants and oral therapies as indicated. Side effects and toxicities differ. The use of ganciclovir often requires discontinuing zidovudine or modifying trimethoprim-sufamethoxazole therapy because of a risk of bone marrow suppression. The renal toxicity potential of foscarnet requires careful monitoring and IV hydrations before or concomitant with treatment. Ongoing monitoring must take place to detect disease progression despite therapy.[42]

Most health care financing systems have determined that CMV treatment (including induction and maintenance) must be provided as outpatient therapy. Both ganciclovir and foscarnet require central venous access devices and teaching the patient or caregiver to maintain the line and administer drug.

Gynecologic Manifestations

Management of HIV disease in women poses many challenges to nurses: inadequate and insufficient research, perception of women as disease vectors rather than persons at risk in their own right, and women's tendency to focus on their children and partners rather than on themselves.[27,30] Since 70% of women with AIDS in the United States are women of color, the confluence of racism, sexism, poverty, and drug addiction demands informed, skilled, and highly sensitive nursing practice.[30]

Many women find out about their (and their sexual partner's) HIV infection during pregnancy or following an AIDS diagnosis of their newborn children.[27,49] Nurses working in family planning, drug clinics, or sexually transmitted disease (STD) clinics play an important role in helping assess women's risk of HIV infection and educating about HIV prevention.[49]

Although women are thought to have clinical manifestations of HIV disease similar to those in men, they also experience gynecologic symptoms that are severe, recurring, and debilitating. These include menstrual irregularities, vaginal infections (candidiasis, herpes), cervical dysplasia (cervical neoplasia associated with human papilloma virus [HPV], infection), pelvic inflammatory disease (PID), genital ulcers, and other STDs.[48] Nurses need to advocate for thorough gynecologic workups and challenge the common practice of deferring gynecologic and rectal examinations during routine physical examinations. A detailed gynecologic history, including sexual, contraceptive, pregnancy, and childbirth histories, should be included. Pap smears are recommended every 6 months, with more accurate diagnostics done with colposcopy whenever possible.[48]

Since the highest prevalence of HIV infection in women occurs during childbearing years, intensive counseling and education about contraception, STDs, and pregnancy options are essential components of quality care for HIV-infected women.[49] Nurses must support women with accurate information and a nonjudgmental approach through the difficult decision-making process surrounding pregnancy.[27] The field of genetic counseling has much to offer by way of a framework that evaluates relative risk in pregnancy decision making and can be useful in training and assisting health care workers to clarify their own values regarding the reproductive rights of their patients and the impact these values and beliefs have on their relationship with their patients.

PAIN MANAGEMENT

Pain management is an area of clinical practice in which nurses can exercise the full weight of their advocacy and clinical skills. Recent studies describing the prevalence of pain in advanced HIV disease reported that between 52% and 97% of patients with HIV disease registered complaints of non–procedure-related pain.[20,26] Differentiating between acute and chronic pain, the pain associated with drug withdrawal, and HIV-related pain and appreciating each patient's unique experience and expressions of pain are essential to planning effective interventions.

Pain is always subjective. Communication between caregivers and their patients is key to assessment and effective intervention.[29] The response of health care providers to complaints of pain will determine the degree of trust that patients will have and their willingness to participate fully in their own care.

Given the high proportion of persons with AIDS who also suffer from chemical dependency, a knowledge of management of withdrawal and detoxification is essential to being able to provide effective pain management. Sensitivity is needed to the concerns of patients in recovery from prior drug use who fear relapse with prescribed analgesics. Patients with chronic pain and those with a history of chemical dependency benefit greatly from having a single provider in charge of their pain management.[29]

Studies have reported that excluding procedure-related pain, abdominal and neuropathic pain are the most frequent types for both drug users and nondrug users with HIV disease.[26] Etiologies for abdominal pain include nonspecific gastritis, lymphoma, gastrointestinal Kaposi's sarcoma, cryptosporidiosis, MAC, and pancreatitis. Neuropathic pain may be due to HIV infection itself or may be a serious side effect of such medications as the newer antiretroviral nucleosides (ddI, ddC, 3TC), vincalkaloids used in the treatment of Kaposi's sarcoma, or isoniazid used in tuberculosis. Drugs that may cause neuropathy need to be reevaluated if patients are experiencing these symptoms.[44]

Other pain syndromes reported in persons with HIV disease include esophagitis; headaches due to meningitis, toxoplasmosis, or CNS lymphoma; skin pain due to cutaneous Kaposi's sarcoma; back, bone, and joint pain; and post-herpetic pain.[26]

The consistent use of a pain assessment tool to determine location, intensity, quality, causes, and contributing factors is essential to track progression and effectiveness of pain control techniques.[47] Keep in mind that other factors will influence a patient's pain threshold, such as insomnia, nausea, anxiety, anger, shame, depression, and fear. Listening to a patient's choice of words to describe symptoms will give clues as to the etiology and, thus, to the interventions. Patients with neuropathic pain often will use words like "tingling," "burning," or "numbness." In one study, 50% of patients with neuropathic pain also experienced other types of pain (either abdominal pain or headaches). Abdominal pain is often described as "sharp" or "crampy," and is usually intermittent.[5,26]

Using the World Health Organization's three-step analgesic ladder provides the framework for progressing from nonopioid analgesics to stronger opioids, with the use of adjuvant drugs at each step. Interventions must be highly individualized. Chronic pain is best dealt with by maintaining routine, around-the-clock scheduling rather than on an as-needed (PRN) basis.[5,20,29] There is no excuse for uncontrolled procedural pain. Effective premedication is essential to give patients the courage to follow through on diagnostic workups and treatments. At San Francisco General Hospital, we have developed a protocol for preprocedural analgesia that involves giving fentanyl 50 to 100 μg flow intravenous push (IVP) every 5 to 10 minutes (up to a maximum of 300 to 500 μg without additional order) prior to and during painful procedures (including chest tube insertion and manipulation, bone marrow biopsy, wound packing and débridement, pleurodesis).

When working with patients who have a history of drug use, nurses should assume that the patient's report of pain is true. They should obtain an accurate assessment and document the patient's drug use history, type, amount, frequency, route, and when last use occurred, and prevent heroin withdrawal with methadone and alcohol withdrawal with benzodiazepines.[29] Patients with drug use histories often have a lower threshold for pain[39]; therefore, providing adequate premedication for painful procedures will assist the patient in tolerating and completing the procedure.

The first sign of tolerance is shorter duration of effect. The nurse should compensate with higher doses rather than more frequent administration. Routine administration rather than PRN helps diminish the need for negotiations and renegotiations. The patient should be informed that the treatment goals are to relieve pain and provide comfort, not to get him or her high. Oral pain medications should be used as much as possible to decrease drug craving that might occur with the sight of needles and mimicking of the drug high experience.[29]

In the event of a sudden onset of cognitive deficit, nurses should proceed judiciously when evaluating a possible pharmacologic-related etiology.[5,29] End-organ disease (renal or liver abnormal function) should be evaluated as contributing to an enhanced drug effect. If stopping pain medications is absolutely necessary for the purpose of evaluation, nurses should proceed quickly to obtain a differential diagnosis. Naloxone should be avoided; severe pain will not be manageable until its effects wear off.[28,29] Holding doses may be more humane.

PSYCHOSOCIAL CONSIDERATIONS

How nurses approach the challenging psychosocial issues facing persons with AIDS will often be key to both patient satisfaction and the ability of patients to follow through with the many treatment demands during the course of the illness. To be effective, nurses must understand the sociopolitical ramifications of their patients disease. In particular, one needs to recognize that an AIDS diagnosis forces identification with stigmatized minority groups of society.[16] This means that patients often enter the health care system with long histories of rejection.[24] Acknowledging that there has been little healthy and rational discussion in society about what AIDS represents—a sexually transmitted, communicable, drug-use-related, and fatal disease—goes a long way in establishing a caring and trusting relationship between nurses and patients. Nurses can acknowledge patients as sexual beings who most people are now afraid to even touch. They can be willing to have an honest dialogue with their patients about death. It is essential, and few people will have both the courage and the skills needed to address this.

Because many people with AIDS have nontraditional family configurations, effective care must include a patient-centered definition of who the patient considers his or her family and who will be involved in the care.[12] This might mean changing hospital visiting policies to allow patients to have access to whomever they consider their significant others. Staff can be given adequate training about sexual orientation and drug use. This is essential in creating a foundation of respect and understanding for patients.

Interventions will differ at the various points along the illness spectrum, from initial diagnosis, first-time opportunistic infection, to recurrence and relapse, and terminal illness. Nurses must be alert to the psychologic impact of a disease characterized by uncertainty.[16] Psychologic interventions include assessment for risk of suicide, advocating for psychiatric evaluation, pharmacologic interventions for depression, and referrals for support groups and individual counseling.

The care of active drug users requires the development of new models and strategies, as we have failed in our efforts at AIDS prevention and care in this at-risk population.[38] The traditional chemical dependency approach has made abstinence from drugs the only goal of treatment and prevention efforts. However, the insufficient number of drug treatment programs combined with their meager success rates challenge us to find intermediate goals that will allow for both HIV transmission prevention and improved quality of care for drug users.[35,38]

Harm-reduction strategies are being used by more and more community-based programs and medical institutions. The driving principle is that continued drug use does not preclude access to quality medical care. Examples of harm-reduction techniques include: needle exchange, HIV testing, community support systems (food, housing, urgent medical care), methadone and other drug treatment programs, and teaching safer injection techniques and sexual practices.[35]

COMANAGEMENT

This second decade of HIV/AIDS has produced a multitude of new treatment options, but has also presented extreme challenges in caring for increasing numbers of patients with special social problems. Both inpatient settings and ambulatory care clinics experience increased numbers of clients with dual and triple diagnoses and many clients who "don't follow the rules." A multidisciplinary approach for working with patients who are challenged by

the system is being implemented at San Francisco General Hospital under a program of comanagement. Many patients with HIV/AIDS experience multiple impediments to care when overwhelmed by social problems such as substance abuse, homelessness, violence, and sick children and/or a partner. Many have had past negative experiences with the health care system. Patients who have special needs can be identified by any member of the health care team. Candidates who qualify for comanagement include those with a disorganized social situation, patients who frequently miss appointments or who use the clinic frequently, and those with multiple medical and/or social problems. The comanagement team can be composed of a nurse, social worker, physician, nurse practitioner, physician assistant, receptionist, etc. The point person on the team is the person with the best rapport with the patient. "Problems" that prompted the need for team management are identified and clearly spelled out. Team members identify attainable goals and establish a plan with the patient. The patient should be comfortable and have rapport with all team members. This ensures consistency in "issue management" and comforts the patient with a sense of ongoing familiarity with her/his case. Staff can be insulated from "burning out" with a patient by simply asking another team member to intervene with a problem. Documentation on established comanagement forms is essential. The climate of comanagement should be one of compassion and concern that is not contingent upon a person being clean and sober or a model patient. The goal is to improve access and help patients attain the level of engagement in their care of which they are capable. Good medical and nursing care can happen only when there is an air of trust, dignity, and respect. Eye contact and physical touch are imperative. Use of language that is clear and understandable will enhance the therapeutic relationship. Information must be gathered in a nonjudgmental way, by avoiding labels such as "difficult," "noncompliant," or "drug-seeking." These terms generate hostile and negative interactions. For patients with drug abuse problems, effective development of a contract (written) can create a partnership between the patient and medical provider to create a plan regarding pain control, insomnia, and anxiety. Effective comanagement can assure patients and staff that challenges in care can be a shared responsibility.

SOCIAL AND ENVIRONMENTAL CONSIDERATIONS

AIDS has as much impact on a person's financial economic status as it has on the immune system; bank balances often fall as precipitously as CD4 cell counts. A careful assessment of a patient's social network and reevaluation at various stages of illness is essential. During the course of the illness, the patient will require progressively greater amounts of care. Often, the care requirements will demand major adjustments in the living situation based on the availability of support in the home. Nurses will need to provide constant and ongoing assessment of a patient's functional status, as well as the ability to follow through on a plan of care that might include administration of complex IV medications in the home setting.

Many AIDS service agencies require abstinence from drugs as a prerequisite for accessing services. Given the difficulty that most patients will have in achieving abstinence, health care providers will need to advocate on behalf of their drug-using patients while reevaluating systems to provide user-friendly services that keep the drug-using patient in contact with the health care providers.[38]

Advocacy for timely execution of advance directives, such as durable power of attorney (DPOA), for health care and clarification of code status will help ease the complexities of management of later stages of AIDS and assist in organizing a patient's social situation. This provides the patient with greater influence and control over treatment decisions when he or she is not extremely ill and can make informed, person-centered decisions. Often, patients will wait too long to execute a DPOA, and cognitive impairment will preclude a legally valid document.

PATIENT–CAREGIVER TEACHING

The management of HIV disease imposes a terrible burden on patients. They and their caregivers must become experts along a broad spectrum ranging from tracking the state of their immune system to administering cytotoxic drugs via a central venous device. Although a wide variety of teaching methods may be used (e.g., verbal, written, audiovisual), constant reinforcement is needed at all stages of illness. Culturally specific approaches are essential, given the subject matters of sex, drugs, and food.

A survey of patients on the inpatient AIDS unit at SFGH showed that medications and nutrition were the top two topics of interest and concern to patients. With the polypharmacy of HIV disease treatment, drug–drug and drug–food interactions are common. Table 33–1 shows some of the factors that must be taken into consideration by patients and caregivers alike.

Other aspects of HIV disease to be addressed in patient educational programs include transmission prevention (safer sex, clean needles, how to inject drugs safely), disease processes and treatments, infection control in the home, medications and their administration, symptom management strategies, importance of ongoing primary care, nutrition, community resources,

TABLE 33–1. DRUG–DRUG AND DRUG–FOOD INTERACTIONS IN THE TREATMENT OF HIV DISEASE

ddI (needs alkaline environment for absorption)	Never give with food or citrus juices
	Give at least 1 hour ac or 2 hours pc
	Never give at the same time as dapsone, ketoconazole, tetracycline, ciprofloxacin, or ofloxacin
	Dose should be given in 2 tablets for sufficient buffering agent, and patient should be advised to chew tablets
	Do not give with IV pentamidine, 2-degree risk of pancreatitis
Dapsone, ketoconazole, itraconazole (need acidic environment for absorption)	May be given with meals
	Do not give within 2 hours of ddI
	Never give with antacids, H_2 blockers
Atovaquone (Mepron) (needs adequate fat, food intake for absorption)	Always given at mealtime or with whole milk or ice cream
	Get nutrition consultation if poor appetite or malabsorption problems or both
Azithromycin, ciprofloxacin, isoniazid, rifampin, ddC, zidovudine	Should not be given with meals

ac, before meals; pc, after meals; IV, intravenously.

patient's rights, and comfort care for the terminally ill.[16]

ETHICAL ISSUES

Historically, nurses have been the members of the health care team to spend the most time with the patient. The progressive nature of HIV disease involves the nurse in the primary care of the patient through many stages of illness and frequently for many years. As advocates for our patients, we may have to examine previously learned professional responses to issues that we may never have confronted before in our professional or personal lives.

As it has in so many other areas, HIV/AIDS has provided a lens through which to examine social processes.[22] The refusal to take care of patients with HIV disease is well documented.[10,14] With the threat of occupational transmission of HIV, nurses have been forced to look at the degree of moral and ethical obligation to patient care. The American Nurses' Association (ANA) has taken a stand on both the professional obligation to provide care and the rights of nurses. The ANA ethical code states "Nurses provide services with respect for human dignity and the uniqueness of the client, unrestricted by considerations of social or economic status, personal attributes, or the nature of the health problem."[2] In 1986, the ANA issued a "Statement Regarding Risk vs. Responsibility in Providing Nursing Care." This document clarifies the circumstances in which a nurse is morally justified to refuse to participate in the care of a patient.[3] These include (1) when the nurse refuses care for reasons of patient advocacy (providing care would violate the rights or wishes of the patient) and (2) when the nurse has a moral objection to a specific intervention. The document further states: "Accepting personal risk which exceeds the limits of duty is not morally obligatory, it is a moral option."[3] Because the risk of occupational exposure to HIV is extremely low, most institutions and professional organizations would not support a nurse's refusal to care for a patient with HIV. Exploring fears about risk of contagion and educating staff is a more effective tool than criticism of perceived risk.

Part of the ethical code of ANA speaks to the issue of refusing to care for a patient if doing so would violate the wishes of the patient. With the perceived futility of the search for a cure and the endurance of physical pain and disability, many patients have considered suicide as a treatment option for advanced HIV disease. Certainly, our immediate obligation is to facilitate a mental health examination to rule out depression. However, nurses have been asked frequently to advocate on behalf of patients who believe in physician-assisted suicide. In an initial study in 1992 regarding this subject, 28% of physicians in a San Francisco–based group of community physicians would be likely to grant a patient's initial request for assistance in committing suicide.[36] A follow-up survey of this same group done in 1995 revealed that 48% of the physicians were likely to grant this request.[41] Many nurses have been asked to refer patients to physicians who are supportive regarding this subject. More direct dialogue between health care providers is essential so that this subject can be discussed and specific guidelines can be established to respond to the concerns of our patients. Nurses also need support in honoring their feelings regarding their emotional response to a patient requesting euthanasia. While society debates the legal and ethical components of physician-assisted suicide, nurses may hear about it on a daily basis from their patients and need to acknowledge that this dialogue exists. A survey of nurses at facilities serving AIDS patients in the San Francisco Bay Area was conducted by the Community Consortium, University of California San Francisco AIDS Program at San Francisco General Hospital to determine nurses' attitudes toward assisted suicide in AIDS. Preliminary data from this survey reveal that a majority of nurses working with AIDS patients would be supportive of a patient's decision to end his/her life (see Table 33–2).

TABLE 33–2. NURSES' ATTITUDES TOWARD ASSISTED SUICIDE IN AIDS*

Reported having been asked indirectly to assist in patient suicide = 54%

Reported having been asked directly to assist in patient suicide = 38%

Reported they would help obtain lethal dose of narcotics for patients = 59%

Reported they would be at the bedside of patient who had taken a lethal dose of narcotics = 73%

* N = 216 nurses.
From Leiser R, et al: Community Consortium, University of California San Francisco, 1996, with permission.

REFERENCES

1. Allen MA, Ownby K: Tuberculosis: The other epidemic. J Assoc Nurses AIDS Care 2(4):20–21, 1991
2. American Nurses' Association: Code for nurses with interpretive statements. Kansas City, MO, ANA, 1985
3. American Nurses' Association: Code for nurses with interpretive statements. Kansas City, MO, ANA, 1986
4. Anaastasio CJ: HIV and tuberculosis: Noncompliance revisited. J Assoc Nurses AIDS Care 6(2):11–23, 1995
5. Brody R, Shofferman J: Pain in far advanced AIDS. Adv Pain Res Ther 16:379–385, 1990
6. Carroll J: Attitudes of professionals to drug abusers. Br J Nurs 2:705–711, 1993
7. Cello JP: Gastrointestinal tract manifestations of AIDS. In Sande MA, Volberding PA, eds. The Medical Management of AIDS, ed 4. Philadelphia, WB Saunders Co, 1994, p 241
8. Centers for Disease Control: The second 100,000 cases of AIDS. MMWR 41:28–29, 1992
9. Cheitlin MD: Cardiac improvement in AIDS. In Cohen PT, Sande MA, Volberding PA, eds. The AIDS Knowledge Base. Waltham, MA, Medical Publishing Group, 1990, p 5.6.1
10. Cooke M: Ethical issues related to AIDS. In Cohen PT, Sande MA, Volberding PA, eds. The AIDS Knowledge Base. Waltham, MA, Medical Publishing Group, 1990, p 12.1.1
11. Daley C: Epidemiology of tuberculosis in the AIDS era. AIDS File 6(4), 1992
12. Dilley J: Management of neuropsychiatric disorders in HIV spectrum patients. In Sande MA, Volberding PA, eds. The Medical Management of AIDS, ed 3. Philadelphia, WB Saunders Co, 1992, pp 218–227
13. Drew L, Buhles W, Erlich K: Management of the herpes virus infections. In Sande MA, Volberding PA, eds. The Medical Management of AIDS, ed 4. Philadelphia, WB Saunders Co, 1994, p 512
14. Eisenberg L: The genesis of fear: AIDS and the public's response to science. Law Med Health Care 14:243–249, 1986
15. Fegan C: Cryptosporidial disease in the adult HIV-infected patient. J Assoc Nurses AIDS Care 3:17, 1992
16. Flaskerud JA: Psychosocial aspects. In Flaskerud JH, Ungvarski PJ, eds. HIV/AIDS: A Guide to Nursing Care, ed 3. Philadelphia, WB Saunders Co, 1994, pp 308–338
17. Grady C: HIV disease: Pathogenesis and treatment. In Flaskerud JH, Ungvarski PJ, eds. HIV/AIDS: A Guide to Nursing Care, ed 2. Philadelphia, WB Saunders Co, 1992, p 44
18. Grady C: Ethical aspects. In Flaskerud JH, Ungvarski PJ, eds. HIV/AIDS: A Guide to Nursing Care, ed 2. Philadelphia, WB Saunders Co, 1992, p 429
19. Hopewell PC: *Pneumocystis carinii* pneumonia—current concepts. In Sande MA, Volberding PA, eds. The Medical Management of AIDS, ed 4. Philadelphia, WB Saunders Co, 1994, pp 367–401
20. Lbovits A, Lefkowitz M, McCarth D, et al: The prevalence and management of pain in patients with AIDS. Clin J Pain 5:245–248, 1989
21. Lee B, Safrin S: Drug interactions and toxicities in patients with HIV disease. In Cohen PT, Sande MA, Volberding PA, eds. The AIDS Knowledge Base. Waltham, MA, Medical Publishing Group, 1994, p 4.6.8
22. Levine C, Dublen N, Levine R: Building a new consequence: Ethical principles and policies for clinical research in HIV/AIDS. AIDS Patient Care 6:67–85, 1992
23. Mac Kenzie WR, Hoxie NJ, Proctor ME, et al: A massive outbreak in Milwaukee of cryptosporidium infection transmitted through the public water supply. N Engl J Med 331:61–67, 1994
24. Martin J: Issues in providing care for advanced HIV disease. In Cohen PT, Sande MA, Volberding PA, eds. The AIDS Knowledge Base. Waltham, MA, Medical Publishing Group, 1994, p 4.16.6
25. McGuire D: Pathogenesis of brain injury in HIV disease. AIDS File 7:1–2, 1993
26. Newshan G, Wainapel S: Pain characteristics and their management in persons with AIDS. J Assoc Nurses AIDS Care 4(2):53–54, 1993
27. Nokes K: HIV infection in women. In Flaskerud JH, Ungvarski PJ, eds. HIV/AIDS: A Guide to Nursing Care, ed 3. Philadelphia, WB Saunders Co, 1994, pp 243–259
28. Paice J, Publiese J, Fitzpatrick J: Opioid use in HIV patients with neurological changes. J Assoc Nurses AIDS Care 6(4):34, 1995
29. Pain Management Guide: San Francisco General Hospital Pain Management Committee, San Francisco, April 1993
30. Rose M: Concerns of women with HIV/AIDS. J Assoc Nurses AIDS Care 4(3):40–44, 1993
31. San Francisco Department of Public Health AIDS Office: Questions and answers about cryptosporidium. Educational Pamphlet, 1996
32. Schecter G: Preventing TB in the health care setting. AIDS File 6(4), 1992
33. Schmidt J: Case management problems and home care. J Assoc Nurses AIDS Care 3:38, 1992
34. Shepard K: Dyspnea in cancer patients. Palliative Care Lett 2: insert 1, 1990
35. Shernoff M, Springer E: Substance abuse and AIDS: Report from the front lines (the impact of professional). J Chem Depend Treat 5(1):141–144, 1992
36. Slome L, Moulton J, Huffine C: Physician's attitude toward assisted suicide in AIDS. J Acquir Immune Defic Syndr 5:712–718, 1992
37. Small PM, Hopewell P: Respiratory system: A general approach. In Cohen PT, Sande MA, Volberding PA, eds. The AIDS Knowledge Base. Waltham, MA, Medical Publishing Group, 1994, p 5.10
38. Springer E: Effective AIDS prevention with active drug users: The harm reduction model. J Chem Depend Treat 4(2):37, 1991
39. Staats JA: Nursing of chemically dependent clients. In Flaskerud JH, Ungvarski PJ, eds. HIV/AIDS: A Guide to Nursing Care, ed 3. Philadelphia, WB Saunders Co, 1994, pp 260–279
40. Stansell JD: Cardiac endocrine and renal complications of HIV infection. In Sande MA, Volberding PA, eds. The Medical Management of AIDS, ed 3. Philadelphia, WB Saunders Co, 1992, p 249
41. Synopsis, Minutes of the Community Consortium's General Business Meeting: Physician assisted suicide survey results. June 1995, p 1
42. Ungvarski PJ: Nursing care of the adult client with

AIDS and cytomegalovirus infection. J Assoc Nurses AIDS Care 3(1):13–14, 1992

43. Ungvarski PJ: Nursing management of the adult client. In Flaskerud JH, Ungvarski PJ, eds. HIV/AIDS: A Guide to Nursing Care, ed 2. Philadelphia, WB Saunders Co, 1992, pp 146–196

44. Ungvarski PJ, Schmidt S: Community-based and long-term care. In Flaskerud JH, Ungvarski PJ, eds. HIV/AIDS: A Guide to Nursing Care, ed 3. Philadelphia, WB Saunders Co, 1994, p 358

45. Vaccariello J, Funesti J, Laverty M, et al: The administration of didanosine (ddI) in the adult: A nursing perspective. J Assoc Nurses AIDS Care 4:26, 1993

46. Von Roenn JH, Dietrich DT: HIV related weight loss.

Improving the management of HIV disease. IAS-USA 3(5):11, 1995

47. Walent RJ: AIDS nursing: Patient care issues in the hospital setting. ONCL 6(2):131–139, 1992

48. Wofsy C: Gender-specific issues in women. In Sande MA, Volberding PA, eds. The Medical Management of AIDS, ed 4. Philadelphia, WB Saunders Co, 1994, pp 648–664

49. Worth L: HIV infection in women. In Cohen PT, Sande MA, Volberding PA, eds. The AIDS Knowledge Base. Waltham, MA, Medical Publishing Group, 1994, p 4.9

50. Yuen S: Peripheral neuropathies. AIDS File 7:2–4, 1993

INDEX

Note: Page numbers in *italics* refer to illustrations; page numbers
followed by t refer to tables.

503